Adverse Events Associated with
CHILDHOOD VACCINES

Evidence Bearing on Causality

Kathleen R. Stratton, Cynthia J. Howe, and
Richard B. Johnston, Jr., *Editors*

Vaccine Safety Committee

Division of Health Promotion and Disease Prevention

INSTITUTE OF MEDICINE

NATIONAL ACADEMY PRESS
Washington, D.C. 1994

NATIONAL ACADEMY PRESS • 2101 Constitution Avenue, N.W. • Washington, D.C. 20418

NOTICE: The project that is the subject of this report was approved by the Governing Board of the National Research Council, whose members are drawn from the councils of the National Academy of Sciences, the National Academy of Engineering, and the Institute of Medicine. The members of the committee responsible for the report were chosen for their special competences and with regard for appropriate balance.

This report has been reviewed by a group other than the authors according to procedures approved by a Report Review Committee consisting of members of the National Academy of Sciences, the National Academy of Engineering, and the Institute of Medicine.

The Institute of Medicine was chartered in 1970 by the National Academy of Sciences to enlist distinguished members of the appropriate professions in the examination of policy matters pertaining to the health of the public. In this the Institute acts under the Academy's 1863 congressional charter responsibility to be an adviser to the federal government and, upon its own initiative, to identify issues of medical care, research, and education. Dr. Kenneth I. Shine is President of the Institute of Medicine.

The project was supported by funds coordinated through the National Institute of Allergy and Infectious Diseases of the National Institutes of Health (contract no. NO1-AI-15130).

Library of Congress Cataloging-in-Publication Data

Adverse events associated with childhood vaccines : evidence bearing
    on causality / Kathleen R. Stratton, Cynthia J. Howe, and Richard B.
    Johnston, Jr., editors ; Division of Health Promotion and Disease
    Prevention, Institute of Medicine.
        p. cm.
        "The project was supported by funds coordinated through the
    National Institute of Allergy and Infectious Diseases of the
    National Institutes of Health (contract no. NO-AI-15130)"—T.p.
    verso.
        Includes bibliographical references and index.
        ISBN 0-309-04895-8
        1. Vaccination of children—Complications. 2. Vaccines—Health
    aspects. 3. Vaccines—Toxicology. I. Stratton, Kathleen R.
    II. Howe, Cynthia J. III. Johnston, Richard B., 1935- .
    IV. Institute of Medicine (U.S.). Division of Health Promotion and
    Disease Prevention. V. National Institute of Allergy and Infectious
    Diseases (U.S.).
        [DNLM: 1. Vaccines—adverse effects. 2. Immunization—in infancy
    & childhood. WS 135 A244 1993]
    RJ240.A38   1993
    615'.372'083—dc20
    DNLM/DLC   93-32099
    for Library of Congress   CIP

Printed in the United States of America.

The serpent has been a symbol of long life, healing, and knowledge among almost all cultures and religions since the beginning of recorded history. The serpent adopted as a logotype by the Institute of Medicine is a relief carving from ancient Greece, now held by the Staatlichemuseen in Berlin.

VACCINE SAFETY COMMITTEE

PAUL D. STOLLEY,* Professor and Chairman, Department of Epidemiology and Preventive Medicine, University of Maryland School of Medicine, Baltimore, Maryland

Project Staff

Michael A. Stoto, Director, Division of Health Promotion and Disease Prevention
Kathleen R. Stratton, Project Director
Cynthia J. Howe, Program Officer
Dorothy R. Majewski, Project Assistant
Michael K. Hayes, Project Editor
Tamar Lasky, Consultant
Hanaa Elhefni, Consultant

---

*Member, Institute of Medicine.

Preface

Few would question the profound importance of vaccines to public health. Not only have deaths from the most common childhood infections been almost eliminated, but so have the devastating morbidities of diseases like measles, paralytic polio, and congenital rubella. This revolution has occurred within the life spans of middle-aged Americans, and it has led to major savings in medical costs and gains in work productivity, as well as to reductions in death and suffering.

In the United States this success has been achieved through increased public awareness, continued support of basic and applied research, the capacity of the pharmaceutical industry, and the dedication of the public and private health care workers responsible for administration of the vaccines.

In the 1980s, however, a few concerned citizens in this country began to raise questions about the risks of vaccination. In fact, although the benefits to society were obvious, the risks to individual infants and children had not been well defined. Some parents considered not having their children immunized, and manufacturers threatened to shut down vaccine production because of an increasing number of lawsuits.

In response, the U.S. Congress passed the National Childhood Vaccine Injury Act in 1986 and the Vaccine Compensation Amendments in 1987. This legislation established a federal compensation process for persons judged to be injured by a vaccine. In addition, Section 312 of the Act mandated that the Institute of Medicine should conduct a scientific review of the possible adverse consequences of pertussis and rubella vaccines. The results of that review were published in 1991. Section 313 of the Act mandated that a second Institute of Medicine committee review possible adverse events associated with the other vaccines commonly given in childhood. This report comprises the deliberations and conclusions of that committee, the Vaccine Safety Committee.

The principal purpose of the committee's work was to describe as precisely as possible, on the basis of all available evidence, the relationships between the vaccines under review and specific adverse events. This led the committee to ask with each vaccine-adverse event pair, "Can administration of the vaccine cause the adverse event?" All available sources of information were analyzed, from epidemiologic studies to unpublished case reports. Final decisions on causality were made by consensus after group discussion of all of the available evidence. In pursuing its conclusions, the committee adopted a neutral stance and maintained that stance consistently through each step in the process, assuming neither the presence nor the absence of a causal relation between the vaccines and the adverse events until the evidence indicated otherwise.

In reaching a conclusion that the evidence favored *rejection* of a causal relation, the committee used only epidemiologic studies (controlled observational studies and controlled clinical trials). In reaching conclusions favoring *acceptance* of a causal relation, however, the committee most commonly relied on case series and individual case reports. This required that the nature and timing of the adverse event were appropriate for causality and that there were no likely alternative explanations for the event. Biologic plausibility was weighed in the overall balance of the determination but was not in itself considered sufficient evidence to accept or reject a causal relation.

As this report describes in detail, it was possible with some of the vaccine-adverse event pairs to reach a conclusion one way or the other—either that the evidence favored rejection (category 3) or that the evidence weighed more or less heavily for acceptance (categories 4 and 5) of a causal relation (see Chapter 2 for explanations of the five categories). With the majority of vaccine-adverse event pairs the evidence was considered inadequate to accept or reject causality. In some instances, the relation has not been well studied and the data are scarce; in others, the data are abundant but the evidence, on the whole, was not conclusive. Category 2 does not distinguish between these two situations, since the conclusion is the same. It could be argued in these cases that since the body of available evidence did not support causality, a causal relation does not exist. It could also be argued that in the absence of evidence favoring rejection of causality, it is possible that the vaccine could cause the adverse event. Both of these interpretations are possible. The committee regrets that this uncertainty may not make it easier to resolve litigation centered on individual instances of putative causality. However, the stringency of our charge precluded statements beyond what the evidence allowed. Concern about this unfortunate condition of uncertainty has led the committee to urge that more definitive research be done on possible adverse events during the development of new vaccines or vaccine combinations and to urge that efforts to sharpen current postmarketing surveillance systems be accelerated.

This report represents the product of long hard work by committee members and Institute of Medicine staff. The Acknowledgments section lists a large number of other people who contributed to the effort in an important way, including parents who had the courage to remind us that public health measures affect the lives of individual human beings. In addition, the committee has recognized that it owes a special debt to its predecessor, the Committee to Review the Adverse Consequences of Pertussis and Rubella Vaccines. That committee developed a logical system, on the basis of the available evidence, of classifying—and thereby communicating—the nature of the causal relations between vaccines and adverse events. The committee has also recognized that the quality of this report could not have been achieved without the work of the extraordinary staff assigned to us by the Institute of Medicine—Kathleen Stratton, Cynthia Howe, Michael Stoto, and Dorothy Majewski. In particular, Kathleen Stratton, the Project Director, with intelligence, infinite kindness, and untiring persistence, kept the committee to its proper task; and we are deeply grateful.

Whatever its commissioned intent, in the end, the work of the Vaccine Safety Committee will have succeeded if this report contributes to present worldwide efforts to protect children from preventable infections using vaccines that incur the lowest possible risk.

Richard B. Johnston, Jr.
Chairman

Acknowledgments

The committee would like to thank the following individuals who provided us with information or assistance: Kenneth J. Bart, National Vaccine Program; W. J. Bellini, Centers for Disease Control and Prevention; Bruce Berget, University of Chicago; Else Borst-Eilers, Health Council of The Netherlands; Philip A. Brunell, Cedars-Sinai Medical Center; John Brydon, Demler Armstrong & Rowland, Long Beach, California; Christine Buhk, Sturgeon Bay, Wisconsin; Hilary Butler, Tuakau, Auckland, New Zealand; Kim Chapman, Colorado Springs, Colorado; Robert T. Chen, Centers for Disease Control and Prevention; James D. Cherry, UCLA Medical Center; Kathleen Crozier, Infectious Disease News; Colette Cogliandro, Chesapeake, Virginia; Shannon Dixon, Honolulu, Hawaii; Andrew W. Dodd, Torrance, California; Philippe Duclos, Health and Welfare Canada; Paul Dyken, University of Southern Alabama; Hanaa Elhefni, University of Maryland, Baltimore; Jan Erickson, National Vaccine Information Center; Elaine C. Esber, U.S. Food and Drug Administration; Juhani Eskola, National Public Health Institute, Finland; Geoffrey Evans, Division of Vaccine Injury Compensation; Gerald M. Fenichel, Vanderbilt University/Advisory Commission on Childhood Vaccines; Jesse Ferguson, Milwaukee, Wisconsin; Reinhard Fescharek, Behringwerke AG; Harvey V. Fineberg, Harvard School of Public Health; Barbara Loe Fisher, Dissatisfied Parents Together; Bonnie Plumeri Franz, Ogdensburg, New York; James Froeschle, Connaught Laboratories; Robert Fujinami, University of Utah; Vincent A. Fulginiti, Tulane University/National Vaccine Advisory Committee; Susan Garzonio, Brodhead, Wisconsin; Mark Geier, medical/legal consultant, Silver Spring, Maryland; Cynthia Goldenberg, Laguna Niguel, California; Stephen R. Gordon, Vaccine Adverse Events Reporting System, Ogden BioServices Corporation; Dan M. Granoff, St. Louis Children's Hospital; Marjorie Grant, Determined Parents to Stop Hurting Our Tots; Diane Griffin, Johns Hopkins University; Stephen Hadler, Centers for Disease Control and Prevention; Caroline B. Hall, University of Rochester/American Academy of Pediatrics; Neal A. Halsey, The Johns Hopkins University; Carolyn Hardegree, U.S. Food and Drug Administration; Joanne Hatem, National Vaccine Information Center; Sandra Holmes, Centers for Disease Control and Prevention; Michael Hugo, Schlichtman, Conway, Crowley, and Hugo, Boston, Massachusetts; Terry and Kurt Johnson, Mission Viejo, California; Samuel Katz, Duke University Medical Center/Advisory Committee on Immunization Practices; Marcel Kinsbourne, Winchester, Massachusetts; Gloria Koslofsky, Norwood, New York; Saul Krugman, New York University Medical Center; Leonard P. Kurland, Mayo Clinic; Walter Kyle, attorney, Franconia, New Hampshire; John LaMontagne, National Institute of Allergy and Infectious Diseases; Kathleen Lane, Spring City, Pennsylvania; Tamar Lasky, University of Maryland, Baltimore; Rosalyn Leiderman, National Library of Medicine; Donald Lindberg, National Library of Medicine; Noel Maclaren, University of Florida; Ruth Macrides, Naples, Florida; Frank Mahoney, Centers for Disease Control and Prevention; Susan Maloney, Rowley, Massachusetts; Andrea Martin, Woodland, California; Dale McFarlin, National Institute of Neurologic Diseases and Stroke; Ann Millan, National Vaccine Information Center; Sandy Mintz, Parents Concerned about the Safety of Vaccines, Anchorage, Alaska; J. Anthony Morris, The Bell of Atri, Inc.; Edward A. Mortimer, Jr., Case Western Reserve University School of Medicine; Robert Moxley, Gage and Moxley, Cheyenne, Wyoming; John Mullen, Centers for Disease Control and Prevention; David Nalin, Merck Research Laboratories; Neal Nathanson, University of Pennsylvania; Elena O. Nightingale, Carnegie Corporation of New York; Abner Notkins, National Institute of Dental Research; Walter A. Orenstein, Centers for Disease Control and Prevention; Mary Pearce, Philadelphia, Pennsylvania; Georges Peter, Rhode Island Hospital/American Academy of Pediatrics; Stanley A. Plotkin, Pasteur Mérieux Connaught Company; John Pollard, University of Sydney Department of Medicine, Sydney, Australia; Arthur L. Prensky, Washington University School of Medicine; Regina Rabinovich, National Institute of Allergy and Infectious Diseases; Vincent Racaniello, Columbia University; Suresh Rastogi, U.S. Food and Drug Administration; Frederick C. Robbins, Case Western Reserve University; Eugene Robin, Stanford University School of Medicine; Amy Scott, U.S. Food and Drug Administration; Martin Smith, Advisory Commission on Childhood Vaccines; William Stevens, U.S. Food and Drug Administration; Peter M. Strebel, Centers for Disease Control and Prevention; Roland Sutter,

Centers for Disease Control and Prevention; Dirk Teuwen, SmithKline Beecham; Klaus V. Toyka, Neurologische Universitatsklinik und Poliklinik im Kopfklinikum, University of Wurzburg; Claudette Varanko, Demler, Armstrong & Rowland, Long Beach, California; Burton A. Waisbren, Milwaukee, Wisconsin; Joel Ward, UCLA Center for Vaccine Research; Steven G. Wassilak, Centers for Disease Control and Prevention; Curtis Webb, Webb, Burton, Carlson, Ledersen & Webb, Twin Falls, Idaho; Robert Weibel, Division of Vaccine Injury Compensation; Susan Weinberg, Baltimore, Maryland; R. P. Wise, U.S. Food and Drug Administration; Peter F. Wright, Vanderbilt University Hospital; Arthur Zahalsky, Southern Illinois University, Edwardsville, Illinois; and Elizabeth Zell, Centers for Disease Control and Prevention. The committee also appreciates the cooperation of the following organizations or institutions: Advisory Commission on Childhood Vaccines; Bell of Atri, Inc.; Centers for Disease Control and Prevention; Determined Parents to Stop Hurting Our Tots; Dissatisfied Parents Together; National Institute of Allergy and Infectious Diseases; National Library of Medicine; National Vaccine Information Center; National Vaccine Program Office; Parents Concerned About the Safety of Vaccines; U.S. Food and Drug Administration; Vaccine Adverse Event Reporting System.

The committee would also like to thank the Institute of Medicine (IOM) staff members whose work supported its deliberations, principally Kathleen R. Stratton, Study Director; Cynthia J. Howe, Program Officer; Dorothy R. Majewski, Project Assistant; and Michael A. Stoto, Director, Division of Health Promotion and Disease Prevention. Others within the IOM and the National Academy of Sciences who were instrumental in seeing the project to completion were Kenneth I. Shine, President of the IOM; Enriqueta C. Bond, Executive Officer; Gary B. Ellis, Former Director, Division of Health Promotion and Disease Prevention; Christopher P. Howson, Deputy Director, Division of International Health; Linda DePugh, Administrative Assistant; Jennifer Holliday, Project Assistant; Jana Katz, intern; Marcia Lewis, Administrative Assistant; Scott Jones and Robert Albritton, computer analysts; Claudia Carl, Michael Edington, and Betsy Turvene, Reports and Information Office; Sally Stanfield, Estelle Miller, and Francesca Moghari, National Academy Press; and Susan Turner-Lowe, Office of News and Public Information. We greatly appreciate the editorial assistance of Michael Hayes. Finally, special thanks are due for the expert assistance of research librarian Laura Baird and library assistants Yauthary Keo, Eileen Moynihan, and Rhashida Beynum.

Contents

Adverse Events Associated with
CHILDHOOD VACCINES

Evidence Bearing on Causality

1

Executive Summary

"Our aim, therefore, must be to study these [complications] as fully as possible in the confident expectation that, as in other branches of science, knowledge will bring enlightenment" (Wilson, 1967).

Childhood immunization has been one of the foremost public health measures of the twentieth century. It has allowed control and prevention of many diseases from which morbidity and mortality can be staggering. Medical personnel in the United States currently rarely see a case of the infectious diseases against which the vaccines are directed. Yet, recent measles epidemics on college campuses and in inner cities suggest that vaccine-preventable disease is not to be ignored. The first health initiative of the new presidential administration was to increase funding for childhood immunization programs to boost vaccination rates in the United States, particularly for children under age 2 years.

BACKGROUND AND HISTORY

The public policy debate regarding immunization stretches beyond the question of how to meet the goals of universal immunization. Concern over the safety of pertussis vaccine was long-standing in Great Britain by the time of the 1982 airing in the United States of a documentary entitled "DPT: Vaccine Roulette" (WRC-TV, 1982) and the 1985 publication of *DPT: A Shot in the Dark* (Coulter and Fisher, 1985). Concern has stretched to other vaccines and has spawned the formation of groups of interested citizens throughout the United States, for example, National Vaccine Information Center/Dissatisfied Parents Together, Determined Parents to Stop Hurting Our Tots, Concerned Health Professionals and Others, and Parents

Concerned About the Safety of Vaccines. More articles and books have been published (e.g., Coulter, 1990; Miller, 1992) to alert the public to the potential risks of vaccination.

In 1986, the U.S. Congress passed the National Childhood Vaccine Injury Act (NCVIA; P.L. 99-660) in response to worries about the safety of currently licensed childhood vaccines and in response to the economic pressures that were threatening the integrity of childhood immunization programs. The litigation costs associated with claims of damage from vaccines had forced several companies to end their vaccine research and development programs as well as to stop producing already licensed vaccines. The NCVIA was an attempt to encourage and ensure vaccine production by creating a no-fault compensation program (the National Vaccine Injury Compensation Program) as a required first resort for those who believed that they or their children had been injured by certain vaccines. The need for a compensation program had long been recognized, and several groups had proposed possible mechanisms for compensating people believed to be injured by vaccination (Institute of Medicine, 1985; Office of Technology Assessment, 1980). This program was envisioned to alleviate, but not completely eliminate, manufacturer liability and encourage research and development of more and safer vaccines. The compensation program is administered by the federal government and is financed by an excise tax on the sale of vaccines covered by the program (Iglehart, 1987; Mariner, 1992).

In addition to establishing the compensation program, the NCVIA set forth other vaccine-related efforts to be carried out by the U.S. Department of Health and Human Services, including mandatory reporting of specific adverse events following childhood immunizations against diphtheria, tetanus, pertussis, measles, mumps, rubella, and polio (see box entitled The Vaccine Injury Table in Chapter 10); voluntary reporting of any reaction to any immunization to the Vaccine Adverse Event Reporting System (see Chapter 10 for a discussion of this passive surveillance system and Figure B-1 for a copy of the reporting form); the creation of a National Vaccine Program Office to coordinate federal vaccine initiatives and to help meet immunization coverage goals; the establishment of advisory groups to the National Vaccine Program and the National Vaccine Injury Compensation Program; and better communication of the potential risks of vaccines through public information pamphlets that are distributed at the time of vaccination (under the direction of the Centers for Disease Control and Prevention) and changes in vaccine package inserts (under the direction of the U.S. Food and Drug Administration).

The NCVIA also mandated that the Secretary of the U.S. Department of Health and Human Services enlist the help of the Institute of Medicine (IOM) of the National Academy of Sciences to study the adverse effects of childhood vaccines. The NCVIA called for two specific studies. The first, mandated under Section 312 of P.L. 99-660, was to address the serious adverse effects of pertussis and rubella vaccines. The Committee to Review the Adverse Consequences of Pertussis and Rubella Vaccines published its findings in 1991 (Institute of Medicine, 1991). Appendix A contains the Executive Summary of that report.

The second study, mandated under Section 313 of P.L. 99-660, was to review adverse events associated with other vaccines commonly administered during childhood. The Vaccine Safety Committee, which was charged with performing the second study, was convened early in 1992. The results of that inquiry are provided in this report.

THE CHARGE TO THE COMMITTEE

The members of the interdisciplinary, 14-member Vaccine Safety Committee have expertise in such areas as immunology, pediatrics, internal medicine, infectious diseases, neurology, virology, microbiology, epidemiology, and public health. The committee was charged with (1) reviewing the relevant scientific and medical literature on specific risks to children associated with the vaccines or vaccine components directed against tetanus, diphtheria, measles, mumps, polio, *Haemophilus influenzae* type b, and hepatitis B currently licensed for use in the United States and (2) reviewing the available data on specific risk-modifying factors, that is, circumstances under which administration of these vaccines increases the risk of an adverse event, characteristics of groups known to be at increased risk of an adverse event, and timing of vaccination that increases the risk of an adverse event.

Risk-benefit comparisons or recommendations about immunization schedules were not within the charge to the Vaccine Safety Committee. Despite the name of the committee, many aspects of vaccine safety, such as purity standards or production techniques, also were beyond the committee's charge.

Both IOM studies mandated in P.L. 99-660 entailed the evaluation of the weight of scientific and medical evidence bearing on the question of whether a causal relation exists between certain vaccines and specific serious adverse events. Like the Committee to Review the Adverse Consequences of Pertussis and Rubella Vaccines, the Vaccine Safety Committee approached its task from a position of neutrality, presuming neither the presence nor the absence of a causal relation between the vaccines and the adverse events under consideration.

THE STUDY PROCESS

Over the course of 18 months, the committee met six times, reviewed more than 7,000 abstracts of scientific and medical studies, read more than 2,000 published books and articles (including many sources in the non-

English literature), analyzed information from U.S. Public Health Service-administered reporting systems for adverse reactions to vaccines, and considered material submitted by interested parties. The committee solicited input from scientists who were invited to participate in two open scientific meetings and from other interested parties at two open public meetings. Details regarding how the committee gathered information are given in Appendix B. All salient information from those reviews is contained in this report.

P.L. 99-660 stated that the review was to include those vaccines covered by the National Vaccine Injury Compensation Program. *Haemophilus influenzae* type b (Hib) and hepatitis B vaccines were added for consideration because of the increasing use of these vaccines and the supposition that in the near future they could be mandatory vaccines covered by the National Vaccine Injury Compensation Program. The list of adverse events investigated for this report derived primarily from negotiations with representatives of the U.S. Public Health Service. However, preliminary investigations into additional adverse events were prompted by queries from interested parties or committee members. After considering the information from these preliminary investigations, the committee added several vaccine-adverse event relations to the original list. Table B-1 in Appendix B contains a complete listing of the specific vaccine-adverse event relations under study.

The report begins with background information. Chapter 2 contains an in-depth discussion of the approach used by the committee to weight the evidence and assess causality. Information on the neurologic disorders and immunologic reactions discussed in much of the report is contained in Chapters 3 and 4. Chapters 5 through 9 include the vaccine-specific evidence and conclusions. All information (evidence, causality argument, and conclusions) regarding death as an adverse event associated with vaccination is contained in Chapter 10.

Adverse Effects of Pertussis and Rubella Vaccines (Institute of Medicine, 1991), the report of the predecessor IOM committee, provides an in-depth review of the literature concerning the adverse events associated with diphtheria and tetanus toxoids and pertussis vaccine (DPT), as well as pertussis vaccine, and should be referred to for conclusions regarding DPT. Appendix A contains the Executive Summary of that report. The charge to the Vaccine Safety Committee was to examine adverse events associated with tetanus toxoid as well as tetanus and diphtheria toxoid combination preparations. The committee reviewed data concerning DPT if the data also concerned diphtheria and tetanus toxoids for pediatric use (DT); however, it was beyond the committee's scope to make conclusions about pertussis vaccine or DPT.

The IOM Committee to Review the Adverse Consequences of Pertussis and Rubella Vaccines made determinations of causality only for rubella vaccine and the rubella vaccine component of multivalent vaccines, but not for measles-mumps-rubella vaccine (MMR). Thus, the Vaccine Safety Committee reviewed data regarding immunization with MMR as well as data on monovalent measles and mumps preparations. The committee has made separate determinations of causality for the measles and mumps vaccine components for the adverse events for which data were available, particularly if measles or mumps vaccine-strain virus was isolated from the patient. In circumstances in which a causality assessment specific to monovalent measles or mumps vaccine was not possible, this is stated in the conclusion regarding that specific adverse event.

In circumstances in which the committee determined that a component of a multivalent preparation was causally related to a specific adverse event, but there is no direct experience of such an adverse event being caused by the multivalent preparation, the committee states this, but judges that the combined preparation also is causally related to that adverse event.

Many case reports described an adverse event(s) in a patient who received more than one vaccine. A common combination, as a result of the immunization schedules recommended in the United States, is DPT, oral polio vaccine, and Hib vaccine. Assessment of causality in those reports was more difficult than if the patient had received only one vaccine or vaccine component, but the committee considered that the reports could be theoretically supportive of causality for the combination but not in themselves sufficient to allow a firm judgment regarding causality.

CAUSALITY AND WEIGHT OF EVIDENCE

As discussed in detail in Chapter 2, the committee considered four types of evidence: biologic plausibility; case reports, case series, and uncontrolled observational studies; controlled observational studies; and controlled clinical trials. The committee used qualitative and quantitative approaches to weigh each type of evidence. Table 1-1 contains a summary of the different types of evidence for every vaccine-adverse event relation studied. The committee believes that although it is plausible that there is a causal relation between any of the vaccine-adverse event associations under review, plausibility has been demonstrated only for certain ones of these. Therefore, information on the plausibility of a causal relation was classified in Table 1-1 as either theoretical only or as demonstrated. The other types of evidence were classified in Table 1-1 as nonexistent, indeterminate, or as weighing, on the whole, for or against a determination of a causal relation. The consideration of all four types of evidence as a whole led to a conclusion of the final weight of evidence regarding causality. Table 1-2 contains these conclusions.

TABLE 1-1 Summary of the Evidence For or Against a Determination of a Causal Relation[a]

Vaccine and Adverse Event	Biologic Plausibility[b]	Case Reports, Case Series, and Uncontrolled Observational Studies	Controlled Observational Studies and Controlled Clinical Trials
Diphtheria and Tetanus Toxoids[c]			
Encephalopathy	Demonstrated	Indeterminate	Against (DT) No data (Td, T)
Infantile spasms[d] (DT only)	Theoretical only	No data	Against
Residual seizure disorders other than infantile spasms	Theoretical only	Indeterminate (DT, T) No data (Td)	No data
Demyelinating diseases of the central nervous system	Demonstrated	For	No data
Guillain-Barré syndrome	Demonstrated	For (T) Indeterminate (DT, Td)	No data
Mononeuropathy	Theoretical only	Indeterminate (T, Td) No data (DT)	No data
Brachial neuritis	Theoretical only	For (T) Indeterminate (Td) No data (DT)	No data

Arthritis	Theoretical only	Indeterminate	No data
Erythema multiforme	Theoretical only	Indeterminate (DT, Td) No data (T)	No data
Anaphylaxis	Demonstrated	For (T) Indeterminate (DT, Td)	No data
Death from SIDS (DT only)[e]	Theoretical only	Indeterminate	Against
Measles Vaccine[f]			
Encephalopathy	Demonstrated	Indeterminate	Indeterminate
Subacute sclerosing panencephalitis	Demonstrated	Indeterminate	Indeterminate
Residual seizure disorder	Demonstrated	Indeterminate	No data
Sensorineural deafness	Theoretical only	Indeterminate (MMR)	No data
Optic neuritis	Demonstrated	Indeterminate	No data
Transverse myelitis	Demonstrated	Indeterminate	No data
Guillain-Barré syndrome	Demonstrated	Indeterminate	No data
Thrombocytopenia	Demonstrated	Indeterminate (measles) For (MMR)	Indeterminate (measles) No data (MMR)
Insulin-dependent diabetes mellitus	Theoretical only	Indeterminate	Indeterminate

continued

TABLE 1-1 (*continued*)

Vaccine and Adverse Event	Biologic Plausibility[b]	Case Reports, Case Series, and Uncontrolled Observational Studies	Controlled Observational Studies and Controlled Clinical Trials
Anaphylaxis	Theoretical only	For	No data
Death from vaccine-strain viral infection[e]	Demonstrated	For	No data
Mumps Vaccine[f]			
Encephalopathy	Demonstrated	Indeterminate	No data
Aseptic meningitis	Demonstrated	Indeterminate	No data
Residual seizure disorder	Theoretical only	No data	No data
Neuropathy	Theoretical only	No data	No data
Sensorineural deafness	Demonstrated	Indeterminate (MMR)	No data
Insulin-dependent diabetes mellitus	Demonstrated	Indeterminate	Indeterminate
Sterility	Demonstrated	No data	No data
Thrombocytopenia	Demonstrated	Indeterminate	No data
Anaphylaxis	Theoretical only	Indeterminate (MMR)	No data

continued

Polio Vaccine (OPV and IPV)[g]

Guillain-Barré syndrome	Demonstrated (OPV) Theoretical only (IPV)	For (OPV) Indeterminate (IPV)	For (OPV) No data (IPV)
Transverse myelitis	Demonstrated (OPV) Theoretical only (IPV)	Indeterminate (OPV) No data (IPV)	No data
Poliomyelitis (OPV only)	Demonstrated	For	No data
Thrombocytopenia (IPV)	Theoretical only	No data	No data
Anaphylaxis (IPV)	Theoretical only	No data	No data
Death from SIDS[e]	Theoretical only	Indeterminate	Indeterminate
Death from vaccine-strain viral infection, including from paralytic polio-myelitis (OPV only)[e]	Demonstrated	For	No data

Hepatitis B Vaccine

Guillain-Barré syndrome	Demonstrated	Indeterminate	No data
Demyelinating diseases of the central nervous system	Demonstrated	Indeterminate	No data
Arthritis	Demonstrated	Indeterminate	No data
Anaphylaxis	Theoretical only	For	No data
Death from SIDS[e]	Theoretical only	Indeterminate	No data

TABLE 1-1 (continued)

Vaccine and Adverse Event	Biologic Plausibility[b]	Case Reports, Case Series, and Uncontrolled Observational Studies	Controlled Observational Studies and Controlled Clinical Trials
Haemophilus influenzae type b Vaccine			
Guillain-Barré syndrome	Theoretical only	Indeterminate	No data
Transverse myelitis	Theoretical only	Indeterminate	No data
Thrombocytopenia	Theoretical only	Indeterminate	Indeterminate
Susceptibility to early Hib disease[h]	Demonstrated	Indeterminate	For (PRP) Against (conjugated)
Anaphylaxis	Theoretical only	Indeterminate	No data
Death from SIDS[e]	Theoretical only	Indeterminate	No data

[a]*Indeterminate* indicates that there is evidence in this category, but the committee did not consider that, on the whole, it weighed either for or against a causal relation. *No data* indicates that the committee did not find data of this type directly bearing on a causal relation between the vaccine and the adverse event.

[b]The committee considered all adverse events to be theoretically plausible and, therefore, classified plausibility in support of causality as either theoretical only or demonstrated. Demonstrated biologic plausibility refers to information on the known effects of the natural disease against which the vaccine is given and the results of animal experiments and in vitro studies.

[c]Unless noted otherwise, the classification for tetanus toxoid (T), diphtheria-tetanus toxoid for pediatric use (DT), and tetanus-diphtheria toxoid for adult use (Td) is the same. The committee was not charged with assessing monovalent diphtheria toxoid or the combined diphtheria and tetanus toxoids and pertussis vaccine (DPT). In Appendix A, see the Executive Summary of *Adverse Effects of Pertussis and Rubella Vaccines* for conclusions about DPT.

[d]Infantile spasms occur only in the age group that receives DT but not Td or T. A possible causal relation between infantile spasms and Td and T was not examined.

[e]In this table, the committee summarizes the data regarding the causal relation between the vaccine and only those deaths that are classified as sudden infant death syndrome (SIDS) or that are a consequence of vaccine-strain viral infection. SIDS occurs primarily in infants too young to receive tetanus and diphtheria toxoids for adult use, measles vaccine, mumps vaccine, or usually, tetanus toxoid. Therefore, a relation between these vaccines and SIDS was not assessed. If the evidence favors the acceptance of (or establishes) a causal relation between a vaccine and an adverse event, and if that adverse event can be fatal, then in the committee's judgment the evidence favors the acceptance of (or establishes) a causal relation between the vaccine and death from the adverse event. Direct evidence regarding death in association with a potentially fatal adverse event that itself is causally related to the vaccine is limited to tetanus–diphtheria toxoid for adult use and Guillain-Barré syndrome, tetanus toxoid and anaphylaxis, and oral polio vaccine (OPV) and poliomyelitis. Direct evidence regarding death in association with a potentially fatal adverse event that itself is causally related to the vaccine is lacking for measles vaccine and anaphylaxis, MMR and anaphylaxis, OPV and Guillain-Barré syndrome, hepatitis B vaccine and anaphylaxis, and *Haemophilus influenzae* type b unconjugated PRP vaccine and early-onset *Haemophilus influenzae* type b disease in children age 18 months or older who receive their first Hib immunization with unconjugated PRP vaccine. See Chapter 10 for details. The data are indeterminate regarding the causal relation between the vaccine and causes of death other than those discussed above. Data regarding death as an adverse consequence of the vaccines under review are discussed in Chapter 10 rather than in the vaccine-specific chapters.

[f]The committee was charged with assessing the causal relation between several adverse events and measles vaccine or mumps vaccine. The committee was not charged with assessing monovalent rubella vaccine. In Appendix A, see the Executive Summary of *Adverse Effects of Pertussis and Rubella Vaccines* for conclusions regarding rubella vaccine. (MMR) indicates that the data derive exclusively from the multivalent preparation.

[g]OPV is oral polio vaccine; IPV is inactivated polio vaccine.

[h]The committee assessed data regarding the increased susceptibility to *Haemophilus influenzae* type b disease within 7 days of immunization with *Haemophilus influenzae* type b vaccine. For this adverse event only, the committee was able to separate the data regarding the unconjugated (PRP) vaccine from the data regarding the conjugated vaccines.

12

TABLE 1-2 Conclusions Based on the Evidence Bearing on Causality

DT/Td/T	Measles[a]	Mumps[a]	OPV/IPV[b]	Hepatitis B	H. influenzae type b
Category 1: No Evidence Bearing on a Causal Relation					
			Transverse myelitis (IPV)		
			Thrombocytopenia (IPV)		
			Anaphylaxis (IPV)		
Category 2: The Evidence Is Inadequate to Accept or Reject a Causal Relation					
Residual seizure disorder other than infantile spasms	Encephalopathy	Encephalopathy	Transverse myelitis (OPV)	Guillain-Barré syndrome	Guillain-Barré syndrome
	Subacute sclerosing panencephalitis	Aseptic meningitis	Guillain-Barré syndrome (IPV)	Demyelinating diseases of the central nervous system	Transverse myelitis
Demyelinating diseases of the central nervous system	Residual seizure disorder	Sensorineural deafness (MMR)	Death from SIDS[c]		Thrombocytopenia
	Sensorineural deafness (MMR)	Insulin-dependent diabetes mellitus		Arthritis	Anaphylaxis
Mononeuropathy	Optic neuritis	Sterility		Death from SIDS[c]	Death from SIDS[c]
Arthritis					

Erythema multiforme   Transverse myelitis   Thrombocytopenia

Guillain-Barré syndrome   Anaphylaxis[d]

Thrombocytopenia

Insulin-dependent diabetes mellitus

Early onset *H. influenzae* b disease (conjugate vaccines)

Category 3: The Evidence Favors Rejection of a Causal Relation

Encephalopathy[e]

Infantile spasms (DT only)[f]

Death from SIDS (DT only)[f,g]

Category 4: The Evidence Favors Acceptance of a Causal Relation

Guillain-Barré syndrome[h]   Anaphylaxis[d]   Guillain-Barré syndrome (OPV)

Brachial neuritis[h]

Early-onset *H. influenzae* b disease in children age 18 months or older who receive their first Hib immunization with unconjugated PRP vaccine

continued

TABLE 1-2 (continued)

DT/Td/T	Measles[a]	Mumps[a]	OPV/IPV[b]	Hepatitis B	H. influenzae type b
Category 5: The Evidence Establishes a Causal Relation					
Anaphylaxis[h]	Thrombocytopenia (MMR)		Poliomyelitis in recipient or contact (OPV)	Anaphylaxis	
	Anaphylaxis (MMR)[d]				
	Death from measles vaccine-strain viral infection[c,i]		Death from polio vaccine-strain viral infection[c,i]		

[a]If the data derive from a monovalent preparation, then in the committee's judgment the causal relation extends to multivalent preparations. If the data derive exclusively from MMR, that is so indicated by (MMR). In the absence of any data on the monovalent preparation, in the committee's judgment the causal relation determined for the multivalent preparations does not extend to the monovalent components.

[b]For some adverse events, the committee was charged with assessing the causal relation between the adverse event and only oral polio vaccine (OPV) (paralytic and nonparalytic poliomyelitis) or only inactivated polio vaccine (IPV) (anaphylaxis and thrombocytopenia). If the conclusions are different for OPV than for IPV for the other adverse events, that is so noted.

[c]This table lists weight-of-evidence determinations only for deaths that are classified as SIDS and deaths that are a consequence of vaccine-strain viral infection. However, if the evidence favors the acceptance of (or establishes) a causal relation between a vaccine and an adverse event, and that adverse event can be fatal, then in the committee's judgment the evidence favors the acceptance of (or establishes) a causal relation between the vaccine and death from the adverse event. Direct evidence regarding death in association with a vaccine-associated adverse event is limited to tetanus-diphtheria toxoid for adult use (Td) and Guillain-Barré syndrome, tetanus toxoid and anaphylaxis, and OPV and poliomyelitis. Direct evidence regarding death in association with a potentially fatal adverse event that itself is causally related to the vaccine is lacking for measles vaccine and anaphylaxis, MMR and anaphylaxis, OPV and anaphylaxis, hepatitis B vaccine and anaphylaxis, and H. influenzae type b unconjugated PRP vaccine and early-onset H. influenzae type b disease in children age 18 months or older who receive their first Hib immunization with unconjugated PRP vaccine. See Chapter 10 for details.

[d]The evidence that establishes a causal relation for anaphylaxis derives from MMR. The evidence regarding monovalent measles vaccine favors acceptance of a causal relation, but are less convincing, mostly because of incomplete documentation of symptoms or the possible attenuation of symptoms by medical intervention.

[e]The evidence derives from studies of diphtheria-tetanus toxoid for pediatric use (DT). If the evidence favors rejection of a causal relation between DT and encephalopathy, then in the committee's judgment the evidence favors rejection of a causal relation between Td and tetanus toxoid and encephalopathy.

[f]Infantile spasms and SIDS occur only in an age group that receives DT but not Td or tetanus toxoid.

[g]The evidence derives mostly from DPT. Because there are supportive data favoring rejection of a causal relation between DT and SIDS as well, if the evidence favors rejection of a causal relation between DPT and SIDS, then in the committee's judgment the evidence favors rejection of a causal relation between DT and SIDS.

[h]The evidence derives from tetanus toxoid. If the evidence favors acceptance of (or establishes) a causal relation between tetanus toxoid and an adverse event, then in the committee's judgment the evidence favors acceptance of (or establishes) a causal relation between DT and Td and the adverse event as well.

[i]The data come primarily from individuals proven to be immunocompromised.

The committee organized these conclusions into five categories. Because some confusion has arisen over the meaning of the category descriptions used by the Committee to Review the Adverse Consequences of Pertussis and Rubella Vaccines, despite extensive explanations in both the footnotes and the text, the Vaccine Safety Committee adopted some minor modifications in wording intended to help in the interpretation of the present report. To facilitate reading by those familiar with the report of the previous committee, the present committee maintained both the number of categories (five) and the order of those categories but modified the wording in an attempt to clarify its meaning. However, the Vaccine Safety Committee (which has some overlap in committee membership and staff with the earlier committee) believes that the categories represent the same concepts intended by the predecessor committee. The categories are:

1. No evidence bearing on a causal relation.
2. The evidence is inadequate to accept or reject a causal relation.
3. The evidence favors rejection of a causal relation.
4. The evidence favors acceptance of a causal relation.
5. The evidence establishes a causal relation.

Chapter 2 contains a discussion of the criteria used by the committee for each determination of the final weight of evidence.

The evidence favors rejection of, favors acceptance of, or establishes a causal relation between a vaccine and an adverse event in approximately one-third of the relations studied. For the other relations the evidence was inadequate to accept or reject a causal relation or there was no evidence bearing on the relation. It is important to note that the use of the term *inadequate* does not necessarily imply that the data were scarce. In some cases the committee identified an abundance of data. However, as a whole, it did not favor either acceptance or rejection of a causal relation. In the lists below, the superscript letters refer to the appropriate notes in Table 1-2. The notes in Tables 1-1 and 1-2 are integral to interpretation of the findings. The committee reached the following conclusions regarding causality.

The evidence favors rejection of a causal relation between:

- diphtheria and tetanus toxoids and encephalopathy,[e] infantile spasms,[f] and death from sudden infant death syndrome (SIDS),[f,g] and
- conjugate Hib vaccines and early-onset Hib disease.

The evidence favors acceptance of a causal relation between:

- diphtheria and tetanus toxoids and Guillain-Barré syndrome[h] and brachial neuritis,[h]
- measles vaccine and anaphylaxis,[d]

• oral polio vaccine and Guillain-Barré syndrome, and

• unconjugated (PRP) Hib vaccine and early-onset Hib disease in children age 18 months or older who receive their first Hib immunization with unconjugated (PRP) vaccine.

The evidence establishes a causal relation between:

• diphtheria and tetanus toxoids and anaphylaxis,[h]
• measles vaccine and death from measles vaccine-strain viral infection,[c,i]
• measles-mumps-rubella vaccine and thrombocytopenia and anaphylaxis,
• oral polio vaccine and poliomyelitis and death from polio-vaccine-strain viral infection,[c,i] and
• hepatitis B vaccine and anaphylaxis.

For the vast majority of vaccine-adverse event relations studied, the data came predominantly from uncontrolled studies and case reports. Most of the pathologic conditions studied are rare in the general population. The risk of developing these conditions because of vaccination would *seem* to be low. Without age-specific incidence rates and relative risk estimates, however, it is not possible to calculate the proportion of individuals whose condition is causally related to a vaccine. When the data permitted, such calculations (i.e., the risk difference or excess risk) were made and can be found in the conclusions in Chapters 5 through 9. Because age-specific incidence rates were not available for many of the pathologic conditions studied and because controlled epidemiologic studies of these relations are lacking, few such estimates could be made.

NEED FOR RESEARCH AND SURVEILLANCE

During its attempt to find evidence regarding causality, the committee identified needs for research and surveillance of adverse events. Work in these areas will help to ensure that all vaccines used are as free from the risk of causing adverse events as possible. Some of the needs identified are for increased surveillance of reports of demyelinating disease and arthritis following hepatitis B vaccination, better follow-up of reports of death and other serious adverse events following vaccination, increased use of large databases (currently used only on a small scale) to supplement passive surveillance reporting systems, and disease registries for the rare pathologic conditions studied by the committee.

REFERENCES

Coulter HL. Vaccination, Social Violence, and Criminality: The Medical Assault on the American Brain. Berkeley, CA: North Atlantic Books; 1990.

Coulter HL, Fisher BL. DPT: A Shot in the Dark. San Diego: Harcourt Brace Jovanovich; 1985.

Iglehart JK. Compensating children with vaccine-related injuries. New England Journal of Medicine 1987;316:1282-1288.

Institute of Medicine. Adverse Effects of Pertussis and Rubella Vaccines. Washington, DC: National Academy Press; 1991.

Institute of Medicine. Vaccine Supply and Innovation. Washington, DC: National Academy Press; 1985.

Mariner WK. The National Vaccine Injury Compensation Program: update. Health Affairs 1992(Spring):255-265.

Miller NZ. Vaccines: Are They Really Safe and Effective? A Parent's Guide to Childhood Shots. Santa Fe, NM: New Atlantean Press, 1992.

Office of Technology Assessment. Compensation for Vaccine-Related Injuries: A Technical Memorandum. Washington, DC: U.S. Government Printing Office; 1980.

Wilson GS. The Hazards of Immunization. London: The Athlone Press; 1967.

WRC-TV. DPT: Vaccine Roulette. Washington, DC: WRC-TV; 1982.

2

Causality and Evidence

CAUSALITY

Definitions

The concept of causality is of cardinal importance in health research, clinical practice, and public health policy. It also lies at the heart of this committee's charge: to make causal inferences about the relation between vaccines routinely administered to children in the United States and several specific adverse health outcomes. Despite its importance, however, causality is not a concept that is easy to define or understand (Kramer and Lane, 1992). Consider, for example, the relation between vaccine x and Guillain-Barré syndrome (GBS). Does the statement "Vaccine x causes GBS" mean that (1) all persons immunized with vaccine x will develop GBS, (2) all cases of GBS are caused by exposure to vaccine x, or (3) there is at least one person whose GBS was caused or will be caused by vaccine x?

The first interpretation corresponds to the notion of a *sufficient cause*; vaccine x is a sufficient cause of GBS if all vaccine x recipients develop the disease. Vaccine x is a *necessary cause* of GBS if the disease occurs only among vaccine x recipients (second interpretation above). Although the idea that a "proper" cause must be both necessary and sufficient underlies Koch's postulates of causality (see Glossary in Appendix C), it is now generally recognized that for most exposure-outcome relations, exposure (i.e., the putative cause) is neither necessary nor sufficient to cause the outcome (third interpretation above). In other words, most health outcomes of interest have *multifactorial* etiologies.

A good example is coronary heart disease (CHD). It has been amply demonstrated that smoking, high blood pressure, lack of exercise, and high serum cholesterol levels are all causally related to the development of CHD. Nonetheless, many people with one or more of these risk factors do not develop CHD, and some cases of CHD occur in people without any of the risk factors. Most of the adverse events considered by the committee have *multifactorial* etiologies.

Types of Causal Questions

The causal relation between a vaccine and a given adverse event can be considered in terms of three different questions (Kramer and Lane, 1992):

1. *Can It? (potential causality):* Can the vaccine cause the adverse event, at least in certain people under certain circumstances?
2. *Did It? ("retrodictive" causality):* Given an individual who has received the vaccine and developed the adverse event, was the event caused by the vaccine?
3. *Will It? (predictive causality):* Will the next person who receives the vaccine experience the adverse event because of the vaccine? Or equivalently: How frequently will vaccine recipients experience the adverse event as a result of the vaccine?

Each of these causality questions has a somewhat different meaning, and for each, there are different methods of assessment. In the section below, each question will be discussed in turn, with reference to how it relates to the committee's charge and how the committee attempted to answer it.

Can It?

The committee has been charged with answering the *Can It?* causality question for the relations between vaccines routinely administered to children and several specific adverse events. The question is conventionally approached through controlled epidemiologic studies. (The term *epidemiologic studies* is used throughout this report in its broad sense to denote studies of disease and other health-related phenomena in groups of human subjects. The term thus includes many clinical studies but excludes animal and in vitro studies on the one hand and individual case reports on the other. See below the section Sources of Evidence for Causality for a more detailed description of epidemiologic studies.) *Can It?* is generally answered in the affirmative if the relative risk (the ratio of the rate of occurrence of the adverse event in vaccinated persons to the rate in otherwise comparable unvaccinated persons) is greater than 1, provided that systematic error (bias) and random error (sampling variation) can be shown to be improbable explanations for the findings. In other words, if a statistically significant relative risk has been obtained in an epidemiologic study (or a meta-analysis of several epidemiologic studies) and is unlikely to be due to systematic bias, *Can It?* causality can be accepted.

Much of the epidemiologic literature on causality has focused on *Can It?*, and a widely used set of criteria has evolved for *Can It?* causality assessment (Hill, 1965; Stolley, 1990; Susser, 1973; U.S. Department of Health, Education, and Welfare, 1964). These criteria are as follows:

1. *Strength of association:* A relative risk (or odds ratio) of 1.0 indicates no association between the vaccine and the adverse event. Relative risks of between 1.0 and 2.0 are generally regarded as indicating a weak association, whereas higher values indicate a moderate or strong association. In general, the higher the relative risk, the less likely the vaccine-adverse event association is to be entirely explained by one or more sources of analytic bias.

2. *Analytic bias:* Analytic bias is a systematic error in the estimate of association between the vaccine and the adverse event. It can be categorized under four types: selection bias, information bias, confounding bias, and reverse causality bias. *Selection bias* refers to the way that the sample of subjects for a study has been selected (from a source population) and retained. If the subjects in whom the vaccine-adverse event association has been analyzed differ from the source population in ways linked to *both* exposure to the vaccine *and* development of the adverse event, the resulting estimate of association will be biased. *Information bias* can result in a bias toward the null hypothesis (no association between the vaccine and the adverse event), particularly when ascertainment of either vaccine exposure or event occurrence has been sloppy; or it may create a bias away from the null hypothesis through such mechanisms as unblinding, recall bias, or unequal surveillance in vaccinated versus nonvaccinated subjects. *Confounding bias* occurs when the vaccine-adverse event association is biased as a result of a third factor that is both capable of causing the adverse event and associated with exposure to the vaccine. Finally, *reverse causality bias* can occur unless exposure to the vaccine is known to precede the adverse event.

3. *Biologic gradient (dose-response effect):* In general, *Can It?* causality is strengthened by evidence that the risk of occurrence of an outcome increases with higher doses or frequencies of exposure. In the case of vaccines, however, dose and frequency tend to be fixed. Moreover, since some of the adverse events under consideration by the committee could represent hypersensitivity or another type of idiosyncratic reaction, the absence of a dose-response effect might not constitute strong evidence against a causal relation.

4. *Statistical significance:* Might chance—that is, sampling variation—be responsible for the observed vaccine-adverse event association? The magnitude of the *P* (probability) value (or the width of the confidence interval) associated with an effect measure such as the relative risk or risk difference is generally used to estimate the role of chance in producing the observed association. This type of quantitative estimation is firmly founded in statistical theory on the basis of repeated sampling. No similar quantitative approach is usually possible, however, for assessing nonrandom errors (bias) in estimating the strength of the association.

5. *Consistency: Can It?* causality is strengthened if the vaccine-adverse event association has been detected in more than one study, particularly if the studies employed different designs and were undertaken in different populations.

6. *Biologic plausibility and coherence:* The vaccine-adverse event association should be plausible and coherent with current knowledge about the biology of the vaccine and the adverse event. Such information includes experience with the naturally occurring infection against which the vaccine is given, particularly if the vaccine is a live attenuated virus. Animal experiments and in vitro studies can also provide biologic plausibility, either by demonstrating adverse events in other animals that are similar to the ones in humans or by indicating pathophysiologic mechanisms by which the adverse event might be caused by receipt of the vaccine.

Although *Can It?* causality is usually addressed from epidemiologic studies, an affirmative answer can occasionally be obtained from individual case reports. Thus, if one or more cases have clearly been shown to be caused by a vaccine (i.e., *Did It?* can be answered strongly in the affirmative), then *Can It?* is also answered, even in the absence of epidemiologic data. In several circumstances, for example, the committee based its judgment favoring acceptance of a causal relation solely on the basis of one or more convincing case reports.

In this regard, however, it must also be added that the *absence* of convincing case reports cannot be relied upon to answer *Can It?* in the negative. If a given vaccine has an extremely long history of use and no cases of occurrence of a particular adverse event have been reported following its administration, doubt is inevitably cast on a possible causal relation. Given an extremely rare adverse event and the notorious problems of underreporting in passive surveillance systems, however, the absence of such reports is insufficient to *reject* a causal relation. The committee acknowledges that that which has not been reported might indeed have occurred.

Instead, the committee relied on epidemiologic studies to reject a causal relation. On the basis of the combined evidence from one or more controlled epidemiologic studies of high methodologic quality and sufficient statistical power (sample size), failure to detect an association between a vaccine and a particular adverse event was judged as favoring rejection of a causal relation.

Did It?

Even though the committee was not specifically charged with assessing the causal role of vaccines in individual cases, such assessments can be useful in evaluating *Can It?* causality. For many of the vaccine-adverse event associations under consideration, no epidemiologic studies have been reported, and individual case reports provide the only available evidence. As discussed above, if that evidence strongly suggests that the vaccine *did* cause the adverse event in one or more cases, then it is logical to conclude that it *can* cause the event.

In fact, many of the associations that the committee was charged with examining were first suggested because one or more cases of adverse events were found to occur following receipt of the vaccine. Some of these originated from case reports in the published medical literature; others originated from reports by physicians, nurses, parents, or vaccine recipients who observed the adverse event following exposure to the vaccine. The arousal of one's suspicions that a vaccine might be the cause of an adverse event that occurs within hours, days, or weeks following receipt of the vaccine is natural and understandable. But the mere fact that *B* follows *A* does not mean that *A* caused *B*; inferring causation solely on the basis of a proper temporal sequence is the logical fallacy of *post hoc ergo propter hoc* (literally, "after this, therefore because of this").

Many factors go into evaluating the causal relation between vaccine exposure and adverse events from individual case reports. Much of the literature in this area has come from postmarketing surveillance programs that monitor adverse drug reactions, such as those programs maintained by the U.S. Food and Drug Administration and comparable agencies in other countries (Venulet, 1982). Such passive, "spontaneous reporting" programs have been shown to have problems with both false-negative and false-positive results; that is, many of the reported cases are probably not caused by exposure to the drug or vaccine, whereas many drug- or vaccine-caused events go unreported (Faich, 1986; Péré, 1991; Tubert et al., 1992).

The information from case reports that is useful in assessing causality can be considered under the following seven headings (Kramer, 1981):

1. *Previous general experience with the vaccine:* How long has it been on the market? How many individuals have received it? How often have vaccine recipients experienced similar events? How often does the

event occur in the absence of vaccine exposure? Does a similar event occur more frequently in animals exposed to the vaccine than in appropriate controls?

2. *Alternative etiologic candidates:* Can a preexisting or new illness explain the sudden appearance of the adverse event? Does the adverse event tend to occur spontaneously (i.e., in the absence of known cause)? Were drugs, other therapies, or diagnostic tests and procedures that can cause the adverse event administered?

3. *Susceptibility of the vaccine recipient:* Has he or she received the vaccine in the past? If so, how has he or she reacted? Does his or her genetic background or previous medical history affect the risk of developing the adverse event as a consequence of vaccination?

4. *Timing of events:* Is the timing of onset of the adverse event as expected if the vaccine is the cause? How does that timing differ from the timing that would occur given the alternative etiologic candidate(s)? How does the timing, given vaccine causation, depend on the suspected mechanism (e.g., immunoglobulin E versus T-cell-mediated)?

5. *Characteristics of the adverse event:* Are there any available laboratory tests that either support or undermine the hypothesis of vaccine causation? For live attenuated virus vaccines, has the vaccine virus (or a revertant) been isolated from the target organ(s) or otherwise identified? Was there a local reaction at the site at which the vaccine was administered? How long did the adverse event last?

6. *Dechallenge:* Did the adverse event diminish as would be expected if the vaccine caused the event? Is the adverse event of a type that tends to resolve rapidly regardless of cause (e.g., a febrile seizure)? Is it irreversible (e.g., death or a permanent neurologic deficit)? Did specific treatment of the adverse event cloud interpretation of the observed evolution of the adverse event?

7. *Rechallenge:* Was the vaccine readministered? If so, did the adverse event recur?

Three ways to assess *Did It?* causality from case reports could be applied to reports of adverse events following receipt of vaccines. The most common is *global introspection* (Lane, 1984). The assessor attempts to take the relevant aforementioned factors into account and to weigh them appropriately in arriving at an overall decision, which is usually expressed as "yes" or "no." Although causality in individual cases is occasionally obvious, it may be difficult or impossible to consider and properly weigh all the relevant facts simultaneously, let alone to possess those facts (Kramer, 1986).

A second method for assessing *Did It?* causality is based on the construction of algorithms (branched logic trees) (Venulet, 1982). Such algorithms have been shown not only to improve the reproducibility and validity of causality assessments but also to make those assessments more *account-able* (Hutchinson and Lane, 1989). In other words, it is easier to see how the assessment methods were used to reach the conclusions. Most algorithms are presented in the form of a flowchart or a questionnaire, which asks a series of questions and assigns a score on the basis of the assessor's answers to those questions. The score is then used to assign a categorical probability rating such as definite, probable, possible, or unlikely.

The third approach is Bayesian analysis (Lane et al., 1987). It is based on Bayes' theorem and calculates the posterior probability of vaccine causation (the probability that the event was caused by the vaccine) from estimates of the prior probability (the probability that the vaccine caused the adverse event prior to observing the particular facts of the individual case) and a series of likelihood ratios for each pertinent element of the observed case. Each likelihood ratio is calculated by dividing the probability of observing what actually occurred, under the hypothesis that the vaccine was the cause, by the probability of observing the same occurrence given nonvaccine causation. The Bayesian approach not only provides a direct estimate of the *Did It?* probability for a given case but it is also accountable in terms of documenting the component estimates that go into calculating the posterior probability. The prior probability relates to the first two headings of information from cases reported above and is often based on epidemiologic data, when available, whereas individual case information is used to construct the likelihood ratios for the third through seventh headings. Full Bayesian analyses are often complicated and time-consuming. Moreover, because the data necessary to estimate the component prior probabilities and likelihood ratios may be unavailable, quantitative expression of the assessor's uncertainty is often highly subjective, even if based on expert opinion.

In evaluating the case reports available to the committee, the committee adopted an informal Bayesian approach. The main elements of the case reports used in the committee's assessments included the individual's medical history, the timing of onset of the adverse event following vaccine administration, specific characteristics of the adverse event, and follow-up information concerning its evolution. Each relevant piece of case information was assessed for its strength of evidence for vaccine versus nonvaccine causation. When such information (particularly concerning timing) was unavailable, the committee usually found it difficult or impossible to infer causality for that case.

The individual's medical history was taken into account in considering the role of alternative etiologic candidates (which affects the prior probability of vaccine causation). For example, a history of abnormal neurologic development or seizures prior to receipt of a vaccine reduces the probability that the encephalopathy or residual seizure disorder that developed after vaccination was caused by the vaccine.

The committee attempted to establish objective criteria for the expected timing of onset for each type of adverse event under consideration. For example, data on experimental acute demyelinating encephalomyelitis and postinfectious GBS were used to establish a time window of 5 days to 6 weeks for the likely occurrence of a vaccine-caused case of GBS, with those cases occurring 7 to 21 days postvaccination judged as being especially likely to be caused by the vaccine. In the absence of reliable age- and sex-specific background (i.e., in the absence of vaccine exposure) incidence rates for GBS, however, the mere occurrence of a case of GBS 2 weeks after receipt of a vaccine becomes interpretable only when compared with the background number of cases that would be expected to occur in individuals of that age and sex in the absence of vaccination. Because of the rather diffuse time window and the lack of reliable descriptive epidemiologic information, therefore, appropriate timing of onset, in and of itself, is insufficient to infer causality for an individual case. A useful contrast is provided by anaphylaxis, which is caused by exposure to a foreign antigen or drug. Given the occurrence of a clinically and pathologically typical case of anaphylaxis within minutes of receipt of a vaccine, it is very difficult to blame anything else.

The characteristics of the adverse event can also be helpful. Thus, the committee tried to ensure that cases of GBS or anaphylaxis met established clinical and laboratory criteria for those conditions. But mere confirmation that a case is "true GBS," although necessary, is insufficient to infer vaccine causation, because such cases do not differ from background cases that occur after a viral infection or spontaneously. On the other hand, clinical and pathologic findings consistent with the diagnosis of anaphylaxis are helpful in distinguishing sudden collapse or death caused by anaphylaxis from sudden collapse or death caused by myocardial infarction, stroke, or some other sudden catastrophic event.

Dechallenge, that is, discontinuing the suspected vaccine or reducing its dose, rarely contributes useful information. Unlike drugs, vaccines are administered at a single point in time, and their immunologic effects tend to persist well after the vaccine antigen(s) has been eliminated. Thus, the evolution of the adverse event is often not helpful in assessing vaccine causation.

Rechallenge is unusual, because physicians are unlikely to readminister a vaccine previously associated with an adverse event. When rechallenge does occur, however, the recurrence or nonrecurrence of the adverse event will often have a major impact on the causality assessment.

Will It?

The *Will It?* causality question refers to how frequently a vaccine causes a specific adverse event and can relate to either individuals or populations.

For individuals, the question refers to the probability that a given vaccine recipient will experience the adverse event because of the vaccine. For populations, *Will It?* refers to the proportion of vaccinees who will experience the adverse event as a result of the vaccine. For either individuals or populations, the answer to *Will It?* is best estimated by the magnitude of the *risk difference* (*attributable risk*): the incidence of the adverse event among vaccine recipients minus the incidence of the adverse event among other otherwise similar nonrecipients. This entity is often confused with the etiologic fraction, probably because the latter is also referred to as the *population attributable risk.*

The risk difference depends on both the background incidence of the adverse event (i.e., among nonrecipients of the vaccine) and the relative risk of its occurrence in vaccine recipients versus nonrecipients. Thus, even when the relative risk is high, the risk difference will be low if the event is extremely rare.

Will It? causality assessments are essential for risk-benefit considerations, because the risk difference expresses the probability of the risk of an adverse event caused by the vaccine. But *Will It?* depends on *Can It?*; if the evidence is insufficient to conclude whether a vaccine *can* cause a given adverse event, then it is also insufficient to conclude whether it *will.* Moreover, when an affirmative answer to the *Can It?* question is based only on case reports rather than epidemiologic studies, no quantitative estimate of *Will It?* is possible.

Even though the *Will It?* question was not part of the committee's specific mandate, estimates of the risk difference (attributable risk) are provided, whenever possible, for those associations for which the committee judged the evidence to favor acceptance of a (*Can It?*) causal relation and for which epidemiologic data provide information on the incidence of the adverse event among nonvaccinees and the relative risk of its occurrence among vaccinees.

SOURCES OF EVIDENCE FOR CAUSALITY

The sources of evidence for causality examined by the committee include demonstrated biologic plausibility, reports of individual cases or series of cases, and epidemiologic studies. In an epidemiologic study, the investigators measure one or more health-related attributes (exposures, outcomes, or both) in a defined sample of human subjects and make inferences about the values of those attributes or the associations among them (or about both the values and associations) in the source population from which the study sample originates. Epidemiologic studies can be either uncontrolled (descriptive) or controlled (analytic), observational (survey) or experimental (clinical trial). These sources of evidence are discussed in greater detail below in the same order in which they will be considered within each of the vaccine- and adverse event-specific chapters.

Biologic Plausibility

All of the vaccine-adverse event associations assessed in this report have some biologic plausibility, at least on theoretical grounds. That is, a knowledgeable person could postulate a feasible mechanism by which the vaccine could cause the adverse event. Actual *demonstration* of biologic plausibility, however, was based on the known effects of the natural disease against which the vaccine is given and the results of animal experiments and in vitro studies. Only demonstrated biologic plausibility was considered by the committee in reaching its causality judgments.

Case Reports, Case Series, and Uncontrolled Observational Studies

The committee obtained reports of individual cases of adverse events following receipt of vaccine through the published medical literature as well as from passive, spontaneous surveillance systems established by the vaccine manufacturers, the U.S. Food and Drug Administration, and the Centers for Disease Control and Prevention. These include the Monitoring System for Adverse Events Following Immunization and the Spontaneous Reporting System, as well as the more recent Vaccine Adverse Event Reporting System (VAERS). Appendix B identifies the material from these systems obtained and reviewed by the committee. Chapter 10 includes a discussion of the limitations of passive surveillance systems such as these, as well as an analysis of the data contained within VAERS regarding reports of deaths following vaccination.

Uncontrolled observational studies are usually based on a cohort design, in which an identified group of vaccinees is followed for some period of time to detect the occurrence of one or more adverse events. These studies often incorporate more active surveillance than is the case in the passive, spontaneous reporting systems mentioned above, although a clear distinction from case series emanating from defined population bases is often difficult. Because no nonexposed control group is included in such studies, however, the rates of occurrence of the adverse events under consideration can usually be interpreted only descriptively, and the evidence derived therefrom is rarely helpful in either accepting or rejecting a causal relation. Also included under uncontrolled observational studies are reports of vaccine exposure in a representative group of individuals experiencing the adverse event. Such studies can also overlap with case series, although the authors of case series often attempt to make causal inferences (or hypotheses) concerning exposure to vaccines and/or other factors and, hence, usually provide considerably more detail about alternative etiologic candidates, the timing of the onset of the adverse event following vaccine administration, and clinical and pathologic descriptions of the adverse event.

Uncontrolled epidemiologic studies do not yield direct estimates of the effect of vaccine exposure on the risk of developing the adverse event. Sometimes, however, the existence of reliable data on the risk in unexposed subjects can form the basis of an external (to the study) control group and, hence, an indirect estimate of the vaccine effect.

Controlled Observational Studies

Controlled observational studies permit a direct estimate of the effect of vaccine exposure on the occurrence of the adverse event. Most are based on either a cohort or a case-control design. In controlled *cohort studies*, a defined group of individuals exposed to a given vaccine are followed longitudinally for the occurrence of one or more adverse events of interest, and the rate of such occurrence is compared with the rate in an otherwise similar group of nonexposed individuals by using either the ratio of rates (relative risk) or their difference (risk difference). In many populations, however, exposure to vaccines is virtually universal; exposure can then be defined within a rather narrow time window; that is, the rate of occurrence of an adverse event within 2 weeks of vaccine administration can be compared with the rate of occurrence of an adverse event several weeks or months thereafter. In *case-control studies*, rates of prior exposure to the suspected vaccine between individuals with (the cases) and without (the controls) the adverse event are compared. No direct calculation of relative risk or risk difference can be made from a case-control study, but the exposure odds ratio (the odds of exposure among the cases divided by the odds of exposure among the controls) can be shown to be a very good estimate of the true relative risk when the adverse event is rare. In fact, the case-control design is often the only feasible epidemiologic research design for rare events (e.g., GBS, transverse myelitis, optic neuritis, and Stevens-Johnson syndrome). As with cohort studies, the time window of exposure (prior to the occurrence of the adverse event) should be defined narrowly to reflect the biologic latent period corresponding to the pathogenesis of the suspected adverse event.

Other types of controlled epidemiologic studies can also provide useful information. In *ecologic studies*, for example, the rates of a given adverse event are compared among otherwise similar regions or countries with different policies for administering a suspected vaccine. Such studies assess the vaccine-adverse event association at the population level, and therefore provide only indirect evidence of the association among individuals.

Controlled Clinical Trials

The epidemiologic study designs discussed up to this point are all observational. Allocation of exposure (receipt or nonreceipt of a given vaccine) was decided either by the vaccine recipients, by their parents, or by their physicians—not by the study investigators. The investigators merely attempted to observe the effect of vaccine exposure; they did not control who did or did not receive the vaccine. This absence of control over who gets exposed is what makes observational studies differ from *experimental studies*, which are also called *clinical trials*. In a controlled clinical trial of a vaccine, outcomes are compared in subjects who are allocated by the investigator to receive or not receive the vaccine. The controlled clinical trial design provides the strongest scientific evidence bearing on the causal relation between a vaccine and an adverse event, particularly when exposure versus nonexposure to a vaccine is assigned in a random fashion. The study design is then referred to as a *randomized clinical trial*. As with observational cohort studies, the effect of vaccine exposure on the occurrence of the adverse event is usually expressed as the relative risk or risk difference. Unfortunately, many of the adverse events under consideration by the committee are so rare that even large, multicenter randomized trials would be too small to detect differences in the incidences of a rare adverse event.

Combining the Evidence

When two or more epidemiologic studies that bear on a given vaccine-adverse event association were located by the committee (particularly when they shared a similar design), the committee used meta-analysis to pool the results from those studies and thereby gain both increased statistical power and enhanced generalizability (Dickersin and Berlin, 1992). Even a meta-analysis of epidemiologic studies, however, does not help in combining the evidence from *different* sources of evidence. Because no generally accepted rules exist for combining such evidence, the committee adopted its own operational criteria.

Although randomized clinical trials are generally accepted as providing the most scientifically valid assessment of causal relations, most have been too small to contribute any useful evidence bearing on the vaccine-adverse event associations under consideration by the committee. Thus, case reports, case series, and uncontrolled observational studies and controlled observational epidemiologic studies were often the main basis for the committee's judgment. As mentioned above, *only* epidemiologic studies were used to conclude that the evidence favored rejection of a causal relation. In the absence of epidemiologic studies favoring acceptance of a causal relation, individual case reports and case series were relied upon, provided that the nature and timing of the adverse event following vaccine administration and the absence of likely alternative etiologic candidates were such that a reasonable certainty of causality could be inferred (as described above) from one or more case reports. The presence or absence of demonstrated biologic plausibility was also considered in weighing the overall balance of evidence for and against a causal relation. In the absence of convincing case reports or epidemiologic studies, however, the mere demonstration of biologic plausibility was felt to constitute insufficient evidence to accept or reject a causal relation.

Acceptance and rejection of a causal relation between any exposure and outcome are inherently asymmetric. Very strong evidence in favor of such a causal relation can be said to *establish* a causal relation, although 100 percent "proof," in the mathematical sense, is never possible. It is almost never possible, however, to be as sure about rejecting such a causal relation because even the largest population-based epidemiologic studies have insufficient statistical power to detect extremely rare causes of an outcome (e.g., an excess risk of 1 per 1 million population). Hence, the categories in which the committee has summarized the evidence for causality (see below) reflect this essential asymmetry.

Despite the committee's attempts at objectivity, the interpretation of scientific evidence always retains at least some subjective elements. Use of such "objective" standards as P values, confidence intervals, and relative risks may convey a false sense that such judgments are entirely objective. However, judgments about potential sources of bias, although based on sound scientific principles, cannot usually be quantitated. This is true even for the scientific "gold standard" in evaluating causal relations, the randomized clinical trial.

For each vaccine-adverse event association under consideration, the committee started from a neutral position, presuming neither the presence nor the absence of a causal relation between the vaccines and the adverse events under consideration. Each category of evidence was then assessed and weighted (as described above) to arrive at an overall judgment as to whether the balance of evidence favored acceptance or rejection of a causal relation between the vaccine and the adverse event. To enhance scientific accountability, the committee's judgment of causality for each vaccine-adverse event association considered is accompanied by an explanation of the evidentiary basis for that judgment.

SUMMARIZING THE EVIDENCE FOR CAUSALITY

The committee attempted to build on the methods and procedures used by the Committee to Review the Adverse Consequences of Pertussis and

Rubella Vaccines (Institute of Medicine, 1991). The pertussis and rubella vaccine committee summarized the evidence bearing on those vaccines using the following five categories: (1) no evidence bearing on a causal relation, (2) evidence insufficient to indicate a causal relation, (3) evidence does not indicate a causal relation, (4) evidence is consistent with a causal relation, and (5) evidence indicates a causal relation. They then assigned each vaccine-adverse event association under their consideration to one of these five categories.

Because some confusion has arisen over the meaning of the category descriptions used by the pertussis and rubella vaccine committee, despite extensive explanation both in footnotes and the text, the Vaccine Safety Committee adopted some minor modifications in wording intended to help in the interpretation of the present report. To facilitate reading by those familiar with the report of the previous committee, the present committee maintained both the number of categories (five) and the order of those categories but modified the wording in an attempt to clarify its meaning.

The names and descriptions of the categories used in this report are as follows:

1. *No evidence bearing on a causal relation.*

Putative associations between vaccine and adverse events for which the committee was unable to locate any case reports or epidemiologic studies were placed in this category. Demonstrated biologic plausibility alone was considered insufficient to remove a given vaccine-adverse event association from this category.

2. *The evidence is inadequate to accept or reject a causal relation.*

One or more (in some instances there were many) case reports or epidemiologic studies were located by the committee, but the evidence for a causal relation neither outweighed nor was outweighed by the evidence against a causal relation. The presence or absence of demonstrated biologic plausibility was considered insufficient to shift this balance in either direction.

3. *The evidence favors rejection of a causal relation.*

Only evidence from epidemiologic studies was considered as a basis for possible rejection of a causal relation. Such evidence was judged as favoring rejection only when a rigorously performed epidemiologic study (or a meta-analysis of several such studies) of adequate size (i.e., statistical power) did not detect a significant association between the vaccine and the adverse event. The absence of demonstrated biologic plausibility was considered supportive of a decision to reject a causal relation but insufficient on its own to shift the balance of evidence from other sources.

4. *The evidence favors acceptance of a causal relation.*

The balance of evidence from one or more case reports or epidemiologic studies provides evidence for a causal relation that outweighs the evidence against such a relation. Demonstrated biologic plausibility was considered supportive of a decision to accept a causal relation but insufficient on its own to shift the balance of evidence from other sources.

5. *The evidence establishes a causal relation.*

Epidemiologic studies and/or case reports provide unequivocal evidence for a causal relation, and biologic plausibility has been demonstrated.

REFERENCES

Dickersin K, Berlin JA. Meta-analysis: state-of-the-science. Epidemiological Reviews 1992;14:154-176.

Faich GA. Adverse drug reaction monitoring. New England Journal of Medicine 1986;314:1589-1592.

Hill AB. The environment and disease: association or causation. Proceedings of the Royal Society of Medicine 1965;58:295-300.

Hutchinson TA, Lane DA. Assessing methods for causality assessment of suspected adverse drug reactions. Journal of Clinical Epidemiology 1989;42:5-16.

Institute of Medicine. Adverse Effects of Pertussis and Rubella Vaccines. Washington, DC: National Academy Press; 1991.

Kramer MS. Difficulties in assessing the adverse effects of drugs. British Journal of Clinical Pharmacology 1981;11:105S-110S.

Kramer MS. Assessing causality of adverse drug reactions: global introspection and its limitations. Drug Information Journal 1986;20:433-437.

Kramer MS, Lane DA. Causal propositions in clinical research and practice. Journal of Clinical Epidemiology 1992;45:639-649.

Lane D. A probabilist's view of causality assessment. Drug Information Journal 1984;18:323-330.

Lane DA, Kramer MS, Hutchinson TA, Jones JK, Naranjo C. The causality assessment of adverse drug reactions using a Bayesian approach. Journal of Pharmaceutical Medicine 1987;2:265-268.

Péré J-C. Estimation du numérateur en notification spontanée. In: Bégaud B, ed. Analyse d'Incidence en Pharmacovigilance: Application à la Notification Spontanée. Bordeaux, France: ARME-Pharmacovigilance Editions; 1991.

Stolley PD. How to interpret studies of adverse drug reactions. Clinical Pharmacology and Therapeutics 1990;48:337-339.

Susser M. Causal Thinking in the Health Sciences. New York: Oxford; 1973.

Tubert P, Bégaud B, Péré JC, Haramburu F, Lellouch J. Power and weakness of spontaneous reporting: a probabilistic approach. Journal of Clinical Epidemiology 1992;45:283-286.

U.S. Department of Health, Education, and Welfare. Smoking and Health: Report of the Advisory Committee to the Surgeon General. PHS Publication No. 1103. Washington, DC: U.S. Public Health Service, U.S. Department of Health, Education, and Welfare; 1964.

Venulet J, ed. Assessing Causes of Adverse Drug Reactions with Special Reference to Standardized Methods. London: Academic Press; 1982.

3

Neurologic Disorders

The possibility of adverse neurologic events has fueled much of the concern about the safety of vaccines. This chapter presents a detailed discussion of the neurologic events considered by the committee. The chapter is organized into two main sections, demyelinating disease and non-demyelinating disease. Specific reports on the association of the vaccines under consideration and the neurologic disorders discussed in this chapter can be found in the subsequent chapters specific to each vaccine or vaccine component.

DEMYELINATING DISEASE

Acute demyelinating disease of the central and peripheral nervous systems can follow viral and some bacterial infections and can complicate the administration of inactivated antiviral vaccines. The acute monophasic central nervous system disease is variably known as postvaccinal encephalomyelitis, postinfectious encephalomyelitis, or acute disseminated encephalomyelitis (ADEM). The peripheral nervous system complication is known as postinfectious neuritis, acute inflammatory demyelinating polyneuritis, or the Guillain-Barré syndrome (GBS) and is characterized by the rapid onset of flaccid motor weakness with depression of tendon reflexes and inflammatory demyelination of peripheral nerves.

Both of these demyelinating complications were noted after the introduction of rabies vaccines grown in animal brain or spinal cord. Pasteur's first rabies vaccine of the 1880s was produced from desiccated infected rabbit spinal cord, and occasional cases of acute encephalomyelitis were seen following multiple injections of the vaccine. These were initially thought to result from inadequate attenuation or inactivation of the virus or the activation of some endogenous agent in the human brain. Because early attenuated or inactivated rabies vaccines were prepared in animal nervous system tissue, the question that the causal factor might be some factor within animal tissues was also raised (Hemachudha et al., 1987a,b). On rare occasions, a clinically and histologically similar encephalomyelitis also complicated injection of the vaccinia virus used for the prevention of small-pox, although this vaccine contained no animal neural tissue. ADEM also has been seen after natural infections with measles, varicella, mumps, rubella, and other viruses (Johnson et al., 1985).

Experimental Models

Thomas Rivers, the father of American virology, worked extensively with vaccinia virus and was intrigued by the similarity of the demyelinating complication of vaccination and the histopathologic changes seen after administration of rabies vaccines. With Schwenker, he carried out multiple inoculations of normal brain tissue into monkeys, and in 1935, they reported the induction of acute, experimental, allergic (autoimmune) encephalomyelitis (EAE) (Rivers and Schwenker, 1935). Subsequently, Kabat et al. (1947) found that EAE could consistently be induced by a single inoculation of brain tissue if it was mixed with adjuvant. Disease developed in 7 to 21 days in some species, and detailed studies of the pathogenesis of EAE were possible. Although multiple brain antigens have been implicated, myelin basic protein most readily induces the disease, and since EAE can be passively transferred with immune cells but not serum, cell-mediated immunity appears to be of primary pathogenetic importance. In drawing analogies to human diseases, it should be noted that different inbred strains of animals show different susceptibilities, and although myelin basic protein is similar between species, the encephalitogenic region of myelin basic protein differs between different species (Martin et al., 1992).

In Latin America, a rabies vaccine was prepared in unmyelinated neo-natal mouse brains to avoid the use of central nervous system myelin. Multiple injections of these preparations into humans, however, were complicated in some cases by an acute polyneuritis similar to GBS (Held and Adaros, 1972). It was assumed that the induction of autoimmunity to a peripheral nerve antigen might be the mechanism. In 1955, Waksman and Adams reported that rabbits injected with peripheral nerve tissue in adjuvant developed an experimental allergic (autoimmune) neuritis (EAN) resembling GBS. The predominant protein related to EAN is a peripheral neurospecific polypeptide protein of the peripheral nerve, and the disease appeared to depend largely on cell-mediated immunity.

Acute Disseminated Encephalomyelitis

ADEM is characterized by acute depression of consciousness and multifocal neurologic findings that usually occur a few days or weeks following vaccine administration or virus-like disease. It is characterized pathologically by diffuse foci of perivenular inflammation and demyelination that are most prominent in the white matter of the brain and spinal cord. A definitive diagnosis of ADEM can be made only pathologically. However, recent imaging studies with enhanced magnetic resonance imagers have defined a characteristic pattern of multiple enhancing white matter lesions in patients with ADEM, and in the future, magnetic resonance imaging findings may give better data on nonfatal, nonbiopsied cases of suspected postimmunization ADEM.

Multiple Sclerosis

The establishment of a relation between acute central and peripheral nervous system demyelinating disease and infections and vaccines has opened the question of a possible relation to chronic demyelinating disease, specifically, multiple sclerosis. When mean levels of antibody to measles virus are assayed in the serum and spinal fluid of patients with multiple sclerosis, they are consistently higher than those in controls, and in some studies elevated levels of antibodies to a variety of different viruses have been found in serum and spinal fluid (Johnson et al., 1985). The persistence of these agents in patients with multiple sclerosis has not been established. In the diagnosis of multiple sclerosis, demyelinating lesions not only must occur in multiple locations within the nervous system but must also occur at different times. A prospective study of patients with multiple sclerosis showed that exacerbations appeared to be more frequent after nonspecific viral illnesses (Sibley et al., 1985). Therefore, it would be feasible that vaccines also might precipitate an exacerbation either in a patient who was predisposed to develop the disease or in a patient with already established disease. However, there is no clear-cut causal relation between any virus or vaccine and multiple sclerosis.

Focal Lesions

Both optic neuritis and transverse myelitis often are components of diffuse demyelinating diseases, both ADEM and multiple sclerosis. When they occur in isolation, their mechanisms and pathologies are usually unknown, although it is suspected that they represent unifocal, acute episodes of demyelination. Transverse myelitis is characterized by the acute onset of signs of spinal cord disease, usually involving the descending motor tracts and the ascending sensory fibers, suggesting a lesion at one level of the spinal cord. By enhanced magnetic resonance imaging, the apparent lesion in the spinal cord extends over many segments of the spinal cord. The annual incidence of transverse myelitis in Rochester, Minnesota, from 1970 to 1980 was 7.4 per 100,000 people (Beghi et al., 1982). The authors noted that this incidence is approximately sixfold higher than a rate calculated for Israel. They attributed this to differences in how successful the two studies were at identifying all cases of transverse myelitis.

Optic neuritis represents a lesion in the optic nerve behind the orbit but anterior to the optic chiasm. This cranial nerve is an extension of the central nervous system, and so when there is demyelinating disease, it represents central demyelination, not peripheral nerve demyelination. When the lesion is central to the orbit, the optic disk appears normal; this clinical form of optic neuritis is called *retrobulbar neuritis*. When the lesion or inflammation is very near the orbit, swelling of the optic disk can be seen on fundoscopic examination; this clinical form is called *papillitis*. This clinical distinction does not imply a different pathogenesis or pathology. Retrobulbar neuritis or papillitis in young adults is a very common early symptom of multiple sclerosis. Optic neuritis may occur as a solitary unexplained monophasic disease, and it may accompany the acute monophasic disease ADEM. No population-based incidence rates were identified.

Guillain-Barré Syndrome

Historical Background

Instances of acute ascending paralysis have been on record since the early nineteenth century, but it was the description by Guillain, Barré, and Strohl in 1916 of two cases (including cerebrospinal fluid findings) that was critical and discriminating enough to delineate a new syndrome. Those authors described acute areflexic weakness without fever, meningismus, or constitutional symptoms in two young infantrymen who both made a complete and rapid recovery. Using the newly introduced diagnostic technique of lumbar puncture, Guillain, Barré, and Strohl showed that the spinal fluid protein level was elevated but without an accompanying pleocytosis. These are the essential elements of GBS. Now, more than 75 years later, a great deal of descriptive and phenomenologic information has been added to the original observations, all of which indicate that this disorder is immune system mediated and targets peripheral nerves. Nevertheless, the critical questions as to the nature and regulation of this abnormal immune response, the nosologic limits of the disorder, and the identities of the specific antigens that were responsible for the syndrome are still not known.

Clinical and Laboratory Features

Guillain-Barré syndrome has recently been fully reviewed in several publications (Arnason and Soliven, 1992; Asbury and Gibbs, 1990; Hughes, 1990; Ropper, 1992; Ropper et al., 1991). The symptoms of GBS usually appear over the course of a single day and may continue to progress for from as few as 3 or 4 days up to 3 or 4 weeks. The symptoms in over 90 percent of the patients plateau by 4 weeks. The major symptom is weakness, generally symmetrical, usually ascending, and usually affecting the legs more than the arms. In a smaller proportion of patients, the symptoms begin in the arms or cranial nerves and descend. About 30 percent of all patients require respiratory support at some stage of the illness, and weakness of the tongue, swallowing, and facial muscles is common in up to 50 percent of all patients with GBS. Paresthesias and even painfulness are experienced in a majority of the patients, but major sensory deficits are not frequent. Ataxia of stance and gait may be an early sign. Reflexes disappear early and return only late in the recovery phase. Fever and constitutional symptoms are generally not present, although in children a degree of meningismus may be noted in a quarter to a third of the patients. The mortality rate is 5 percent or less. For survivors, recovery is the rule, requiring anywhere from a few weeks to well over a year. Some 15 to 20 percent of survivors manifest some residual findings, and 5 percent or more have serious residual disabilities.

Factors affecting prognosis are age (older people do more poorly), the fulminance and severity of the neuropathy, the severity of the electrodiagnostic findings early in the disease, and early treatment, either plasmapheresis or high-dose intravenous immunoglobulin (Cornblath et al., 1988; McKhann et al., 1988; van der Meché et al., 1992).

Cerebrospinal fluid is normal in the first few days of illness, but the protein content rises toward the end of the first week and remains elevated for several months in over 90 percent of patients. Spinal fluid cell counts are below 10 cells, mostly lymphocytes, per mm^3, but in human immunodeficiency virus (HIV)-positive individuals, spinal fluid cell counts may be as high as 100 to 200/mm^3.

The characteristic electrodiagnostic features are those of demyelination with variable degrees of admixed, presumably secondary, axonal degeneration. These abnormalities include prolongation of distal latencies and F-wave latencies, particularly as early features; slowing of nerve conduction velocity, frequently in a multifocal pattern; conduction block; and chronodispersion of evoked compound action potentials. In some cases axonal degeneration predominates, as determined by electrodiagnostic criteria and, when studied, by pathologic observation (Feasby et al., 1986, 1993). Whether axonal degeneration may be a primary event in GBS is controversial. At worst, nerve trunks may be completely inexcitable. Widespread axonal degeneration is associated with prolonged and incomplete recovery.

Diagnostic Criteria

In 1978, diagnostic criteria for GBS were promulgated in response to a request from the National Institutes of Health (Asbury et al., 1978). These criteria continue to be in general use and are reproduced in the box entitled Definition of Guillain-Barré Syndrome and Criteria for Diagnosis; recently proposed electrodiagnostic criteria are given in the box entitled Proposed Electrodiagnostic Criteria for Demyelination of Peripheral Nerve (Asbury and Cornblath, 1990). The features required for diagnosis include progressive motor weakness and areflexia. The features that are strongly supportive of the diagnosis include progression for less than 4 weeks, relative symmetry, mild sensory symptoms or signs, frequent cranial nerve involvement, a high proportion of functional recovery, some autonomic dysfunction, and the absence of fever at the onset of neuropathy. Electrodiagnostic and spinal fluid findings are also included in the criteria. In addition, a number of features that either cast doubt on the diagnosis or rule it out are elaborated. Efforts to refine and detail these criteria, including electrodiagnostic criteria (Asbury and Cornblath, 1990), have continued (Arnason and Soliven, 1992; Asbury, 1981).

Antecedent Events

Over half of all patients with GBS have a history of a preceding acute infectious illness, either respiratory or gastrointestinal, in the 1 to 4 weeks prior to the onset of neuropathic symptoms. Although the basis for the preceding illness remains unidentified in many patients, several infectious agents are strongly associated with GBS. Nonviral infectious agents include *Campylobacter jejuni*, which is perhaps the most common, and *Mycoplasma pneumoniae*. Certain viral infections are also strongly associated with GBS, including cytomegalovirus and Epstein-Barr virus, vaccinia virus used for smallpox vaccination, and HIV. A host of other viral infections, including measles, mumps, and hepatitis B, have been reported as antecedent events, but it is unclear whether their occurrence preceding GBS exceeds that from chance alone. Less commonly, vaccines, surgical procedures, and malignant disorders, particularly Hodgkin's disease and other lymphomas, are either antecedent events or underlying conditions.

Definition of Guillain-Barré Syndrome and Criteria for Diagnosis

Guillain-Barré syndrome is a recognizable entity for which the basis for diagnosis is descriptive on the basis of the present state of knowledge. The features that allow a diagnosis include clinical, laboratory, and electrodiagnostic criteria. The problem is not with the recognition of a typical case but with knowing the boundaries by which the core disorder is delimited. The following criteria are established, in light of current knowledge and opinion, to define those limits.

The presence of preceding events is frequent, but they are not essential to the diagnosis. Most commonly, preceding events are viral infections, but the association of Guillain-Barré syndrome with preceding surgery, inoculations, and *Mycoplasma* infections is also known. In addition, Guillain-Barré syndrome occurs more frequently than by chance in the setting of preexisting illnesses such as Hodgkin's disease, lymphoma, or lupus erythematosus. Many patients with Guillain-Barré syndrome have no history of any of these events, and the diagnosis should be made independently of them.

I. Features Required for Diagnosis

  A. Progressive motor weakness of more than one limb. The degree ranges from minimal weakness of the legs, with or without mild ataxia, to total paralysis of the muscles of all four extremities and of the trunk, bulbar and facial paralysis, and external ophthalmoplegia.

  B. Areflexia (loss of tendon jerks). Universal areflexia is the rule, although distal areflexia with definite hyporeflexia of the biceps and knee jerks suffices if other features are consistent.

II. Features Strongly Supportive of the Diagnosis

  A. Clinical features (ranked in order of importance)

   1. Progression. Symptoms and signs of motor weakness develop rapidly but cease to progress by 4 weeks into the illness. Approximately 50 percent of patients will reach the nadir by 2 weeks, 80 percent by 3 weeks, and more than 90 percent by 4 weeks.

   2. Relative symmetry. Symmetry is seldom absolute, but usually, if one limb is affected, the opposite limb is affected as well.

   3. Mild sensory symptoms or signs.

   4. Cranial nerve involvement. Facial weakness occurs in approximately 50 percent of patients and is frequently bilateral. Other cranial nerves may be involved, particularly those innervating the tongue and muscles of deglutition and sometimes the extraocular motor nerves. On occasion (less than 5 percent), the neuropathy may begin in the nerves to the extraocular muscles or other cranial nerves.

   5. Recovery. Recovery usually begins 2 to 4 weeks after progression

Source: Adapted from Asbury et al. (1978).

stops. Recovery may be delayed for months. Most patients recover functionally.

6. Autonomic dysfunction. Tachycardia and other arrhythmias, postural hypotension, hypertension, and vasomotor symptoms, when present, support the diagnosis. These findings may fluctuate. Care must be exercised to exclude other bases for these symptoms, such as pulmonary embolism.
7. Absence of fever at the onset of neuritic symptoms.

Variant clinical features (not ranked in order of importance)

1. Fever at the time of onset of neuritic symptoms.
2. Severe sensory loss with pain.
3. Progression beyond 4 weeks. Occasionally, a patient's disease will continue to progress for many weeks longer than 4 weeks or the patient will have a minor relapse.
4. Cessation of progression without recovery or with major permanent residual deficit remaining.
5. Sphincter function. Usually, the sphincter is not affected, but transient bladder paralysis may occur during the evolution of symptoms.
6. Central nervous system involvement. Ordinarily, Guillain-Barré syndrome is thought of as a disease of the peripheral nervous system. Evidence of central nervous system involvement is controversial. In occasional patients, such findings as severe ataxia interpretable as cerebellar in origin, dysarthria, extensor plantar responses, and ill-defined sensory levels are demonstrable, and these need not exclude the diagnosis if other features are typical.

B. Cerebrospinal fluid (CSF) features strongly supportive of the diagnosis

1. CSF protein. After the first week of symptoms, CSF protein levels are elevated or have been shown to rise on serial lumbar punctures.
2. CSF cells. Counts of 10 or fewer mononuclear leukocytes/mm^3 of CSF.

Variant CSF features supportive of diagnosis

1. No increase in the level of CSF protein in the period from 1 to 10 weeks after the onset of symptoms (rare).
2. Counts of 11 to 50 mononuclear leukocytes/mm^3 of CSF.

C. Electrodiagnostic features strongly supportive of the diagnosis. Approximately 80 percent of patients will have evidence of nerve conduction slowing or blockage at some point during the illness. Conduction velocity is usually less than 60 percent of normal, but the

continued

process is patchy and not all nerves are affected. Distal latencies may be increased to as much as three times normal. Use of F-wave responses often gives a good indication of slowing over proximal portions of the nerve trunks and roots. Up to 20 percent of patients will have normal conduction study results. Results of conduction studies may not become abnormal until several weeks into the illness.

III.   Features Casting Doubt on the Diagnosis

1. Marked, persistent asymmetry of weakness.
2. Persistent bladder or bowel dysfunction.
3. Bladder or bowel dysfunction at onset.
4. More than 50 mononuclear leukocytes/mm^3 in CSF.
5. Presence of polymorphonuclear leukocytes in CSF.
6. Sharp sensory level.

IV.   Features That Rule out the Diagnosis

1. A current history of hexacarbon abuse (the volatile solvents *n*-hexane and methyl *n*-butyl ketone). This includes huffing of paint lacquer vapors or addictive glue sniffing.
2. Abnormal porphyrin metabolism indicating a diagnosis of acute intermittent porphyria. This would manifest as increased excretion of porphobilinogen and δ-aminolevulinic acid in the urine.
3. A history or finding of recent diphtheritic infection, either faucial or wound, with or without myocarditis.
4. Features clinically consistent with lead neuropathy (upper limb weakness with prominent wrist drop; may be asymmetrical) and evidence of lead intoxication.
5. The occurrence of a purely sensory syndrome.
6. A definite diagnosis of a condition such as poliomyelitis, botulism, hysterical paralysis, or toxic neuropathy (e.g., from nitrofurantoin, dapsone, or organophosphorus compounds), which occasionally may be confused with Guillain-Barré syndrome.

Vaccinations are an infrequent antecedent event in patients with GBS, probably occurring in less than 1 to 5 percent of all cases. In most large series of GBS, recent vaccination either is not mentioned or is described in an occasional person. Hankey (1987) noted that 5 of 109 subjects had recently been vaccinated (two with diphtheria and tetanus toxoids and pertussis vaccine [DPT] and one each with rubella vaccine, tetanus toxoid, and cholera and typhoid vaccines). Winer and colleagues (1988) noted six recent vaccinees in a series of 100 consecutive cases of GBS, but they also found five recent vaccinees in the 100 case controls.

Vaccinations have also had major public policy implications in relation to GBS. In the swine flu incident of 1976-1977 (Langmuir et al., 1984;

**Proposed Electrodiagnostic Criteria
for Demyelination of Peripheral Nerve**

These criteria concern nerve conduction studies (including proximal nerve segments) in which the predominant process is demyelination.
Must have three of the following features:

I. Reduction in conduction velocity in two or more motor nerves.

    A. <80 percent of the lower limit of normal (LLN) if the amplitude is >80 percent of LLN.
    B. <70 percent of LLN if the amplitude is <80 percent of LLN.

II. Conduction block or abnormal temporal dispersion in one or more motor nerves: either the peroneal nerve between the ankle and below the fibular head, median nerve between the wrist and elbow, or the ulnar nerve between the wrist and below the elbow.

    Criteria for partial conduction block:

    A. >15 percent change in duration between proximal and distal sites and >20 percent drop in the negative-peak area or peak-to-peak amplitude between the proximal and distal sites.

III. Prolonged distal latencies in two or more nerves.

    A. >125 percent of the upper limit of normal (ULN) if the amplitude is >80 percent of LLN.
    B. >150 percent of ULN if the amplitude is <80 percent of LLN.

IV. Absent F-waves or prolonged minimum F-wave latencies (10-15 trials) in two or more motor nerves.

    A. >120 percent of ULN if the amplitude is >80 percent of LLN.
    B. >150 percent of ULN if the amplitude is <80 percent of LLN.

Source: Adapted from Asbury and Cornblath (1990).

Safranek et al., 1991; Schonberger et al., 1979), the risk of developing GBS in the 6 weeks following vaccination was some six- to eightfold greater than that for those who were not vaccinated, even though the overall incidence was only about 1 per 100,000 vaccinees. What it was about the swine flu vaccine that led to GBS on rare occasions has never been discovered; nevertheless, the capacity of that particular vaccine to trigger excess cases of GBS is thoroughly documented. In addition, the clinical features of GBS following swine flu vaccination resembled in all respects those

TABLE 3-1   Demyelinating Disorders Encountered with Rabies Vaccines

Vaccine Components	Incidence of Neuroparalytic Events	Distribution Pattern of Neuroparalytic Events	Type of Event	
			Encephalomyelitis (%)	GBS (%)
Mature brain and spinal cord (Semple vaccine)	1:300-1:3,000	Uniform	85	15
Suckling mouse brain	1:7,500	Clustered	0	100
Human diploid cell vaccine	0		0	0

following other antecedent events or no antecedent events. Monitoring for GBS following the administration of other influenza vaccines in the years subsequent to the 1976-1977 swine flu vaccine incident did not disclose any excess cases of GBS (Hurwitz et al., 1981; Kaplan et al., 1983; Roscelli et al., 1991).

It has been known for decades that GBS occurs following the administration of another vaccine, namely, rabies vaccine produced from the nervous tissue of an infected animal (Table 3-1). Because they are inexpensive, these vaccines are still made and used in certain parts of the world, including Asia and South America. Vaccine made from mature sheep or goat brain and then inactivated with phenol (Semple vaccine) causes encephalomyelitis as its main neurologic adverse event, and the reported incidence of such events is from 1 per 300 to 1 per 3,000 vaccinees (Hemachudha et al., 1987b, 1988). A small proportion, perhaps 15 percent, of Semple vaccinees who develop a neuroparalytic adverse event have characteristic GBS. Of interest, these patients develop high levels of antibody to myelin basic protein, a central myelin constituent in serum and cerebrospinal fluid (Hemachudha et al., 1987a, 1988). In contrast, rabies vaccine produced from infected suckling mouse brain induces, on occasion (approximately 1 in 7,500 vaccinees), a GBS-like syndrome (Lopez Adaros and Held, 1971). The clinical features tend to be unusually severe (Cabrera et al., 1987). These individuals rarely develop antibody titers to myelin basic protein (Hemachudha et al., 1988), which is consistent with the fact that the suckling mouse brain is unmyelinated. It is not clear what the basis for GBS might be following the administration of either Semple rabies vaccine or suckling mouse brain rabies vaccine, but most authorities believe that the neuroparalytic events that occur following receipt of these two rabies vaccines are related to an immune response to admixed neural constituents in the inoculum.

As discussed elsewhere in this chapter, the expected latency between an antecedent event (when infection or administration of antigen occurs) and the first symptoms of GBS is mainly between 7 and 21 days. Occasional cases appear to have latencies of between 22 and 42 days. All evidence indicates that GBS is immune mediated via a delayed-type hypersensitivity mechanism. Taken together, these two observations allow a range of latencies to be stated for GBS, that is, 5 days to 6 weeks. Similarly, ADEM is widely believed to be the human counterpart of experimental allergic encephalomyelitis, and EAE has an observed latency of about 10 to 20 days. ADEM has a similar clinical latency, and its pathologic features also have all of the hallmarks of a delayed-type hypersensitivity response. On the basis of these observations and inferences, a conservative estimate of the limits of the latencies for both GBS and ADEM is considered to be from 5 days to 6 weeks throughout this report.

Pathology and Pathogenesis

A characteristic pathologic feature of GBS is the presence of mononuclear cell infiltrates in peripheral nerves and roots in both a diffuse and a perivenular distribution (Arnason and Soliven, 1992; Asbury et al., 1969). Lesions are patchy and variable, and some patients may show almost no cellular inflammation (Honavar et al., 1991). Lesions are most prominent in the proximal plexuses and roots, particularly the ventral root, but may be found scattered throughout the peripheral nervous system, including the autonomic trunks and intramuscular twigs. Demyelination often corresponds to the distribution of cellular infiltration, but demyelination is quite extensive even in those patients in whom cellular infiltration is minimal. Axonal degeneration occurs, presumably as a secondary event at sites where lesions are intense, but the extent and distribution of axonal degeneration vary widely from patient to patient. The extent of axonal degeneration has a strong effect on the rate and completeness of recovery.

Lymphocytes in the infiltrate are primarily T cells, with CD4-positive cells predominating in early lesions and CD8-positive cells being the most plentiful in mature lesions. Bone marrow-derived macrophages swarm into the lesions and constitute by far the most numerous pathologic cell types in nerves. Myelin destruction appears to be macrophage mediated, either by myelin lamellar stripping by macrophage processes or by vesicular disruption of myelin. The role of lymphocytes in myelin destruction is unclear. The pathologic appearance of GBS is characteristic of a delayed-type hypersensitivity response and closely resembles the lesions of experimental allergic neuritis (Waksman and Adams, 1955). In addition, there is abundant evidence of immune system activation in patients with GBS, including greatly increased levels of circulating soluble interleukin-2 receptor and cytokines such as tumor necrosis factor and evidence of complement activation both in peripheral blood and in cerebrospinal fluid. The specific epitopes and their origins, whether derived from the host or the infectious agent, or both, remain uncertain. Numerous anti-nerve antibodies that bind to various protein, glycoprotein, and glycolipid moieties have been described in patients with GBS, but none occur in more than a fraction of cases. Whereas the P2 myelin protein, which is specific for peripheral nerve, and selected peptide fragments of it are capable of inducing experimental allergic neuritis under appropriate conditions, the P2 myelin protein does not appear to play a role in GBS.

Descriptive Epidemiology

A large number of studies have examined the incidence of GBS in many parts of the world. These show a relatively uniform occurrence of about 1 to 2 cases per 100,000 population per year in all populations examined, mainly occurring throughout the year and in all age groups. Epidemic outbreaks have been rare and imperfectly documented. The swine flu incident of 1976-1977 is, perhaps, the most completely described outbreak (Langmuir et al., 1984; Safranek et al., 1991; Schonberger et al., 1979). The unusual circumstances of the swine flu incident should be noted. Over 40 million people were vaccinated in a period of a few weeks, an unprecedented mass vaccination program. It is likely that the excess cases of GBS might not have been detected if the numbers of people vaccinated had not been so large. A seasonal incidence of clinical GBS occurs annually in children and young adults in the northern part of the People's Republic of China (McKhann et al., 1991, in press), although the electrodiagnostic and pathologic features in these cases indicate a severe axonal lesion and not the usual demyelinating process with inflammation of the delayed hypersensitivity type.

A persistent problem has been the uncertainty about the expected incidence of GBS unrelated to vaccination in the cohort under 5 years of age. There is reasonably good information to suggest that the overall incidence of GBS for all ages is about 1 case per 1,000,000 population per month. Many authorities have suggested that the incidence of GBS in the pediatric age group (0-16 years of age) is lower than that in adults. For a number of years, the literature has provided data indicating that the incidence of GBS in the cohort under the age of 5 years is higher than that in children older than that (Beghi et al., 1985b; Coe, 1989; Soffer et al., 1978) and one study found a high incidence in preschool children of 5.4 cases per 100,000 per year (Kibel et al., 1983). Other observers have found a lower incidence of GBS in children, with the incidence distributed evenly from infancy to the teenage years (Hurwitz et al., 1981; Rantala et al., 1991; Uhari et al., 1989).

Recently, several population-based studies of the incidence of GBS applied strict criteria for the diagnosis of GBS, and relatively full case ascertainment appears to have been achieved (Hankey, 1987; Roman et al., unpublished observations, 1993; Winner and Evans, 1990). All of these studies indicate an incidence of GBS in the preschool age group of between 1.0 and 1.5 cases per 100,000 children per year, which is similar to the expected incidence in adults. The annual incidence of GBS in children in these studies is on the order of 0.1 cases per 100,000 children between the ages of 5 and 14 years (Winner and Evans, 1990) and 0.62 per 100,000 children and teenagers between the ages of 10 and 19 years (Hankey, 1987).

To obtain an idea of whether excess cases of GBS in relation to childhood vaccination occur each year, the following paradigm might be considered. Approximately 3,000 cases of GBS occur in the United States each year. If the preschool-age cohort makes up about 9 percent of the population, that would account for 270 cases per year if the incidence rate was uniform. As indicated above, the incidence of GBS in preschool children may well approximate the overall expected incidence in adults. Using some other assumptions, one can arrive at an estimate that about 6 percent of preschool-age children are within 5 days to 6 weeks of their most recent vaccination. If this is true, then one would expect about 16 cases of GBS per year in recently vaccinated preschool-age children. It is uncertain how many of these cases of GBS would be by chance alone and would be unrelated to vaccination. Nevertheless, excess cases of GBS occurring 5 days to 6 weeks after vaccination of preschool-age children have not been noted in the population-based studies mentioned above. This issue was also considered above in the section Antecedent Events. The data from the Monitoring System for Adverse Events Following Immunization show fewer cases of GBS per year, but such an analysis does not allow for the systematic underreporting that probably occurred.

Summary of Demyelinating Diseases

In evaluating the vaccines considered in this report for a causal relation with demyelinating disease, several facts need to be considered:

- Natural infections with measles and mumps viruses have been associated with ADEM.
- ADEM and GBS in humans, similar to EAE or EAN in experimental animals, generally occur after an interval of 5 days to 6 weeks following infection (not clinical disease) or injection of antigen.
- ADEM and GBS can occur after the administration of either live attenuated or killed vaccines (in the case of vaccinia virus and the swine influenza vaccines, respectively).

Thus, it is biologically plausible that injection of an inactivated virus, bacterium, or live attenuated virus might induce in the susceptible host an autoimmune response by deregulation of the immune response, by nonspecific activation of the T cells directed against myelin proteins, or by autoimmunity triggered by sequence similarities of proteins in the vaccine to host proteins such as those of myelin. The latter mechanism might evoke a response to a self-antigen, so-called molecular mimicry (Fujinami and Oldstone, 1989).

NON-DEMYELINATING DISEASE

Encephalopathy

Historically, encephalopathy has been a vague term that is difficult to define. Encephalopathy has been used in the literature to characterize a constellation of signs and symptoms reflecting a generalized disturbance in brain function (Institute of Medicine, 1991). Encephalopathy has been defined as "a diffuse interference with brain function resulting from a generalized or multifocal insult that causes a widespread disorder in the function of neurons" (Dodson, 1978, p. 416). Fenichel (1982) noted that the terms *encephalopathy* and *encephalitis* are used interchangeably to denote a variety of symptoms including alterations in behavior or state of consciousness, convulsions, headache, and focal neurologic deficit. In general, when pleocytosis in cerebrospinal fluid is present, the term *encephalitis* is used, implying an inflammatory response within the brain. The term *encephalopathy* is used when an illness clinically appears like an encephalitis but no inflammatory response is evident (Cherry et al., 1988). Encephalitis is a type of encephalopathy. That is, every case of encephalitis is also a case of encephalopathy, but not every case of encephalopathy is due to an inflammatory response, and thus is not a case of encephalitis.

There are both clinical and pathologic definitions of encephalopathy. For a patient to be considered to have a case of encephalopathy, the patient must have clinical signs and there must be reason to assume there is an underlying pathologic, structural, or persistent biochemical abnormality. For example, seizures can result from extremes of temperature or metabolic changes with no underlying pathologic, structural, or persistent biochemical change. Recurrent seizures without any known precipitating event, on the other hand, could imply a pathologic change sufficient to use the term *encephalopathy*. Alternatively, there may be pathologic changes in the brain without clinically detectable signs. For example, an increase in size or number of astrocytes may be detectable pathologically, but be sufficiently mild to have only a subclinical association.

Recently, in proposed changes to the Aids to Interpretation of the Vaccine Injury Table, encephalopathy has been strictly defined (U.S. Department of Health and Human Services, 1992). The Vaccine Injury Table defines the vaccines and adverse events that are covered under the National Vaccine Injury Compensation Program. Health care providers must report the occurrence of an adverse event listed in the table if it falls within the specified latencies from vaccination. The box in Chapter 10 includes the current Vaccine Injury Table and Aids to Interpretation. Some proposed changes are reproduced in this chapter in the box entitled Changes Proposed by DHHS in the Definition of Encephalopathy in the Aids to Interpretation of the Vaccine Injury Table.

This definition of acute and chronic encephalopathy is useful because of its precision, and the committee considered this proposed definition as it reviewed the evidence. As is made clear throughout the report, the evidence reviewed by the committee varied greatly in both the quality and quantity of clinical details provided. Very few studies provided enough detail to ascertain whether the cases of encephalopathy reported meet the criteria proposed in the Vaccine Injury Table. The committee read and considered all reports of encephalopathy, regardless of the extent of documentation of the adverse event. Although a 24-hour period for the duration of stupor or coma associated with encephalopathy is a widely accepted and reasonable standard based on a unit of time (a day), the committee felt that it is not an absolute. However, this distinction regarding the time period did not affect the final conclusions regarding encephalopathy.

The occurrence of encephalopathy in a child does not imply a particular severity or duration of illness, nor does it indicate that a child will have irreversible brain injury. Many children do recover from serious neurologic illnesses and therefore may not have permanent neurologic sequelae (Institute of Medicine, 1991). The annual incidence of encephalitis in Olmsted County, Minnesota, from 1950 to 1981 was 7.4 per 100,000 people (Beghi et al., 1984). The incidence in children less than age 1 year was 22.5, in children between age 1 and 4 years it was 15.2, and in children between ages 5 and 9 years it was 30.2 per 100,000. There was a case fatality rate of 3.8 percent.

Aseptic meningitis refers to inflammation of the meninges, not of the brain. It can result from a variety of infectious, toxic, chemical, or physical agents. No bacterial organism can be identified in or isolated from the cerebrospinal fluid, but serologic studies often implicate a viral etiology. Mumps virus and polioviruses can cause aseptic meningitis. The annual incidence of aseptic meningitis in Olmsted County, Minnesota, from 1950 to 1981 was 10.9 per 100,000 population (Nicolosi et al., 1986). The incidence was markedly higher in children under age 1 year (82.4 per 100,000) and slightly higher in children between 1 and 4 years old (16.2 per 100,000). No deaths occurred in any of the 183 individuals with aseptic meningitis.

Changes Proposed by DHHS in the Definition of Encephalopathy in the Aids to Interpretation of the Vaccine Injury Table

- The term *encephalopathy* means any acute or chronic significant acquired abnormality of, or injury to, or impairment of function of, the brain.

  - *Acute encephalopathy shall be defined as follows:*
    An acute encephalopathy should be sufficiently severe to require health care intervention and hospitalization.

    - *For children less than 24 months of age* who present without an associated seizure event, an acute encephalopathy shall be defined as a significantly decreased level of consciousness, specifically stupor or coma, lasting for at least 24 hours. Those children less than 24 months of age who present following a seizure shall be viewed as having an acute encephalopathy if their stupor or coma persists beyond 24 hours and cannot be attributed to a postictal state or medication.
    - *For children 24 months of age or older,* an acute encephalopathy is one that persists for at least 24 hours and that is characterized by at least two of the following:

      — a significant change in mental status that is not medication related; specifically a confusional state or a delirium, or a psychosis;
      — a significantly decreased level of consciousness, which is independent of a seizure and cannot be attributed to the effects of medication; or
      — a seizure associated with loss of consciousness.

    - Increased intracranial pressure may be a clinical features of acute encephalopathy in any age group.
    - The following clinical features alone, or in combination, do not qualify as evidence of an acute encephalopathy or a significant change in either mental status or level of consciousness as described above: Sleepiness, irritability (fussiness), high-pitched and unusual screaming, persistent inconsolable crying, and bulging fontanelle. Seizures in themselves are not sufficient to constitute a diagnosis of encephalopathy. In the absence of other evidence of an acute encephalopathy, seizures shall not be viewed as the first symptom or manifestation of the onset of an encephalopathy.

  - *Chronic encephalopathy* is defined as persistence of the acute findings over an extended period, usually several months to years beyond the acute episode. Individuals who return to a normal neurologic state after the acute encephalopathy shall not be presumed to have suffered residual neurologic damage from the vaccine; any subsequent chronic encephalopathy shall not be presumed to be a sequela of the acute encephalopathy. Children with evidence of a chronic encephalopathy secondary to genetic, prenatal, or perinatal factors shall not be considered to have a condition set forth in the Vaccine Injury Table.

Source: Adapted from U.S. Department of Health and Human Services (1992).

Subacute Sclerosing Panencephalitis

Clinical and Laboratory Features

Subacute sclerosing panencephalitis (SSPE) is a rare form of panencephalitis primarily affecting children and adolescents. It is characterized by the insidious onset of a progressive cerebral dysfunction developing over the course of weeks or months. Initially, there usually is an alteration in personality and a deterioration in school performance. Myoclonic jerks follow some 2 months later. These jerks are involuntary, but the affected patient remains conscious and is frequently thought to be stumbling or simply clumsy. The jerks tend to disappear during sleep. As the disease progresses, so does the myoclonus, often reaching a frequency of 1 every 10 seconds. Ultimately, extrapyramidal dyskinesias such as athetosis, chorea, ballismus, and dystonic posturing develop. The patient becomes extremely spastic and has difficulty swallowing. There is a progressive loss of vision resulting from focal chorioretinitis, cortical blindness, or optic atrophy. In the terminal stages of SSPE, the patient becomes unresponsive and vegetates in a decorticate state, compounded by hypothalamic dysfunction with vasomotor instability, hypothermia, and alterations in blood pressure and pulse rate. An encephalographic pattern of paroxysmal bursts of two- to three-cycle-per-second high-voltage slow waves with associated spike discharges and then a short period of flattened activity—the so-called burst-suppression pattern—is characteristic. The myoclonic jerks tend to coincide with the paroxysmal electroencephalographic bursts. The entire course of SSPE is quite variable, lasting from weeks to years with periods of remission. The average patient dies within 2 years of the onset of this disease, but in rare cases, patients have remained in the vegetative state for 10 or more years.

The diagnosis is suggested by the clinical presentation and is strengthened by the detection of high titers of serum antibodies against measles virus and the presence of oligoclonal measles virus antibodies in the cerebrospinal fluid. The ultimate confirmation is based on the classical appearance of Cowdry type A inclusion bodies as well as the detection of measles antigen in the brain tissue obtained by biopsy or at autopsy.

Pathology and Pathogenesis

The neuropathology of SSPE—involving both the grey and the white matter—is that of a subacute encephalitis accompanied by demyelination. There are lesions in the cerebral cortex, hippocampus, cerebellar cortex, basal ganglia, brainstem, and spinal cord. Eosinophilic intranuclear and intracytoplasmic inclusion bodies are seen in the neurons and glia. Immunocytochemical studies show the presence of measles virus antigen.

SSPE is a result of an aberrant measles virus infection. The nature of the aberration is not well understood, but viruses isolated from the brains and lymphoid tissues of these patients are not typical measles viruses. They show various degrees of defectiveness, which in some cases require complex techniques of "rescue" before they would replicate in tissue culture. The central question that remains is whether the original measles virus infection involved a defective measles virus or whether the virus became altered during the prolonged period of latency in the host. If the former is the case, this would suggest a wholly exogenous etiology of SSPE. If the latter is the case, then one would have to consider the possibility of an a priori abnormality in the host.

Although SSPE has had several original descriptions, Dawson is usually credited with the identification of this disease when he described the inclusion bodies in the neurons in 1933 (Dawson, 1933, 1934). Van Bogaert identified the lesions in the white matter in 1945 (Van Bogaert, 1945). Bouteille and coworkers (1965) identified the ultrastructural pattern resembling the nucleocapsids of a paramyxovirus, which led Connolly and coworkers to the immunological identification of measles virus within the lesions (Connolly et al., 1967). Tissue cultures derived from the brains of patients with SSPE were shown to contain similar inclusions bearing measles virus antigen (Baublis and Payne, 1968). They also contained structures resembling paramyxovirus nucleocapsids (Katz et al., 1969). Measles virus was finally cultured from a patient's brain tissue by cocultivation of the brain cells with indicator cells (Horta-Barbosa et al., 1969; Payne et al., 1969) and by a deliberate fusion with indicator cells (Barbanti-Brodano et al., 1970). Later, Horta-Barbosa et al. (1971) also isolated the virus from lymph node biopsy specimens from patients in the early stages of the disease.

Descriptive Epidemiology

SSPE usually affects children younger than 12 years of age, but cases of SSPE in young adults in their 20s have been reported. Boys are more frequently affected than girls. The incidence of SSPE has decreased dramatically since the beginning of immunization with the live attenuated measles virus vaccine (Modlin et al., 1977). Estimates of the incidence of SSPE after natural measles infection range from 5 to 20 cases per 1 million children with clinical measles infection per year (Halsey et al., 1978).

Residual Seizure Disorder

Seizures are paroxysmal neurologic events that can occur with or without a loss of consciousness and can include a variety of sensory experiences (e.g., auditory seizures), motor manifestations (e.g., focal motor or tonic-clonic seizures), or both. The terms *fits* and *convulsions* are frequently used synonyms for motor seizures. In addition, seizures can occur with or without fever. Febrile seizures are well-defined, relatively common events that are precipitated by fever in children under 5 years of age who do not harbor an underlying seizure disorder. If more than one seizure occurs within 24 hours or if the seizures last longer than 10 minutes or are accompanied by transient focal neurologic features, they are termed *complex febrile seizures*. Acute symptomatic seizures are those that occur in association with an acute process that affects the brain, such as head trauma or a bacterial infection. Afebrile seizures are those that occur in the absence of fever or other acute provocation. Recurrent afebrile seizures are referred to as *epilepsy*. Infantile spasms are a type of epileptic disorder in young children and are characterized by flexor, extensor, and mixed flexor-extensor seizures that tend to occur in clusters (Kellaway et al., 1979). The earliest manifestations of infantile spasms are subtle and are easily missed, making it difficult to identify the precise age at onset.

Recently, the National Vaccine Injury Compensation Program proposed clarification of its definition of residual seizure disorder as a seizure occurring within 72 hours of vaccination followed by two or more afebrile seizures over the next 12 months, with the seizures separated by at least 24 hours (U.S. Department of Health and Human Services, 1992). Continuing seizures in subsequent years would be anticipated. The clarifications define an afebrile seizure as one that occurs with a temperature of <101°F (rectally) or <100°F (orally). This definition is considered in the remainder of this report. When a definition for a seizure in a specific study being evaluated varies from those stated above, the definition used in the study is given.

Sensorineural Deafness

Sensorineural deafness is a form of hearing loss resulting from pathologic changes in the end organ structures within the cochlea or in the neural connections between the cochlea and the cochlear nuclei in the brainstem. This usually arises from toxic, metabolic, or ischemic events. Viral infection of the cochlea can lead to sensorineural deafness as well. It is plausible that the live attenuated viruses used in vaccines can infect the cochlea, but there is no evidence that this occurs. No population-based incidence rates were identified.

Neuropathy

The term *neuropathy* as used here designates those disorders of peripheral nerve other than GBS that have, on occasion, been described in relation to vaccine administration. Most reports fall into two clinical categories, mononeuropathy and brachial neuritis. Diagnosis in both instances rests upon the clinical and electrodiagnostic features.

Mononeuropathy

Mononeuropathy means a dysfunction limited to the distribution of a single peripheral nerve that is large enough to be named. The deficit may be motor, sensory, or both and may be either partial or complete. When mononeuropathy occurs in association with vaccination, the onset is usually acute or subacute. In some instances, mononeuropathy is clearly related to intraneural injection of vaccine, as with radial nerve palsy with wrist drop following a misdirected deltoid injection (Ling and Loong, 1976). Inadvertent intraneural administration of any injectable is likely to produce a mononeuropathy and is usually painful in nature (Combes and Clark, 1960; Scheinberg and Allensworth, 1957; Sunderland, 1968).

In other cases, the affected nerve trunk lies at a distance from the injection site. The basis for this type of mononeuropathy is unclear. Patients with mononeuropathies tend to recover, but usually after many weeks or months. Latencies of greater than 4 weeks between vaccination and the onset of mononeuropathy render an association between mononeuropathy and vaccine administration highly unlikely.

Brachial Neuritis

Brachial neuritis, also known as brachial plexus neuropathy or, in the United Kingdom, as neuralgic amyotrophy, has been linked to vaccination or administration of antiserum since brachial neuritis was first described a half century ago. Clinically, most cases of brachial neuritis are heralded by a deep, steady, often severe aching pain in the shoulder and upper arm. Patients usually wish to lie still with the arm in the position of least pain. As the pain subsides in days or weeks, weakness and marked atrophy of selected arm and shoulder muscles are noted, usually unilaterally. Particularly commonly affected muscles (and nerves) are the serratus anterior with scapular winging (long thoracic nerve), the deltoid muscle (axillary nerve), and the infraspinatus muscle (suprascapular nerve). A patch or patches of sensory involvement are present in half or more of the patients. In as many as one-third of the patients, the distribution of muscle weakness and atrophy is bilateral (Tsairis et al., 1972). By clinical and electrodiagnostic criteria, lesions are focal or multifocal and localize in the brachial plexus and sometimes in the more distal nerve trunks. The character of the lesion is axonal without conduction block. Recovery, which occurs mainly as a result of regeneration and collateral reinnervation, is slow and often requires from 12 to 30 months. About 15 percent of all cases of brachial neuritis occur following vaccination or antiserum administration (Tsairis et al., 1972). Brachial neuritis may be present on the same side as or the opposite side of the injection. The latency ranges from a few days to 3 or at most 4 weeks. Little is known of the basis or mechanism of brachial neuritis. The annual incidence of brachial neuritis in Rochester, Minnesota, from 1970 to 1981 was estimated to be 1.64 per 100,000 individuals (Beghi et al., 1985a).

REFERENCES

Arnason BG, Soliven B. Acute inflammatory demyelinating polyradiculoneuropathy. In: Dyck PJ, et al., eds. Peripheral Neuropathy, 3rd edition. Philadelphia: W.B. Saunders; 1992.

Asbury AK. Diagnostic considerations in Guillain-Barré syndrome. Annals of Neurology 1981;9(Suppl.):1-5.

Asbury AK, Cornblath DR. Assessment of current diagnostic criteria for Guillain-Barré syndrome. Annals of Neurology 1990;27(Suppl.):S21-S24.

Asbury AK, Gibbs CJ Jr, eds. Autoimmune neuropathies: Guillain-Barré syndrome. Annals of Neurology 1990;27(Suppl.):S1-S79.

Asbury AK, Arnason BG, Adams RD. The inflammatory lesion in idiopathic polyneuritis. Medicine 1969;48:173-215.

Asbury AK, Arnason BG, Karp HR, McFarlin DE. Criteria for diagnosis of Guillain-Barré syndrome. Annals of Neurology 1978;3:565-566.

Barbanti-Brodano G, Oyanagi S, Katz M, Koprowski H. Presence of two different viral agents in brain cells of patients with subacute sclerosing panencephalitis (SSPE). Proceedings of the Society for Experimental Biology and Medicine 1970;134:230-236.

Baublis JV, Payne RE. Measles antigen and syncytium formation in brain cell cultures from subacute sclerosing panencephalitis (SSPE). Proceedings of the Society for Experimental Biology and Medicine 1968;19:543-597.

Beghi E, Kurland LT, Mulder DW. Incidence of acute transverse myelitis in Rochester, Minnesota, 1970-1980, and implications with respect to influenza vaccine. Neuroepidemiology 1982;1:176-188.

Beghi E, Nicolosi A, Kurland LT, Mulder DW, Hauser WA, Shuster L. Encephalitis and aseptic meningitis, Olmsted County, Minnesota, 1950-1981. I. Epidemiology. Annals of Neurology 1984;16:283-294.

Beghi E, Kurland LT, Mulder DW, Nicolosi A. Brachial plexus neuropathy in the population of Rochester, Minnesota, 1970-1981. Annals of Neurology 1985a;18:320-323.

Beghi E, Kurland LT, Mulder DW, Wiederholt WC. Guillain-Barré syndrome: clinicoepidemiologic features and effect of influenza vaccine. Archives of Neurology 1985b;42:1053-1057.

Bouteille M, Fontaine C, Vedredd CL, Delarue J. Sur un cas d'encephalite subaigue a inclusions: etude anatomo-clinique et ultrastructurate. Revue Neurologique 1965;113:454-458.

Bussens P, Pilette J. Complications meconnues de la vaccination antipoliomyelitique par voie orale. [Unrecognized complications of oral antipoliomyelitis vaccination.] Revue Medicale de Liege 1976;31:608-611.

Cabrera J, Griffin DE, Johnson RT. Unusual features of the Guillain-Barré syndrome after rabies vaccine prepared in suckling mouse brain. Journal of Neurological Science 1987;81:239-245.

Cherry JD, Brunell PA, Golden GS, Karzon DT. Report of the task force on pertussis and pertussis immunization—1988. Pediatrics 1988;81(6, Pt 2):939-984.

Clark C, Hashim G, Rosenberg R. Transverse myelitis following rubeola vaccination. Neurology 1977;27:360.

Coe CJ. Guillain-Barré syndrome in Korean children. Yonsei Medical Journal 1989;30:81-87.

Combes MA, Clark WK. Sciatic nerve injury following intragluteal injection: pathogenesis and prevention. American Journal of Diseases in Children 1960;100:579.

Connolly JH, Allen IV, Hurwitz LJ, Miller JH. Measles-virus antibody and antigen in subacute sclerosing panencephalitis. Lancet 1967;1:542-544.

Connolly JH, Allen IV, Hurwitz LJ, Millar JH. Subacute sclerosing panencephalitis: clinical, pathological, epidemiological, and virological findings in three patients. Quebec Journal of Medicine 1968;37:625-644.

Cornblath DR, Mellits ED, Griffin JW, and the GBS Study Group. Motor conduction studies in the Guillain-Barré syndrome: description and prognostic value. Annals of Neurology 1988;23:354-359.

Dawson JR. Cellular inclusions in cerebral lesions of lethargic encephalitis. American Journal of Pathology 1933;9:7-15.

Dawson JR. Cellular inclusions in cerebral lesions of epidemic encephalitis (second report). Archives of Neurology and Psychiatry 1934;31:685-700.

Dodson WE. Metabolic encephalopathies in neurological pathophysiology. In: Eliasson SG, Prensky AL, Hardin WB Jr, eds. Neurological Pathophysiology. New York: Oxford; 1978.

Feasby TE, Gilbert JJ, Brown WF, Bolton CF, Hahn AF, Koopman WF, et al. An acute axonal form of Guillain-Barré polyneuropathy. Brain 1986;109:1115-1126.

Feasby TE, Hahan AF, Brown WF, Bolton CF, Gilbert JJ, Koopman WJ. Severe axonal degeneration in acute Guillain-Barré syndrome: evidence of two different mechanisms? Journal of the Neurological Sciences 1993;116:185-192.

Fenichel GM. Neurological complications of immunization. Annals of Neurology 1982;12:119-128.

Fujinami RS, Oldstone MB. Molecular mimicry as a mechanism for virus-induced autoimmunity. Immunological Research 1989;8:3-15.

Guillain G, Barré JA, Strohl A. Sur un syndrome de radiculonevrite avec hyperalbuminose due liquide cephalo-rachidien sans reaction cellulaire: remarques sure les caracteres cliniques et graphiques des reflexes tendineux. Bulletins et Memoires Societé Medicale des Hopitaux de Paris 1916;40:1462-1470.

Halsey NA, Modlin JF, Jabbour JT. Subacute sclerosing panencephalitis (SSPE): an epidemiologic review. In: Stevens JG, et al., eds. Persistent Viruses. New York: Academic Press; 1978:101-114.

Hankey GJ. Guillain-Barré syndrome in Western Australia, 1980-1985. Medical Journal of Australia 1987;146:130-133.

Held JR, Adaros HL. Neurological disease in man following administration of suckling mouse brain antirabies vaccine. Bulletin of the World Health Organization 1972;46:321-327.

Hemachudha T, Griffin DE, Giffels JJ, Johnson RT, Moser AB, Phanuphak P. Myelin basic protein as an encephalitogen in encephalomyelitis and polyneuritis following rabies vaccination. New England Journal of Medicine 1987a;316:369-374.

Hemachudha T, Phanuphak P, Johnson RT, Griffin DE, Ratanavongsiri J, Siriprasomsup W. Neurologic complications of Semple-type rabies vaccine: clinical and immunologic studies. Neurology 1987b;37:550-556.

Hemachudha T, Griffin DE, Chen WW, Johnson RT. Immunologic studies of rabies vaccination-induced Guillain-Barré syndrome. Neurology 1988;38:375-378.

Honavar M, Tharakan JK, Hughes RA, Leibowitz S, Winer JB. A clinicopathological study of the Guillain-Barré syndrome: nine cases and literature review. Brain 1991;114:1245-1269.

Horta-Barbosa L, Fucillo DA, Sever JL. Subacute sclerosing panencephalitis: isolation of measles virus from a brain biopsy. Nature 1969;221:974.

Horta-Barbosa L, Hamilton R, Wittig B, Fuccillo DA, Sever JL. Subacute sclerosing panencephalitis: isolation of suppressed measles virus from lymph node biopsies. Science 1971;173:840-841.

Hughes RA. Guillain-Barré Syndrome. London: Springer-Verlag; 1990.

Hurwitz ES, Schonberger LB, Nelson DB, Holman RC. Guillain-Barré syndrome and the 1978-1979 influenza vaccine. New England Journal of Medicine 1981;304:1557-1561.

Institute of Medicine. Adverse Effects of Pertussis and Rubella Vaccines. Washington, DC: National Academy Press; 1991.

Johnson, RT. Viral aspects of multiple sclerosis. Handbook of Clinical Neurology 1985;3:319-336.

Johnson RT, Griffin DE, Gendelman HE. Postinfectious encephalomyelitis. Seminars in Neurology 1985;5:180-190.

Kabat EA, Wolf A, Bezer AE. The rapid production of acute disseminated encephalomyelitis in rhesus monkey by injection of heterologous and homologous brain tissue with adjuvants. Journal of Experimental Medicine 1947;85:117-130.

Kaplan JE, Schonberger LB, Hurwitz ES, Katona P. Guillain-Barré syndrome in the United States, 1978-1981: additional observations from the national surveillance system. Neurology 1983;33:633-637.

Katz M, Oyanagi S, Koprowski H. Structures resembling myxovirus nucleocapsids in cells cultures from brains. Nature 1969;222:888-890.

Kellaway P, Krachoby RA, Frost JD, Zion T. Precise characterization and quantification of infantile spasms. Annals of Neurology 1979;6:214-218.

Kibel MA. Guillain-Barré syndrome in childhood. South African Medical Journal 1983;63:715.

Langmuir AD, Bregman DJ, Kurland LT, Nathanson N, Victor M. An epidemiologic and clinical evaluation of Guillain-Barré syndrome reported in association with the administration of swine influenza vaccines. American Journal of Epidemiology 1984;119:841-879.

Ling CM, Loong SC. Injection injury of the radial nerve. Injury 1976;8:60-62.

Lopez Adaros H, Held JR. Guillain-Barré syndrome associated with immunization against rabies: epidemiological aspects. Research Publications of the Association for Research in Nervous and Mental Disease 1971;49:178-186.

Martin R, McFarland H, McFarlin D. Immunological aspects of demyelinating diseases. Annual Review of Immunology 1992;10:153-183.

McKhann GM, Griffin JW, Cornblath DR, Mellits ED, Fisher RS, Quaskey SA. Plasmapheresis and Guillain-Barré syndrome: analysis of prognostic factors and the effect of plasmapheresis. Annals of Neurology 1988;23:347-353.

McKhann GM, Cornblath DR, Ho TW, Li CY, Bai AY, Wu HS, Yei QF, et al. Clinical and electrophysiological aspects of acute paralytic disease of children and young adults in northern China. Lancet 1991;38:593-597.

McKhann GM, Cornblath DR, Griffin JW, Ho TW, Li CY, Jiang Z, et al. Acute motor axonal neuropathy: a frequent cause of acute flaccid paralysis in China. Annals of Neurology, In press.

Modlin JF, Jabbour JT, Witte JJ, Halsey NA. Epidemiologic studies of measles, measles vaccine, and subacute sclerosing panencephalitis. Pediatrics 1977;59:505-512.

Nicolosi A, Hauser WA, Beghi E, Kurland LT. Epidemiology of central nervous system infections in Olmsted County, Minnesota, 1950-1981. Journal of Infectious Diseases 1986;154:399-408.

Payne FE, Baublis JV, Itabashi HH. Isolation of measles virus from cell cultures of brain from a patient with subacute sclerosing panencephalitis. New England Journal of Medicine 1969;281:585-589.

Pollard JD, Selby G. Relapsing neuropathy due to tetanus toxoid: report of a case. Journal of Neurological Science 1978;37:113-125.

Rantala H, Uhari M, Niemela M. Occurrence, clinical manifestations, and prognosis of Guillain-Barré syndrome. Archives of Disease in Childhood 1991;66:706-709.

Rivers TM, Schwenker FF. Encephalomyelitis accompanied by myelin destruction experimentally produced in monkeys. Journal of Experimental Medicine 1935;61:689-702.

Ropper AH. The Guillain-Barré syndrome. New England Journal of Medicine 1992;326:1130-1136.

Ropper AH, Wijdicks EF, Truax BT. Guillain-Barré syndrome. Philadelphia: F.A. Davis; 1991.

Roscelli JD, Bass JW, Pang L. Guillain-Barré syndrome and influenza vaccination in the US Army, 1980-1988. American Journal of Epidemiology 1991;133:952-955.

Safranek TJ, Lawrence DN, Kurland LT, Culver DH, Wiederholt WC, Hayner NS, et al. Reassessment of the association between Guillain-Barré syndrome and receipt of swine influenza vaccine in 1976-1977: results of a two-state study. Expert Neurology Group. American Journal of Epidemiology 1991;133:940-951.

Scheinberg L, Allensworth M. Sciatic neuropathy in infants related to antibiotic injections. Pediatrics 1957;19:261-265.

Schonberger LB, Bregman DJ, Sullivan-Bolyai JZ, Keenlyside RA, Ziegler DW, Retailliau HF, et al. Guillain-Barré syndrome following vaccination in the National Influenza Immunization Program, United States, 1976-1977. American Journal of Epidemiology 1979;110:105-123.

Sibley WA, Bamford CR, Clark K. Clinical viral infections and multiple sclerosis. Lancet 1985;1:1313-1315.

Soffer D, Feldman S, Alter M. Epidemiology of Guillain-Barré syndrome. Neurology 1978;28:686-690.

Sunderland S. Nerves and Nerve Injuries. Baltimore: The Williams & Wilkins Company; 1968.

Tsairis P, Dyck PJ, Mulder DW. Natural history of brachial plexus neuropathy: report on 99 patients. Archives of Neurology 1972;27:109-117.

Uhari M, Rantala H, Niemela M. Cluster of childhood Guillain-Barré cases after an oral poliovaccine campaign (letter). Lancet 1989;2:440-441.

U.S. Department of Health and Human Services. U.S. Public Health Service, National Vaccine Injury Compensation Program; Revision of the Vaccine Injury Table; Proposed Rule. Federal Register, 42 CFR Part 100, August 14, 1992;57(158):36877-36885.

Van Bogaert L. Une leucoencephalite sclerosante subaigue. Journal de Neurologie de la Psychiatrie 1945;8:101-120.

van der Meché FG, Schmitz PI, Dutch Guillain-Barré Study Group. A randomized trial comparing intravenous immune globulin and plasma exchange in Guillain-Barré syndrome. New England Journal of Medicine 1992;326:1123-1129.

Waksman BH, Adams RD. Allergic neuritis: an experimental disease of rabbits induced by the injection of peripheral nervous tissue and adjuvants. Journal of Experimental Medicine 1955;102:213-235.

Winer JB, Hughes RA, Anderson MJ, Jones DM, Kangro J, Watkins RP. A prospective study of acute idiopathic neuropathy. II. Antecedent events. Journal of Neurology, Neurosurgery and Psychiatry 1988;51:613-618.

Winner SJ, Evans G. Age-specific incidence of Guillain-Barré syndrome in Oxfordshire. Quarterly Journal of Medicine 1990;77(New Series):1297-1304.

4

Immunologic Reactions

Since the beneficial effects of vaccines are a result of changes in the immune system, it would not be surprising if some of the adverse effects were also. A classification of immunologic reactions that can cause disease has been proposed by Coombs and Gell (1968). Four reactions make up the classification: type I, immediate hypersensitivity, the most serious clinical manifestation of which is anaphylaxis; type II, reaction of antibody with tissue antigens; type III, Arthus-type reaction, caused by deposition of antigen-antibody complexes in tissues, leading to the tissue-damaging effects of complement and leukocytes; and type IV, delayed-type hypersensitivity, which is mediated largely by T lymphocytes and macrophages. In clinical reactions to foreign antigens, these categories frequently overlap. These reactions are a by-product of the body's capacity to reject foreign invasion, particularly by microorganisms. If these reactions are responsible for causing adverse events to vaccines, then these reactions would be extensions of the beneficial responses to vaccines, which are mediated by protective immunoglobulin G (IgG) antibodies and T-lymphocyte responses.

ANAPHYLAXIS

Anaphylaxis (a type I reaction) was described in some detail in the Institute of Medicine's report *Adverse Effects of Pertussis and Rubella Vaccines* (Institute of Medicine, 1991, Chapter 6). The discussion in that chapter applies equally to this report. The term *anaphylaxis* generally re-

59

fers to a sudden, potentially life-threatening, systemic condition mediated by highly reactive molecules released from mast cells and basophils. Mediators include histamine, platelet-activating factor, and products of arachidonic acid metabolism (Fisher, 1987). Release of mediators depends typically upon the interaction of antigen with specific antibodies of the IgE class that are bound to the mast cells and basophils. Antibodies of other immunoglobulin classes are thought to mediate anaphylaxis on occasion. By definition, the antibodies are formed by prior exposure to the same or a closely related antigen. Anaphylaxis results from widespread release of mediators that enter the circulation, and thus, anaphylaxis is an expression of allergy that is systemic. At a cellular level, the reaction begins within seconds of exposure to the inciting antigen. However, depending upon the degree of sensitization (IgE antibody formation), and presumably upon the rate with which the antigen enters the circulation, localized or systemic symptoms may not be expressed for minutes or a few hours (Dolovich et al., 1973; Pearlman and Bierman, 1989). In proposed changes to the Vaccine Injury Table, which is used by the Vaccine Injury Compensation Program to determine eligibility for compensation for vaccine-induced injuries, the time frame for the onset of anaphylaxis/anaphylactic shock following vaccination has been set at 4 hours (U.S. Department of Health and Human Services, 1992). Classic symptoms include pallor and then diffuse erythema, urticaria and itching, subcutaneous edema, edema and spasm of the larynx, wheezing, tachycardia, hypotension, and hypovolemic shock (Kniker, 1988; Pearlman and Bierman, 1989). These symptoms are due to leaking of fluid from blood vessels, constriction of smooth-muscle in certain viscera, and relaxation of vascular smooth muscle. If death occurs, it is most commonly from airway obstruction caused by laryngeal edema or bronchospasm, or from cardiovascular collapse from arterial smooth-muscle relaxation and transudation of fluids from the intravascular space (Pearlman and Bierman, 1989). Tissues at autopsy show primarily widespread edema.

Less severe manifestations of immediate hypersensitivity that do not qualify as anaphylaxis under the above definition occur commonly. These may be expressed as urticaria and generalized pruritus, wheezing, or more alarming symptoms such as facial and other edemas. However, hypotension, shock, and collapse do not occur either because the reactions are naturally less severe or because they are aborted by intervention with epinephrine or antihistamines.

The clinical presentation of anaphylaxis can also be produced by intravascular antigen-antibody reactions that activate the complement system. In this case, the antibodies may be of the IgG or IgM class. Peptides that are split from activated complement components act on mast cells and basophils to induce the release of the same mediators (Kniker, 1988). This reaction is recognized most clearly after intravenous administration of antigen; it has been hypothesized to occur rarely after intramuscular or subcutaneous injection through rapid entry (within 1 to 5 minutes) of large amounts of the antigen into the venous circulation. This reaction in an infant presumably could be mediated by IgG antibody received transplacentally from the mother; such antibody would be expected to persist for the first 6 months of life and possibly longer (Benacerraf and Kabat, 1950; Cohen and Scadron, 1946). Anaphylaxis also can occur without an obvious cause (Wiggins et al., 1989).

INTERACTION OF ANTIBODY WITH NORMAL TISSUE ANTIGENS

In type II reactions, antibody combines with an antigen expressed on normal tissue cells, complement is activated, and the resultant inflammation damages the tissue. It is not clear whether this type of reaction is triggered by alteration in the expression of a tissue antigen or by the formation of an antibody to an antigen in food or an invading microorganism that then cross-reacts with a host antigen. Antigens in a vaccine could theoretically mimic a tissue antigen and elicit such a cross-reacting response, but this has not been shown. On first exposure to such an antigen, any resultant tissue reaction would be expected to develop in about 2 or 3 weeks; on reexposure, a tissue reaction might occur within a few days. (These estimates are hypothetical and are based on what is known about primary and secondary antibody responses to foreign antigens.) The basis for type II reactions is not understood.

ARTHUS REACTION

The Arthus reaction (Arthus, 1903) is mediated differently from either anaphylaxis or type II reactions. Basic to this type III or Arthus reaction is the formation of antigen-antibody complexes, with a moderate excess of antigen, with deposition in the walls of blood vessels, and consequent organ damage. This is not an acute, immediately overwhelming condition. It generally develops over 6 to 12 hours if antibody levels are already high, or it can develop over several days (e.g., in serum sickness) as antibody levels increase and antigen persists. In this reaction, immune complexes in the walls of blood vessels initiate an inflammatory reaction involving complement and leukocytes, particularly neutrophils. Tissue sections show acute inflammation, and profound tissue destruction can occur.

Localized Arthus reactions have been reported to be common at the site of injection of some vaccines and occur when reimmunization is performed in the presence of high levels of circulating IgG antibody (Facktor et al., 1973). They are characterized by pain, swelling, induration, and edema beginning several hours after immunization and usually reaching a peak 12 to 36 hours after immunization. They are self-limited, resolving over the course of a few days. Their frequency and severity can be lessened by spacing immunizations more widely, as has been recommended for tetanus-diphtheria toxoid booster injections.

Generalized Arthus reactions of a serum sickness-like character have also been invoked following vaccine administration. Such generalized serum sickness-like reactions were common in the era when horse serum was used to treat or prevent many infectious diseases and when very large quantities of immunogenic foreign protein were infused (sometimes repeatedly). These reactions require both IgG antibody and circulating excess antigen. Considering the small quantity of protein in present-day vaccines that is injected, it is not clear that such reactions could occur as a result of immunization. In animal models, symptoms and pathology tend to localize in the kidney, skin, joints, lung, and brain (Henson, 1982). The manifestations after vaccination most commonly ascribed to serum sickness-like mechanisms are arthritis and fever.

DELAYED-TYPE HYPERSENSITIVITY

Delayed-type hypersensitivity (type IV reaction) results from the stimulation of antigen-specific lymphocytes with the resultant replication of these cells at the site of exposure to antigen. This stimulation induces the release of lymphokines, migration of macrophages to the site, further immunologic stimulation, and resultant tissue damage. As with IgG antibody responses, this form of hypersensitivity represents the normal immunologic response to certain types of foreign antigen, and it is seen commonly after recovery from natural infections. On first exposure, the response peaks after about 3 weeks; on reexposure, the response typically peaks after 24 to 48 hours.

Delayed-type hypersensitivity has been thought to be involved in the development of neurologic complications of vaccination, particularly the development of neurologic disease after receipt of the early rabies vaccines (no longer in use) because of the large quantities of contaminating nervous system antigens in the vaccines. The possible involvement of delayed-type hypersensitivity in reactions to contemporary vaccines is discussed in the chapters on the specific vaccines and adverse events.

EFFECT OF VACCINES ON THE IMMUNE SYSTEM

The capacity of the injection of capsular polysaccharide (PRP) from *Haemophilus influenzae* type b to transiently decrease antibody specific to (and only to) *H. influenzae* type b is discussed in Chapter 9. A different question has been raised, that is, the possibility of a generalized immunologic suppression from simultaneous administration of more than one vaccine or vaccine component. Exposure to multiple foreign antigens is a common part of normal extrauterine life. During a single episode of upper respiratory viral infection, humans are exposed, depending on the particular virus involved, to between 4 and 10 foreign proteins, and during a routine "strep throat" infection, to between 25 and 50. Moreover, acquisition of a single new bacterium in the gastrointestinal tract, a common and normal event in consumption of everyday foods, or acquisition of one of the apparently harmless bacteria that inhabit the mouth and nose exposes the immune system to at least 50 potential antigens (Goldblatt et al., 1990). Each one of these foreign molecules typically contains numerous epitopes (antigenic determinants), each of which evokes a separate immune response. Moreover, each of the proteins is broken down in the body to expose still other epitopes, which may be antigenic depending on the genetic background of the host. The normal child may not respond to each of these proteins/epitopes, but in the case of *Branhamella catarrhalis*, a bacterium that inhabits the nasopharynxes of all normal children, antibodies to 17 different proteins can be detected after colonization (Goldblatt et al., 1990).

Infants, since they are born out of a germ-free environment into a world replete with microorganisms, undergo constant exposure to foreign antigens as their mucosal surfaces are populated with normal bacterial flora and as they are exposed to potentially more pathogenic microorganisms in the environment. During such encounters, the microorganisms would be expected to shed large amounts of their antigens for a period of days. The gradual rise in the levels of circulating immunoglobulins represents one part of the total immunologic response to this onslaught.

In the face of these normal events, it seems unlikely that the number of separate antigens contained in childhood vaccines, whether given orally or by injection, would represent an appreciable added burden on the immune system that would be immunosuppressive. Nevertheless, it is theoretically possible that some vaccine constituent might predispose an individual to infection through its action as an antigen or some other means. The combination of diphtheria-pertussis-tetanus vaccine has been the object of some research, in this regard, in part because pertussis toxin modulates certain immune functions in experimental animals. Fears that four deaths from bacterial infection after a trial of acellular pertussis vaccine in Sweden might have been due to the vaccine were allayed by a subsequent study (Storsaeter et al., 1988) that failed to find an increase in the number of patients hospitalized with bacterial infections after receipt of the vaccine. A report from Israel described an increase in minor infectious illnesses in the 30 days after administration of diphtheria and tetanus toxoids and pertussis vaccine (DPT) (Jaber et al., 1988). However, it is not possible to evaluate these results because of a combination of reporting bias, learning effect, and modification of illness incidence by season. Subsequently, three investigations have reported a lower or unchanged incidence of both minor and major infections after immunizations (Black et al., 1991; Davidson et al., 1991; Joffe et al., 1992). All three studies included a case-control design to examine serious infections. Two studies were conducted in the Kaiser Permanente health maintenance organization, and in both of these, a statistically significant *decrease* in infections after immunization was demonstrated. There were, however, potential confounding covariants, such as breast-feeding, frequency of well-child visits, and attendance at day care, so that a protective effect could not be unequivocally assigned to DPT. The conclusion of all three studies was, nevertheless, that no association of increased susceptibility to infection could be demonstrated in the weeks following DPT and oral polio vaccine immunizations. Since several hundred individuals were examined in the three studies, an infrequent association between immunization and infectious disease was not excluded.

It is also well known that many natural viral infections, particularly measles, can temporarily suppress components of the immune system (Starr and Berkovich, 1964; Ward et al., 1991), and there have been concerns that live attenuated viral vaccines might have a similar effect. Soon after the live attenuated measles vaccine was developed, it was shown that immunization temporarily suppressed the delayed-type hypersensitivity skin test response to purified protein derivative, an index of cell-mediated immunity to *Mycobacterium tuberculosis* (Brody and McAlister, 1964; Starr and Berkovich, 1964). The suppression was, however, less consistent and less prolonged than that following natural measles infection, presumably because of the attenuation of growth of the vaccine virus at all levels. Other viral vaccines, both live attenuated and inactivated, have been shown to have similar, although often mild and inconstant, effects on skin test responses to various antigens (Berkovich et al., 1972; Brody et al., 1964; Ganguly et al., 1976; Kupers et al., 1970). In addition, more recent studies have shown that, after measles immunization or reimmunization, certain lymphocyte functions, such as the ability to replicate when stimulated with phytohemagglutinin or to excrete certain chemotactic factors, are mildly but measurably depressed (Hirsch et al., 1981), and the number of CD8-positive lymphocytes falls slightly (Nicholson et al., 1992).

It may be asked, then, whether use of combination viral vaccines might exacerbate the potential problem of immune system suppression. The committee found no report of a systematic comparison of the effects of monovalent and polyvalent live attenuated vaccines on immunity. Combined measles-mumps-rubella vaccine (MMR) has been reported to have a temporary suppressive effect on neutrophil function (Toraldo et al., 1992) and on the ability of lymphocytes to proliferate in response to phytohemagglutinin or *Candida albicans* stimulation (Munyer et al., 1975), but neither study compared monovalent and trivalent vaccines. MMR vaccination was included in one of the large health maintenance organization case-control studies of possible serious bacterial infection after immunization (Black et al., 1991); although there was a trend toward fewer infections in vaccinees than in controls, none of the differences was significant.

At present, the data are insufficient to answer with certainty whether immunosuppression in the form of laboratory and skin test abnormalities after the receipt of a vaccine does, in fact, indicate a decrease in the capacity to resist infection. Therefore, as new vaccines are developed and as the old ones are used at different dosages or in different combinations or are administered at different ages, this question should continue to be a concern. To date, studies of current vaccines suggest that if immunization leads to an infection, it must do so infrequently.

REFERENCES

Arthus M. Injections répétées de sérum de cheval chez le lapin. Comptes Rendus des Séances de la Société de Biologie et ses Filiales (Paris) 1903;55:817-820.

Benacerraf B, Kabat EA. A quantitative study of the Arthus phenomenon induced passively in the guinea pig. Journal of Immunology 1950;64:1-19.

Berkovich S, Fikrig S, Brunell PA, Portugalaza C, Steiner M. Effect of live attenuated mumps vaccine virus on the expression of tuberculin sensitivity. Journal of Pediatrics 1972;80:84-87.

Black SB, Cherry JD, Shinefield HR, Fireman B, Christenson P, Lampert D. Apparent decreased risk of invasive bacterial disease after heterologous childhood immunization. American Journal of Diseases of Children 1991;145:746-749.

Brody JA, McAlister R. Depression of tuberculin sensitivity following measles vaccination. American Review of Respiratory Diseases 1964;90:611-617.

Brody JA, Overfield T, Hammes LM. Depression of the tuberculin reaction by viral vaccines. New England Journal of Medicine 1964;271:1294-1296.

Cohen P, Scadron SJ. Effects of active immunization of mother upon offspring. Journal of Pediatrics 1946;29:609-619.

Coombs RR, Gell PG. Classification of allergic reactions responsible for clinical hypersensitivity and disease. In: Gell PG, Coombs RR, eds. Clinical Aspects of Immunology, 2nd edition. Oxford: Blackwell; 1968.

Davidson M, Letson W, Ward JI, Ball A, Bulkow L, Christenson P, et al. DTP immunization and susceptibility to infectious diseases. American Journal of Diseases of Children 1991;145:750-754.

Dolovich J, Hargreave FE, Chalmeis R, Shier KJ, Cauldie J, Bienenstock J. Late cutaneous allergic responses in isolated-IgE-dependent reactions. Journal of Allergy and Clinical Immunology 1973;52:38-46.

Facktor MA, Bernstein RA, Fireman P. Hypersensitivity to tetanus toxoid. Journal of Allergy and Clinical Immunology 1973;52:1-12.

Fisher M. Anaphylaxis. Diseases of Man 1987;33:433-479.

Ganguly R, Cusumano CL, Waldman RH. Suppression of cell-mediated immunity after infection with attenuated rubella virus. Infection and Immunity 1976;13:464-469.

Goldblatt D, Turner MW, Levinsky RJ. *Branhamella catarrhalis*: antigenic determinants and the development of the IgG subclass response in childhood. Journal of Infectious Diseases 1990;162:1128-1135.

Henson PM. Antibody and immune-complex-mediated allergic and inflammatory reactions. In: Lachmann PJ, Peters DK, eds. Clinical Aspects of Immunology, 4th edition. Oxford: Blackwell; 1982.

Hirsch RL, Mokhtarian F, Griffin DE, Brooks BR, Hess J, Johnson RT. Measles virus vaccination of measles seropositive individuals suppresses lymphocyte proliferation and chemotactic factor production. Clinical Immunology and Immunopathology 1981;21:341-350.

Institute of Medicine. Adverse Effects of Pertussis and Rubella Vaccines. Washington, DC: National Academy Press; 1991.

Jaber L, Shohat M, Mimouni M. Infectious episodes following diphtheria-pertussis-tetanus vaccination: a preliminary observation in infants. Clinical Pediatrics 1988;27:491-494.

Joffe LS, Glode MP, Gutierrez MK, Wiesenthal A, Luckey DW, Harken L. Diphtheria-tetanus toxoids-pertussis vaccination does not increase the risk of hospitalization with an infectious illness. Pediatric Infectious Disease Journal 1992;11:730-735.

Kniker WT. Anaphylaxis in children and adults. In: Bierman CW, Pearlman DW, eds. Allergic Diseases from Infancy to Adulthood. Philadelphia: W.B. Saunders Co.; 1988.

Kupers TA, Petrich JM, Holloway AW, St. Geme JW, Jr. Depression of tuberculin delayed hypersensitivity by live attenuated mumps virus. Journal of Pediatrics 1970;76:716-721.

Munyer TP, Mangi RJ, Dolan T, Kantor FS. Depressed lymphocyte function after measles-mumps-rubella vaccination. Journal of Infectious Diseases 1975;134:75-78.

Nicholson JKA, Holman RC, Jones BM, McDougal JS, Sprauer MA, Markowitz LE. The effect of measles-rubella vaccination on lymphocyte populations and subpopulations in HIV-infected and healthy individuals. Journal of Acquired Immune Deficiency Syndromes 1992;5:528-537.

Pearlman DS, Bierman CW. Allergic disorders. In: Stiehm ER, ed. Immunologic Disorders in Infants and Children, 3rd edition. Philadelphia: W.B. Saunders Co.; 1989.

Starr S, Berkovich S. Effects of measles, gamma-globulin-modified measles and vaccine measles on the tuberculin test. New England Journal of Medicine 1964;270:386-391.

Storsaeter J, Olin P, Renemar B, Lagergard T, Norberg R, Romanus V, Tiru M. Mortality and morbidity from invasive bacterial infections during a clinical trial of acellular pertussis vaccines in Sweden. Pediatric Infectious Disease Journal 1988;7:637-645.

Toraldo R, Tolone C, Catalanotti P, Ianniello R, D'Avanzo M, Canino G, et al. Effect of measles-mumps-rubella vaccination on polymorphonuclear neutrophil functions in children. Acta Paediatrica 1992;81:887-890.

U.S. Department of Health and Human Services. U.S. Public Health Service, National Vaccine Injury Compensation Program; Revision of the Vaccine Injury Table; proposed rule. Federal Register, 42 CFR Part 100, August 14, 1992;57(158):36877-36885.

Ward BJ, Johnson RT, Vaisberg A, Jauregui E, Griffin DE. Cytokine production *in vitro* and the lymphoproliferative defect of natural measles virus infection. Clinical Immunology and Immunopathology 1991;61:236-248.

Wiggins CA, Dykewicz MS, Patterson R. Idiopathic anaphylaxis: a review. Annals of Allergy 1989;62:1-4.

5

Diphtheria and Tetanus Toxoids

BACKGROUND AND HISTORY

Tetanus

The causative agent of tetanus, *Clostridium tetani*, is a gram-positive, spore-forming anaerobic bacillus. *C. tetani* produces two exotoxins, tetanolysin and tetanospasmin. Tetanus results from the latter toxin, one of the most potent toxins on a weight basis (Wassilak and Orenstein, 1988). Tetanus toxin enters the nervous system at peripheral nerve endings. The toxin binds to a receptor, is internalized by endocytosis, and is transported to nerve cell bodies, primarily motoneurons, in the central nervous system (Fishman and Carrigan, 1988). Tetanus toxin appears to work presynaptically to affect neurotransmitter release (Bergey et al., 1987). The mode of action of tetanus toxin is similar to that of another well-known toxin, botulinum toxin, which is also produced by an anaerobic organism (Simpson, 1986). The mechanisms of action of these toxins have not been fully elucidated.

Early studies in experimental animals demonstrated that protective neutralizing antibodies could be elicited by repeated inoculations with a minute amount of toxin (Wassilak and Orenstein, 1988). These antisera also could provide passive protection when administered to nonimmune recipients. In 1926, Ramon and Zoeller immunized human subjects with a toxoid prepared by formaldehyde and heat treatment of the toxin. Although the protective level of antibody could not be assessed directly in human subjects (by challenge with active toxin), two early workers in this field immunized themselves with the tetanus toxoid and then challenged themselves with two to three fatal doses of tetanus toxin. They were protected by their prechallenge serum levels of 0.007 and 0.01 American units of tetanus toxoid per ml (Wolters and Dehmel, 1942). In 1950, the World Health Organization (WHO) reset the international unit (IU) to equal the American unit (see the section Biologic Events Following Immunization below).

Two types of tetanus toxoid are available in the United States: fluid and adsorbed. The adsorbed vaccines contain less than 1.25 mg of aluminum and 4 to 10 flocculation units (Lf) of toxoid per 0.5-ml dose. (The quantity of toxoid is measured by in vitro flocculation when toxoid is mixed with a known amount of antitoxin, and the results are recorded as the limit of flocculation [Lf].) The fluid preparations contain 4 to 5 Lf of toxoid. All tetanus toxoids in the United States contain 0.02 percent formaldehyde and 0.1 percent thimerosal. Some investigators have noted an increased rate of severe local reactions and abscess formation when adsorbed diphtheria toxoid or diphtheria and tetanus toxoids for pediatric use (children under 7 years of age) (DT) were used (e.g., 30 percent adsorbed versus 8 percent fluid) (Collier et al., 1979; Holden and Strang, 1965). However, others have not corroborated these findings and note that adsorbed toxoids have similar reaction rates as long as the injections are given intramuscularly rather than subcutaneously. In addition, adsorbed toxoids offer the benefit of enhanced immunogenicity (Jones et al., 1985; Relihan, 1969; Trinca, 1965; White, 1980; White et al., 1973).

Diphtheria

Diphtheria is an acute respiratory infection caused by *Corynebacterium diphtheriae*. In a nontoxigenic form, the organism may colonize the throat of asymptomatic individuals or may produce mild pharyngitis. However, when the bacterium is infected with a bacteriophage carrying the structural gene for biosynthesis of the toxin responsible for clinical disease, classic diphtheria can result. The clinical presentation includes a fibrinous, adherent pharyngeal membrane and complications of severe systemic toxicity, myocarditis, and peripheral neuritis. Case fatality rates were commonly in the range of 50 percent prior to the availability of antitoxin therapy. It is now known that diphtheria toxin is one of a family of A and B toxins. The A and B fragments of diphtheria toxin are part of a single polypeptide chain. Fragment A ("active") is a potent enzyme that acts intracellularly to block protein synthesis. The only known substrate for fragment A is elongation factor 2, which is involved in catalyzing the movement of ribosomes on eukaryotic messenger RNA. A single molecule of fragment A can kill a cell. Fragment B ("binding") is responsible for the recognition of receptors on mammalian cells and the translocation of fragment A into cells (Uchida, 1986). Protective human antibodies against diphtheria are directed against fragment B (Mortimer, 1988). The protective role of antisera against the toxin was documented by Behring in the late nineteenth century (Holmes, 1940), and the use of diphtheria antiserum raised in horses to treat human diphtheria was introduced a few years later. Active immunization with inactivated toxin in experimental animals was adapted to immunization of humans.

Early in the history of immunization against diphtheria, active toxin and antitoxin (prepared in horses) were administered as a mixture. In several reports, fatalities caused by the toxic effects of inadequately neutralized diphtheria toxin occurred in children given these mixtures (Dittmann, 1981b; Wilson, 1967). Following the introduction of toxin neutralization by chemical means (formalin), one report of incomplete detoxification appeared. In Kyoto, Japan, in 1948, 68 of 606 children died following inoculation with a formalin-detoxified vaccine. Free toxin was detected in one batch of the vaccine (Dittmann, 1981b). Currently licensed toxoids produced in the United States are now prepared and tested by procedures specified in the *Code of Federal Regulations*, and no cases of toxin-related disease have been reported since 1948.

Because of the severity of clinical diphtheria and the early recognition that protection was safely induced by immunization with diphtheria toxoid, controlled clinical trials of the efficacy of diphtheria toxoid were never performed. Early in the history of immunization against diphtheria, Schick (1913) introduced a test that correlated with protective immunity, thus making it possible to study both naturally acquired and toxoid-induced immunity. This test consists of the intradermal injection of a small amount of purified toxin. In nonimmune individuals who lack circulating antitoxin, a red, slightly hemorrhagic area appears at the injection site within 48 hours. Individuals with protective levels of antitoxin antibody (>0.01 U/ml) have no local reaction. On the basis of the correlation of a negative Schick test with protective immunity and a correlation between negative Schick test results and a serum antitoxin titer of 0.01 to 0.02 U/ml, one or both of these tests have been used to measure the efficacy of diphtheria immunization protocols that utilize various doses and administration schedules.

In the United States, children receive vaccines according to schedules determined by the American Academy of Pediatrics and the Advisory Committee on Immunization Practices. These groups recommend that diphtheria and tetanus toxoids and pertussis vaccine (DPT) be given at ages 2, 4, and 6 months, between ages 15 and 18 months, and between ages 4 and 6 years. The acellular pertussis-containing (DTaP) preparation can be substituted for

DPT for the fourth and fifth doses. Diphtheria and tetanus toxoids for pediatric use (DT) should be used in children younger than age 7 years in whom DPT is contraindicated. Tetanus and diphtheria toxoids for adult use (Td) should be used in individuals older than age 7 years. They should be administered every 10 years following the last DPT or DT vaccination.

BIOLOGIC EVENTS FOLLOWING IMMUNIZATION

Tetanus

Following an injection of tetanus toxoid, the recipient develops neutralizing antibodies that prevent the effects of toxin on the nervous system. Antibody levels are now reported in comparison with an international standard set by the WHO as international units per milliliter, and it is generally agreed that a level of 0.01 IU/ml or greater is protective (Wassilak and Orenstein, 1988). Protective levels of antibody are achieved in most children and adults after two doses of tetanus toxoid given 4 or more weeks apart, although children under 1 year of age may require three doses of tetanus toxoid (Barkin et al., 1984, 1985a). However, protective levels are relatively short-lived, particularly in infants and older adults, and thus, a reinforcing (booster) dose is given 6 to 12 months after the primary series of immunizations. Following this booster, long-term immunity usually exceeding 10 years develops (Peebles et al., 1969).

Minor local reactions (pain, erythema, swelling of less than 1 cm) occur within 48 hours following 1-80 percent of immunizations with tetanus toxoid (Collier et al., 1979; Jones et al., 1985; White, 1980). The reaction rate varies with the dose and type of toxoid, the number of prior doses of toxoid received, and the method of injection. Severe reactions (>8 cm of erythema or induration) are much less common and are often accompanied by a sore, swollen arm and systemic manifestations such as fever and malaise. Severe reactions occur much more frequently with larger doses of toxoid (McComb and Levine, 1961; Schneider, 1964), and in several studies, severe reactions have been found to correlate with high antibody levels prior to immunization (Collier et al., 1979; Facktor et al., 1973; Korger et al., 1986; Levine and Edsall, 1981; Levine et al., 1961; McComb and Levine, 1961; Relihan, 1969; White et al., 1973). Prior to the recognition of the long duration of immunity, frequent booster doses given after minor wounds or as prophylaxis for factory employees or children attending summer camps led to high levels of antibody.

The correlation between severe local reactions and high antibody levels prior to immunization strongly suggests that these reactions may be caused by immune complex formation between antibodies and antigen. In the case of severe local reactions, this is classified as an Arthus reaction, in which immune complexes form locally in the walls of small arteries (Edsall et al., 1967; Eisen et al., 1963; Facktor et al., 1973). In rare cases, it is possible that the immune complexes may form in the circulation, deposit in tissues, and activate complement. This would result in the clinical syndrome of serum sickness. These patients may develop glomerulonephritis, arthritis, and vasculitis. However, some investigators have been unable to confirm a consistent correlation between more severe local reactions and high antibody levels (Holden and Strang, 1965; Jones et al., 1985; White et al., 1973), and thus, it is likely that other factors such as toxoid variables, adjuvants, dose, and host factors may also play a role in the development of severe local reactions.

Routine immunization with tetanus toxoid also induces a cellular immune response, and intradermal skin testing with tetanus toxoid frequently is used as a screen for anergy (Gordon et al., 1983; Grabenstein, 1990; Steele et al., 1976). The absence of a delayed-type hypersensitivity response does not imply a lack of protective immunity, and conversely, a positive response does not appear to correlate with clinically important hypersensitivity reactions to the toxoid (Eisen et al., 1963; Facktor et al., 1973; Gold, 1941; Vellayappan and Lee, 1976).

Diphtheria

In the preimmunization era, many people acquired immunity to diphtheria (and a negative Schick test) presumably by asymptomatic colonization. Also, protective immunity was observed in young infants, most likely on the basis of the presence of transplacentally acquired antibody (Schick, 1913).

Diphtheria toxoid adsorbed with aluminum hydroxide or phosphate was shown to be more immunogenic and to produce fewer local reactions than fluid toxoid. The minimum schedule for children was found to be three doses, with the first two doses spaced by 1-2 months and the third dose given 6-12 months later. Booster doses were found to be necessary, particularly in countries where widespread immunization markedly decreased the opportunity for asymptomatic colonization (Bjorkholm et al., 1986; Christenson and Bottiger, 1986; James et al., 1951; Karzon and Edwards, 1988; Rappouli et al., 1988). To maintain protective levels of antitoxin antibody against diphtheria, recall immunization is suggested in older children and adults at 10-year intervals.

Early studies of the immune response to immunization against diphtheria revealed that some immune individuals responded to a Schick test with immediate hypersensitivity reactions (wheal and erythema within minutes) or delayed-type hypersensitivity reactions that were maximal at 24-72 hours (Zingher and Park, 1923). An important consequence of this observation was that interpretation of a "positive" Schick reaction to toxin required a control test with purified toxoid. Another implication was that pseudoreactions might predict clinically relevant hypersensitivity to further immunization with diphtheria toxoid (Pappenheimer, 1984). However, not all investigators found a high degree of correlation between Schick test results and adverse reactions (Settergren et al., 1986), and routine testing prior to immunization is impractical. Pappenheimer et al. (1950) demonstrated that a significant proportion of the delayed-type hypersensitivity reactions in previously immunized subjects were against the contaminants in the crude toxoid rather than against the highly purified diphtheria toxin. The role of bacterial cellular fractions in adverse reactions has been confirmed by Relyveld and colleagues (1979, 1980).

The problems of high rates of severe local and systemic reactions (fever, malaise, myalgia, headaches, and chills) noted in earlier studies with diphtheria toxoid in older children and adults have been alleviated by (1) the use of improved methods for purifying toxins, (2) reduction of the dose of toxoid (<2 Lf of diphtheria toxoid in Td versus 10-20 Lf in DPT and 10-12 Lf in DT), and (3) the use of adsorbed vaccine (Edsall et al., 1954; Levine et al., 1961; Myers et al., 1982; Smith, 1969). By this approach, the rates of adverse reactions related to hypersensitivity have been very low (Middaugh, 1979; Mortimer et al., 1986; Myers et al., 1982; Sheffield et al., 1978). Mild local reactions (tenderness and swelling at the injection site) occurred in 16 to 27 percent of vaccinees. Erythema, marked swelling, or systemic symptoms occurred in fewer than 2 percent of individuals.

ENCEPHALOPATHY

Clinical Description

Encephalopathy has been used in the literature to characterize a constellation of signs and symptoms reflecting a generalized disturbance in brain function often involving alterations in behavior or state of consciousness, convulsions, headache, and focal neurologic deficit. The annual incidence of encephalitis for the years 1950 to 1981 in Olmsted County, Minnesota was 7.4 per 100,000 (Beghi et al., 1984; Nicolosi et al., 1986). The incidence in children less than 1 year of age was 22.5, in children between 1 and 4 years of age it was 15.2, and in children between 5 and 9 years of age it was 30.2 per 100,000. Other estimates of encephalopathy for children less than age 2 years were somewhat lower than those reported by Beghi et al. (1984) and Nicolosi et al. (1986). Other estimates for annual incidence range from 5 per 100,000 children younger than age 2 years (Walker et al., 1988) to 10 per 100,000 children younger than age 2 years (Gale et al., 1990). For a more complete discussion of encephalopathy, see Chapter 3.

History of Suspected Association

Diphtheria toxin causes a toxic peripheral neuropathy in about 20 percent of cases (Mortimer, 1988), but diphtheria toxin has not been found to be associated with central nervous system (CNS) disease such as encephalopathy. Tetanus is a neurologic disease characterized by severe lower motor neuron hyperexcitability with consequent muscle spasms produced by the potent neurotoxin tetanospasmin (Wassilak and Orenstein, 1988).

Diphtheria and tetanus toxoids are generally given together as Td in adults and as DT or DPT (a combination that includes vaccine directed against pertussis) in children. DT and Td differ because of the lower concentration of diphtheria toxoid in the preparation for adults. Monovalent diphtheria and monovalent tetanus toxoids are also available. Pertussis as a clinical disease has long been known to cause encephalopathy, as discussed in detail by the Institute of Medicine (1991). The possibility that immunization against pertussis was responsible for serious adverse neurologic events leading to encephalopathy was raised as early as 1933, with concerns continuing to be reported through the present. Several large epidemiologic studies were designed to study the association between DPT and acute neurologic events in children. From those studies, information regarding DT was also obtained because of the lack of universal acceptance of DPT. The National Childhood Encephalopathy Study (Alderslade et al., 1981) and the North West Thames study (Pollock and Morris, 1983) provide some information on encephalopathy and DT. Additionally, two case-control studies in Italy (Crovari et al., 1984; Greco, 1985) were carried out to investigate a clinical observation that encephalopathy in several children was temporally related to DT immunization.

Evidence for Association

Biologic Plausibility

Although tetanus toxin can reach the CNS, it is not clearly associated with encephalopathy. The neurologic sequelae of tetanus have been described. Symptoms experienced by patients after recovery from tetanus include irritability, sleep disturbances, myoclonus, decreased libido, postural hypotension, and abnormalities on electroencephalograms (Illis and Taylor, 1971). The symptoms disappeared within 2 years of recovery from tetanus. These were attributed by the author as secondary to the action of tetanus toxin on inhibitory synapses in the CNS. The neurologic consequences of diphtheria are primarily peripheral neuropathy.

Case Reports, Case Series, and Uncontrolled Observational Studies

The North West Thames study by Pollock and Morris (1983), an uncontrolled cohort study, was a collection of reports of all reactions to vaccines in the North West Thames region of England and Wales. It was designed to intensify the reporting of severe manifestations, particularly neurologic complications, after childhood immunization between January 1975 and December 1981. Of 400,500 doses of DT and oral polio vaccine (OPV) (133,500 children completing a primary series of three doses of vaccine) and 221,000 single booster doses of DT given at school entry, seven children had seizures without neurologic damage and were well at follow-up. Three children with other neurologic conditions were identified; one child (9 months old) had infantile spasms predating vaccination, another child (9 years old) had a seizure with hemiplegia 1 day after receipt of DT but was normal on follow-up, and another child (7 months old) developed hemiparesis 14 days after receipt of DT and was normal on follow-up. None of these neurologic events was considered to be encephalopathic.

Because it was felt that reactions that occurred after vaccination with DT were being underreported in the first part of the North West Thames study (compared with the reporting of reactions that occurred after vaccination with DPT), an alternative method of study was undertaken on the basis of a hospital activity analysis of hospitals in the North West Thames region during 1979. Children under 2 years of age were included in the study if their diagnosis at the time of discharge included a neurologic event. No control group was used. Of 18,000 children who completed a primary series of DT (approximately 54,000 doses of DT were administered), 18 children had seizures (all febrile) within 28 days of DT immunization and 3 children had some other neurologic disease that developed within 28 days of DT immunization. Two of these children had focal seizures at 22 and 24 days after DT immunization, and the other child died of encephalopathy 28 days after DT immunization. Insufficient detail was given to describe the case of encephalopathy.

Several clinical trials compared DT and DPT (therefore, they are considered uncontrolled cohort studies for DT), and they showed that there were no serious neurologic adverse events after receipt of DT. Those studies, by Cody et al. (1981) and Barkin et al. (1985b), had only very small samples of those immunized with DT (784 and 40 subjects, respectively) and therefore do not provide much additional knowledge of the adverse events following immunization with DT.

Quast and colleagues (1979) found in the records of Behringwerke (a pharmaceutical firm in the former West Germany) a case report of a 36-year-old female who developed polyneuromyeloencephalopathy 5 days after receiving her first dose of aluminum-adsorbed tetanus toxoid in 1976. The authors provided no clinical information other than the fact that she recovered completely.

Several small case series described in the literature looked for adverse events following immunization with both DPT and DT (Feery, 1982; Waight et al., 1983). Those studies showed no adverse neurologic events following receipt of DT, although the sample sizes in those two studies were small (335 and 221 subjects, respectively).

The following cases were reported in the Vaccine Adverse Event Reporting System (VAERS) between November 1990 and July 1992: a 50-year-old male who developed syncope, visual disturbance, and hypoglycemia 1 day after receiving tetanus toxoid; a 14-year-old male who developed encephalitis and transverse myelitis 2.5 months following Td administration; and a 17-year-old male who developed lymphocytic meningoencephalitis 10 days following receipt of Td and measles-mumps-rubella vaccine (MMR).

Controlled Observational Studies

The best observational case-control study that provides information about immunization with DT and association with neurologic illness is the National Childhood Encephalopathy Study (NCES) (Alderslade et al., 1981), which was undertaken because of concerns about possible adverse events following receipt of pertussis vaccine. That study identified children aged 2-36 months who were admitted to a hospital with neurologic illness during the 3 years from July 1976 to June 1979 in England, Scotland, and Wales. The first 1,000 of 1,182 cases identified during that time were studied. For each case there were two "at-home" controls matched for age, sex, and area of residence. No statistically significant association with DT immunization and neurologic adverse events was found in cases compared with controls. On the basis of the data in Table V.15 on page 122 of the NCES (Alderslade et al., 1981), the odds ratio (OR) is 0.92 (95 percent confidence interval [CI], 0.64-1.30). However, as with infantile spasms, a nonsignificantly higher rate of exposure to DT was observed within the 7 days prior to the date of onset of illness in the case patients, and a correspondingly lower rate of exposure was observed between more than 7 and less than 28 days prior to onset. Because nearly one-third of the cases had prolonged febrile convulsions, the excess rate of exposure to DT within 7 days, if real, may merely reflect the tendency of DT vaccination to cause fever.

Greco (1985) carried out a case-control study in the Campania (Naples) region of Italy from January 1980 to February 1983 to test the association between encephalopathy and immunization with DT. The Italian Ministry of Health had received reports that described several cases of encephalopathy in children who had received DT within the week prior to illness, and those reports were the impetus for the study. A case was defined as a patient between the ages of 3 and 48 months who was admitted to the Santobono Hospital intensive care unit during the study period with one or more of the following diagnoses: coma of unknown cause, Reye syndrome, convulsions of unknown cause, respiratory distress with coma from an unknown cause, and death or stupor from an unknown cause. Forty-five patients that met the case definition were identified, and for each case there were four matched controls: two hospital controls and two residential controls. Hospital controls were matched to cases by age, sex, and date of admission; residential controls were matched by age, sex, and place of residence. The authors found that 64 percent of the case patients had been immunized with DT during the month prior to hospitalization, whereas 10 percent of hospital controls and 13 percent of residence controls had been immunized with DT. The reported ORs were 40.9 (95 percent CI, 6.3-102.5) for immunization with DT within the month prior to hospitalization and 92.6 (95 percent CI, 35.1-244.1) within the week prior to hospitalization.

The study by Greco (1985) has many methodologic problems. First and foremost, the cases leading to the Italian Ministry of Health's alert concerning the possible association between DT vaccination and encephalopathy served as part of the case group for the study. Additionally, cases were selected without blinding with respect to their prior immunization status. As described in the article, many of the case patients had elevated transaminase and ammonia levels but had normal cerebrospinal fluid (CSF) findings, suggesting the diagnosis of Reye syndrome. To the extent that DT may have been given to children with concomitant influenza or other viral illnesses, the occurrence of local or febrile reactions may have led to treatment with aspirin and, secondarily, the development of Reye syndrome. No information on aspirin use was given in the article describing the study. In addition, case DT recipients were twice as likely as control DT recipients to have received OPV simultaneously.

In response to the same reports that led to the study by Greco (1985), another case-control study (Crovari et al., 1984) was undertaken in the Luguria (Genoa) region of Italy to assess the association between recent DT immunization and coma or complicated convulsions. The study of Crovari et al. (1984) drew its cases from admissions to the intensive care unit, infectious disease ward, and general ward of the hospital of the Istituto G. Gaslini in Genoa between January 1980 and June 1983. The case patients were between 3 and 48 months of age and were admitted with coma, complicated convulsions of unknown etiology, or both. Children with known epilepsy or febrile convulsions were supposedly excluded from the case group, but the authors later state (in the results) that the majority of patients presented with "hyperpyrexia." Twenty-nine cases were identified, and each case was matched with four controls (two inpatient and two outpatient) by sex and age for inpatient controls and by age, sex, and residence for outpatient controls. The study did not show a statistically significant association between receipt of DT and coma or complicated convulsions (matched OR, 1.6; 95 percent CI, 0.54-4.74). However, the outpatient controls were randomly selected from records of vaccinated children. This would inflate exposure rates among the outpatient control group and perhaps create a negative bias in the odds ratio. Unpublished information provided by the authors permitted a separate (unmatched) analysis for the cases and inpatient controls, which revealed an unmatched OR of 2.16 (95 percent CI, 0.37-12.49). A meta-analysis combining the data from the NCES and the cases and inpatient controls from the study of Crovari et al. (1984) yields a Mantel-Haenszel OR of 0.95 (95 percent CI, 0.68-1.34).

Controlled Clinical Trials

No controlled clinical trials have compared DT recipients with an appropriate control.

Causality Argument

There is some biologic plausibility that tetanus toxoid-containing preparations might cause encephalopathy, on the basis of the evidence of Illis and Taylor (1971) that tetanus toxin has been associated with CNS sequelae. The case reports and case series reviewed above offer no convincing evidence for the occurrence of encephalopathy following immunization with DT. Three case-control studies addressed the question of a possible relation between DT immunization and encephalopathy. The best of the controlled observational studies is the NCES (Alderslade et al., 1981). The authors of that study did not detect an association between the occurrence of acute neurologic illness and receipt of DT (OR, 0.92; 95 percent CI, 0.64-1.30), nor did a meta-analysis combining the NCES results with those based on cases and inpatient controls in the study by Crovari et al. (1984) (OR, 0.95; 95 percent CI, 0.68-1.34). Therefore, the combined evidence strongly suggests that no relation exists between immunization with DT and the onset of acute neurologic illness. The possibility of lot-specific reactions to DT, as has been demonstrated for DPT preparations (Baraff et al., 1989), suggests that studies could be more revealing if the vaccines were tracked by lot. (See Chapter 11 for suggestions for further research.)

If the evidence favors rejection of a causal relation between DT and acute encephalopathy, then in the committee's judgment the evidence favors rejection of a causal relation between DT and chronic encephalopathy and between Td and tetanus toxoid alone and encephalopathy.

Conclusion

The evidence favors rejection of a causal relation between DT, Td, or tetanus toxoid and encephalopathy (acute or chronic).

RESIDUAL SEIZURE DISORDER

Clinical Description

Seizures are neurologic events that may occur with or without the loss of consciousness and can include a variety of sensory experiences (e.g., auditory seizures), motor manifestations (e.g., focal motor or tonic-clonic seizures), or both. In addition, seizures can occur with or without fever. Febrile seizures are well-defined, relatively common events that are precipitated by fever in children without a seizure disorder. Afebrile seizures are those that occur in the absence of fever. Recurrent afebrile seizures are referred to as epilepsy and are synonymous with residual seizure disorder. Approximately 0.5 to 2 percent of the population experiences epilepsy. It can occur at any age. Infantile spasms are a type of epileptic disorder in young children characterized by flexor, extensor, and mixed flexor-extensor seizures that tend to occur in clusters or flurries (Kellaway et al., 1979). The earliest manifestations of infantile spasms are subtle and are easily missed, making it difficult to identify the precise age at onset. Incidence rates of infantile spasms range from 0.25 to 0.4 per 1,000 live births. The vast majority of studies report a peak onset between ages 4 and 6 months. Approximately 65 percent of children with infantile spasms go on to have other types of seizures. For a more complete discussion of the definition of seizures, see Chapter 3.

History of Suspected Association

Diphtheria toxin causes a toxic peripheral neuropathy in about 20 percent of cases (Mortimer, 1988), but diphtheria toxin has not been associated with CNS disease. Tetanus is a neurologic disease characterized by severe muscle spasms produced by the potent neurotoxin tetanospasmin (Wassilak and Orenstein, 1988). This neurotoxin can produce three clinical syndromes: (1) localized, (2) generalized (80 percent of cases), and (3) cephalic. In patients with generalized tetanus, the neurotoxin makes its way to the CNS and can then cause spasm of any muscle as well as autonomic nervous system disturbances. Tetanospasms (generalized tonic-tetanic seizure-like activity) can occur, but cognitive functions are not affected. Tetanospasms are generalized muscle spasms, not generalized seizures in which the level of consciousness is affected. Cephalic tetanus is rare and is associated with cranial nerve palsies. Therefore, clinical diphtheria disease and tetanus disease have not been associated with seizures.

Inasmuch as DT, Td, tetanus toxoid, and DPT have been known to cause fever, they have been associated with the occurrence of acute febrile seizures. Febrile seizures alone do not lead to a residual seizure disorder. There are a paucity of case reports in the literature describing seizures (other than febrile) that have occurred in association with diphtheria and tetanus toxoids. However, several large epidemiologic studies were designed to investigate the association between receipt of DPT and acute neurologic events in children. From those studies, information regarding DT was also obtained because there was not universal acceptance of DPT. Bellman et al. (1983) examined a subset of the NCES data for a relation between the onset of infantile spasms and recent vaccination with DT and DPT. Pollock et al. (1984, 1985) and Pollock and Morris (1983) examined the relation between the onset of neurologic events (including seizures) and vaccination with DT and DPT in several different studies.

Evidence for Association

Biologic Plausibility

There are no data directly bearing on the biologic plausibility of a relation between diphtheria or tetanus toxoid and residual seizure disorder.

Case Reports, Case Series, and Uncontrolled Observational Studies

Three uncontrolled observational (cohort) studies provide descriptive information. The North West Thames study (Pollock and Morris, 1983 [see previous section on encephalopathy]), an uncontrolled cohort study, also offers some information regarding seizures following DT immunization. In the voluntary reporting part of the study, of 133,500 children who received a primary series of three immunizations (400,500 doses) of DT (and OPV), and 221,000 single booster doses of DT given at school entry, seven children had seizures, and all were normal on follow-up. Two of these were febrile seizures associated with respiratory illness and possible fever, and three were in children with personal or family histories of seizures. In the hospital activity analysis, of 18,000 children who received a primary series of DT (and OPV) (54,000 doses), 18 children had seizures, all of which were febrile, within 28 days of immunization. Of the children who presented with neurologic disease after DT immunization, two patients with convulsions with focal signs presenting at 22 and 24 days postimmunization, respectively, were reported. Long-term follow-up of these two patients was not presented in the report, but the relatively long period of time between receipt of DT and seizures (22 and 24 days, respectively) makes a causal inference between receipt of the toxoids and the adverse event much less plausible.

In another uncontrolled study (for the purposes of DT immunization), Pollock et al. (1984, 1985) examined the symptoms that were reported to occur after primary immunization with DT and DPT (and OPV). Infants attending the Hertfordshire Area Health Authority, England, were recruited during a 3-year period beginning in January 1978. They were followed through their primary immunization series, and parents were questioned within 2 weeks and again at 6-8 weeks after each immunization. Of 4,024 children administered 10,601 doses of DT, seizures were reported in 2 children at the first follow-up. One child had a febrile seizure 8 hours after injection of DT, and the other child had a respiratory infection and seizure 5 days after injection of DT. The latter child's sibling had a history of febrile seizures. Neither of these children had residual sequelae. At the 6-week follow-up, three cases of febrile convulsions were reported to have occurred 3-6 weeks postvaccination in three children who received DT but who did not have a personal or family history of seizures, and a fourth case of febrile convulsions was reported in a child with a previous history of convulsions. Neurologic disorders were diagnosed as arising between the first and second follow-up examinations in three children in the group that received DT. Epilepsy was diagnosed in two children; one child had a seizure 8 days after immunization, and another child had a seizure 6 weeks after immunization. The third child had a convulsion and then transitory hemiplegia 5 weeks after immunization. Two of the three children and a sibling of the third child had a prior history of convulsions, therefore implying prior neurologic illness. That study did not show any evidence for residual seizure disorder de novo following receipt of DT.

Hirtz and colleagues (1983) described the results of the National Collaborative Perinatal Project (NCPP), which followed the children born to 54,000 women in 1959 until 1966, when the children were 7 years of age. Medical histories of neurologic events (including seizures) were obtained at regular intervals, and developmental examinations were done at certain intervals. Thirty-nine children in the study experienced a seizure within 2 weeks of immunization (DPT, polio, measles, influenza, smallpox, tetanus booster, or unspecified). All but one of the seizures were febrile. Three children experienced seizures with a latency of longer than 2 weeks following vaccination. One child received DPT, but the vaccines administered to the other two children were not specified. One of those children had a seizure 1 day after receiving a tetanus booster. The child had a prior neurologic history, in that several months earlier he had sustained a skull fracture in a car accident and had been in a coma but had apparently recovered. The data do not make clear whether this child had a febrile seizure or if he had a residual seizure disorder at the 7-year follow-up.

No reports in VAERS submitted between November 1990 and July 1992 describe residual seizure disorders in association with receipt of tetanus toxoid alone, DT or Td alone, or tetanus toxoid, DT, or Td in combination with other vaccines.

Controlled Observational Studies

The most methodologically sound of the observational studies is the case-control study by Bellman et al. (1983), which examined a subset of the NCES data (Alderslade et al., 1981) for the relation between the onset of infantile spasms and recent DT or DPT immunization. They analyzed all 1,182 cases in the NCES (as opposed to the first 1,000, as was done in the larger NCES study [Alderslade et al., 1981]). Cases and controls were compared for their exposure to either DPT or DT in the 7 or 28 days before the onset of spasms. Of the 269 cases of infantile spasms reported to the NCES, there were 19 cases of infantile spasms whose onset was within 28 days of DT immunization. Infantile spasms were positively associated with receipt of DT within the week prior to the date of onset, but were negatively associated with receipt of DT between 1 and 4 weeks prior to the date of onset. The OR for all cases of infantile spasms with exposure to DT within the 28 days prior to the onset of this condition was 0.83 (95 percent CI, 0.46-1.50). This provides strong evidence suggesting that DT does not cause infantile spasms. The authors concluded that DT does not cause the development of infantile spasms but may trigger their onset in those children in whom the disorder is destined to develop.

Controlled Clinical Trials

None.

Causality Argument

There is no demonstrated plausibility that diphtheria or tetanus toxoids can cause residual seizure disorder. The case reports available for review are those in VAERS. No reports in VAERS described seizures after receipt of tetanus toxoid, DT, or Td alone or in combination with other vaccines. There are VAERS reports of seizures in patients following receipt of DPT. Because in these cases DT was given with pertussis vaccine (as DPT) and other vaccines, it is impossible to know which, if any, of the cases of seizures could be attributed to vaccine.

One case-control study (Bellman et al., 1983) examined the question of a possible relation between DT immunization and seizures. Bellman et al.

(1983) examined a subset of the NCES data for the relation between the onset of infantile spasms and recent DT and DPT immunizations. Infantile spasms were positively associated with receipt of DT within the week prior to the date of onset but were negatively associated with receipt of DT between 1 and 4 weeks prior to the onset. The unmatched OR for all patients with infantile spasms who were exposed to DT within the 28 days prior to the onset of this condition was 0.83 (95 percent CI, 0.46-1.50). This provides strong evidence suggesting that DT does not cause infantile spasms.

The other studies in the literature that addressed this issue were uncontrolled observational studies. In the North West Thames study (Pollock and Morris, 1983), only two seizures (other than febrile seizures) were reported in association with DT immunization. These cases were found in the hospital activity analysis (case review) part of the study. Two patients with seizures with focal signs presented at 22 and 24 days, respectively, after DT immunization. Long-term follow-up of these patients was not described in the report; therefore, no information describing whether a residual seizure disorder developed was provided. However, the relatively long period of time between the receipt of DT and the development of seizures in both patients (22 and 24 days) makes a causal relation between vaccine and the event much less biologically plausible. In other uncontrolled observational studies by Pollock et al. (1984, 1985), no evidence of residual seizure disorder in association with DT was seen in children who were neurologically normal prior to immunization with DT. In the NCPP uncontrolled cohort study by Hirtz et al. (1983), no cases of residual seizure disorder were seen in association with immunization with tetanus toxoid. The one seizure recorded in temporal association with tetanus toxoid administration occurred in a child with a previous neurologic condition; the data do not make it clear whether he had residual seizure disorder.

Conclusion

The evidence favors rejection of a causal relation between DT and infantile spasms.

The evidence is inadequate to accept or reject a causal relation between DT and residual seizure disorder other than infantile spasms.

The evidence is inadequate to accept or reject a causal relation between tetanus toxoid or Td and residual seizure disorder.

DEMYELINATING DISEASES OF THE CENTRAL NERVOUS SYSTEM

Clinical Description

Demyelinating diseases of the CNS can be categorized into disseminated and focal lesions. Acute disseminated encephalomyelitis (ADEM) is characterized by acute depression of consciousness and multifocal neurologic findings occurring within days to weeks (5 days to 6 weeks) following an inciting event. It is characterized pathologically by diffuse foci of perivenular inflammation and demyelination most prominent in the white matter of the brain and spinal cord (Johnson et al., 1985). Optic neuritis and transverse myelitis are focal demyelinating lesions that can occur in isolation or as components of diffuse demyelinating diseases such as ADEM and multiple sclerosis. Transverse myelitis is characterized by the acute onset of signs of spinal cord disease, usually involving the descending motor tracts and the ascending sensory fibers, suggesting a lesion at one level of the spinal cord. The annual incidence of transverse myelitis in Rochester, Minnesota, from 1970 to 1980 was 7.4 per 100,000 individuals (Beghi et al., 1982). Optic neuritis represents a lesion in the optic nerve behind the orbit but anterior to the optic chiasm. No population-based incidence rates were identified. For a more complete description of demyelinating diseases of the CNS, see Chapter 3.

History of Suspected Association

Demyelinating disease of the CNS has long been known to follow viral and some bacterial infections and the administration of live attenuated and inactivated antiviral vaccines. Demyelinating complications following vaccination were first noted after the introduction of rabies vaccine grown in animal brain or spinal cord in the 1880s. On rare occasions, encephalomyelitis also complicated the injection of vaccinia virus, which is used for the prevention of smallpox. For a more complete discussion of the history of the suspected association between vaccines and the development of demyelinating lesions of the CSF, see Chapter 3. In the more recent literature, several case reports of ADEM in association with tetanus toxoid have been described (Schlenska, 1977; Schwarz et al., 1988), but there has not been a pathologically proven case of ADEM following administration of tetanus toxoid, DT, DPT, or Td. Case reports of transverse myelitis (Read et al., 1992; Whittle and Roberton, 1977) and optic neuritis (Quast et al., 1979; Topaloglu et al., 1992) have been presented in the literature as well.

Evidence for Association

Biologic Plausibility

Chapter 3 provided a detailed discussion of the historic and scientific evidence that establishes a relation between vaccines and the development of demyelinating diseases of the CNS. In summary, it is biologically plausible that injection of an inactivated virus, bacterium, or live attenuated virus might induce an autoimmune response in the susceptible host, either by deregulation of the immune response, by nonspecific activation of T cells directed against myelin proteins, or by autoimmunity triggered by sequence similarities to host proteins such as those of myelin. The latter mechanism might evoke a response to a self-antigen (molecular mimicry) (Fujinami and Oldstone, 1989).

Case Reports, Case Series, and Uncontrolled Observational Studies

Reports in the literature of cases that clinically resemble ADEM include one described by Schlenska (1977). A 36-year-old woman developed lethargy, slurred speech, nystagmus, hemihypesthesia, decreased sensation along several thoracic dermatomes, and pyramidal tract signs 5 days after receiving a tetanus toxoid booster. She had good recovery over an 11-month period with no further episodes. Another report by Schwarz et al. (1988) describes a 21-year-old man who developed coma with midbrain signs after tetanus toxoid administration on two occasions 2.5 years apart. Latencies from the time of toxoid administration to the onset of symptoms were 7 and 8 days, respectively.

Several case reports describing transverse myelitis after tetanus booster administration were found in the literature. In 1977, Whittle and Roberton described a 7-month-old girl who developed flaccid paraparesis 6 days after receiving DT and OPV. Read et al. (1992) described a 50-year-old man who developed flaccid legs, areflexia, and a sensory level at T-6 12 days after receiving a tetanus booster. A magnetic resonance imaging study showed no lesions in the brain, suggesting that this lesion was indeed limited to the spinal cord. In a case described by Topaloglu et al. (1992), an 11-year-old girl developed spastic paraparesis, bilateral papillitis, and visual defects 3 days after receiving a booster of tetanus toxoid. An 11-month follow-up showed no recurrence of symptoms, and there was total recovery except for the persistence of pale optic disks. This does suggest disease in multiple foci, as is seen in ADEM, but the time interval between immunization and disease was too brief to suggest a mechanism analogous to experimental allergic encephalomyelitis. Two pertinent case reports of transverse myelitis were found in VAERS (submitted between November

1990 and July 1992). In one patient transverse myelitis developed after administration of Td, and in another patient transverse myelitis developed after administration of Td and hepatitis B vaccine. The temporal and clinical details provided in these reports from VAERS are insufficient for proper evaluation of the cases.

Well-documented cases of optic neuritis following vaccine administration are even rarer than cases of transverse myelitis. Quast et al. (1979) reported a 46-year-old man who developed acute optic neuritis 10 days after receiving a tetanus booster. As discussed above, Topaloglu et al. (1992) described an 11-year-old girl who developed transverse myelitis and optic neuritis 3 days after receipt of a tetanus booster. No cases of solitary optic neuritis in association with tetanus toxoid, DT, or Td were found in VAERS (submitted between November 1990 and July 1992).

Controlled Observational Studies

None.

Controlled Clinical Trials

None.

Causality Argument

There is biologic plausibility for a causal relation between vaccines and demyelinating disorders. The reports in the literature that describe a possible association between demyelinating diseases of the CNS (ADEM, transverse myelitis, and optic neuritis) are case reports. There are at least two case reports in the literature for each of the above-mentioned demyelinating diseases of the CNS. The case reports describe the demyelinating disease that occurs within the biologically plausible latency period of 5 days to 6 weeks, and the case reports provide enough clinical detail that one can be relatively certain of the neurologic diagnosis. What the case reports cannot address is whether the frequency of the cases that occurred was greater than the expected background rate for these specific demyelinating diseases. Annual incidence rates have been estimated for transverse myelitis (Beghi et al., 1982). These data were calculated for Rochester, Minnesota, for the years 1970 to 1980. The estimated rate of 0.83 per 100,000 individuals is much higher than a rate calculated for Israel, presumably because of differences in how successful the two studies were at identifying all cases of transverse myelitis. No population-based incidence rates for ADEM or optic neuritis were identified. This question is difficult at best for rare adverse events and can be answered only if both good *age-specific* background rates for the specific disease in question are known and aggressive surveillance of adverse events is carried out or if large controlled observational studies are done. None of this specific information is available when considering the relation between tetanus toxoid, DT, or Td and the occurrence of ADEM, transverse myelitis, or optic neuritis.

Conclusion

The evidence is inadequate to accept or reject a causal relation between tetanus toxoid, DT, or Td and demyelinating diseases of the CNS (ADEM, transverse myelitis, and optic neuritis).

GUILLAIN-BARRÉ SYNDROME

Clinical Description

Guillain-Barré syndrome (GBS), also known as acute inflammatory demyelinating polyneuritis, is characterized by the rapid onset of flaccid motor weakness with depression of tendon reflexes and elevation of protein levels in CSF without pleocytosis. The annual incidence of GBS appears to be approximately 1 per 100,000 for adults. The data are not definitive, but the annual incidence of GBS in children under age 5 years appears to be approximately the same. The annual incidence of GBS in children over age 5 years and teenagers appears to be lower. Chapter 3 contains a detailed description of GBS.

History of Suspected Association

Demyelinating disease of the peripheral nervous system has long been known to follow viral and some bacterial infections and can complicate the administration of live attenuated and inactivated viral vaccines. However, vaccinations are an infrequent antecedent event in patients with GBS, probably occurring in less than 1 to 5 percent of all patients. In most large case series of GBS, recent vaccination either is not mentioned or is described in only an occasional person (Hankey, 1987; Winer et al., 1988). For a more complete discussion of the history of the suspected association between vaccines and the development of GBS, see Chapter 3. A number of case reports in the medical literature have described GBS following receipt of tetanus toxoid. These are discussed in the following section.

Evidence for Association

Biologic Plausibility

Chapter 3 provides a detailed discussion of the historical and scientific evidence establishing the biologic plausibility of a relation between vaccines and the development of GBS. In summary, it is biologically plausible that injection of an inactivated virus, bacterium, or live attenuated virus might induce an autoimmune response to peripheral nerve and root in the susceptible host, either by deregulation of the immune response, by nonspecific activation of T cells directed against myelin proteins, or by autoimmunity triggered by sequence similarities to host proteins such as those of myelin. The latter mechanism might evoke a response to a self-antigen, so-called molecular mimicry (Fujinami and Oldstone, 1989).

Case Reports, Case Series, and Uncontrolled Observational Studies

In surveying the medical literature, 29 instances of adverse events labeled as either GBS or polyneuritis were found in association with diphtheria or tetanus toxoids (Dittmann, 1981b; Holliday and Bauer, 1983; Hopf, 1980; Newton and Janati, 1987; Onisawa et al., 1985; Pollard and Selby, 1978; Quast et al., 1979; Reinstein et al., 1982; Robinson, 1981; Rutledge and Snead, 1986; Schlenska, 1977). These occurred primarily in the European literature. The majority of reported cases were in adults who had received either tetanus toxoid alone (21 individuals) or who had received tetanus toxoid and anti-tetanus toxin serum (4 individuals). Anti-tetanus toxin serum is known to induce GBS in its own right (Miller and Stanton, 1954). In most of the case reports describing what was labeled as GBS or polyneuritis, clinical details are lacking or, when present, are inconsistent with the diagnostic criteria for GBS. Three of the 25 cases following receipt of tetanus toxoid are described in enough detail and fall within the diagnostic criteria to be acceptable as documented cases of GBS with an appropriate latency (5 days to 6 weeks) following vaccination (Hopf, 1980; Newton and Janati, 1987; Pollard and Selby, 1978). One patient (Newton and Janati, 1987) received tetanus toxoid made by a U.S.-licensed manufacturer. All these patients were adults.

One particular case reported by Pollard and Selby (1978) is particularly relevant for a possible causal relation between tetanus toxoid and GBS for that case. A 42-year-old male laborer received tetanus toxoid on three separate occasions over a period of 13 years, and following each vaccination a self-limited episode of clear-cut, well-documented polyneuropathy of the GBS variety ensued. The latencies for each episode were 21, 14, and 10 days, respectively. He had minimal residual neurologic signs following the second episode, and made a full functional recovery following the third episode (J. D. Pollard, University of Sydney, Sydney, Australia, personal communication, 1993). A well-studied sural nerve biopsy during the third episode showed demyelination, onion bulb formation, and incipient hypertrophic neuropathy. The patient's lymphocytes could be induced to proliferate upon exposure to tetanus toxoid and to elaborate the lymphokine macrophage inhibition factor upon exposure to peripheral nerve homogenate, although these responses can be seen in vaccinees without GBS. Other studies of hypersensitivity to peripheral nerve antigens were not done. The immunologic basis for his sensitivity to tetanus toxoid was not demonstrated. Subsequently, since 1981, this man has experienced multiple recurrences of demyelinating polyneuropathy, most following acute viral illnesses. Plasmapheresis administered at 3-week intervals was initiated in 1986 and has continued until the time of this writing. In recent years he has remained functionally normal, but has minor residual sensory findings on examination (J. D. Pollard, University of Sydney, Sydney, Australia, personal communication, 1993).

Few cases of GBS following receipt of DT have been reported. Dittmann (1981b) noted that three instances of acute polyneuritis, presumably GBS, were reported as adverse events following administration of this vaccine. These data were based on passive reporting following the distribution of approximately 5.5 million doses of vaccine between 1950 and 1976 in the former East Germany.

The Monitoring System for Adverse Events Following Immunization (MSAEFI) lists four cases of GBS between 1979 and 1990 following vaccination with DT. VAERS lists two cases of GBS in temporal association with Td submitted between November 1990 and July 1992. Both patients simultaneously received DT and MMR.

Controlled Observational Studies

None.

Controlled Clinical Trials

None.

Causality Argument

There is biologic plausibility for a causal relation between vaccines and demyelinating disorders. The literature describing a possible association between GBS and tetanus toxoid, DT, or Td consists of case reports. The most convincing case in the literature is that reported by Pollard and Selby

(1978), who described a 42-year-old man who developed GBS on three separate occasions (over a 13-year period) following receipt of tetanus toxoid. The relation between tetanus toxoid and GBS is convincing at least for that one individual, even though this man has subsequently experienced multiple recurrences of demyelinating polyneuropathy, most following acute viral illnesses (J. D. Pollard, University of Sydney, Sydney, Australia, personal communication, 1993). Of the other cases relating receipt of tetanus toxoid to the development of GBS, two others (Hopf, 1980; Newton and Janati, 1987) are recorded in enough detail to be accepted as GBS; one of these patients (Newton and Janati, 1987) received tetanus toxoid made by a U.S.-licensed manufacturer. Both patients were adults. Aside from the data in MSAEFI and VAERS, which generally do not provide sufficient clinical descriptions to establish the diagnosis, there is little information in the literature relating DT or Td to the development of GBS. The case series by Dittmann (1981b) describes three cases of polyneuritis following administration of Td. What the case reports cannot address is whether the frequency of cases is higher than the expected background rate of GBS. This question is difficult at best for rare adverse events and can be done only if (1) good age-specific background rates for the specific disease in question are known, (2) aggressive surveillance of adverse events is done, or (3) large controlled observational studies are done. None of this specific information is available when considering the relation between tetanus toxoid, DT, or Td and the occurrence of GBS. However, because the case by Pollard and Selby (1978) demonstrates that tetanus toxoid *did* cause GBS, in the committee's judgment tetanus toxoid *can* cause GBS.

Conclusion

The evidence favors a causal relation between tetanus toxoid and GBS.

If the evidence favors a causal relation between tetanus toxoid and GBS, then in the committee's judgment the evidence favors a causal relation between vaccines containing tetanus toxoid (DT and Td) and GBS.

Because the conclusions are not based on controlled studies, no estimate of incidence or relative risk is available. It would seem to be low.

Risk-Modifying Factors

GBS, as a separate discrete attack, recurs in a small percentage of those previously afflicted, perhaps 2 to 3 percent, and some individuals have been known to have three or four separate episodes. Other than the patient described by Pollard and Selby (1978), who experienced three attacks, each within 10-21 days of receipt of tetanus toxoid, cases of recurrence after vaccination are not documented. Nevertheless, if GBS occurs within 5 days to 6 weeks of a vaccination, subsequent vaccinations with either the same or different immunogens could be associated with a greater risk of GBS than if the person had never had GBS. A previous history of GBS unrelated to vaccination as an antecedent event is even more uncertain as a risk factor.

NEUROPATHY

Clinical Description

The term *neuropathy* as used here designates those disorders of peripheral nerves other than GBS and has, on occasion, been described in relation to vaccine administration. Most reports fall into two clinical categories, mononeuropathy and brachial neuritis. Diagnosis in both instances rests upon the clinical and electrodiagnostic features. A mononeuropathy implies dysfunction limited to the distribution of a single peripheral nerve large enough to be named. In some instances, mononeuropathy is clearly related to direct injection of vaccine into or near the nerve trunk, as with radial nerve palsy with wrist drop following a misdirected deltoid injection (Ling and Loong, 1976). Brachial neuritis is also known as brachial plexus neuropathy or, in the United Kingdom, as neuralgic amyotrophy. Brachial neuritis is frequently heralded by deep, steady aching pain in the shoulder and upper arm. The annual incidence of brachial neuritis in Rochester, Minnesota, from 1970 to 1981 was 1.64 per 100,000 people (Beghi et al., 1985). For a more complete description, see Chapter 3.

History of Suspected Association

Mononeuropathies, particularly those resulting from direct injection of a substance into the nerve trunk, have been described in the literature in relation to injection of vaccines as well as other therapeutic agents (Ling and Loong, 1976). Brachial neuritis has also been linked to vaccination. A review of brachial neuritis by Tsairis and colleagues (1972) states that about 15 percent of all cases of brachial neuritis occurred following administration of vaccine or antiserum, with tetanus toxoid being the most frequently cited.

Evidence for Association

Biologic Plausibility

Injury of a peripheral nerve by intramuscular injection can result from the needle or injection of the solution into a nerve (Scheinberg and Allensworth, 1957). Nerve damage may also result from chemical irritation and the toxic action of the injected solution (Combes and Clark, 1960; Sunderland, 1968), or neuritis may develop from progressive inflammatory and fibrotic changes (Tarlov et al., 1951). If the injury results from progressive inflammatory and fibrotic changes, there is usually a latent period before the onset of paralysis. The severity of neural damage is determined by the internal structure of the nerve at the site of injury and the amount of toxicity of the injected material (Sunderland, 1968). Most therapeutic agents in use could cause paralysis if injected into the wrong site (Ling and Loong, 1976). The committee did not consider such injuries to be adverse events associated with the toxoid.

The pathogenesis of brachial neuritis is not well understood. It has been suggested that this form of neuropathy may be a manifestation of a systemic or localized infectious disorder, possibly viral, or the result of an allergic or hypersensitivity reaction, such as that which may occur after vaccination, but this is far from conclusive (Tsairis et al., 1972). Although the pathogenesis of brachial neuritis is unclear, it is a well-defined clinical syndrome, and its occurrence following administration of tetanus toxoid has been described in the literature numerous times (Baust et al., 1979; Bensasson et al., 1977; Dittmann, 1981c; Gersbach and Waridel, 1976; Kiwit, 1984; Tsairis et al., 1972).

Case Reports, Case Series, and Uncontrolled Observational Studies

Two case reports in the literature link administration of tetanus toxoid to a peripheral mononeuropathy. Ling and Loong (1976) described a 47-year-old male who developed a left radial nerve palsy 2 weeks following a painful injection of tetanus toxoid into his left arm. This case was felt to be caused by direct injection of tetanus toxoid directly into the radial nerve. Blumstein and Kreithen (1966) described a 23-year-old who developed a complete radial nerve paralysis 7 hours following injection of tetanus toxoid into the right deltoid muscle. Cranial mononeuropathies have been described in three separate case reports. Eicher and Neundorfer (1969) reported a reversible paralysis of the left recurrent laryngeal nerve 8 days after receipt of a booster injection of tetanus toxoid. von Wirth (1965) described a patient who developed reversible deafness resulting from cochlear neuritis 5 days following receipt of a booster of tetanus toxoid. Harrer et al. (1971) described a 21-year-old man who developed deglutition paralysis and accommodation paresis 10 days following receipt of a tetanus toxoid booster. All of these cases, except those in which tetanus toxoid was injected directly into the nerve, were considered to have an allergic basis.

A number of case reports in the literature associate the development of brachial neuritis with administration of tetanus toxoid. Dittmann (1981c) provides an uncritical review of 12 cases of "neuritis" following receipt of tetanus toxoid reported in the former East Germany from 1963 to 1976. The average latency was 14 days. Two of the eleven cases that fulfilled all diagnostic criteria of brachial neuritis reported by Beghi and colleagues (1985) listed tetanus toxoid as an antecedant event. One of those two patients also had an antecedent influenzal illness. The latency from vaccination to onset of symptoms was not described for either case. Four separate case reports of brachial plexus neuropathy have also been described (Baust et al., 1979; Bensasson et al., 1977; Gersbach and Waridel, 1976; Kiwit, 1984) in adults (ages 20-48), all following receipt of booster doses of tetanus toxoid, with latencies ranging from 4 days to 3 weeks.

Other cases of probable or unclassified neuropathies are on record as occurring after tetanus toxoid vaccination, sometimes in association with other vaccines (Deliyannakis, 1971; Dieckhofer et al., 1978; Ehrengut, 1986; Paradiso et al., 1990). The significance of these cases is uncertain.

Three case reports of possible neuropathy following tetanus toxoid or Td administration were found in VAERS (submitted between November 1990 and July 1992). The documentation of the clinical and laboratory findings from these cases is sketchy at best; therefore, the correct diagnosis was difficult to determine. One report described a 47-year-old man who developed a probable brachial neuritis 1 year following receipt of tetanus toxoid. The long latency prior to the onset of symptoms makes this case unlikely to be related to tetanus toxoid. Another report described a 37-year-old man who had pain in his hand immediately after injection of Td into the deltoid muscle; this is probably a case of direct injection into the radial nerve. The last report described a 41-year-old man who developed what was probably brachial neuritis 12 days following receipt of Td.

Tsairis and colleagues (1972) reviewed 99 patients with brachial plexus neuropathy seen at the Mayo Clinic in Rochester, Minnesota, between 1954 and 1968. Of the 99 patients, 14 had immunizations in the month prior to the development of brachial plexus neuropathy (4 patients had received tetanus toxoid alone, 1 had received tetanus toxoid and influenza vaccine, and a 3-month-old had received DPT). Latencies for the group that received tetanus toxoid alone ranged from 6 to 21 days. The authors indicate that some of the affected limbs were contralateral to the injection.

Controlled Observational Studies

None.

Controlled Clinical Trials

None.

Causality Argument

All of the available information in the literature regarding mononeuropathies and brachial neuritis and their relation with tetanus toxoid, DT, or Td come from case reports or uncontrolled observational studies. The evidence found in the literature relating receipt of tetanus toxoid, DT, or Td and mononeuropathy caused by direct injection into the radial nerve comes from two case reports (Ling and Loong, 1976; VAERS). This type of injury is most likely due to the intraneural nature of the injection rather than to some characteristic of the vaccine itself. The committee does not consider this an adverse event related to the vaccine.

The evidence for peripheral mononeuropathy in association with administration of tetanus toxoid, DT, or Td not related to direct injection into the nerve is less clear. Three case reports of transient cranial mononeuropathies that developed 5, 8, and 10 days following administration of tetanus toxoid have been reported in the literature. The authors speculated that these neuropathies were related to a "neuroallergic" phenomenon following injection of tetanus toxoid. Less is known about the etiology or pathogenesis of this type of phenomenon, rendering the evidence for this type of association solely on the basis of three case reports more speculative than conclusive.

Although little is understood regarding the pathogenesis of brachial neuritis as a distinct clinical syndrome, it is well described in the literature. In a large case series a significant portion of the cases were temporally related to vaccine administration, particularly to tetanus toxoid (Tsairis et al., 1972). Likewise, review of individual case reports revealed four well-documented case reports of brachial plexus neuropathy following administration of tetanus toxoid (Baust et al., 1979; Bensasson et al., 1977; Gersbach and Waridel, 1976; Kiwit, 1984), with latencies ranging from 4 to 21 days. Although the mechanisms of brachial neuritis are not well understood, there is biologic plausibility that vaccines could cause an allergic or hypersensitivity reaction that manifests as brachial neuritis. This provides reasonably good, although sparse, evidence that brachial neuritis can occur in relation to tetanus toxoid, although controlled epidemiologic studies designed to look at this relation do not exist.

If one presumes that, on average, the predominantly adult population of Rochester, Minnesota, was receiving tetanus toxoid approximately once every 10 years (120 months) during the periods covered by the Tsairis et al. and Beghi et al. studies, then an "expected" rate of receipt of tetanus toxoid within the month prior to onset of brachial plexus neuropathy can be estimated as 1/120. Based on reported exposure to tetanus toxoid alone in the Tsairis et al. study, the exposure odds ratio (OR) can be roughly estimated as 4.8. For the Beghi et al. study, the corresponding OR is 10.1. Thus the relative risk of brachial plexus neuropathy is on the order of 5 to 10. Given the population-based background incidence reported by Beghi et al. of 1.64 per 100,000 per year, or 0.14 per 100,000 per month, the one-month attributable incidence (excess risk) can be estimated as 0.5 to 1 case per 100,000 tetanus toxoid recipients.

Conclusion

The evidence is inadequate to accept or reject a causal relation between tetanus toxoid, DT, or Td and peripheral mononeuropathy (other than those caused by direct intraneural injection).

The evidence favors acceptance of a causal relation between tetanus toxoid and brachial neuritis.

If the evidence favors acceptance of a causal relation between tetanus toxoid and brachial neuritis, then in the committee's judgment the evidence favors acceptance of a causal relation between DT and Td and brachial neuritis. The relative risk for brachial neuritis following vaccination with tetanus toxoid-containing vaccines can be estimated as on the order of 5 to 10 and the one-month attributable incidence (excess risk) on the order of 0.5 to 1 case per 100,000 tetanus toxoid recipients.

Risk-Modifying Factors

None.

ARTHRITIS

Clinical Description

Arthritis is inflammation of one or more joints detectable as swelling, redness, and tenderness. Arthralgia is pain in a joint or joints. According to the 1988 National Health Interview Survey, approximately 13 percent of respondents surveyed reported currently having "arthritis of any kind or rheumatism." Prevalence rates increased with age, with approximately 0.2 percent of persons under age 18 years reporting arthritis of any kind or arthralgia.

History of Suspected Association

None.

Evidence for Association

Biologic Plausibility

A causal relation between immunization with tetanus or diphtheria toxoid and arthritis is biologically plausible on the basis of the toxoid's potential to induce a systemic form of immune complex disease (serum sickness). However, generalized serum sickness-like reactions require excess circulating antigen, an unlikely occurrence in view of the small amount of protein contained in currently used vaccines. No studies in animals or human subjects suggest an association between tetanus or diphtheria toxoid and arthritis on the basis of any other mechanism.

The immune response to tetanus toxoid is commonly used as a model system to investigate patients suspected of having immunologic abnormalities, either deficiencies of their immune responsiveness or exaggerated, uncontrolled immune responsiveness. Thus, in many studies of diseases thought to be caused by abnormally high inflammatory responses, such as rheumatoid arthritis or systemic lupus erythematosus, the immune responses to tetanus toxoid have been studied in detail. The response to tetanus toxoid also is measured as a control in assessing the response to antigens from infectious agents known to cause disease associated with arthritis in humans (*Borrelia* species, group A streptococci, and *Yersinia* species) or in animals (mycobacteria). In patients with these infections, antigens from the infectious agents are suspected of triggering abnormally high responses to self-antigens, such as the components of joint tissue (collagen). Tetanus toxoid is used as a control because most subjects have immunity to this antigen induced by prior immunization. In the extensive literature reporting the results of those studies (Desai et al., 1989; Devey et al., 1987; Herman et al., 1971; Höyeraal and Mellbye, 1974; Yu et al., 1980), no examples of enhanced reactivity specific for tetanus toxoid have been found. Under some experimental conditions, subjects with rheumatoid arthritis had increased reactivities to all antigens to which they had been exposed (Burmester et al., 1991), but when compared with other antigens, tetanus toxoid was also a poor stimulator of synovial cell inflammation (Pope et al., 1989; Söderströn et al., 1990). One study showed that immune complexes containing tetanus toxoid were only weak activators of neutrophils (Langholz and Nielsen, 1990).

Case Reports, Case Series, and Uncontrolled Observational Studies

Jawad and Scott (1989) described a previously healthy 34-year-old woman who developed rheumatoid arthritis following immunization with tetanus toxoid. She received two doses of tetanus toxoid 1 month apart, and 1 week after receipt of the second dose, she developed a severe local reaction at the site of injection that lasted for 10 days. As the local reaction faded, she developed a symmetric inflammatory polyarthritis that persisted and met the clinical and laboratory criteria for rheumatoid arthritis. In a letter to the editor, Daschbach (1972) mentioned a case of what he termed "typical serum sickness" that occurred in a 7-year-old boy 3 days after receipt of an injection of diphtheria and tetanus toxoids. The child responded to treatment with corticosteroids and antihistamines. Serum obtained 6 weeks later had precipitins for tetanus, but none for diphtheria. No further clinical details were given. One case report entitled "Reactive arthritis and immune vasculitis with cardiovascular shock after triple (diphtheria-pertussis-tetanus) vaccination" was found in the literature (Sell and Katzmann, 1990). A 4-month-old infant developed lymphadenopathy, fever, urticaria, and swelling of both wrists within 24 to 28 hours after the initial DPT immunization. All signs of clinical illness resolved in 5 days. The attending physician reported this case in the form of a question to a column in a pediatrics journal. The reply emphasized the importance of attempting to make a scientific determination of the cause of illness. The importance of these efforts became apparent when virologic and serologic tests revealed that the cause of illness was an acute parvovirus type B19 infection. The infant received subsequent DPT immunizations without incident. In a review of the adverse effects of tetanus toxoid that included 740 individuals (Jacobs et al., 1982), no cases of arthritis were reported. Seven persons had arthralgias (1 percent of the reactions). In a review of the experience in the former West Germany with 100 million doses of tetanus toxoid given over 15 years (Korger et al., 1986), 13 of 2,674 adverse events were listed as "swelling and inflammatory changes of joints." No details or follow-up were provided. Dittmann (1981a,b) reported no cases of arthritis in an extensive review of diphtheria toxoids (DT or diphtheria toxoid alone) covering 15 years in the former East Germany. In a prospective evaluation of reactions to tetanus and diphtheria toxoids carried out in Denmark between 1952 and 1970, no cases of arthritis were reported in association with 2.5 million injections of monovalent tetanus toxoid and 3.7 million injections of combined diphtheria and tetanus toxoids (Christensen, 1972).

No cases of arthritis associated with receipt of tetanus toxoid alone were reported in VAERS (submitted between November 1990 and July 1992). Three cases of arthritis were reported in adults who received Td. In one individual, myalgia, headache, and nausea developed within 1 hour after immunization, and then swelling of multiple joints developed 13 days after receipt of vaccine. The second individual had arthritis (proximal interphalangeal) in one hand that developed immediately after immunization, persisted for 6 weeks, and then resolved. The third patient developed septic arthritis of the left shoulder 6 days after immunization; the septic arthritis was most likely related to the laceration for which tetanus prophylaxis had been given. Seven cases of "joint pain and tenderness radiating to the shoulder with redness and swelling at the site of immunization" after Td immunization were reported on one form. No additional clinical information was provided. One case of erythema multiforme and migratory polyarthritis was reported in a child aged 1.5 years. Symptoms developed 5 days after immunization with *Haemophilus influenzae* type b (Hib) vaccine, DT, and OPV, but they resolved after 6 weeks; the child also had received acetaminophen. MSAEFI reports from 1979 to 1990 of individuals receiving one vaccine included four reports of joint inflammation (arthralgia or arthritis) following administration of DT. Follow-up was available for two of these individuals, and both recovered. Ninety-nine cases of joint inflammation were reported following Td immunization; of 39 patients available for follow-up, 27 recovered. Two cases of joint inflammation were reported following tetanus toxoid immunization; no follow-up information was available.

Controlled Observational Studies

None.

Controlled Clinical Trials

None.

Causality Argument

The biologic plausibility for a causal relation between diphtheria and tetanus toxoids and arthritis is based on the toxoid's *potential* to induce serum sickness. Arthritis is fairly common in the nonpediatric population who receives tetanus toxoid or Td. Evidence for an association between diphtheria or tetanus toxoid and arthritis is limited to case reports and case series. The inconclusive nature of the reports of arthritis observed in association with receipt of tetanus and diphtheria toxoids given either alone or in combination provides insufficient evidence for a causal relation. None of the cases included clinical, laboratory, or pathologic evidence for a mechanism of association.

Conclusion

The evidence is inadequate to accept or reject a causal relation between tetanus or diphtheria toxoid and arthritis.

ERYTHEMA MULTIFORME

Clinical Description

Erythema multiforme (EM) is an inflammatory eruption characterized by symmetric erythematous, macular, bullous, papular, nodular, or vesicular lesions of the skin or mucous membranes. The characteristic lesion is an iris (or bull's eye or target) lesion that consists of a central papule with two or more concentric rings. Stevens-Johnson syndrome is a severe form of EM with involvement of at least two mucosal surfaces in addition to the skin eruption. A hypersensitivity reaction to a number of substances, including infectious agents, is a proposed mechanism, but the pathophysiology has not been defined. No population-based incidence rates were identified.

History of Suspected Association

There is no particular history of suspected association between EM and either diphtheria or tetanus toxoid. Two cases of EM following DPT immunization were identified by Leung (1984b). Leung and Szabo (1987) reported two additional cases following administration of DPT in 1987.

Evidence for Association

Biologic Plausibility

In 1980, Shelley produced the classic iris lesions of EM by intradermal injection of a variety of heat-killed bacteria or their common endotoxin, lipopolysaccharide W, into a patient who was recovering from erythema multiforme bullosum of unknown etiology. Biopsy of the lesions induced by injection of bacterial products showed immunoglobulin A (IgA), IgM, fibrin, and complement deposition that duplicated the findings in the patient's spontaneous lesions. In addition, the patient's peripheral leukocytes produced fibrin thrombi in vitro when exposed to gram-negative bacterial antigens and endotoxin. It is biologically plausible that similar bacterial antigens in diphtheria or tetanus toxoid could induce EM.

Case Reports, Case Series, and Uncontrolled Observational Studies

In 1988, Griffith and Miller reported a case of EM following administration of diphtheria and tetanus toxoids. Eight hours after his third immunization with DT and OPV, a 9-month-old infant developed a generalized maculopapular dermatitis that progressed to vesicular lesions after 4 days.

Several were hemorrhagic and some were target-like. Biopsy revealed "a partially necrotic epidermis with subepidermal vesicles, scattered mononuclear infiltrate in the papillary and reticular dermis, and some exocytosis" (p. 758). Those authors stated that, to their knowledge, this was the first case of EM following DT immunization. They reported that they contacted all current and previous manufacturers of diphtheria and tetanus toxoids and could confirm no other cases.

Two cases of EM following Td immunization were reported to VAERS (submitted between November 1990 and July 1992). One case occurred in a woman who was also treated with silver sulfadiazine cream for a burn. The other case occurred in a woman who was allergic to iodine, but no details about the indication for immunization or the use of antiseptics or antibacterial agents for wound care were provided. One case of EM was reported in a child 5 days after she received Hib, DT, OPV, and acetaminophen. This child also had migratory polyarthritis that lasted for 6 weeks, and a diagnosis of serum sickness was made (see section on arthritis above).

Controlled Observational Studies

None.

Controlled Clinical Trials

None.

Causality Argument

There is biologic plausibility for a relation between diphtheria and tetanus toxoids and EM on the basis of a hypersensitivity mechanism and an investigation of bacterial injection in one human subject. The direct evidence in humans for an association between diphtheria or tetanus toxoid and EM is limited to one published case report of EM occurring after the administration of DT and three case reports made to VAERS (two Td, one DT). However, in one of the cases reported to VAERS, the patient had been exposed to another likely cause of EM, and in another, the patient had been immunized with multiple vaccines.

Conclusion

The evidence is inadequate to accept or reject a causal relation between tetanus or diphtheria toxoid and EM.

ANAPHYLAXIS

Clinical Description

Anaphylaxis is a sudden, potentially life-threatening, systemic condition mediated by highly reactive molecules from mast cells and basophils. The clinical manifestations of anaphylaxis include pallor and then diffuse erythema, urticaria, and itching, subcutaneous edema, edema and spasm of the larynx, wheezing, tachycardia, hypotension, and hypovolemic shock, usually occurring within minutes of intramuscular or subcutaneous exposure to antigen. For this review, cases of anaphylaxis occurring within 4 hours of vaccine administration were included (Table 5-1). Chapter 4 contains a more complete discussion of anaphylaxis.

History of Suspected Association

Induction of active immunity to tetanus in human subjects was first demonstrated in 1927 by Ramon and Zoeller. Widespread use of tetanus toxoid as a vaccine began in 1938, and initially, there were few reports of side effects. However, in 1940, Whittingham reported 12 cases of "constitutional symptoms" and two cases of anaphylaxis occurring after receipt of initial or subsequent doses of vaccine made up of either fluid or alum-precipitated preparations. Parish et al. (1940) reported an additional case of anaphylaxis, and Regamey (1965) reported fatal anaphylaxis in a man immunized in 1933. A probable association between the reactions and beef proteins in the culture broth was demonstrated by scratch testing with Witte peptone, a medium supplement made from beef and pork fibrins (Gold, 1941; Whittingham, 1940). When these components were removed, no further anaphylactic reactions were reported until 1973 (Staak and Wirth, 1973). Since that time, an interval when hundreds of millions of doses have been administered, nine cases of anaphylaxis meeting the definition given above could be found in literature from throughout the world.

Concern over the possibility of serious hypersensitivity reactions in association with diphtheria immunization was raised because of the high rate of local reactivity in adults, the frequent reactions to control toxoid in the Schick test (Kuhns and Pappenheimer, 1952; Pappenheimer, 1984), and the frequent development of IgE antibodies after immunization with tetanus and diphtheria toxoids (Nagel et al., 1977).

Evidence for Association

Biologic Plausibility

A study by Kovalskaya (1967) demonstrated that it is possible to sensitize mice with large intraperitoneal doses of DT or DPT to fatal anaphylactic reactions with large doses of the monovalent tetanus, diphtheria, or pertussis antigen.

Several studies in humans have demonstrated the frequent development of tetanus and diphtheria IgE antibodies after booster immunization (Cogne et al., 1985; Nagel et al., 1977). However, a study of in vitro basophil degranulation in subjects with tetanus-specific serum IgE was entirely negative (Miadonna, 1980). Miadonna examined the role of IgG antibodies that might block binding of antigen to IgE on basophils. However, added IgG did not seem to affect the degranulation of basophils after exposure to tetanus toxoid, and the authors concluded that, in their system, the IgE receptor on basophils has a low affinity for tetanus-specific IgE antibodies, thus explaining the very low rate of allergic reactions (0.06 percent) that they observed in a study of 25,000 children immunized with tetanus toxoid (Miadonna and Falagiani, 1978). Facktor et al. (1973) and Vellayappan and Lee (1976) studied 70 and 38 individuals, respectively, who had no clinical history of reactions to tetanus toxoid and found a high incidence of immediate cutaneous hypersensitivity reactions (63 percent in both studies). Conversely, Jacobs et al. (1982) skin tested and challenged with tetanus toxoid 740 individuals with a history of adverse reactions to tetanus toxoid, including 95 individuals who reported an "anaphylactoid" reaction. Ninety-four of the 95 individuals with anaphylactoid reactions had negative skin tests. The one patient with a positive skin test tolerated full tetanus toxoid challenge without adverse effects. Thus, although a small number of cases of anaphylaxis apparently related to tetanus toxoid have been observed (see below), the relation between these reactions and specific IgE antibodies and the accepted measurements of immediate hypersensitivity remains unclear.

In a study of 158,230 airmen who received two injections of alum-precipitated Td (<2 Lf of diphtheria toxoid), 101 were referred for evaluation for an allergic reaction or any reaction (local or systemic) severe enough to interfere with normal activities (Smith and Wolnisty, 1962). No apparent relation between the symptoms and the immunization was found in 53 of the airmen; all 53 received boosters of Td without adverse effects. Forty-eight were skin tested intradermally for immediate wheal and flare reactions. None had a reaction to diphtheria toxoid, but two had a reaction to tetanus toxoid. These two individuals had a history of urticaria that developed within hours after receiving Td. They were immunized with diphtheria toxoid without adverse effects. The remaining 46 subjects each received

TABLE 5-1   Case Reports of Anaphylaxis Following Vaccination with Diphtheria or Tetanus Toxoid

Study; Vaccines	Time of First Symptom (h)	Generalized Urticaria	Generalized Pruritis	Flush	Edema	Collapse
Whittingham, 1940; tetanus	1	No	Yes	Yes	Yes	Yes
Whittingham, 1940; tetanus	0.1	Yes	Yes	Yes	Yes	No
Parish and Oakley, 1940; tetanus	0.1	Yes	Yes	Yes	No	Yes
Regamey, 1965; tetanus	2	?	?	?	?	?
Staak and Wirth, 1973; tetanus	0.1	No	No	No	?	Yes
Lleonart-Bellfill et al., 1991; tetanus; typhoid	0.1	No	Yes	Yes	No	Yes
Ratliff and Burns-Cox, 1984; tetanus and lignocaine	1	No	No	No	No	Yes
Zaloga and Chernow, 1982; tetanus	0.1	No	No	No	No	Yes
Chanukoglu et al., [a] 1975; tetanus	0.1	No	Yes	No	No	Yes
Fischmeister, 1974; tetanus	0.1	No	No	No	No	Yes

Hypotension	Wheezing	Upper Airway Obstruction	Other	Epinephrine	Analphylaxis
?	? Dyspnea	?	Improved in 20 min	Yes	Yes; skin test +; Witte peptone
No	? Dyspnea	?	Normal in 15 min	Yes	Yes; skin test +; Witte peptone
No	No	No	Back, abdominal pain	Yes	Yes
?	?	?	Immunized in 1933; Death/ autopsy; "extreme bronchospasm"	No	Yes
?	No	?	Death/autopsy; peribronchial eosinophils	No	Yes
Yes	? Dyspnea	No	3 mo later serum IgE increased; skin test: tetanus +, typhoid -	Yes	Yes
?	Yes	?	Respiratory arrest; asystole seizures; recovered	Yes	Yes
Yes	Yes	Yes	Normal in 24 h	Yes	Yes
Yes	Yes	?	Vomiting; normal in 24 h	Yes	Yes
?	Yes	Yes	Normal in 10 min; edema, itching 12 days later	No; prednisone calcium	Yes

continued

TABLE 5-1   *(Continued)*

Study; Vaccines	Time of First Symptom (h)	Generalized Urticaria	Generalized Pruritis	Flush	Edema	Collapse
Bilyk and Dubchik, 1978; tetanus	0.1	Yes	No	No	Yes	?
Mansfield et al., 1986; prick skin test; tetanus	0.1	Yes	?	No	Yes	No
Ovens, 1986; diphtheria; tetanus; polio	0.1	Yes	No	No	No	Yes
Mandal, 1980; tetanus	0.1	Yes	Yes	Yes	Yes	Diaphore-sis
Werne and Garrow, [a,b] 1946; diphtheria; pertussis	Unknown but <4 h	No	No	No	?	Yes
Werne and Garrow,[a,b] 1946; diphtheria; pertussis	Unknown but <4 h	No	No	No	?	Yes

[a]All patients studied were adults except: Chanukoglu et al. (1975), age = 4 years; and Werne and Garrow (1946), age = 10 months.
[b]Each entry is for one member of a pair of identical twins.

two injections of Td without difficulty. In that study, the investigators found a much lower rate of severe reactions than the 10 percent reported by Edsall et al. in 1954, but the authors noted that many reacting substances had been eliminated from the toxoid since that time.

Case Reports, Case Series, and Uncontrolled Observational Studies

Thirteen cases of anaphylaxis meeting the criteria of a life-threatening systemic reaction occurring within 4 hours of immunization with tetanus toxoid have been reported in the literature. These cases are summarized in

Hypotension	Wheezing	Upper Airway Obstruction	Other	Epinephrine	Analphylaxis
Yes	Dyspnea, "tightness" in chest	No	Better in hours	Yes	Yes
Yes	Yes	No	Urticaria 7 yr ago after tetanus + antitoxin	Yes	Yes
Yes	Yes	Yes	Resolved	Yes	Yes
?	No	Yes	Resolved in 12 h with antihistamines, dexamethasone	No	Yes
Probable	No	Yes	Death/autopsy; arterial narrowing and infiltration with polymorphonuclear leukocytes, eosino-phils; brain, lungs, liver	No	Yes
Probable	No	Yes	Same	No	Yes

Table 5-1. One of the 13 cases of anaphylaxis from 1933 was described in a review by Regamey (1965). Three occurred in 1940 and were presumed (by skin testing) to be related to contamination of the vaccine by Witte peptones (Parish and Oakley, 1940; Whittingham, 1940). Two deaths occurred in association with tetanus toxoid administered as a single antigen. In the 1965 review, Regamey reported a fatality in a 20-year-old man 2 hours after he received his third tetanus toxoid injection. This patient had a history of an episode of collapse and convulsions after receiving his second dose of tetanus toxoid. In 1973, Staak and Wirth reported the death of a 24-year-old woman 30 minutes after receiving an injection of tetanus toxoid.

The cause of death was thought to be an anaphylactic reaction. Postmortem examination revealed emphysema of the lungs with bronchial hypersecretion and peribronchial infiltration with eosinophils, findings consistent with anaphylaxis. No local reaction was present at the site of injection. The woman had a history of chronic bronchitis and had tolerated previous immunizations with tetanus toxoid well. Her last immunization had occurred 14 years earlier. Two letters to the editor questioning the assumption of causality followed publication of that report. Spiess and Staak (1973) raised the possibility of inadvertent intravascular injection, and Ehrengut and Staak (1973) noted that vaccine was given "in both arms," raising the issue that equine antiserum might have been given in addition to vaccine. They noted that in the previous report of death following immunization with tetanus toxoid, Regamey (1965) believed the reaction may have been related to the use of blood components from horses during toxoid production (the patient was immunized in 1933). Since the report by Staak and Wirth in 1973, no case report of death following immunization with tetanus toxoid alone has been reported.

One patient with anaphylaxis (Ratliff and Burns-Cox, 1984) received 4 ml of 2 percent lignocaine in addition to tetanus toxoid. The young man reported by Lleonart-Bellfill et al. (1991) received tetanus toxoid and typhoid vaccine simultaneously, but intradermal skin testing with a 1:10 dilution of aluminum-adsorbed tetanus toxoid performed 3 months later elicited an immediate positive wheal reaction, whereas similar testing with typhoid vaccine was negative. Patch testing with thimerosal and aluminum hydrochloride also was negative. The patient had elevated total serum IgE levels, although the authors noted that even the presence of specific anti-tetanus IgE in the serum correlates poorly with severe anaphylaxis because elevated levels of IgE are found in many healthy individuals without a clinical history of hypersensitivity to tetanus toxoid (see above). Four additional patients (Kittler et al., 1966; Leung, 1984a; Mansfield et al., 1986) had features strongly suggestive of anaphylaxis, but they received epinephrine promptly, and thus, the full clinical syndrome may not have developed.

In the report by Korger et al. (1986) concerning data on adverse reactions collected in the former West Germany over 15 years (1970-1984), during which time 100 million doses of tetanus toxoid were dispensed, no cases of anaphylactic shock after receipt of tetanus toxoid were reported.

In 1946, Werne and Garrow reported fatal anaphylactic shock in identical twin infants, aged 10 months, following immunization with their second injection of both diphtheria toxoid and pertussis antigen. It was recorded that the infants cried "considerably" after reaching home, drank large amounts of water, and "fell asleep." Later, they were arousable only by loud noises, and one infant was noted to be "cold and wringing wet with perspiration." The following morning, the infants were taken to the hospital, where one was pronounced dead on arrival and the other was in shock and died several hours later. No free diphtheria toxin was found in the vaccine, and the histopathology was consistent with death from anaphylactic shock. One additional case of anaphylaxis associated with diphtheria toxoid has been reported (Ovens, 1986). That report described a 32-year-old woman who also received inactivated polio vaccine and tetanus toxoid (Table 5-1). She denied a prior history of immunization, so the possibility of a reaction to another vaccine component could not be ruled out, and no further analysis was performed.

Two cases of anaphylaxis following Td immunization were reported through VAERS (submitted between November 1990 and July 1992). Neither case met the committee's criteria for anaphylaxis. In one instance, the patient developed dyspnea alone 3 hours after immunization; in the other, the patient had an apparent vasovagal reaction that lasted 15 minutes. In the MSAEFI reports of adverse events with follow-up information following administration of single vaccines, 1 case of anaphylaxis was reported following administration of DT, 16 were reported following Td, and none were reported following tetanus toxoid. All 17 patients recovered. Clinical details for assessing whether these cases met the criteria for anaphylaxis described above were not available.

In the previous Institute of Medicine report on the adverse effects of DPT (Institute of Medicine, 1991), the available evidence indicated a causal relation between one or more of the vaccine components and anaphylaxis. The pertussis component could not be implicated specifically.

Christensen (1972) reported the results of a prospective review of all side reactions to diphtheria and tetanus toxoids administered in Denmark between 1952 and 1970. In that country, the author notes that a centralized reporting system and a single vaccine supplier (State Serum Institute, Copenhagen) provide a mechanism for a "fairly good estimate" of the frequency of serious reactions to vaccine. Among 2.5 million adults who received monovalent tetanus toxoid and 1.1 million children who received DT, two cases of "acute collapse" were reported. Both reactions occurred in children (4 and 11 years of age) after receiving their first dose of tetanus toxoid. Each child developed "shock" but recovered completely after treatment with epinephrine. Although the reactions were reported as anaphylactic, the author noted that neither patient had "specific stigmata" of anaphylaxis.

In a prospective study comparing adverse events after primary immunization with DPT (6,004 infants) and DT (4,024 infants) (Pollock et al., 1984), 13 children developed pallor and cyanosis within 5 minutes to 24 hours. Nine cases occurred following administration of DPT and four occurred following administration of DT. The episodes did not resemble anaphylaxis and resolved spontaneously. In the 7-year survey of vaccine reactions in the North West Thames region conducted by Pollock and Morris

(1983), two cases of anaphylaxis or collapse were reported during the primary series of DT immunizations (133,500 children; each child completed a course of three doses), six followed booster DT immunization (221,000 children; one dose), and one followed immunization with tetanus toxoid (the number immunized was not given). Five of these children were described as becoming cold, clammy, and pulseless, but all "recovered rapidly." The other four children were said to have mild manifestations, including slight facial swelling, pallor, and vasovagal attacks, from which they recovered. From the available descriptions, none of the events in either study resembled anaphylaxis as defined for the present analysis.

Controlled Observational Studies

None.

Controlled Clinical Trials

None.

Causality Argument

Studies in experimental animals and data collected from human subjects suggest that both tetanus and diphtheria toxoids can induce immediate hypersensitivity reactions. Although elevated levels of tetanus- and diphtheria-specific IgE antibodies are frequently demonstrated in immunized individuals, neither these antibodies nor immediate skin reactivity correlates well with clinical manifestations of hypersensitivity to the toxoids. Nine cases of anaphylaxis temporally related to immunization with tetanus toxoid alone have been reported since the removal of contaminating proteins. Thus, it appears that tetanus toxoid can cause anaphylaxis. No cases of anaphylaxis associated with administration of diphtheria toxoid alone have been reported.

Conclusion

The evidence establishes a causal relation between tetanus toxoid and anaphylaxis.

If the evidence establishes a causal relation between tetanus toxoid and anaphylaxis, then in the committee's judgment the evidence establishes a causal relation between DT or Td and anaphylaxis.

Because the conclusions are not based on controlled studies, no estimate of incidence or relative risk is available. It would seem to be low.

Risk-Modifying Factors

Individuals with a history of immediate hypersensitivity reactions to previous doses of vaccines containing tetanus toxoid may be at increased risk of subsequent reactions. In such individuals, special precautions have been suggested (American Academy of Pediatrics, Committee on Infectious Diseases, 1991; Jacobs et al., 1982; Wassilak and Orenstein, 1988).

DEATH

A detailed discussion of the evidence regarding death following immunization can be found in Chapter 10. Only the causality argument and conclusions follow. See Chapter 10 for details.

Causality Argument

The evidence favors rejection of a causal relation between DPT and sudden infant death syndrome (SIDS) (Institute of Medicine, 1991). Pollock et al. (1984) presented data suggesting that the relative risk of SIDS after DPT versus that after DT is not significantly different from 1. In the committee's judgment the evidence favors rejection of a causal relation between DT and SIDS.

The evidence favors acceptance of a causal relation between DT, Td, and tetanus toxoid and GBS. The evidence establishes a causal relation between DT, Td, and tetanus toxoid and anaphylaxis. Both GBS and anaphylaxis can be fatal. The only well-documented cases of death causally related to immunization with tetanus toxoid, DT, or Td are attributable to anaphylaxis; the evidence regarding death as a consequence of GBS that temporally followed administration of one of these toxoids is very limited. In the committee's judgment DT, Td, or tetanus toxoid may rarely cause fatal GBS or anaphylaxis. There is no evidence or reason to believe that the case fatality rate from vaccine-associated GBS or anaphylaxis would differ from the case fatality rate for these adverse events associated with any other cause.

Reports of death from all other causes are not clearly linked to the preceding immunization. No cases of death were reported by Christensen (1972) in Denmark between 1952 and 1970, a time during which 2.5 million doses of monovalent tetanus toxoid, 2.67 million doses of DT, and 1.1 million doses of Td were given. No cases of death associated with tetanus toxoid, DT, or Td were reported through MSAEFI between 1979 and 1990. During that time, approximately 1.3 million doses of DT and 29 million doses of Td were distributed.

Conclusion

The evidence establishes a causal relation between DT, Td, and tetanus toxoid and death from anaphylaxis. Although this conclusion is based on direct evidence, it is not based on controlled studies and no relative risk can be calculated. However, the risk of death from anaphylaxis following DT, Td, or tetanus toxoid would appear to be extraordinarily low.

The evidence favors acceptance of a causal relation between DT, Td, and tetanus toxoid and death from GBS. This conclusion is not based on controlled studies and no relative risk can be calculated. However, the risk of death from GBS following DT, Td, or tetanus toxoid would seem to be extraordinarily low.

The evidence favors rejection of a causal relation between DT and SIDS.

The evidence is inadequate to accept or reject a causal relation between tetanus toxoid, DT, or Td and death from causes other than those listed above.

REFERENCES

Alderslade R, Bellman MH, Rawson NS, Ross EM, Miller DL. The National Childhood Encephalopathy Study: a report on 1000 cases of serious neurological disorders in infants and young children from the NCES research team. In: Department of Health and Social Security. Whooping Cough: Reports from the Committee on the Safety of Medicines and the Joint Committee on Vaccination and Immunisation. London: Her Majesty's Stationery Office; 1981.

American Academy of Pediatrics, Committee on Infectious Diseases. The Red Book. Report of the Committee on Infectious Diseases, 22nd edition. Elk Grove, IL: American Academy of Pediatrics; 1991.

Baraff LJ, Manclark CR, Cherry JD, Christenson P, Marcy SM. Analyses of adverse reactions to diphtheria and tetanus toxoids and pertussis vaccine by vaccine lot, endotoxin content, pertussis vaccine potency and percentage of mouse weight gain. Pediatric Infectious Disease Journal 1989;8:502-507.

Barkin RM, Samuelson JS, Gotlin LP. DTP reactions and serologic response with a reduced dose schedule. Journal of Pediatrics 1984;105:189-194.

Barkin RM, Pichichero ME, Samuelson JS, Barkin SZ. Pediatric diphtheria and tetanus toxoids vaccine: clinical and immunologic response when administered as the primary series. Journal of Pediatrics 1985a;106:779-781.

Barkin RM, Samuelson JS, Gotlin LP, Barkin SZ. Primary immunization with diphtheria-tetanus toxoids vaccine and diphtheria-tetanus toxoids-pertussis vaccine adsorbed: comparison of schedules. Pediatric Infectious Disease 1985b;4:168-171.

Baust W, Meyer D, Wachsmuth W. Peripheral neuropathy after administration of tetanus toxoid. Journal of Neurology 1979;222:131-133.

Beghi E, Kurland LT, Mulder DW. Incidence of acute transverse myelitis in Rochester, Minnesota, 1970-1980, and implications with respect to influenza vaccine. Neuroepidemiology 1982;1:176-188.

Beghi E, Nicolosi A, Kurland LT, Mulder DW, Hauser WA, Shuster L. Encephalitis and aseptic meningitis, Olmsted County, Minnesota, 1950-1981. I. Epidemiology. Annals of Neurology 1984;16:283-294.

Beghi E, Kurland LT, Mulder DW, Nicolosi A. Brachial plexus neuropathy in the population of Rochester, Minnesota, 1970-1981. Annals of Neurology 1985;18:320-323.

Bellman MH, Ross EM, Miller DL. Infantile spasms and pertussis immunisation. Lancet 1983;1:1031-1034.

Bensasson M, Lanoe R, Assan R. Un cas de syndrome algodystrophique du membre superieur survenu apres vaccination antitetanique. [A case of algodystrophy of the upper limb occurring after tetanus vaccination.] Semaine des Hopitaux de Paris 1977;53:2965-2966.

Bergey GK, Bigalke H, Nelson PG. Differential effects of tetanus toxin on inhibitory and excitatory synaptic transmission in mammalian spinal cord neurons in culture: a presynaptic locus of action for tetanus toxin. Journal of Neurophysiology 1987;57:121-131.

Bilyk MA, Dubchik GK. Anafilakticheskaia reaktsiia posle podkozhnogo vvedeniia stolbmiachnogo anatoksina. [Anaphylactic reaction following subcutaneous administration of tetanus anatoxin.] Klinicheskaia Meditsina 1978;56:137-138.

Bjorkholm B, Bottiger M, Christenson B. Antitoxin antibody levels and the outcome of illness during an outbreak of diphtheria among alcoholics. Scandinavian Journal of Infectious Diseases 1986;18:235-239.

Blumstein GI, Kreithen H. Peripheral neuropathy following tetanus toxoid administration. Journal of the American Medical Association 1966;198:1030-1031.

Burmester GR, Altstidl U, Kalden JR. Stimulatory response towards the 65 kDa heat shock protein and other mycobacterial antigens in patients with rheumatoid arthritis. Journal of Rheumatology 1991;18:171-176.

Chanukoglu A, Fried D, Gotlieb A. [Anaphylactic shock due to tetanus toxoid]. Harefuah 1975;89:456-457.

Christensen PE. Side reactions to tetanus toxoid. Scientific Publication, Pan American Health Organization 1972;253:36-43.

Christenson B, Bottiger M. Serological immunity to diphtheria in Sweden in 1978 and 1984. Scandinavian Journal of Infectious Diseases 1986;18:227-233.

Cody CL, Baraff LJ, Cherry JD, Marcy SM, Manclark CR. Nature and rates of adverse reactions associated with DTP and DT immunizations in infants and children. Pediatrics 1981;68:650-660.

Cogne M, Ballet JJ, Schmitt C, Bizzine B. Total and IgE antibody levels following booster immunization with aluminum absorbed and nonabsorbed tetanus toxoid in humans. Annals of Allergy 1985;54:148-151.

Collier LH, Polakoff S, Mortimer J. Reactions and antibody responses to reinforcing doses of adsorbed and plain tetanus vaccines. Lancet 1979;1:1364-1368.

Combes MA, Clark WK. Sciatic nerve injury following intragluteal injection: pathogenesis and prevention. American Journal of Diseases in Children 1960;100:579.

Crovari P, Gasparini R, D'Aste E, Culotta C, Romano L. Studio caso-controllo sulla associazione tra sindromi neurologiche e vaccinazioni obbligatorie in Liguria nel periodo Gennaio 1980-Febbraio 1983. [Case-control study on the association of neurological syndromes and compulsory vaccinations in Liguria during the period January 1980-February 1983.] Bollettino dell Istituto Sieroterapico Milanese 1984;63:118-124.

Daschbach RJ. Serum sickness and tetanus immunization (letter). Journal of the American Medical Association 1972;220:1619.

Deliyannakis E. Peripheral nerve and root disturbances following active immunization against smallpox and tetanus. Military Medicine 1971;136:458-462.

Desai BV, Dixit S, Pope RM. Limited proliferative response to type II collagen in rheumatoid arthritis. Journal of Rheumatology 1989;16:1310-1314.

Devey ME, Bleasdale K, Isenberg DA. Antibody affinity and IgG subclass of responses to tetanus toxoid in patients with rheumatoid arthritis and systemic lupus erythematosus. Clinical Experimental Immunology 1987;68:562-569.

Dieckhoefer K, Scholl R, Wolf R. Neurologische Storungen nach Tetanusschutzimpfung. [Neurological disorders after protective tetanus vaccination.] Medizinische Welt 1978;29:1710-1712.

Dittmann S. Die Diphtherieschutzimpfung und Ihre atypischen Verlaufsformen. [Diphtheria immunization: atypical course.] Beitrage zur Hygiene und Epidemiologie 1981a;25:143-154.

Dittmann S. Diphterieschutzimpfung. [Diphtheria immunization.] Beitrage zur Hygiene und Epidemiologie 1981b;25:237-239.

Dittmann S. Tetanusschutzimpfung. [Tetanus immunization.] Beitrrage zur Hygiene und Epidemiologie 1981c;25:239-240.

Edsall G, Altman JS, Gaspar AJ. Combined tetanus-diphtheria immunization of adults: use of small doses of diphtheria toxoid. American Journal of Public Health 1954;44:1537-1545.

Edsall G, Elliott MW, Peebles TC, Eldred MC. Excessive use of tetanus toxoid boosters. Journal of the American Medical Association 1967;202:111-113.

Ehrengut W. Neurale Komplikastionen nach Diphtherie-Schutzumpfung und Impfungen mit Diphtherietoxoid-Mischimpfstoffen. [Neural complications following immunization against diphtheria.] Deutsche Medizinische Wochenschrift 1986;111:939-942.

Ehrengut W, Staak M. Anaphylaktische Reaktion nach Tetanustoxoid-Injektion. [Anaphylactic reaction following injection of tetanus toxoid.] Deutsche Medizinische Wochenschrift 1973;98:517.

Eicher W, Neundorfer B. Rekurrenslahmung nach Tetanustoxoid-Auffrischimpfung (mit allergischer Lokalreaktion). [Paralysis of the recurrent laryngeal nerve following a booster injection of tetanus toxoid (associated with local allergic reaction).] Münchener Medizinische Wochenschrift 1969;111:1692-1695.

Eisen AH, Cohen JJ, Rose B. Reaction to tetanus toxoid. New England Journal of Medicine 1963;269:1408-1411.

Facktor MA, Bernstein RA, Fireman P. Hypersensitivity to tetanus toxoid. Journal of Allergy and Clinical Immunology 1973;52:1-12.

Feery BJ. Incidence and type of reactions to triple antigen (DTP) and DT (CDT) vaccines. Medical Journal of Australia 1982;2:511-515.

Fischmeister M. Akute Reaktion nach Tetanustoxoi-Injektion. [Acute reaction following injection with tetanus toxoid (letter).] Deutsche Medizinische Wochenschrift 1974;99:850.

Fishman PS, Carrigan DR. Motoneuron uptake from the circulation of the binding fragment of tetanus toxin. Archives of Neurology 1988;45:558-561.

Fujinami RS, Oldstone MB. Molecular mimicry as a mechanism for virus-induced autoimmunity. Immunological Research 1989;8:3-15.

Gale JL, Thapa PB, Bobo JK, Wassilak SG, Mendelman PM, Foy HM. Acute neurological illness and DTP: report of a case-control study in Washington and Oregon. Sixth International Symposium on Pertussis Abstracts. DHHS Publication No. (FDA) 90-1162. Bethesda, MD: U.S. Public Health Service, U.S. Department of Health and Human Services; 1990.

Gersbach P, Waridel D. Paralysie apres preevention antitetanique. [Paralysis after tetanus prevention.] Schweiz Medizinische Wochenschrift 1976;106:150-153.

Gold H. Sensitization induced by tetanus toxoid, alum precipitated. Journal of Laboratory and Clinical Medicine 1941;27:26-36.

Gordon EH, Krouse HA, Kinney JL, Stiehm JR, Klaustermeyer WB. Delayed cutaneous hypersensitivity in normals: choice of antigens and comparison to in vitro assays of cell-mediated immunity. Journal of Allergy and Clinical Immunology 1983;72:487-494.

Grabenstein JD. Delayed-hypersensitivity testing: guide to product selection. Hospital Pharmacy 1990;25:1102-1107.

Greco D. Case-control study on encephalopathy associated with diphtheria-tetanus immunization in Campania, Italy. Bulletin of the World Health Organization 1985;63:919-925.

Griffith RD, Miller OF III. Erythema multiforme following diphtheria and tetanus toxoid vaccination. Journal of the American Academy of Dermatology 1988;19:758-759.

Hankey GJ. Guillain-Barré syndrome in Western Australia, 1980-1985. Medical Journal of Australia 1987;146:130-133.

Harrer G, Melnizky U, Wendt H. Akkommodationsparese und Schlucklahmung nach Tetanus-Toxoid-Auffrischungsimpfung. [Accommodation paresis and swallowing paralysis following tetanus toxoid booster inoculation.] Wien Medizinische Wochenschrift 1971;121:296-297.

Herman JH, Bradley J, Ziff M, Smiley JD. Response of the rheumatoid synovial membrane to exogenous immunization. Journal of Clinical Investigation 1971;50:266-273.

Hirtz DG, Nelson KB, Ellenberg JH. Seizures following childhood immunizations. Journal of Pediatrics 1983;102:14-18.

Holden JM, Strang DU. Reactions to tetanus toxoid: comparison of fluid and adsorbed toxoids. New Zealand Medical Journal 1965;64:574-577.

Holliday PL, Bauer RB. Polyradiculoneuritis secondary to immunization with tetanus and diphtheria toxoids. Archives of Neurology 1983;40:56-57.

Holmes WH. Diphtheria: History. Bacillary and Rickettsial Infections. New York: Macmillan; 1940.

Hopf HC. Guillain-Barré-Syndrom nach Tetanus-Schutzimpfung: Übersicht und Fallmitteilung. [Guillain-Barré syndrome following tetanus toxoid administration: survey and report of a case.] Aktuelle Neurologie 1980;7:195-200.

Höyeraal HM, Mellbye OJ. Humoral immunity in juvenile rheumatoid arthritis. Annals of Rheumatic Disease 1974;33:248-253.

Illis LS, Taylor FM. Neurological and electroencephalographic sequelae of tetanus. Lancet 1971;1:826-830.

Institute of Medicine. Adverse Effects of Pertussis and Rubella Vaccines. Washington, DC: National Academy Press; 1991.

Jacobs RL, Lowe RS, Lanier BQ. Adverse reactions to tetanus toxoid. Journal of the American Medical Association 1982;247:40-42.

James G, Longshore WA, Hendry JL. Diphtheria immunization studies of students in an urban high school. American Journal of Hygiene 1951;53:178-201.

Jawad AS, Scott DG. Immunisation triggering rheumatoid arthritis? (letter). Annals of Rheumatic Disease 1989;48:174.

Johnson RT, Griffin DE, Gendelman HE. Postinfectious encephalomyelitis. Seminars in Neurology 1985;5:180-190.

Jones AE, Melville-Smith M, Watkins J. Adverse reactions in adolescents to reinforcing doses of plain and adsorbed tetanus vaccines. Community Medicine 1985;7:99-106.

Karzon D, Edwards K. Diphtheria outbreaks in immunized populations. New England Journal of Medicine 1988;318:41-43.

Kellaway P, Krachoby RA, Frost JD, Zion T. Precise characterization and quantification of infantile spasms. Annals of Neurology 1979;6:214-218.

Kittler FJ, Smith PJ, Hefley BF, Cazort AG. Reactions to tetanus toxoid. Southern Medical Journal 1966;59:149-153.

Kiwit JC. Neuralgic amyotrophy after administration of tetanus toxoid. Journal of Neurology, Neurosurgery and Psychiatry 1984;47:320.

Korger G, Quast U, Dechert G. Tetanusimpfung: Vertraglichkeit und Vermeidung von Nebenreaktionen. [Tetanus vaccination: tolerance and avoidance of adverse reactions.] Klininische Wochenschrift 1986;64:767-775.

Kovalskaya SI. Anafilaktogennye svoistva adsorbipovannoi i neadsorbirovannoi kokliusnodifterino-stolbniachnoi vaktsin. [The anaphylactogenic properties of absorbed and non-absorbed pertussis-diphtheria-tetanus vaccines.] Zhurnal Mikrobiologii, Epidemiologii, i Immunobiologii 1967;44:105-109.

Kuhns WJ, Pappenheimer AM. Immunochemical studies of antitoxin produced in normal and allergic individuals hyperimmunized with diphtheria toxoid. Journal of Experimental Medicine 1952;95:363-374, 375-392.

Langholz E, Nielsen OH. Induction of endogenous arachidonic acid metabolism in human neutrophils with snake venom phospholipase A2, immune complexes, and A23187. Prostaglandins, Leukotrienes and Essential Fatty Acids 1990;39:227-229.

Leung A. Anaphylaxis to tetanus toxoid. Irish Medical Journal 1984a;77:306.

Leung AK. Erythema multiforme following DPT vaccination. Journal of the Royal Society of Medicine 1984b;77:1066-1067.

Leung AK, Szabo TF. Erythema multiforme following diphtheria-pertussis-tetanus vaccination. Kobe Journal of Medical Science 1987;33:121-124.

Levine L, Edsall G. Tetanus toxoid: what determines reaction proneness? Journal of Infectious Diseases 1981;144:376.

Levine L, Ibsen J, McComb JA. Adult immunization: preparation and evaluation of combined fluid tetanus and diphtheria toxoids for adult use. American Journal of Hygiene 1961;73:20-35.

Ling CM, Loong SC. Injection injury of the radial nerve. Injury 1976;8:60-62.

Lleonart-Bellfill R, Cistero-Bahima A, Cerda-Trias MT, Olive-Perez A. Tetanus toxoid anaphylaxis. DICP Annals of Pharmacotherapy 1991;25:870.

Mandal GS, Mukhopadhyay M, Bhattacharya AR. Adverse reactions following tetanus toxoid injection. Journal of the Indian Medical Association 1980;74:35-37.

Mansfield LE, Ting S, Rawls DO, Frederick R. Systemic reactions during cutaneous testing for tetanus toxoid hypersensitivity. Annals of Allergy 1986;757;135-137.

McComb J, Levine L. Adult immunization. II. Dosage reduction as a solution to increasing reactions to tetanus toxoid. New England Journal of Medicine 1961;265:1152.

Miadonna A. Caratteristiche biologiche delle IgE specifiche per il tossoide tetanico. [Biological characteristics of specific IgE for tetanus toxoid.] Bollettino del Istituto Sieroterapico Milanense 1980;59:554-559.

Miadonna A, Falagiani P. Determinazione delle IgE specifiche in 15 soggetti con sospetta allergia al tossoide tetanico. [Specific IgE determination in 15 subjects with suspected tetanus toxoid allergy.] Folia Allergologica Immunologica Clinica 1978;25:609-611.

Middaugh JP. Side effects of diphtheria-tetanus toxoid in adults. American Journal of Public Health 1979;69:246-249.

Miller HG, Stanton JB. Neurological sequelae of prophylactic inoculation. Quarterly Journal of Medicine 1954;23:1-27.

Mortimer EA. Diphtheria toxoid. In: Plotkin SA, Mortimer EA, eds. Vaccines. Philadelphia: W.B. Saunders; 1988.

Mortimer J, Melville-Smith M, Sheffield F. Diphtheria vaccine for adults. Lancet 1986;2:1182-1183.

Myers MG, Beckman CW, Vosdingh RA, Hankins WA. Primary immunization with tetanus and diphtheria toxoids: reaction rates and immunogenicity in older children and adults. Journal of the American Medical Association 1982;248:2478-2480.

Nagel J, Svec D, Waters T, Fireman P. IgE synthesis in man. I. Development of specific IgE antibodies after immunization with tetanus diphtheria (TD) toxoids. Journal of Immunology 1977;118:334-341.

Newton NJ, Janati A. Guillain-Barré syndrome after vaccination with purified tetanus toxoid. Southern Medical Journal 1987;80:1053-1054.

Nicolosi A, Hauser WA, Beghi E, Kurland LT. Epidemiology of central nervous system infections in Olmsted County, Minnesota, 1950-1981. Journal of Infectious Diseases 1986;154:399-408.

Onisawa S, Sekine I, Ichimura T, Homma N. Guillain-Barré syndrome secondary to immunization with diphtheria toxoid. Dokkyo Journal of Medical Science 1985;12:227-229.

Ovens H. Anaphylaxis due to vaccination in the office. Canadian Medical Association Journal 1986;134:369-370.

Pappenheimer AM Jr. Diphtheria. In: Germanier R, ed. Bacterial Vaccines. Orlando, FL: Academic Press; 1984.

Pappenheimer AM Jr, Edsall G, Lawrence HS, Banton JJ. A study of reactions following administration of crude and purified diphtheria toxoid in an adult population. American Journal of Hygiene 1950;52:353-370.

Paradiso G, Micheli F, Fernandez Pardal M, Casas Parera I. Neuropatia desmielinizante multifocal siguiendo vacunacion antitetanica. [Multifocal demyelinating neuropathy after tetanus vaccine.] Medicina 1990;50:52-54.

Parish HJ, Oakley CL. Anaphylaxis after injection of tetanus toxoid. British Medical Journal 1940;1:294-295.

Peebles TC, Levine L, Eldred ML. Tetanus-toxoid emergency boosters: a reappraisal. New England Journal of Medicine 1969;280:575-581.

Pollard JD, Selby G. Relapsing neuropathy due to tetanus toxoid: report of a case. Journal of Neurological Science 1978;37:113-125.

Pollock TM, Morris J. A 7-year survey of disorders attributed to vaccination in North West Thames region. Lancet 1983;1:753-757.

Pollock TM, Miller E, Mortimer JY, Smith G. Symptoms after primary immunisation with DTP and with DT vaccine. Lancet 1984;2:146-149.

Pollock TM, Miller E, Mortimer JY, Smith G. Post-vaccination symptoms following DTP and DT vaccination. Developments in Biological Standardization 1985;61:407-410.

Pope RM, Pahlavani MA, LaCour E. Antigenic specificity of rheumatoid synovial fluid lymphocytes. Arthritis and Rheumatism 1989;32:1371-1380.

Quast U, Hennessen W, Widmark RM. Mono- and polyneuritis after tetanus vaccination (1970-1977). Developments in Biological Standardization 1979;43:25-32.

Ramon G, Zoeller C. Médecine Expérimentale—De la valeur antigène l'anatoxine tétanique chez l'homme. Comptes Rendues Hebdomadaires des Séances de l'Académie des Sciences 1926;182:245-247.

Ramon G, Zoeller C. L'anatoxine tétanique et l'immunisation active de l'homme vis-à-vis du tétanos. Annales Institut Pasteur 1927;41:803-833.

Rappouli R, Perugini M, Falsen E. Molecular epidemiology of the 1984-1986 outbreak of diphtheria in Sweden. New England Journal of Medicine 1988;318:12-14.

Ratliff DA, Burns-Cox CJ. Anaphylaxis to tetanus toxoid. British Medical Journal 1984;288:114.

Read SJ, Schapel GJ, Pender MP. Acute transverse myelitis after tetanus toxoid vaccination (letter). Lancet 1992;339:1111-1112.

Regamey RH. Die Tetanus-Schutzimpfung. [Tetanus immunization in Handbook of Immunization.] In: Herrlick A, ed. Handbuch der Schutzimpfungen. Berlin: Springer; 1965.

Reinstein L, Pargament JM, Goodman JS. Peripheral neuropathy after multiple tetanus toxoid injections. Archives of Physical Medicine and Rehabilitation 1982;63:332-334.

Relihan M. Reactions to tetanus toxoid. Journal of the Irish Medical Association 1969;62:430-434.

Relyveld EH. Current developments in production and testing of tetanus and diphtheria vaccines. Progress in Clinical and Biological Research 1980;47:51-76.

Relyveld EH, Henocq E, Bizzini B. Studies on untoward reactions to diphtheria and tetanus toxoids. Developments in Biological Standardization 1979;43:33-37.

Robinson IG. Unusual reaction to tetanus toxoid (letter). New Zealand Medical Journal 1981;94:359.

Rutledge SL, Snead OC. Neurologic complications of immunizations. Journal of Pediatrics 1986;109:917-924.

Scheinberg L, Allensworth M. Sciatic neuropathy in infants related to antibiotic injections. Pediatrics 1957;19:261-265.

Schick B. Die diphtherietoxin-Hautreaktion des Menschen als Vorprobe der prophylaktischen Diphtherieheilseruimnektion. Münchener Medizinische Wochenschrift 1913;60:2606.

Schlenska GK. Unusual neurological complications following tetanus toxoid administration. Journal of Neurology 1977;215:299-302.

Schneider CH. Reactions to tetanus toxoid: a report of five cases. Medical Journal of Australia 1964;1:303-305.

Schwarz G, Lanzer G, List WF. Acute midbrain syndrome as an adverse reaction to tetanus immunization. Intensive Care Medicine 1988;15:53-54.

Sell E, Katzmann GW. Reaktive Arthritis und Immunvasculitis mit cardiovascularem Schock nach Dreifach-(Diphtherie-Pertussis-Tetanus) Schutzimpfund? [Reactive arthritis and immune vasculitis with cardiovascular shock after triple (diphtheria-tetanus-pertussis) vaccination.] Kinderarztliche Praxis 1990;58:547-549.

Settergren B, Broholm KA, Norrby SR, Christenson B. Schick test as a predictor of immunity to diphtheria and of side effects after revaccination with diphtheria vaccine. British Medical Journal 1986;292:524-525.

Sheffield FW, Ironside AG, Abbott JD. Immunisation of adults against diphtheria. British Medical Journal 1978;2:249-250.

Shelley WB. Bacterial endotoxin (lipopolysaccharide) as a cause of erythema multiforme. Journal of the American Medical Association 1980;243:58-60.

Simpson LL. Molecular pharmacology of botulinum toxin and tetanus toxin. Annual Review of Pharmacology and Toxicology 1986;26:427-453.

Smith JW. Diphtheria and tetanus toxoids. British Medical Bulletin 1969;25:177-182.

Smith RE, Wolnisty C. Allergic reactions to tetanus, diphtheria, influenza and poliomyelitis immunization. Annals of Allergy 1962;20:809-813.

Söderströn K, Halapi E, Nilsson E. Synovial cells responding to a 65-kDa mycobacterial heat shock protein have a high proportion of TcR-gamma-delta subtype uncommon in peripheral blood. Scandinavian Journal of Immunology 1990;32:503-515.

Spiess H, Staak M. Anaphylaktische Reaktionen nach aktiver Tetanus-Immunisierung. [Anaphylactic reaction following active tetanus immunization.] Deutsche Medizinische Wochenschrift 1973;98:682.

Staak M, Wirth E. Zur problematik anaphylaktischer Reaktionen nach aktiver Tetanus-Immunisierung. [Anaphylactic reactions following active tetanus immunization.] Deutsche Medizinische Wochenschrift 1973;98:110-111.

Steele RW, Suttle DE, LeMaster PC. Screening for cell-mediated immunity in children. American Journal of Diseases of Children 1976;130:1218-1221.

Sunderland S. Nerves and Nerve Injuries. Baltimore: The Williams & Wilkins Company; 1968.

Tarlov IM. Paralysis caused by penicillin injection; mechanism complication—a warning. Journal of Neuropathology and Experimental Neurology 1951;10:158-176.

Topaloglu H, Berker M, Kansu T, Saatci U, Renda Y. Optic neuritis and myelitis after booster tetanus toxoid vaccination (letter). Lancet 1992;339:178-179.

Trinca JC. Active immunization against tetanus: the need for a single all-purpose toxoid. Medical Journal of Australia 1965;2:116-120.

Tsairis P, Dyck PJ, Mulder DW. Natural history of brachial plexus neuropathy: report on 99 patients. Archives of Neurology 1972;27:109-117.

Uchida T. Diphtheria toxin. In: Dorner F, Drews J, eds. Pharmacology of Bacterial Toxins. IEPT Section 199. Oxford: Pergamon Press; 1986.

Vellayappan K, Lee CY. Tetanus toxoid hypersensitivity. Journal of the Singapore Paediatric Society 1976;18:17-19.

von Wirth G. Reversible kochlearisschadigung nach Tetanol-Injektion? Münchener Medizinische Wochenschrift 1965;107:379-381.

Waight PA, Pollock TM, Miller E, Coleman EM. Pyrexia after diphtheria/tetanus/pertussis and diphtheria/tetanus vaccines. Archives of Disease in Childhood 1983;58:921-923.

Walker AM, Jick H, Perera DR, Knauss TA, Thompson RS. Neurologic events following diphtheria-tetanus-pertussis immunization. Pediatrics 1988;81:345-349.

Wassilak SG, Orenstein WA. Tetanus. In: Plotkin SA, Mortimer EA, eds. Vaccines. Philadelphia: W.B. Saunders; 1988.

Werne J, Garrow I. Fatal anaphylactic shock occurrence in identical twins following second injection of diphtheria toxoid and pertussis antigen. Journal of the American Medical Association 1946;131:730-735.

White WG. Reactions after plain and adsorbed tetanus vaccines (letter). Lancet 1980;1:42.

White WG, Barnes GM, Barker E, Gall D, Knight P, Griffith AH, et al. Reactions to tetanus toxoid. Journal of Hygiene 1973;71:283-297.

Whittingham HE. Anaphylaxis following administration of tetanus toxoid. British Medical Journal 1940;1:292-293.

Whittle E, Roberton NR. Transverse myelitis after diphtheria, tetanus, and polio immunisation. British Medical Journal 1977;1:1450.

Wilson GS. The Hazards of Immunization. London: The Athlone Press; 1967.

Winer JB, Hughes RA, Anderson MJ, Jones DM, Kangro J, Watkins RP. A prospective study of acute idiopathic neuropathy. II. Antecedent events. Journal of Neurology, Neurosurgery and Psychiatry 1988;51:613-618.

Wolters KL, Dehmel H. Abschliessende untersuchungen über die Tetanus Prophylaxe durch active Immunisierung. Zeitschrift für Hygeitschrift 1942;124:326-332.

Yu DT, Winchester RJ, Fu SM, Gibofsky A, Ko HS, Kunkel HG. Peripheral blood Ia-positive T cells: increases in certain diseases and after immunization. Journal of Experimental Medicine 1980;151:91-100.

Zaloga GP, Chernow B. Life-threatening anaphylactic reaction to tetanus toxoid. Annals of Allergy 1982;49:107-108.

Zingher A, Park HW. Immunity results obtained in school children with diphtheria toxoid (modified toxin) and with 1/10 L+ mixtures of toxin-antitoxin. Proceedings of the Society for Experimental and Biological Medicine 1923;21:383-385.

6

Measles and Mumps Vaccines

BACKGROUND AND HISTORY

Measles

Measles formerly afflicted virtually all children before they reached adolescence. It is a viral infection caused by a member of the paramyxovirus group. Conventionally, the diagnosis of measles is made clinically on the basis of its signs and symptoms, which include a characteristic rash. The diagnosis can be confirmed by a laboratory test that detects antibodies to the measles virus. It is also possible to isolate the measles virus, but this effort often fails. Therefore, failure to isolate the virus is not an argument against the diagnosis. A diagnosis of measles based solely on clinical appearance could be erroneous, because a number of other exanthematous diseases can resemble measles.

The disease can be quite debilitating, and its complications are among the most serious consequences of childhood exanthematous infections (Robbins, 1962). These include otitis media, croup, diarrhea, hemorrhagic rash, pneumonia, parainfectious encephalitis, and subacute sclerosing panencephalitis. Whatever its toll in industrialized countries, where the measles fatality rate is 1 per 10,000 cases (Babbott and Gordon, 1954), measles has been a far greater scourge in developing countries, with case fatality rates as high as 1,000 per 10,000 cases (Morley, 1974).

For these reasons, efforts to prevent measles have been extraordinary.

The initial method of prevention depended on postexposure prophylaxis with immune gamma globulin (Stokes et al., 1944). This method, although quite effective, was marred by several difficulties. It required vigilance with respect to exposure and almost immediate action, because if gamma globulin was given more than 4 days after the exposure, it was no longer effective at preventing disease, although it did attenuate it. Moreover, the prevention it afforded was short-lived, because the injected antibodies tended to disappear within about 2 months. An effort to allow the infection to take place, but in an attenuated form, by injecting less immune globulin was usually successful. The consequence of this was a milder case of clinical measles and a resulting lifelong immunity. However, the titration was not always perfect, and in some children the disease was inadvertently prevented, and therefore, they were soon susceptible again, whereas other children developed nearly full-blown measles, with all the risks of serious morbidity and complications.

The next step in prevention efforts was the development of a killed vaccine. The killed vaccine was derived from the Edmonston strain, which was originally isolated in 1954 (Enders and Peebles, 1954). The component antigen was the virus inactivated by formalin and precipitated by alum. Although this vaccine was in use for nearly 4 years (1963 to 1967), it was abandoned when analysis indicated that it provided only short-lived immunity and it was found that formerly vaccinated children developed severe reactions called "atypical measles" after their immunity waned and they became infected with the wild-type measles virus (Centers for Disease Control, 1967).

Development of a live attenuated measles vaccine began a new era in the prevention of this disease. The initial vaccine was derived from the Edmonston strain, which was attenuated by serial passage in various tissue cultures and ultimately grown in chicken embryo cells. The resulting variant was named the Edmonston B strain. It was quite immunogenic, but it was not free of side effects. One-third of the recipients developed high fever, and half of the recipients had a rash. Nevertheless, none of the recipients acted ill. Administration of the vaccine with immune globulin of the proper titer attenuated the reaction without interfering with the induction of permanent immunity.

In the meantime, two vaccines derived from the Edmonston B strain were developed by additional serial passage in chicken embryo cells that were maintained at a lower than optimal temperature. The resulting more-attenuated Enders strain (Hilleman et al., 1968a,b) was the product of an additional 40 passages of the Edmonston B strain; the Schwarz strain was the product of an additional 85 passages of the Edmonston B strain (Schwarz, 1964). Each vaccine induced immunity, and the side effects from these further attenuated vaccines were substantially reduced. The more-attenu-

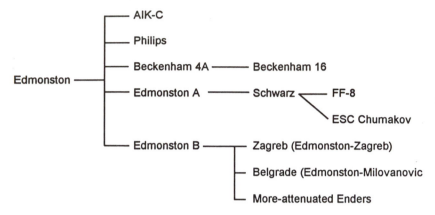

FIGURE 6-1   Derivation of measles vaccine strains. Sources: Adapted from Plotkin and Mortimer (1988, p. 189) and Hirayama M. (1983).

ated Enders strain vaccine is currently in use in the United States; the
Schwarz strain is used elsewhere in the world.   Other strains have been
developed and used in various smaller population groups. Figure 6-1 illustrates the derivation of many measles vaccines from the Edmonston strain.
Table 6-1 lists the measles vaccines used in the United States.

TABLE 6-1 Measles Vaccines Used in the United States

Attenuation	Strain	Trade Name	Manufacturer	Years in Use
Live attenuated	Edmonston B	Rubeovax	Merck Sharpe & Dohme	1963-1975
		M-Vac	Lederle	1963-1975
		Pfizer-vax; Measles-L	Pfizer	1963-1975
		Generic	Lilly, Parke Davis, Philips Roxane	1963-1975
Live, more attenuated	Schwarz (derived from Edmonston A)	Lirugen	Pitman Moore-Dow	1965-1976
	More-attenuated Enders (derived from Edmonston B)	Attenuvax	Merck Sharp & Dohme	1968-present

Source: Adapted from Plotkin and Mortimer (1988, p. 189).

Mumps

Unlike measles, mumps is not considered a globally devastating disease. Nevertheless, because of its complications, it was targeted for prevention by use of a vaccine. The complications that prompted this were epididymoorchitis, aseptic meningitis, meningoencephalitis, and deafness (usually, but not exclusively, unilateral) (Coll, 1974).

Before a vaccine was developed, there was no effective means of preventing this disease. Mumps is rare in the first year of life, and its rarity has been attributed to the passive protection rendered by maternal antibodies (Meyer, 1962). Nevertheless, immune globulin injections administered after exposure do not prevent mumps (Reed et al., 1967).

Development of mumps vaccine had two stages. Initially, there was an inactivated vaccine (Enders, 1946). It was not sufficiently effective, in that it offered protection only to some 80 percent of the recipients and the protection lasted for less than 1 year. Therefore, investigators undertook efforts to develop an attenuated strain of mumps virus that could be used as a live vaccine.

The Jeryl Lynn strain, the mumps virus strain used in mumps vaccines in the United States, came about by numerous passages in vitro, first in embryonated hen's eggs and then in chicken embryo cells (Buynak and Hilleman, 1966). The seroconversion rate was nearly 97 percent. Subsequently, two other strains were developed by similar attenuation of a wild-type isolate. They are Leningrad-3-Parkow and Urabe AM9, which were generated in the former Soviet Union and Japan, respectively.

The American Academy of Pediatrics recommends that measles-mumps-rubella vaccine (MMR) be given at age 15 months and at entry into middle or junior high school. The Advisory Committee on Immunization Practices recommends that MMR be administered at 15 months and then again at school entry at age 4 to 6 years. ("MMR" is used in this report to indicate any multivalent vaccine preparation directed against measles, mumps, and rubella. No association with a specific manufacturer is intended or should be inferred.)

BIOLOGIC EVENTS FOLLOWING IMMUNIZATION

Measles

Although the measles vaccine is administered by injection rather than by the natural, respiratory route of infection, the host response is similar to that evoked by the wild-type virus in all but two respects. The immunized subject develops humoral and cellular immune responses some 48 hours earlier than the naturally infected host, and the recipient of the vaccine does not develop clinical measles. Three classes of immune globulin (IgA, IgG, and IgM) are produced and are detectable in the serum and nasal mucus of vaccinated subjects (Bellanti et al., 1969).

The standard test of immunity to measles is based on the detection of serum antibodies by the enzyme-linked immunosorbent assay method. Although the titers of these antibodies induced by the vaccine tend to be somewhat lower than those resulting from natural infection (Schwarz and Anderson, 1965), immunity acquired by vaccination is long-lasting (Krugman, 1983).

Mumps

Following the administration of mumps vaccine, seroconversion is slower and the antibody titers achieved are lower than those following natural infection. A neutralizing antibody response can be detected in some recipients 2 weeks after vaccine administration; in others, it can be delayed for up to 6 weeks (Hilleman et al., 1968a,b). It is assumed that this immunity is long-lasting, but this has not yet been established.

ENCEPHALOPATHY AND ENCEPHALITIS

Clinical Description

Encephalopathy refers to any acute or chronic acquired abnormality of, injury to, or impairment of the function of the brain. Symptoms can include alterations in state of consciousness or behavior, convulsions, headache, and focal neurologic deficits. Encephalitis refers to an encephalopathy caused by an inflammatory response in the brain. This is usually manifested with systemic constitutional symptoms, particularly pleocytosis of the cerebrospinal fluid (CSF). However, the terms encephalopathy and encephalitis have been used imprecisely and even interchangeably in the literature. The discussion that follows uses the terminologies of the authors of the reports. However, if the authors used the term encephalitis, but there was no documentation of pleocytosis in the CSF, "encephalitis" is used in quotation marks.   The annual incidence of encephalitis for the years 1950 to 1981 in Olmsted County, Minnesota, was 7.4 per 100,000 people (Beghi et al., 1984; Nicolosi et al., 1986). The incidence in children less than age 1 year was 22.5, in children between ages 1 and 4 years it was 15.2, and in children between ages 5 and 9 years it was 30.2 per 100,000. Other estimates of encephalopathy for children less than age 2 years were somewhat lower than those reported by Beghi et al. and Nicolosi et al. cited above. Other estimates for annual incidence range from 5 per 100,000 people (Walker et al., 1988) to 10 per 100,000 people (Gale et al., 1990). Chapter 3 contains a discussion of encephalopathy.

History of Suspected Association

The occurrence of encephalitis following a natural measles virus infection is well described. The condition is quite severe, often leading to permanent brain damage or even death. There may be no detectable pathologic lesion, but in most cases some edema and demyelination are noted. Early studies of the adverse events associated with measles vaccine concentrated on "encephalitis." These are described below (Landrigan and Witte, 1973; Nader and Warren, 1968).

The first report of encephalopathy following vaccination with the live attenuated Edmonston B (Rubeovax) measles vaccine appeared in 1967 (Trump and White, 1967). A 2-year-old girl developed unsteadiness 7 days following vaccination. This was followed by pronounced generalized ataxia (diagnosed as cerebellar ataxia), fever, vomiting, and an exanthem. There was pleocytosis in the CSF 1 month after vaccination. The ataxia persisted for at least 8 months. Because of the child's history and physical and laboratory findings, the investigators attributed the condition to measles vaccination. Two early case series investigations of neurologic disorders following measles vaccination included reports of "encephalitis." These are discussed below.

Mumps affects the central nervous system as well, but it is more likely to cause meningitis than encephalitis (Azimi et al., 1969). This condition tends to be self-limited and has a good prognosis. Cases of pure encephalitis following mumps are rare, but they can be quite severe.

Evidence for Association

Biologic Plausibility

Chapter 3 contains a discussion of the biologic plausibility for certain types of encephalopathies and vaccination. As described above, natural (wild-type) measles virus infection is associated with a well-described, frequently very severe encephalitis.

Case Reports, Case Series, and Uncontrolled Observational Studies

Many uncontrolled observational studies in the literature describe the occurrence of encephalopathy after administration of measles vaccine. These are reviewed first. Data from similar studies regarding multivalent preparations are described next. Individual case reports and unpublished case reports from U.S. Public Health Service passive surveillance systems are discussed last. There are no data regarding monovalent mumps vaccine and encephalopathy.

Measles Vaccine   The first published case of encephalopathy (acute cerebellar ataxia) attributed to measles vaccine was discussed above (Trump and White, 1967).   Retrospective analyses of populations who have received measles vaccine have been reported from many countries, including the United States.   These uncontrolled observational studies provide no information on the concurrent background rates of encephalopathy.   Table 6-2 summarizes case series and uncontrolled observational studies in which the incidence rates of encephalopathy or encephalitis following administration of measles vaccine were calculated by the authors.

Two case series addressed early concerns in the United States that measles vaccine might cause encephalitis.   The first was a report of 23 cases of neurologic disease following measles vaccination in the United States from January 1965 to February 1967 (Nader and Warren, 1968).   The authors characterized 18 of the 23 cases as "encephalitis" (described as including disturbances of sensorium, seizure, major loss of motor function, and cerebral edema; no data are provided regarding pleocytosis in the CSF).   The interval from vaccination to the onset of symptoms ranged between 3 and 24 days.   Postmortem findings in one case revealed herpes simplex virus in brain tissue.   There were two cases of aseptic meningitis, two cases of cerebellar ataxia, and one case of extraocular muscle paralysis.   The authors estimated a rate of 1.5 reported cases of "encephalitis" within a 4-week period of vaccination per 1 million doses of vaccine distributed.   They compared this with a background rate of 2.8 cases of encephalitis (unrelated to vaccination or known parainfectious causes) per 1 million children for any 4-week period.   The authors concluded, "No single clinical or epidemiologic characteristic appears consistently in the reports of cases of possible neurologic sequelae of measles vaccination" (p. 998).

A review of 84 patients with neurologic disorders occurring within 30 days of vaccination against measles virus reported to the Centers for Disease Control from 1963 to 1971 revealed 59 patients with extensive neurologic disorders, which included encephalomyelitis (Landrigan and Witte, 1973).   The cases reported by Nader and Warren (1968) and discussed above are a subset of the data of Landrigan and Witte (1973).   Although in all 59 patients the onset of symptoms occurred between 1 and 25 days after vaccination, in 45 it coincided with the period of maximal viral replication (6 to 15 days after vaccination).   Of 50 patients for whom follow-up information was available (follow-up presumably from 1963 to sometime before 1973), 26 recovered fully, 5 died (2 of the 5 had pathologic features of Reye syndrome), and 19 were left with permanent neurologic damage.   Thirteen of the 59 patients were classified as having encephalomyelitis.   Long-term follow-up of 12 of the patients showed residual neurologic signs in 3 patients.   Long-term follow-up was available for 31 of 36 patients considered to have encephalopathy.   Ten of those 31 patients recovered fully, 5 died,

TABLE 6-2 Rates of Encephalitis/Encephalopathy After Measles Vaccination from Uncontrolled Studies

Reference	Years Covered	Measles Vaccine Used	Condition	No. of Cases	Calculated Rate per Million Doses
Nader and Warren, 1968	January 1965 to February 1967	Live attenuated	Encephalitis	18	1.5
Landrigan and Witte, 1973 (overlaps with Nader and Warren, 1968)	1963 to 1971	Live attenuated	Encephalomyelitis (including transverse myelitis)	13	1.2
			Encephalopathy	36	
Hirayama, 1983	1978 to 1982 (?)	Schwarz	Encephalitis/ encephalopathy	8	3.7
		Biken-CAM		4	2.9
White, 1983	1965 to 1976	Unspecified	Encephalitis	7	1.8
Koch et al., 1989	1987	MMR (unspecified)	Meningitis/ encephalitis	5	11
Fescharek et al., 1990	1976 to 1989	More attenuated Enders (measles, measles-mumps, MMR)	Meningitis/ encephalitis	16 (total)	3
				5*	1

* The authors thought that 5 of the 16 cases were possibly causally related to the vaccine.

and 16 were left with neurologic residua. The authors calculated rates of "encephalitis" of 1.16 cases per 1 million doses of vaccine distributed.

Among the recipients of more than 3 million doses of measles vaccine (various strains, but mostly the Schwarz strain) in the United Kingdom between 1968 and 1974, there were 47 cases of "encephalitis" (Beale, 1974). The report does not discuss the criteria used for the diagnosis. Data on the occurrence of encephalitis in temporal relation to administration of measles vaccine for the years 1965-1976 in Canada showed a rate of 1.79 cases of encephalitis per 1 million doses of vaccine distributed (White, 1983). These data are based on hospital admissions associated with International Classification of Diseases codes for "viral encephalitis unspecified" and "acute viral encephalitis."

In a report from the former East Germany (Dietzsch and Kiehl, 1976), there were 7 central nervous system (CNS) complications out of 174,725 immunizations with an unstated vaccine, but it was probably one of the strains from the former Soviet Union. Two febrile seizures, four cases of encephalopathy, and one case of encephalitis (there was pleocytosis in the CSF) were reported. Few clinical details were reported. Two of the patients with encephalopathy and the patient with encephalitis recovered completely, one patient with encephalopathy was left with a residual paralysis, and another died of leukemia.

A report from the former Soviet Union (Ozeretskovskii and Gurvich, 1991) referred to cases of encephalitis and encephalitic reaction caused by a measles vaccine (probably the Smorodintsev strain), but offered no primary data. The authors quote three rates per 100,000 vaccinees: 0.1, 0.02, and 190 cases. The rate of 0.02 is far below the acknowledged background rate of encephalitis and the rate of 190 is far above any rates quoted anywhere for encephalitis/encephalopathy after receipt of measles vaccine. Considering the imprecision of the definition of "encephalitis" and "encephalitic reaction" and the discrepancy of the rates, it is impossible to interpret that report.

A report of adverse events associated with measles vaccine in Japan from 1978 to 1983 cited 12 cases of "encephalitis" or "encephalopathy," without describing them, and derived a rate of 3.7 cases of "encephalitis" per 1 million vaccinees administered the Schwarz vaccine and 2.9 cases per 1 million vaccinees administered the Biken-CAM vaccine (Hirayama, 1983). A follow-up to that report published 5 years later (Isomura, 1988) mentioned 16 cases of "encephalitis" (4 more cases than the earlier report), but provided no details. The incidence rate for "encephalopathy" and "encephalitis" following measles vaccination appeared to be lower than the observed incidence of encephalitis from all causes among age-matched controls (Hirayama, 1983; Isomura, 1988). This comparison was not derived from a controlled cohort study, however.

Measles Vaccine-Containing Preparations In an analysis of 433 spontaneous reports to a vaccine manufacturer in the Federal Republic of Germany (former West Germany) between 1976 and 1989 (Fescharek et al., 1990), 6 of 16 reports of "meningitis" or "encephalitis" were thought by the authors to be possibly related to measles, measles-mumps, or measles-mumps-rubella vaccine, leading to a rate of 1 case per 1 million doses distributed, as calculated by the authors. The vaccine strains are those currently licensed in the United States, that is, the more attenuated measles vaccine and Jeryl Lynn mumps vaccine. Assuming that all 16 reports of cases of "meningitis" and "encephalitis" were causally related to the vaccine, the rate would increase to about 3 cases per 1 million doses distributed, which is within the range reported in other countries, as described above.

A study based on a new passive surveillance system in Canada reported a rate of 1.1 cases of meningitis or encephalitis, without distinguishing between the two, per 100,000 doses of MMR (Koch et al., 1989). (This high rate was probably due to the inclusion of meningitis in the survey.) It was estimated that more than 8 million doses of MMR were distributed in Canada during the reporting period.

A description of 212 adverse events associated with MMR reported to Swedish health authorities from 1982 to 1984 (when an estimated 700,000 doses of MMR were sold) includes 17 reports of transient, serious cases of neurologic symptoms: 3 patients with "encephalitic symptoms" who were treated at the hospital, 7 patients with "encephalitic symptoms" who were not hospitalized, 5 patients with acute symptoms with motor difficulties, 1 patient with seizures and fever, and 1 patient with hemiparesis (Taranger and Wiholm, 1987). "Encephalitic symptoms" included tiredness, whining, irritability, and mood changes with or without fever. No mention of CSF pleocytosis was made. Follow-up of at least 1 year showed that one 18-month-old boy who had developed symptoms of mild encephalitis with balance problems had residua of foot dragging and stumbling when he was tired.

Case Reports Many case reports describe encephalitis or encephalopathy following administration of measles vaccine. Because isolation of measles virus is problematic and exposure to wild-type measles virus is common, it is difficult to assess a possible role of measles or measles vaccine in the occurrence of encephalopathy or encephalitis in an individual case. Typical case reports follow.

A 5-year-old received a live measles vaccine and developed fever two weeks later (Alves et al., 1992). Three days after the onset of fever, the boy presented with hemiparesis, dysarthria, and a generalized rigid-akinetic syndrome. A spinal tap obtained four days later showed pleocytosis. One month later he was diagnosed with postencephalitic parkinsonism. He responded to levodopa therapy. The parkinsonism persisted for the 2 years between the time of vaccination and publication of the report (Alves et al., 1992). A 14-month-old girl received the Wellcome measles vaccine and developed convulsions 12 days later (Barbor and Grant, 1969). She became confused, restless, and then unconscious. Although the authors called this an encephalitis, there was no CSF pleocytosis on days 13 or 21 post-vaccination. She made little progress in the 4 months between hospitalization and publication of the report. An electroencephalographic record of slow waves, which are not characteristic of measles encephalitis, and possible slight head trauma 9 days after vaccination suggested a temporal, not a causal, relation between the convulsions and the measles vaccination. A 13-month-old girl was admitted to the hospital with involuntary jerking movements of her limbs 10 days after receiving a further attenuated Enders live measles vaccine (Jagdis et al., 1975). She was afebrile, although she had fever for 2 days prior to admission. The CSF was turbid and showed pleocytosis. She had a convulsion followed by apnea. She died 13 days after vaccination. Postmortem examination suggested viral encephalitis; Cowdry type A inclusion bodies suggested measles virus as the etiologic agent, but no measles virus was isolated. She had no known exposure to wild-type measles virus, but an epidemic in the community was ending. Haun and Ehrhardt (1973) described a boy age 11 months who developed drowsiness, convulsions, and coma 12 days following vaccination with the L-16 SSW measles vaccine (a variant derived from the Soviet strain Leningrad-16). There was pleocytosis in the CSF. He died the same day as onset of symptoms. Autopsy findings were suggestive of disseminated intravascular coagulation as the cause of death. A boy age 2 years was administered live measles vaccine 10 days before the development of persistent convulsions (Starke et al., 1970). The child suffered convulsions accompanied by unconsciousness until his death a month later. He had experienced convulsions in the first year of life during a bout of pneumonia. The autopsy stated there was CNS death, "encephalitis" following measles inoculation, and septic pulmonary infarction. No further details are given.

Several reports of encephalopathy following measles vaccination can be found in the Vaccine Adverse Event Reporting System (VAERS) (submitted between November 1990 and July 1992). As with many VAERS reports, the information that is supplied is frequently inadequate to support or reject a diagnosis or to exclude the possibility that other factors are responsible for the disorder, if the case was encephalopathy or encephalitis. The committee found that 17 VAERS reports were suggestive of encephalopathy or encephalitis in vaccinees (mostly MMR) from ages 5 months to 16 years. Reported latencies ranged from 1 to 14 days after immunization. The patients presented with symptoms such as fever, ataxia, somnolence, convulsions, and flaccid paralysis. Several reports contained too little information to suggest a diagnosis or to shed light on causality.

A specific type of measles encephalopathy, immunosuppressive measles encephalopathy (IME), has been documented in two immunosuppressed children following vaccination against measles. IME is distinct from acute measles encephalitis and subacute sclerosing panencephalitis. It has an incubation period of 5 weeks to 6 months. In one case of a 7-year-old girl with acute lymphoblastic leukemia (Valmari et al., 1987), measles virus was isolated from her CSF approximately 10 weeks after she received MMR (which contains the more attenuated measles vaccine used in the United States). The authors believed the isolated virus was vaccine strain rather than the wild-type strain because the child had no contact with natural measles during the 5 weeks to 6 months prior to the onset of symptoms. A previously described case of IME in a leukemic child involved the Schwarz strain vaccine virus (Mitus et al., 1962). Measles virus was cultured from throat and conjunctiva, but not from postmortem brain tissue.

Controlled Observational Studies

The National Childhood Encephalopathy Study, a case-control study described in detail in Chapter 5, reported a significant association between measles vaccination and onset of either convulsions or encephalopathy within 7 to 14 days of receiving the vaccine (Alderslade et al., 1981). However, a separate analysis of those diagnosed with encephalitis or encephalopathy was not performed

Controlled Clinical Trials

A report from India (Kumar et al., 1982) described 206 children injected with the Schwarz strain of measles vaccine and 206 children who were not immunized. A 14-month-old girl was diagnosed with encephalitis (fever, vomiting, semi-consciousness, weakness, occasional white blood cells in the CSF) on postvaccination day 10. At the time the report was published, she was reported to be recovering "gradually." There were no cases of encephalitis in the controls, but the numbers are far too small to detect an association.

Causality Argument

There is demonstrated biologic plausibility that measles vaccine might cause encephalopathy. Although there are a number of reports of encephalitis or encephalopathy following immunization with measles vaccines of various strains, the rates quoted are impossible to distinguish from background rates. Good case-control or controlled cohort studies of these conditions in similar unvaccinated populations, which are necessary for determining the causal relation between measles and mumps and encephalopathy and encephalitis, are lacking. No conclusive evidence of the occurrence of encephalopathy or encephalitis resulting from the administration of measles vaccine was identified. There are no data regarding the occurrence of encephalopathy following administration of monovalent mumps vaccine. It is therefore not possible to implicate specifically either the measles or mumps component of MMR.

Conclusion

The evidence is inadequate to accept or reject a causal relation between measles or mumps vaccine and encephalitis or encephalopathy.

ASEPTIC MENINGITIS

Clinical Description

Aseptic meningitis is defined as an inflammation of the meninges associated with pleocytosis of the CSF. In the early stage of aseptic meningitis polymorphonuclear leukocytes predominate, but within 8 to 16 hours this changes to a predominance of mononuclear cells. There may be some elevation of protein, but in general, the glucose level is normal. In patients with aseptic meningitis associated with mumps, there may be hypoglycorrhachia. Bacterial cultures are negative. The description of aseptic meningitis in the wake of mumps vaccine administration follows this pattern, except that hypoglycorrhachia was not mentioned in the reports.

The yearly incidence of aseptic meningitis for the years 1950 to 1981 in Olmsted County, Minnesota, was 10.9 per 100,000 people (Nicolosi et al., 1986). The annual incidence was markedly higher in children less than age 1 year (82.4 per 100,000) and slightly higher in children between ages 1 and 4 years (16.2 per 100,000) and in children between ages 5 and 9 years (18.8 per 100,000).

History of Suspected Association

Mumps disease is clearly associated with aseptic meningitis. The committee was charged with investigating a possible causal relation between only mumps vaccine and aseptic meningitis.

Evidence for Association

Biologic Plausibility

Mumps disease has been found to be clearly associated with aseptic meningitis. Mumps virus (both wild-type and vaccine strains) has been isolated from the CSF of patients with aseptic meningitis.

Case Reports, Case Series, and Uncontrolled Observational Studies

The ability to isolate mumps virus from the CSF of patients presenting with symptoms of meningitis and to determine the type of the isolate as a wild-type or a vaccine strain indicates that mumps vaccine can cause aseptic meningitis. Many case series and observational studies have documented cases of meningitis after vaccination with mumps virus-containing vaccine. Of particular interest are the cases in which the vaccine strain was identified. This has been done extensively with the Urabe strain. Data concerning the Urabe strain mumps vaccine will be presented first. Data related to the Jeryl Lynn strain (that used in the United States) are presented last.

In 1989, Gray and Burns published two letters (Gray and Burns, 1989a,b) in *The Lancet* concerning a 3-year-old girl presenting with aseptic meningitis 21 days after vaccination with MMR. Fluorescent-antibody tests identified the isolated virus as mumps virus (Gray and Burns, 1989a), and soon thereafter, this virus was identified by nucleotide sequencing analysis as the Urabe strain (Gray and Burns, 1989b).

Identification of the mumps virus as the Urabe vaccine strain by nucleotide sequence analysis of the isolates from eight patients with meningitis in Canada led to suspension of the sale of that vaccine in Canada in May 1990 (Brown et al., 1991). Using the polymerase chain reaction to amplify the genetic signal, investigators from Japan also typed mumps virus isolated from patients with meningitis as a vaccine strain, most probably Urabe (Mori et al., 1991; Yamada et al., 1990).

Most recently, the Nottingham (United Kingdom) Public Health Laboratory isolated mumps virus from the CSF of eight children following administration of Urabe-containing MMR (Colville and Pugh, 1992). Seven of the isolates resembled the vaccine strain (the sample from the eighth patient could not be typed). Vaccination occurred 17 to 24 days prior to the lumbar puncture. The rate of virologically confirmed and suspected MMR-associated meningitis was calculated to be 1 case per 3,800 doses. None of the children had severe illness, and no sequelae were seen. Colville and Pugh (1992) reviewed laboratory records from an approximately 3-year period and determined that there were excess cases of lymphocytic meningitis in the group that recently received MMR compared with the incidence in those who had not recently been vaccinated with MMR. More cases of Urabe strain-related meningitis have been identified in the United Kingdom, and use of the Urabe vaccine strain has been suspended in that country.

A Urabe strain-containing MMR was released in Canada in 1986. Soon after that, cases of mumps meningitis began to appear. In an investigation at Montreal Children's Hospital of four patients with meningitis that appeared within 19 to 26 days after receipt of the Urabe-containing vaccine, mumps virus was isolated from the patients' CSF, as detected by hemadsorption inhibition with mumps antisera (McDonald et al., 1989). This did not distinguish the vaccine strain from the wild-type strain; however, none of the four patients were known to have had contact with an individual with natural mumps virus infection. The illnesses were not severe, and all patients recovered without sequelae.

Retrospective studies of mumps-associated meningitis and reports from surveillance systems provide more data regarding a relation between mumps vaccine and meningitis. Cizman et al. (1989) retrospectively reviewed the medical records of 2,418 children hospitalized and treated for aseptic meningitis at University Medical Center in Ljubljana, Yugoslavia, between 1979 and 1986. The etiology of the aseptic meningitis was assessed by serologic tests and isolation of the virus from CSF, urine, feces, or throat swabs. They confirmed the presence of mumps virus strains by the complement fixation test with a specific antiserum. They also tested for poliovirus, Central European tick-borne encephalitis virus, and herpes simplex virus. In 115 children, the onset of aseptic meningitis occurred within 30 days of vaccination against measles and mumps (Leningrad 3 strain), leading to an attack rate of approximately 1 per 1,000 immunized children, as calculated by the authors. Most of the cases occurred between 11 and 25 days after vaccination. The attack rate in immunized 6- to 8-year-old children was 3.5 times greater than that in immunized 1- to 3-year-old children. None of the children had sequelae. Signs of parotitis and virologic findings suggestive of mumps infection were found in 65 of the children, although only 1 child had a history of exposure to mumps. Much more enterovirus was isolated from children with non-vaccine-associated aseptic meningitis than from the 115 children with vaccine-associated aseptic meningitis. Although the authors did not calculate a rate of aseptic meningitis and they did not report how many cases of aseptic meningitis they finally attributed specifically to mumps vaccination, they were clearly concerned about the high incidence and, on the basis of in vitro tests, believed that their vaccine was inadequately attenuated compared with the Jeryl Lynn strain.

Introduction of vaccination for measles, mumps, and rubella (using the Urabe strain mumps vaccine) in Japan in 1989 coincided with early reports of mumps vaccine-associated meningitis. This prompted surveillance efforts in Japan to study the problem. Pediatricians at 24 hospitals in the

Gunma Prefecture were asked to fill out a questionnaire regarding clinical details and laboratory findings for patients with aseptic meningitis without a history of vaccination with MMR and for patients with parotitis and convulsive disorders within 2 months of vaccination with MMR during an 8-month period in 1989 (Fujinaga et al., 1991). There were 35 cases of aseptic meningitis within 2 months of vaccination with MMR. These patients had no history of contact with individuals with natural mumps virus infection. Mumps meningitis was seen in 38 patients with no history of vaccination, and meningitis resulting from other causes was seen in 46 patients. Mumps virus, but no other viral isolates, was detected by indirect immunofluorescence in 13 patients with aseptic meningitis who had been vaccinated within the 2 previous months, but who were negative for contact with wild-type mumps virus. Characterization of virus in samples from 13 patients by the polymerase chain reaction and nucleotide sequence determination or by restriction enzyme analysis determined that all 13 viruses were of the Urabe strain. They referred to these as the virus-positive group. They divided the remaining 22 patients into two groups: 11 patients who seroconverted (the serum-positive group) and 11 patients who had clinical signs of meningitis but from whom virus was not isolated and who had not seroconverted. They calculated incidence rates for the virus-positive group, the serum-positive group, and the clinical meningitis group for the 2-month period of 3, 2.5, and 1.5 cases per 1,000 children vaccinated with MMR, respectively. The estimated background incidence of acute neurologic diseases in the Gunma Prefecture for the years 1987 and 1988, by comparison, was 0.37 per 1,000 children.

A nationwide surveillance of neurologic complications after mumps vaccine administration in Japan during 1989 (which presumably included the data from the report described above [Fujinaga et al., 1991]) revealed 311 suspected cases of vaccine-related meningitis among 630,157 vaccinations with MMR (Sugiura and Yamada, 1991). Of 222 CSF samples examined, 99 samples contained mumps virus, and 96 of these were shown by molecular biology techniques to be the Urabe strain. The incidence rates of suspected or laboratory-confirmed aseptic meningitis were 1 in 2,026 and 1 in 6,564 people administered MMR, respectively. The authors noted that these incidence rates were higher than the estimated incidence rate among those who received monovalent Urabe strain mumps vaccine before or during the survey period. They also noted that all patients with aseptic meningitis recovered without sequelae.

Data concerning aseptic meningitis in association with the Jeryl Lynn strain mumps virus are more scarce than those related to the Urabe strain. Virus was isolated from a patient with symptoms of meningitis beginning 20 days after vaccination with the Jeryl Lynn strain of mumps vaccine (that used in the United States) (Ehrengut and Zastrow, 1989). The isolated virus, obtained from a swab of the orifice of Stenson's duct and from the CSF, was identified as the vaccine strain on the basis of the morphology of the cytopathic effect but not by molecular analysis. Fescharek and colleagues (1990) described the isolation of mumps virus from two patients with meningitis reported to the pharmaceutical firm Behringwerke AG in the former West Germany. The mumps vaccine administered was Jeryl Lynn (that used in the United States), but identification of the virus as wild-type or vaccine strain was not attempted.

Eleven cases of meningitis following receipt of MMR in the United States (the Jeryl Lynn strain of mumps vaccine) reported in VAERS (submitted between November 1990 and July 1992) were examined by the committee. In no case was the strain identified or the virus isolated. The latencies from vaccination to symptoms ranged from 3 days to 2 weeks. In some patients the clinical symptoms seemed supportive of a diagnosis of meningitis, but intercurrent infections were seen in two of the patients, insufficient information was available for three patients, and encephalopathy was possible for another patient.

Controlled Observational Studies

None.

Controlled Clinical Trials

None.

Causality Argument

There is strong biologic plausibility that mumps virus could cause aseptic meningitis. Wild-type mumps virus clearly does so. Isolation of the virus and typing by molecular biologic techniques as the vaccine strain of mumps virus from patients who developed aseptic meningitis following immunization with mumps vaccine provide evidence of a causal relation. This relation is firmly established for the Urabe strain. The incidence appears to be approximately 1 case per few thousand vaccine recipients. The matter is unclear with regard to the Jeryl Lynn strain (that used in the United States), because in the sole reported case in which the virus was identified as the "vaccine strain," the isolated virus was typed by the older morphologic technique and not by molecular analysis. In the two other published cases of Jeryl Lynn-associated mumps meningitis, the virus was not typed as the vaccine or wild-type strain. VAERS contains several reports of what probably is meningitis after administration of Jeryl Lynn mumps vaccine-containing preparations, but the reports do not describe virus isolation or typing. A recent study of various commercial mumps vaccine preparations demonstrates the existence of two populations of Jeryl Lynn strain virus in commercial vaccine preparations, with sequence variation of up to 4.4 percent for some genes (Afzal et al., 1992). Only one population of the Urabe strain was detected. The authors hypothesized that one of the populations could interfere with the growth of the other, thus influencing rates of adverse reactions. There are no data to substantiate this hypothesis directly.

Conclusion

The evidence is inadequate to accept or reject a causal relation between the Jeryl Lynn strain mumps vaccine and aseptic meningitis.

SUBACUTE SCLEROSING PANENCEPHALITIS

Clinical Description

Subacute sclerosing panencephalitis (SSPE) is a rare subacute encephalitis accompanied by demyelination. The entire course of SSPE may be one of slow progressive deterioration, but variable periods of remission can occur. The usual duration is about 12 to 24 months to a vegetative state or death. A more complete discussion of SSPE can be found in Chapter 3.

History of Suspected Association

Laboratory findings implicate a measles-like virus as the cause of SSPE. Epidemiologic data have also linked SSPE to prior measles infection.

The first report of SSPE in a patient with a negative history for measles but a positive history of vaccination with live attenuated measles vaccine was reported in 1968 (Schneck, 1968). The child had received measles vaccine with immune globulin 3 weeks prior to the onset of symptoms. The clinical course accelerated 10 weeks after vaccination, and the child died 18 months after vaccination. Serologic studies were not performed, but post-mortem histologic examination of the brain supported a diagnosis of SSPE. Several more case reports of SSPE in children negative by history for measles but positive for receipt of the measles vaccine followed and are described in more detail below.

The dramatic decline in the number of measles cases in the United States from 1964 to 1968 paralleled a decline in the number of cases of SSPE starting in the early 1970's. Only 4.2 new cases of SSPE per year, on average, were reported from 1982 to 1986 (Dyken et al., 1989). This is in contrast to the 48.6 new cases of SSPE per year, on average, reported from 1967 to 1971. This decline is attributed to the increased use of measles vaccine, introduced in the United States in 1963. However, a report of data from the National Registry for Subacute Sclerosing Panencephalitis showed that the proportion of newly diagnosed cases of SSPE occurring in children identified by history as vaccinated against measles increased approximately threefold from 1967 to 1974 (Modlin et al., 1977). These data are discussed in more detail below.

The first publication in 1972 of data in the newly established National Registry for Subacute Sclerosing Panencephalitis in the United States reported 14 patients (of a total of 219 records in the registry) who had received a measles vaccine prior to the onset between 1960 and 1970 of SSPE (Jabbour et al., 1972). Six of the 14 patients were reported to have had measles prior to the onset of SSPE as well. The interval between vaccination and the onset of SSPE was 1 year or more in all 14 cases. The specific type of measles vaccine administered is not known.

The committee was charged with investigating a possible causal relation between measles vaccine only and SSPE.

Evidence for Association

Biologic Plausibility

SSPE is a recognized sequela of measles infection, and it is biologically plausible that it could occur after administration of the live attenuated viral vaccine. Identification of the cause of SSPE as wild-type or vaccine-strain measles virus has not been possible. The viruses isolated from patients with SSPE differ from the known measles viruses. The viruses may have become altered by the prolonged residence in the brains of the patients, or they may have been different at the time of the original infection.

Case Reports, Case Series, and Uncontrolled Observational Studies

The first published case report of SSPE in a child with a history of vaccination with live attenuated measles vaccine appeared in 1968 and was described above (Schneck, 1968). In the following 5 years, several more reports of SSPE in individuals vaccinated against measles appeared (Cho et al., 1973; Gerson and Haslam, 1971; Jabbour et al., 1972; Klajman et al., 1973; Landrigan and Witte, 1973; Parker et al., 1970; Payne et al., 1969). These reports represented a total of 22 patients with SSPE, 7 of whom had a history of both measles and measles vaccination (Gerson and Haslam, 1971; Jabbour et al., 1972). The other 15 patients had a negative history for measles and a positive history for receipt of live attenuated measles vaccine (Cho et al., 1973; Jabbour et al., 1972; Klajman et al., 1973; Landrigan and Witte, 1973; Parker et al., 1970; Payne et al., 1969; Schneck, 1968). For two of those 15 patients, exposure to measles virus was probable, but clinical measles was not recorded (Landrigan and Witte, 1973; Parker et al., 1970). The latency between vaccination against measles and the onset of SSPE symptoms ranged from 3 weeks (Landrigan and Witte, 1973; Schneck, 1968) to 5 years (Cho et al., 1973).

The absence of prevaccination serology and the inability to characterize the cause of SSPE as wild-type or vaccine-strain measles virus in all cases preclude, as discussed below, a determination that the SSPE was caused by administration of the live attenuated measles vaccine. A negative history of natural measles disease in unimmunized persons is always suspect because measles infection can occur subclinically without rash. No case reports of SSPE definitively show that the cause of SSPE in a specific patient was the vaccine-strain virus and not the wild-type virus.

In 1978 the question about SSPE and measles vaccine surfaced again in response to a report concerning a boy who at age 7 years showed signs of SSPE, including deterioration in school performance, incontinence, and forgetfulness (Dodson et al., 1978). Within a few weeks of receiving live attenuated measles vaccine at age 8 years, the patient's symptoms progressed. At 2.5 to 3 months after vaccination, the patient died. SSPE was diagnosed by high measles virus titers in serum and CSF and a high ratio of immunoglobulin G/albumin in serum and CSF. At age 13 months he had suffered a mild illness considered by history to be measles. The authors hypothesized that the measles vaccine accelerated an already evolving SSPE.

The National Registry for Subacute Sclerosing Panencephalitis was founded in 1969, in response to an interest in the effects of measles vaccine on the incidence of SSPE (Schacher, 1968). Originally housed at the University of Tennessee Center for Health Sciences, it now resides at the University of South Alabama. The registry now includes data on more than 575 patients (Paul R. Dyken, University of South Alabama, Mobile, personal communication, 1993). The number of new cases of SSPE documented in the registry decreased from 46 in 1967 to 33 in 1972 to 13 in 1974 (Modlin et al., 1977). The average number of new reports of SSPE per year from 1982 to 1986 was 4.2 (Dyken et al., 1989) and is now about 1, although underreporting is suspected (Paul R. Dyken, University of South Alabama, Mobile, personal communication, 1993).

Analysis of 375 confirmed cases of SSPE that occurred in the United States from 1960 to 1974 (Modlin et al., 1977) demonstrated a decreasing incidence of SSPE beginning in the early 1970's. From 1967 to 1970 the proportion of new cases of SSPE associated with measles vaccine was less than 13 percent, but it increased to 20.6 percent in 1973 and 38.5 percent in 1974. This prompted the authors to note:

Although far from conclusive, the data presented here suggest that live, attenuated measles vaccine virus may be capable of contributing to the pathogenesis of SSPE. However, the risk of SSPE following vaccination, if any, appears less than the risk following natural measles (Modlin et al., 1977, p. 511).

A review of the data in the registry of patients with SSPE whose onset occurred up to 1986 (Dyken et al., 1989), which included the 375 patients described by Modlin et al. (1977) in the study described above and 200 additional patients, confirmed the continuing decline in the incidence of SSPE and the increase in the proportion of patients with SSPE who had a history of measles vaccination.

Reports of patients with SSPE from other countries after the institution of measles immunization campaigns have supported a role for measles disease in the pathogenesis of SSPE. The very high levels of hemagglutination inhibition (HAI) antibody in the serum and CSF of 100 patients with SSPE observed in Tehran, Iran, between 1977 and 1982 (Mirchamsy, 1983) compared with the HAI antibody levels in patients known to have been vaccinated against measles suggest that these patients had naturally acquired measles. Similarly, all 70 patients with SSPE reported to the Virusdiagnostic Laboratory in Stuttgart, Germany, between 1967 and 1978 were negative for measles vaccination by history (Enders-Ruckle, 1978). Of 26 patients with documented SSPE in Northern Ireland between 1965 and 1985, none had a history of measles vaccination (Morrow et al., 1986). Beersma and colleagues (1988) described 77 patients with SSPE in The Netherlands whose onset of symptoms occurred between 1976 and 1986. Only two of the patients had received a measles vaccine. One of the two patients developed clinical measles 1 week after vaccination and SSPE 9 years later. The other child developed SSPE 1.5 years after vaccination against measles. Prior measles virus infection could not be ruled out. Eleven of 215 patients with SSPE identified in Japan between 1966 and 1985 had received measles vaccine but had not had measles virus infection by history. A total of 184 patients had a history of measles virus infection but not vaccination against measles (Okuno et al., 1989).

There are no reports of SSPE in VAERS (submitted between November 1990 and July 1992), nor is there a discussion of SSPE in the surveillance reports from the data base of the Monitoring System for Adverse Events Following Immunization (MSAEFI), which preceded VAERS.

Controlled Observational Studies

Because SSPE is such a rare condition, study of its etiology is best done by using a case-control design. Patients known to have SSPE are compared with individuals without SSPE to determine whether the proportions of certain characteristics or factors thought to be disease related are similar in the two groups. In this way, a number of possible etiologic factors can be investigated in a single study.

In the years between the two reviews of the data in the SSPE registry discussed above, a case-control study of patients in the SSPE registry was reported (Halsey et al., 1980). Fifty-two patients with SSPE were compared with controls (49 playmates and 49 hospitalized children) matched for age, sex, and race. Children with SSPE were more likely than their age-matched controls to have had measles (odds ratio [OR], 7; 95% confidence interval [95% CI], 2.5 to 19.6), but they were less likely than controls to have received measles vaccine (OR, 0.28; 95% CI, 0.11 to 0.70). The age of infection with measles virus for children with SSPE was significantly less than that for controls who had measles. There was no difference in age at the time of vaccination between those subjects and controls who did not have a prior measles infection. The same proportion of cases as controls had more than one measles vaccination.

If the etiology of SSPE has changed over the years such that a proportion of all cases were due to the vaccine, then the demographic and epidemiologic characteristics of the SSPE cases would be expected to change as well. Two such ecologic studies have been reported. When U.S. patients whose SSPE was diagnosed between 1956 and 1975 were compared with those whose SSPE was diagnosed between 1976 and 1986, there was no difference in the ratio of males to females or in the proportion of African Americans with SSPE (Dyken et al., 1989). The question of latency was assessed by dividing the patients into three groups: those with a history of measles only, those with a history of both measles and measles vaccination, and those with a history of measles vaccination only. The latency to the onset of SSPE for each of the three groups increased between the periods of 1956-1966 and 1980-1986. The latency to the onset of SSPE for the group with a history of measles vaccine only was shorter than the latencies for the groups with a history of measles, but this difference was not statistically significant.

Similar analyses were done for cases of SSPE in Romania. Cernescu et al. (1990) compared 50 patients whose SSPE onset was in 1978-1979 with 62 patients whose SSPE onset was in 1988-1989. The patients in the 1978-1979 cohort were diagnosed before the national measles immunization program in Romania was implemented in 1979. For the 1988-1989 cohort, they found an increased mean age at the time of onset (6.1 versus 12.1 years) and a difference in the ratio of males to females (2.7:1 versus 0.76:1). They also reported that 76 percent of the cases of SSPE from the 1978-1979 cohort reported a primary measles infection at less than 2 years of age, compared with only 47 percent of the 1988-1989 cohort. The mean interval from the time of measles to the onset of SSPE also increased, from 54 to

106 months, as had the proportion of cases with extreme levels of measles antibody (36 versus 88.7 percent).

Controlled Clinical Trials

No controlled clinical trials of measles vaccination have provided data on the incidence of SSPE. The Medical Research Council of the United Kingdom reported follow-up data on the incidence and complications of wild-type measles infection from a randomized trial of 36,000 patients who received either live measles vaccine or killed vaccine followed later by live measles vaccine or no vaccine. Follow-up was for up to 4 years and 9 months (Medical Research Council, 1971). No mention was made of SSPE, indicating either that there were no cases or that it was not an outcome that was examined. Because other neurologic events were noted and because SSPE is such a striking and serious disease, it is likely that any cases of SSPE would have been reported, if they had occurred.

Causality Argument

There is no question that measles virus is causally related to SSPE. Therefore, it is biologically plausible that there is a link between receipt of live attenuated measles vaccine and SSPE. There is strong evidence that if such an association does exist, it would be very weak compared with the association between a naturally acquired measles infection and SSPE. This evidence is mainly temporal; that is, the incidence of SSPE has decreased dramatically in parallel with widespread measles immunization. There have been only two new cases of SSPE in U.S. citizens reported to the National Registry of Subacute Sclerosing Panencephalitis since 1989 (Paul R. Dyken, University of South Alabama, Mobile, personal communication, 1993). Neither patient had a history of natural measles infection. One patient was immunized at 15 months of age.

It is likely that at least some patients with SSPE have had unrecognized measles infection prior to immunization, and that the SSPE is directly related to this measles infection. Evidence for this comes from Krugman et al. (1962), who reported that before the use of measles vaccine, 15 percent of children whose parents reported no history of measles were found to be immune to the infection. In addition, data on 375 children in the National Registry for Subacute Sclerosing Panencephalitis obtained from Modlin et al. (1977) indicated that four children who had SSPE but no history of measles or measles vaccination in fact had elevated measles virus antibody titers.

The data of Cernescu et al. (1990) showing that the characteristics of patients with SSPE onset in 1978-1979 (prior to national measles immunization) differ from those of patients with SSPE onset in 1988-1989 indicate a possible change in the nature of the disease since the introduction of measles vaccine and a concurrent decrease in the incidence of measles. If such a change is confirmed by other studies (and this will be difficult, because there are so few new cases of SSPE), it could indicate a different etiology for current SSPE cases compared with those in the past. It could also merely indicate a change in the time of life at which a child is infected with measles and subsequently develops SSPE (e.g., since the beginning of widespread immunization, perhaps only infants who are too young for immunization are infected with measles virus and only a proportion of these develop SSPE).

It will be difficult to obtain other evidence for a causal relation between measles vaccine and SSPE. First, the number of cases of SSPE in the United States is now so low that detection of even moderately strong associations may be difficult. Second, the period of time between infection with the measles virus and development of SSPE is quite long, and if an association between measles vaccine and SSPE exists, a similarly long latency (perhaps 10 years or more) would be expected. Even if the latencies for the two conditions were different and the difference were moderately large, the difference would be difficult to detect because the range of time from measles infection to SSPE is fairly long and the number of new cases of SSPE is low.

Although application of new scientific methods, such as RNA sequencing, could be used to describe more completely the virus that causes SSPE, the well-known genetic alterations of the virus from wild-type measles virus will confound interpretation of the data and make it unlikely that investigators will be able to determine whether there is an independent association between measles vaccine and the development of SSPE.

There has been some concern as to whether measles vaccine could exacerbate preexisting SSPE (Dodson et al., 1978) and whether a second dose of measles vaccine could more often result in SSPE (Halsey, 1990). After publication of the case report of Dodson et al. (1978) of an 8-year-old boy with SSPE whose condition appeared to have been exacerbated by administration of the measles vaccine, Halsey et al. (1978) reported data suggesting that such a concern was not warranted. The National Registry for Subacute Sclerosing Panencephalitis contained records of nine patients who received attenuated or killed measles vaccine after the onset of SSPE symptoms. Four of the nine patients died an average of 3.6 years after the onset of SSPE symptoms and 2.4 years after vaccination. The remaining five patients on record at that time were still alive an average of 10.5 years after the onset of SSPE symptoms and 9.3 years after vaccination. Halsey and colleagues argued that the variability in the course of SSPE rendered the assertions of Dodson et al. (1978) questionable. The same data set contained evidence that the proportion of SSPE patients who received more than one dose of vaccine was the same as for the control population.

Conclusion

The evidence is inadequate to accept or reject a causal relation between measles vaccine and SSPE.

RESIDUAL SEIZURE DISORDER

Clinical Description

A residual seizure disorder (RSD) caused by vaccination can be defined as a seizure that occurs within 72 hours of vaccination and that is followed by two or more afebrile seizures during the next 12 months (U.S. Department of Health and Human Services, 1992). Subsequent seizures would be anticipated in succeeding years. Approximately 0.5 to 2 percent of the population experience epilepsy. It can occur at any age. Chapter 3 contains a more lengthy discussion of RSD. The cases of RSD reported in this section would not necessarily fit the criteria for RSD presented above. The committee accepted an author's statement that a case was RSD. In addition, the committee considered all cases in which a person experienced repeated (more than one) afebrile seizures to be RSD to not exclude incorrectly any true cases of RSD.

Evidence for Association

Biologic Plausibility

Naturally acquired measles infection is associated with encephalitis, and patients with encephalitis can present with seizures. There are no specific data bearing on the biologic plausibility of an association between measles or mumps vaccine and RSD.

Case Reports, Case Series, and Uncontrolled Observational Studies

The National Collaborative Perinatal Project followed about 54,000 pregnant women, living in 13 cities in the United States, between 1959 and 1966 (Hirtz et al., 1983). Among the children born to those women, 2,766 children experienced at least one seizure within the first 7 years of life. Thirty-nine of those children experienced a convulsion within 2 weeks following an immunization. One child had convulsions following two separate immunizations (against measles and smallpox), so there were a total of 40 seizures. Ten seizures occurred following measles vaccination, generally with a latency of 7 to 10 days. All but one of the seizures were associated with fever; however, the vaccine administered to the child with the afebrile seizures was not specified. The children were followed for up to 7 years, and all 10 children who had received measles vaccination "did well" with no long-term neurologic sequelae.

Nader and Warren (1968) described 23 cases of neurologic disease that followed administration of measles vaccine and that were reported to the U.S. National Communicable Disease Center between 1965 and 1967. During that time, 15 million doses of measles vaccine were distributed throughout the United States. Eleven of the 23 patients were reported to have seizures or convulsions (three of which were noted to be accompanied by fever), and there was one case of persistent spastic quadriplegia. One of the cases of seizures persisted after the acute phase of the illness.

Beale (1974) reported on the measles vaccine experience in the United Kingdom. From 1968 to 1974, more than 3 million children were immunized with Schwarz or Beckenham 31 measles vaccines. Adverse reactions were reported to the governmental Committee on Safety of Medicines. There were 57 febrile convulsions associated with the Schwarz vaccine and 65 associated with the Beckenham 31 vaccine. No other data describing the nature of the seizures or long-term follow-up of the patients were available.

In a study of voluntary reporting of reactions to vaccination in the North West Thames region of England between 1975 and 1981, when approximately 170,000 children received live measles vaccine (as well as other childhood vaccines), there were 26 reports of convulsions without evidence of neurologic damage following measles vaccination (Pollock and Morris, 1983). No further details were provided, except that at follow-up the children were normal.

Maspero and colleagues (1991) reported a case series of 1,148 children immunized in 1990 in Lombardy, Italy, with the Edmonston-Zagreb vaccine strain and compared them with a case series of children in a nearby district immunized from 1980 to 1987 with the Schwarz vaccine strain. The authors reported that they saw no neurologic events following administration of the Edmonston-Zagreb vaccine. There was no comparable statement regarding the incidence of neurologic outcomes in the population immunized with the Schwarz strain.

A 19-month-old Japanese boy was immunized with measles vaccine (Schwarz strain) and 11 days later developed a fever and prolonged (30 minutes) convulsions with loss of consciousness (Abe, 1985). He had four more brief convulsions over the next 6 months, all with fever, and his electroencephalogram exhibited transient abnormalities 14 months later. The report indicated that 2.5 years following the first seizure, the boy's development appeared to be normal.

Haun and Ehrhardt (1973) described an 11-month-old child who developed clonic seizures and CSF pleocytosis within 12 days of receiving the Leningrad-16 SSW measles vaccine strain and died soon thereafter. (This case is discussed again in Chapter 10.)

Griffin and colleagues (1991) examined the records of a cohort of children in Tennessee enrolled in the Medicaid program who had received MMR or measles-rubella vaccine (MR) in their first 3 years of life to estimate the incidence of neurologic outcomes. As determined from computerized records, children who were enrolled in the Medicaid program within 90 days of birth in one of four counties, who had a Tennessee birth certificate indicating a birth date within the study period (approximately 1974 to 1984), and who received during those years at least one diphtheria and tetanus toxoid and pertussis vaccine (DPT) immunization at ages 29-365 days and at least one MMR or MR immunization between 12 and 36 months of age were included in the study. Follow-up began at the time of the first MMR or MR immunization and was restricted to the first 36 months of life. Of the population of 18,364 children enrolled in the Medicaid program who received immunizations, 100 were confirmed to have had a seizure. Of these, 77 had febrile seizures (4 children had seizures between days 7 and 14 postimmunization and none were recurrent), 15 had afebrile seizures (1 child had two seizures at 1 and 3 days postimmunization, and another child had a seizure at 29 days postimmunization), and 8 had seizures associated with other acute neurologic illnesses. Most seizures occurred more than 30 days following the immunization. It is possible that there was underascertainment of seizure cases in this cohort, because only those patients for whom a medical claim was filed were counted. Thus, children who moved, went off the Medicaid program, or whose parents did not file a claim were not counted as seizure cases. The authors made no attempts to follow seizure cases for long-term problems.

Fescharek et al. (1990) described convulsions that occurred in 41 patients following administration of vaccine containing measles antigen, mumps antigen, or both. Seven of the 41 patients had convulsions that were not accompanied by fever. More detailed information was not supplied. It is not clear whether any of the convulsions represented the early signs of an RSD.

A report from the passive surveillance system used to detect adverse events following immunization in Canada provided the rates of occurrence of adverse events but not long-term outcomes (Koch et al., 1989). Included in that report were all adverse events reported prior to the end of 1988 for individuals who had received immunizations at any time in 1987. For the purposes of classification, convulsions/seizures were defined as those involving muscle contractions and a decreased level of consciousness, with or without a fever, and had to have been diagnosed by a physician. Forty-four cases were classified as convulsions/seizures following the administration of MMR; the associated rate was 9.3 cases per 100,000 doses. Although some follow-up beyond 1 year was done to identify residual disorders, the authors did not provide data regarding seizures.

Controlled Observational Studies

The committee was not able to identify any controlled observational studies that reported on the possible association between measles or mumps vaccine and RSD.

Controlled Clinical Trials

As noted above, the Medical Research Council of the United Kingdom reported follow-up data (up to 4 years and 9 months) from a randomized trial of 36,000 patients who received either live attenuated measles vaccine or killed vaccine followed by live attenuated vaccine or no vaccine (Medical Research Council, 1971). Although follow-up was designed to examine the incidence and complications of wild-type measles infection, had an RSD occurred, it might have been noted in such a long-term study. There was no mention of RSD.

Causality Argument

There is evidence that acute seizures are possible sequelae of immunization with measles and mumps vaccines. Therefore, it is biologically plausible that there is a connection between immunization and RSD. However, it would be essential to rule out the possibility that the acute cases described in the literature are not febrile seizures, which are common in children and which would not be expected to lead to an RSD. The available data are from case reports and case series; there are no data from observational studies that would allow the calculation of a risk of RSD for vaccinated as opposed to unvaccinated individuals. Perhaps most important, none of the available cases can be confirmed as RSD on the basis of the report alone.

Conclusion

The evidence is inadequate to accept or reject a causal relation between measles vaccine and residual seizure disorder.

There is no evidence bearing on a causal relation between mumps vaccine and residual seizure disorder.

The evidence is inadequate to accept or reject a causal relation between multivalent measles or mumps vaccines and residual seizure disorder.

SENSORINEURAL DEAFNESS

Clinical Description

Sensorineural deafness refers to hearing impairment resulting from disturbances of the cochlea or auditory nerve. The ability to hear high frequencies is often selectively lost. No population-based incidence rates were identified.

History of Suspected Association

This condition, which can be unilateral or bilateral, is characteristic of natural mumps infection and is reported in about 4 percent of cases of mumps. Partial or complete recovery is common.

Evidence for Association

Biologic Plausibility

Viral infections of the cochlea are known to occur. Sensorineural deafness can be a complication of natural mumps virus infection.

Case Reports, Case Series, and Uncontrolled Observational Studies

A 7-year-old girl who had audiometry 2 years earlier for an unstated reason developed total deafness in the left ear 11 days after an injection of MMR. This was not preceded by any symptoms such as dizziness or earache. There was no recovery of hearing (Nabe-Nielsen and Walter, 1988a,b). A 3-year-old girl was evaluated because of bilateral deafness. At the age of 15 months she received MMR. Ten days later, she developed high fever, headache, ataxia, and irritability, which lasted several days. Nystagmus was noted. She recovered spontaneously, but soon after she was noted to have hearing impairment. On evaluation at the age of 3 years, she had moderate to severe bilateral, unremitting sensorineural deafness (Brodsky and Stanievich, 1985).

Controlled Observational Studies

None.

Controlled Clinical Trials

None.

Causality Argument

There is demonstrated biologic plausibility that mumps vaccine could cause sensorineural deafness, in that wild-type mumps virus is associated with the condition. The biologic plausibility for a causal relation between measles vaccine and sensorineural deafness is less firm. Although cases of sensorineural deafness following administration of mumps and measles vaccines have been reported, the timing of onset and other nonspecific features make it impossible to distinguish vaccine from nonvaccine causation. Virus isolation would be helpful in assessing causality when the data are as scarce as described for the causal relation between measles and mumps vaccines and sensorineural deafness; however, such data are lacking.

Conclusion

The evidence is inadequate to accept or reject a causal relation between measles or mumps vaccines and sensorineural deafness.

OPTIC NEURITIS

Clinical Description

Patients with optic neuritis present with unilateral or bilateral impairment of vision. This process can be transient, with full recovery following, or the loss of vision can be permanent. In most instances the underlying pathogenesis is demyelination involving the optic nerve. Chapter 3 contains a more detailed discussion of optic neuritis. No population-based incidence rates were identified.

History of Suspected Association

Measles virus and measles vaccine have long been studied for their ability to cause demyelinating disorders. The committee was charged with investigating a possible causal relation between only measles vaccine and optic neuritis.

Evidence for Association

Biologic Plausibility

Chapter 3 contains a description of the general biologic plausibility for a role for vaccines, particularly live viral vaccines, in causing demyelinating disorders. There are no data bearing on the biologic plausibility that measles vaccine specifically can cause optic neuritis.

Case Reports, Case Series, and Uncontrolled Observational Studies

There are several reports of optic neuritis following measles vaccination. A 6-year-old boy developed bilateral optic neuritis 18 days after an injection of MMR. He was treated with corticosteroids and experienced a complete resolution after several weeks (Kazarian and Gager, 1978). Marshall et al. (1985) described a 16-month-old girl who experienced an acute loss of vision 16 days after an injection of MMR. Two days earlier she felt warm to the touch and developed a cough, conjunctivitis, and a generalized maculopapular rash. Examination revealed diffuse chorioretinitis and papilledema, which ultimately evolved into a "salt and pepper" pattern. Seven months later she improved, but she had macular scarring. Riikonen (1989) described 18 children with optic neuritis following infection, vaccination, or both. Of those 18, 10 went on to develop multiple sclerosis. Six of these children had been vaccinated between 3 days and 1 month before the onset of optic neuritis, but none had received measles vaccine during that time period. All 18 of the children were reported to have received measles vaccine (unspecified) between 12 and 18 months of age; the age of onset of optic neuritis ranged from 5 years 2 months to 14 years 10 months.

Controlled Observational Studies

None.

Controlled Clinical Trials

None.

Causality Argument

There is demonstrated biologic plausibility of a causal relation between optic neuritis and measles vaccine, in that measles virus is associated with demyelinating disorders. The number of reported cases is too small and the data contained within the reports are too equivocal to support a positive association between measles vaccine and optic neuritis. As discussed in Chapter 3, optic neuritis can result from many causes and is frequently associated with multiple sclerosis.

Conclusion

The evidence is inadequate to accept or reject a causal relation between measles vaccine and optic neuritis.

TRANSVERSE MYELITIS

Clinical Description

Transverse myelitis is a focal, demyelinating lesion that can occur in isolation or as a component of diffuse demyelinating diseases such as acute disseminated encephalomyelitis and multiple sclerosis. Transverse myelitis is characterized by an acute onset of signs of spinal cord disease, usually involving the descending motor tracts and the ascending sensory fibers, suggesting a lesion at one level of the spinal cord. Chapter 3 contains a general discussion of transverse myelitis. The annual incidence of transverse myelitis in Rochester, Minnesota, from 1970 to 1980 was estimated to be 0.83 per 100,000 people (Beghi et al., 1982). The authors noted that this incidence is approximately sixfold higher than the rate calculated for Israel. They attribute this to differences in case ascertainment.

History of Suspected Association

Measles virus is known to be associated with demyelinating disorders. The committee was charged with investigating a possible causal relation between only measles vaccine and transverse myelitis.

Evidence for Association

Biologic Plausibility

Chapter 3 contains an in-depth discussion of the biologic plausibility of a relation between vaccines and demyelinating disorders. Measles virus is associated with central demyelinating diseases.

Case Reports, Case Studies, and Uncontrolled Observational Studies

A case report (in abstract form) linking transverse myelitis with live attenuated measles vaccine was identified (Clark et al., 1977). Thirteen days after vaccination with Schwarz strain measles vaccine, a 16-year-old girl developed symptoms of transverse myelitis. Measles virus was recovered from her throat and stool. The authors hypothesized a relation between vaccine-associated demyelination and cell-mediated responses to measles virus antigens and myelin basic protein.

As mentioned earlier, Landrigan and Witte (1973) used data voluntarily submitted to the Centers for Disease Control regarding neurologic disorders following administration of measles vaccine. From 1963 to 1971, 84 cases of neurologic disorders with onset of less than 30 days after administration of live measles vaccine were reported in the United States. One of the case patients was diagnosed as having transverse myelitis. No further information was provided.

VAERS contains one report (submitted between November 1990 and July 1992) of transverse myelitis developing shortly after MMR vaccination alone and one after MMR given in conjunction with DPT, oral polio vaccine (OPV), and Haemophilus influenzae type b (Hib) vaccine. The temporal and clinical details in those reports are insufficient for proper evaluation.

Controlled Observational Studies

None.

Controlled Clinical Trials

None.

Causality Argument

There is demonstrated biologic plausibility for a causal relation between measles vaccine and transverse myelitis, in that measles virus is well associated with demyelinating disorders. Two cases of transverse myelitis following administration of measles vaccine and two cases following administration of MMR were identified. These cases were temporally associated with administration of the vaccine; there was no other evidence that associated the vaccine and the adverse event. No data from observational or experimental studies lend support to the hypothesized association. The incidence of transverse myelitis unrelated to vaccine is estimated to be about 1 case per 100,000 population (Beghi et al., 1982). Thus, the number of cases identified do not appear to be above background rates, and any study designed to detect an excess number of cases over the background would have to be very large.

Conclusion

The evidence is inadequate to accept or reject a causal relation between measles vaccine and transverse myelitis.

GUILLAIN-BARRÉ SYNDROME

Clinical Description

Guillain-Barré syndrome (GBS) is characterized by the rapid onset of flaccid motor weakness with depression of tendon reflexes and inflammatory demyelination of peripheral nerves (Asbury and Gibbs, 1990). The annual incidence of GBS appears to be approximately 1 per 100,000 people for adults. The data are not definitive, but the annual incidence of GBS in children under age 5 years appears to be approximately the same. The annual incidence of GBS in children over age 5 years and teenagers appears to be lower. Chapter 3 contains a detailed discussion of GBS.

History of Suspected Association

A possible relation between live attenuated viral vaccines and demyelinating disease has been investigated for many years, as described in Chapter 3. There is no specific information suggesting an association between measles vaccine and GBS. The committee was charged with investigating a possible causal relation between only measles vaccine and GBS.

Evidence for Association

Biologic Plausibility

Chapter 3 contains a detailed discussion of the arguments that vaccine can cause demyelination, including GBS. GBS has been described in a few patients following natural (wild-type) measles infection (Lidin-Janson and Straanegard, 1972). Thus, GBS appears to be a rare but possible sequela of measles.

Case Reports, Case Series, and Uncontrolled Observational Studies

Grose and Spigland (1976) reported two cases of GBS that developed in patients within 1 week after immunization with measles vaccine. One of these patients, a 19-month-old girl, was part of a study of 24 patients with GBS for whom serologic studies were performed as part of an effort by the authors to identify possible causal viral agents. She received a combined measles (Moraten strain) and rubella vaccine 5 days before the development of symptoms (unable to stand and support her own weight). The authors eliminated the possibility that the neurologic reaction was unlikely to be related to rubella vaccine, because the rubella virus titers indicated that the child was already immune to rubella virus when she was given the vaccine. Four years later the authors saw a second patient with characteristics similar to those of their first one. A 10-month-old girl was given measles vaccine (Moraten strain), as well as her second doses of DPT and OPV, and 4 days later she developed early symptoms of GBS. Both children had a primary immune response to measles antigen, as demonstrated by the seroconversion following immunization.

Norrby (1984) described a 12-year-old girl who became ill with a disorder diagnosed as GBS soon after being vaccinated with MMR, but her CSF protein levels were normal, which casts doubt on the diagnosis. The other findings were supportive of a diagnosis of GBS. The authors presented summary data from Merck Sharp & Dohme indicating that 1 in 60 million doses of MMR has been associated with GBS. Landrigan and Witte (1973) used data voluntarily submitted to the Center for Disease Control regarding neurologic disorders following administration of measles vaccine. From 1963 to 1971, 84 cases of neurologic disorders with onset less than 30 days after live attenuated measles virus vaccination were reported in the United States, but these did not include GBS. In a review of adverse event reports submitted between 1976 and 1989 to the Behringwerke AG pharmaceutical firm in the former West Germany, Fescharek and colleagues (1990) described three cases of GBS following vaccination with measles or mumps vaccines (the specific vaccines used in the three patients were not identified). Two of the cases were thought to be related to something other than the vaccines; however, this was not elaborated. Assuming that all three cases were causally related, the authors calculated an incidence of 1 in 1.8 million doses of vaccine distributed.

Summary data from MSAEFI record eight cases of GBS following measles immunization reported between 1979 and 1990. One patient received measles-rubella vaccine and seven received MMR. Nine VAERS reports (submitted between November 1990 and July 1992) reviewed by the committee describe the occurrence of GBS after measles immunization. Three of the five VAERS reports indicating the occurrence of GBS after vaccination with MMR alone met the diagnostic criteria for GBS as outlined in Chapter 3. The patients reported in the other four reports received other vaccines in addition to MMR.

Controlled Observational Studies

None.

Controlled Clinical Trials

None.

Causality Argument

There is biologic plausibility for a causal relation between measles vaccine and GBS. GBS has been shown to follow natural measles virus infection. As described in Chapter 3, several vaccines and viruses are suspected of playing a role in GBS. Reports in the literature describing a possible relation between GBS and measles vaccine are case reports, case series, and uncontrolled observational studies. These include at most a total of six cases of GBS reported in the published literature and seven cases from VAERS. These cases were temporally related to vaccination; however, lack of clinical details and other antecedent events preclude a determination of a causal relation.

Conclusion

The evidence is inadequate to accept or reject a causal relation between measles vaccine and GBS.

INSULIN-DEPENDENT DIABETES MELLITUS

Clinical Description

Diabetes mellitus is a genetically determined disease manifested by abnormal metabolism of carbohydrate, protein, and fat (Fajans, 1989; Kaplan, 1990). Type I or insulin-dependent diabetes mellitus (IDDM) is associated with an insufficiency of insulin secretion by pancreatic beta cells and is characterized by an absolute need for injected insulin to sustain life. In most cases the onset of IDDM is in childhood, but it may occur at any age. Almost all diabetes in children is insulin-dependent. Approximately 10 to 15 percent of diabetics in industrialized countries have IDDM. The annual incidence of IDDM in the United States is about 12 to 14 new cases per 100,000 children ages 0 to 16 years. By age 20, approximately 0.3 percent of individuals will have developed IDDM.

History of Suspected Association

Although the pathogenesis of IDDM is not completely understood, most investigators feel that both environmental and genetic factors are involved, and there are compelling data suggesting that viruses may be one of the most important environmental triggers of pancreatic beta cell destruction in individuals with a genetic predisposition for IDDM (Banatvala et al., 1987; Maclaren, 1992). Genetic susceptibility has been associated with certain histocompatibility locus antigens (HLAs) on chromosome 6 (Gutierrez-Lopez et al., 1992; Maclaren, 1992).

Evidence favoring a role for environmental factors such as viral infections in the development of IDDM includes the finding that only about one of every two or three pairs of identical twins who develop IDDM are concordant for the disease, and individuals at highest genetic risk for IDDM, as well as rodents genetically homogeneous for spontaneously developing IDDM, do not always acquire the disease (Gutierrez-Lopez et al., 1992; Lipton et al., 1992; Maclaren, 1992).

Several different mechanisms appear to be involved in the pathogenesis of virus-induced IDDM. These have been summarized by Yoon and colleagues and consist of four main categories: (1) direct destruction of pancreatic beta cells by cytolytic viruses without the stimulation of an autoimmune reaction, (2) viral triggering of an autoimmune response, either by molecular mimicry or by altering the immunologic appearance of beta cell antigens, (3) cumulative insults to beta cells by environmental factors such as viral infections and toxins (Dahlquist, 1991; Tishon and Oldstone, 1987; Yoon et al., 1987b), and (4) persistent viral infection resulting in an altered ability to produce insulin with or without progressive beta cell destruction over a period of time (Oldstone, 1989; Tishon and Oldstone, 1987; Yoon et al., 1987a; Yoon and Ray, 1985).

There is no notable history of a suspected association between monovalent measles vaccine and IDDM. Suspicion of an association between mumps vaccine and IDDM is based on the ability of the wild-type mumps virus to cause pancreatitis (Association for the Study of Infectious Disease, 1974; Craighead, 1975; Prince et al., 1978), individual cases of IDDM with onset shortly following acute clinical mumps infections (Gamble et al., 1980; Harris, 1899; Hinden, 1962; Kremer, 1947; McCrae, 1963; Messaritakis, 1971; Otten et al., 1984; Patrick, 1924; Peig et al., 1981), clusters of IDDM after mumps epidemics (Dacou-Voutetakis et al., 1974), and large epidemiologic studies demonstrating parallel curves between outbreaks of mumps disease and new cases of IDDM (Gunderson, 1927; Sultz et al., 1975). Some cases of IDDM with clinical onset temporally related to immunization with mumps vaccine have been reported in the literature and VAERS (submitted between November 1990 and July 1992) (Blom et al., 1991; Helmke et al., 1986; Otten et al., 1984; Pawlowski and Gries, 1991; Quast et al., 1979; Sinaniotis et al., 1975; Taranger and Wiholm, 1987).

Evidence for Association

Plausibility

Pancreatitis is a well-recognized clinical feature of epidemic parotitis, with an incidence ranging from less than 1 to as high as 25 percent (Association for the Study of Infectious Disease, 1974; Craighead, 1975). Since 1899, there have been many reports of abrupt-onset IDDM in individuals of all ages within a few days to weeks following mumps infection or exposure to mumps infection in household members or close contacts (Harris, 1899; Hinden, 1962; Kremer, 1947; McCrae, 1963; Messaritakis, 1971; Otten et al., 1984; Patrick, 1924; Peig et al., 1981). One study found a significant excess of consultations for mumps in the 6 months before the onset of IDDM, particularly in the month prior to the onset of symptoms, in 1,663 children with recently diagnosed IDDM in Great Britain and Wales ($P <$ 0.001) (Gamble et al., 1980).

There have been reports of clusters of IDDM following epidemics of mumps disease (Dacou-Voutetakis et al., 1974) and cyclic variations in incidence curves for IDDM resembling those seen for epidemics of infectious diseases (Gundersen, 1927; Sultz et al., 1975). Some data demonstrate that the curves of the incidence rates of IDDM in children parallel those for epidemics of parotitis and mumps encephalitis, with a lag of from 2 to 4 years (Gundersen, 1927; Sultz et al., 1975). Some investigators attribute the sharp rise in the incidence of IDDM in boys in 1950 to 1960 to the common practice of purposefully exposing boys to mumps in the 1950s, since mumps orchitis occurs less commonly as a complication of mumps disease in children than adults (Sultz et al., 1975).

There have been numerous case reports of IDDM following infection with viruses other than the mumps virus, the most common being coxsackievirus and rubella virus. One of the most convincing reports of the ability of viruses to induce acute-onset IDDM was published by Yoon and colleagues in 1979. They isolated a variant of coxsackievirus B4 from autopsy specimens of a 10-year-old boy's pancreas. The child had developed diabetic ketoacidosis within 3 days of onset of symptoms of a flu-like illness and died 7 days later. He had lymphocytic infiltration of the islets of Langerhans, necrosis of beta cells, and a rise in the neutralizing antibody titer to this virus. One of several inbred strains of mice inoculated with the human viral isolate developed diabetes, and fluorescein-labeled antiviral antibody staining revealed antigens of the same virus in the mouse beta cells.

Since then other cases of a temporal association between the onset of IDDM and well-documented coxsackievirus B4 and B5 infections have been reported (Champsaur et al., 1982; Gladisch et al., 1976). Additional evidence suggesting that coxsackieviruses may cause pancreatic damage and subsequent IDDM has been provided by a report by Jenson and colleagues who found evidence of insulitis and beta cell damage in pancreatic sections from four of seven neonates who died of coxsackievirus B infection, although this finding does not prove that the infants would have developed IDDM if they had lived (Jenson et al., 1980).

Evidence that persistent viral infection may cause IDDM comes from studies of patients with the congenital rubella syndrome and experimental evidence that rubella infection in rabbit and hamster models causes pancreatic beta cell damage (Menser, 1978; Rayfield et al., 1986). Rubella virus has been isolated from the pancreases of several patients with congenital infections (De Prins et al., 1978; Monif, 1974), and inflammation of the pancreas has been reported in other children with congenital rubella (Bunnell and Monif, 1972; Patterson et al., 1981). Epidemiologic studies have shown that the prevalence of IDDM among children with congenital rubella infection is high in some countries, but not in others, suggesting that only patients with congenital rubella plus a genetic predisposition for developing IDDM are affected (Menser et al., 1978; Rubinstein et al., 1982). Indeed, it has been demonstrated that the frequencies of the HLAs DR2 and DR3 are significantly lower and higher, respectively, in patients with IDDM and congenital rubella than in those without IDDM (Rubinstein et al., 1982).

Experiments in animals have demonstrated that viruses such as coxsackievirus, encephalomyocarditis virus, mengovirus, reovirus, and lymphocytic choriomeningitis virus are capable of inducing IDDM, but most studies have shown that both the strain of the virus and the genetic susceptibility of the animal are important in the development of IDDM (Menser et al., 1978; Rayfield et al., 1986; Tishon and Oldstone, 1987; Yoon and Ray, 1985; Yoon et al., 1978, 1979, 1987a,b). This is illustrated particularly well by the ability of certain strains of lymphocytic choriomeningitis virus to stimulate the onset of IDDM and of others to prevent it (Dyrberg et al., 1988; Oldstone, 1988; Oldstone et al., 1990a,b; Tishon and Oldstone, 1987).

Infection with live (but not inactivated) mumps and rubella viruses, and coxsackievirus B4 has been found to lead to increased expression of HLA class I molecules and minor decreases in insulin secretion in cultured human beta cells (Parkkonen et al., 1992). Several common viruses including mumps virus, coxsackievirus B, and reovirus type 3 can infect human pancreatic beta cells in vitro and destroy them (Parkkonen et al., 1992; Prince et al., 1978; Yoon and Ray, 1985).

Case Reports, Case Series, and Uncontrolled Observational Studies

The case reports implicating measles vaccine as a potential cause of IDDM involve administration of the mumps vaccine at the same time.

There have been several cases of IDDM reported following MMR, measles-mumps, or mumps vaccination. The committee heard presentations at its May 1992 public meeting from two parents whose daughters developed IDDM after receiving MMR (see Appendix B). There have been four cases of IDDM reported to VAERS (submitted between November 1990 and July 1992) following receipt of MMR and one or two following receipt of mumps vaccine (both reports might represent the same child, since both were 6-year-old males who developed IDDM following mumps immunization). The ages have ranged from 1 to 27 years, with one case each being reported at ages 1, 7, 18, and 27 years. There was either one or two cases in a child age 6 years, as explained above. The onset of symptoms of IDDM in these patients ranged from 2 days to 2.3 months after immunization, with one case occurring at 2 days, two at 6 weeks, and one at 2.3 months. The intervals in the others were not specified.

In 1975, Sinaniotis and colleagues reported the onset of IDDM 1 month after receipt of mumps vaccine in a 6.5-year-old boy. In 1991, Pawlowski and Gries described an 11-year-old boy who had mumps disease at age 16 months and then received measles-mumps vaccine 5 months before the onset of IDDM. He had severe abdominal pain and fever 1 week after immunization.

In 1984, Otten and colleagues reported three cases of IDDM, with onset in one case 10 days and in two cases 3 weeks after mumps vaccine in children 3, 2, and 16 years of age, respectively. They noted that the two younger children were positive for HLAs DR3 and DR4 and that the older boy was positive for DR4. In 1986, Helmke and colleagues reported seven children who developed IDDM in the second to fourth week following mumps or measles-mumps vaccination. All seven children were positive for DR4, and three were also positive for DR3.

In 1979, Quast and colleagues noted that in the first 2 years after mumps and measles-mumps vaccines were introduced in the former West Germany, two cases of IDDM with onset 7 and 10 days after immunization with measles-mumps and mumps vaccines, respectively, were reported to the manufacturer, Behringwerke AG.

In 1990, Fescharek and colleagues noted that 20 cases of IDDM were reported to the manufacturer, Behringwerke AG, from 1976 through 1989, a period during which about 5 million doses of mumps vaccine were distributed in the former West Germany, giving a rate of 1 for every 250,000 doses distributed. The two cases of IDDM identified by Quast et al. (1979) are probably part of the more extensive study from the records of Behringwerke AG (Fescharek et al., 1990). For 19 of 20 patients, the interval between immunization and the onset of symptoms was reported, and this ranged from 3 days to 7 months. Twelve cases began within 30 days of immunization. The annual number of new cases of IDDM was assumed to be about

12 per 100,000 on the basis of a mean value of the incidences of IDDM in comparable countries, since no data were available for the former West Germany. It was estimated that for every 5 million children vaccinated against mumps, 50 spontaneous cases of IDDM would have been expected by random coincidence within 30 days after immunization.

In 1987, Taranger and Wiholm noted that three cases of IDDM diagnosed within 1 month of MMR immunization were reported to the pharmaceutical department of the Swedish Health Authorities during the 3-year period (1982 to 1984), when 700,000 doses of the vaccine were sold. All were 12-year-old girls. They noted that one had developed symptoms of IDDM 2 to 3 weeks before being immunized. Prospective data on the incidence of IDDM in children in Sweden since 1977 revealed that one to two girls at that age were expected to develop IDDM during each 1-month period. Thus, they concluded that the number of cases reported after receipt of MMR did not exceed the expected background frequency.

Sultz and colleagues (1975) conducted interviews with 112 parents of diabetic children in Erie County, New York (approximately one-third of all cases identified for the 25 years from 1946 through 1971), and noted that IDDM was preceded by mumps disease or exposure to mumps virus in almost 50 percent of the children and by mumps vaccination in an additional 11 percent. The median lag time was 3 years (mean, 3.8 years).

Controlled Observational Studies

In 1991, Blom and colleagues reported the results of a nationwide controlled study in Sweden evaluating vaccinations, infections, and the use of medicines during the year preceding the diagnosis of IDDM as possible risk determinants for IDDM in children 0 to 14 years of age. The study included 339 children with recent-onset IDDM and 528 control children matched for age, sex, and county. The data were obtained from mailed questionnaires that indicated that the purpose of the study was to reveal possible relations between different childhood diseases and environmental factors. It did not mention that the study was focusing on IDDM. They found no evidence that vaccinations increased the risk of developing IDDM in childhood. Mumps and MMR vaccinations had no significant effect on the relative risk of developing IDDM (for mumps: OR, 1.75; 95 percent CI, 0.54 to 5.70; for MMR: OR, 0.95; 95 percent CI, 0.71 to 1.28). However, measles vaccination was associated with a significantly decreased relative risk of developing IDDM (OR, 0.74; 95 percent CI, 0.55 to 1.00). Other data from that study demonstrated a lack of association between any specific infectious agent and IDDM, although children with IDDM had more infections during the year prior to diagnosis.

Controlled Clinical Trials

None.

Causality Argument

There is no demonstrated biologic plausibility to suggest a causal relation between monovalent measles vaccine and IDDM. Indeed, the available data demonstrate a decreased relative risk for IDDM in individuals who have received measles vaccination (Blom et al., 1991).

There is evidence suggesting that mumps virus infection can trigger the onset of IDDM in some individuals. Biologic plausibility data implicating the mumps virus in the pathogenesis of IDDM include (1) the association between viral infections, including mumps, and IDDM in humans, (2) the detection of circulating autoantibodies against pancreatic antigens, particularly islet cells, during convalescence from mumps infection as well as early in the course of IDDM, and (3) in vitro studies demonstrating that the wild-type mumps virus can infect human pancreatic beta cells.

Data regarding a possible association between mumps vaccine and IDDM are limited to the cases noted above of a temporal relation between mumps immunization and the onset of symptoms of IDDM (Fescharek et al., 1990; Helmke et al., 1986; Otten et al., 1984; Pawlowski and Gries, 1991; Quast et al., 1979; Sinaniotis et al., 1975; Taranger and Wiholm, 1987). It should be noted that because the etiology of IDDM may be multifactorial, any temporal relation with mumps vaccine may be because other factors (such as toxins, nutrients, or other infections) have already destroyed enough pancreatic beta cells that even minor damage by the mumps vaccine virus may trigger the onset of diabetic symptoms.

The incidence of IDDM shortly following mumps immunization of children in Sweden and Germany was at or below expected background levels (Blom et al., 1991; Fescharek et al., 1990). It should be noted, however, that most of the postulated mechanisms of the pathogenesis of IDDM (autoimmune, cumulative environmental effects, or persistent infection) suggest that there may be a prolonged interval between vaccination and the onset of symptoms of IDDM. Even if the vaccine virus were to cause IDDM by direct cytolysis of pancreatic beta cells, it will be difficult to document this by isolating the virus from pancreatic tissue since, currently, there is a very low mortality early in the course of IDDM, when the virus would most likely be present.

Conclusion

The evidence is inadequate to accept or reject a causal relation between measles or mumps vaccine and IDDM.

STERILITY DUE TO ORCHITIS

Clinical Description

Sterility is the inability to produce offspring. Orchitis is inflammation of the testis, which is manifested by swelling and tenderness and is usually of infectious origin, such as tuberculosis, mumps, enterovirus, syphilis, or certain fungal diseases. Orchitis is also referred to as testitis, didymitis, and orchiditis. No population-based incidence rates were identified.

History of Suspected Association

There is no suspected association between measles vaccine alone and orchitis or sterility. The possibility of an association between mumps vaccine and sterility secondary to orchitis has been suspected on the basis of reports of orchitis following infection with wild-type mumps virus.

Evidence for Association

Biologic Plausibility

There are no data bearing directly on the biologic plausibility of an association of orchitis or sterility with measles vaccine. The most compelling argument for biologic plausibility regarding orchitis following mumps vaccine are the reports of orchitis following infection with the wild-type mumps virus. In 1950, Werner (1950a) reported that mumps is complicated by orchitis in one-fifth of all cases of mumps occurring in males after puberty. He also found that mumps orchitis had been the cause of testicular atrophy in 43 percent of 44 cases of obvious testicular atrophy found in an examination of 2,000 random males 14 to 34 years of age. In another study, he analyzed seminal fluid from 49 males with a past history of mumps orchitis (Werner, 1950b). The age of onset of orchitis ranged from 10 to 27 years, with a median age of 16 years. The interval between the onset of orchitis and the study ranged from a few months to 9 years, with a median of 4 years. Some degree of testicular atrophy was apparent in 39 of 49 patients. Some 51 percent of 49 patients from 18 to 27 years of age with a past history of mumps orchitis had semen with mean sperm counts and motilities that were lower than those for semen from control subjects. Only one man had azoospermia. Testicular atrophy was no more common among patients with abnormal semen specimens than it was in the group with orchitis as a whole. Mumps orchitis was felt, on the basis of seminal fluid examination, to have impaired fertility in 13 percent of the individuals with a past history of the disease. Werner (1950b) concluded that since only 1.7

percent of all males with mumps contract orchitis (but 20 percent or more of males who develop mumps after puberty have orchitis) and only 13 percent of those with orchitis had impaired fertility attributable to mumps orchitis, mumps orchitis is not an important cause of sterility in males.

Penttinen and colleagues (1968) found that 15 to 25 percent of men who contracted mumps developed orchitis, and in about 10 to 20 percent of these men it was bilateral and, thus, had the potential to cause sterility. Two other studies have found that 30 to 38 percent of postpubertal males with mumps develop orchitis (Beard et al., 1977; Philip et al., 1959). They reported bilateral involvement in 17 and 37 percent of cases, respectively. Mumps orchitis was found to be most common in the second through fourth decades of life (Beard et al., 1977).

A review of the records of 2,482 patients with mumps (about half of whom were under 15 years of age) admitted to 16 infectious disease units in England and Wales revealed that 333 of 1,513 males developed orchitis and 71 males had orchitis and meningitis or encephalitis (Association for the Study of Infectious Disease, 1974). Interestingly, 5 of 969 females had oophoritis. The authors noted that orchitis was second only to CNS involvement as a complication of mumps. There were no recorded sequelae, but the investigators did not attempt to follow up these patients for sterility because "the practical difficulties associated with such a study are formidable" (p. 555).

In 1954, Sandler reported azoospermia in a 34-year-old male who developed bilateral orchitis following mumps disease. Although his azoospermia persisted for over 1 year, he subsequently fathered a child.

In a retrospective study, McKendrick and Nishtar (1966) found that several men had fathered children following either unilateral or bilateral mumps orchitis.

Several authors concluded that since orchitis is usually unilateral, it is rarely a cause of permanent sterility (Association for the Study of Infectious Disease, 1974; Bendersky-Malbec, 1982; Penttinen et al., 1968; Werner, 1950b).

Case Reports, Case Series, and Uncontrolled Observational Studies

The data regarding mumps vaccine-associated orchitis in the literature are in two reports of surveillance for adverse reactions to immunization in other countries. Three cases of orchitis were reported following administration of MMR in Canada in 1987, for an incidence of 0.5 cases per 100,000 doses of MMR distributed (Koch et al., 1989). Six cases of suspected orchitis were reported following administration of measles or mumps (Jeryl Lynn strain) vaccine in the former West Germany from 1976 through 1989 (Fescharek et al., 1990). During that period of time an estimated 5.5 million doses of measles, mumps, and measles-mumps vaccines and MMR were sold. Two of these patients had hydroceles. The other four patients recovered after 2 to 3 days "with only slight inconvenience to the vaccinee" (p. 447).

There have been 11 reports in VAERS (submitted between November 1990 and July 1992) of orchitis, or possible orchitis, following vaccination with MMR (10 reports) or mumps vaccine (1 report). The ages of the vaccinees ranged from 19 months to 26 years, with a median age of 12 years. The interval from immunization to the onset of symptoms was noted for nine patients and ranged from 1 to 34 days, with a median of 16 days. Six patients recovered, and no outcome was reported for five patients. Five cases were bilateral, and four cases were unilateral (all on the left side); for two cases the laterality was not specified. Seven patients were stated to have orchitis. The diagnosis was questionable in four patients. In one case the patient had been seen in the past for problems with his testicles. Following immunization he had three episodes of testicular swelling and pain, with each episode lasting about 2 hours. In another case, a urologist diagnosed torsion versus mild epididymitis and could not rule out the possibility that the condition was related to MMR. In another case, the patient did not have swollen testicles when examined on two occasions by a physician, although he was reported by his mother to have swollen testicles and swollen legs. In another, the patient had a swollen left testicle that was not red or hot to the touch and was diagnosed as having "testis disease."

In 1976, Borsche reported that after about 1,000 vaccinations with monovalent mumps vaccine, no side effects were noted.

A study of live attenuated mumps vaccine (Rubini strain) in monkeys, 13 adult males, and 60 children aged 15 to 24 months revealed no inflammation, swelling, or pain of the testes (Gluck et al., 1986).

Controlled Observational Studies

Penttinen and colleagues (1968) found that the frequency of orchitis as a complication of mumps was two to three times lower among recipients of mumps vaccine than among nonvaccinated servicemen. Furthermore, they found that the rate of orchitis was 25 times lower among the vaccinees than among nonvaccinated men, suggesting that the vaccine afforded protection from mumps orchitis.

Controlled Clinical Trials

Schwarz and colleagues (1975) looked for, but did not find, orchitis in 1,232 children who received MMR (Jeryl Lynn strain or a placebo).

Causality Argument

There is no evidence bearing on a causal relation between measles vaccine and orchitis or sterility.

Biologic plausibility for a causal relation between mumps vaccine and orchitis stems from the relation between wild-type mumps virus and orchitis (Association for the Study of Infectious Disease, 1974; Bendersky-Malbec, 1982; British Medical Journal, 1980; Sandler, 1954; Werner, 1950a,b) and from the temporal correlation between mumps vaccine and orchitis in several individual cases. Because orchitis is uncommon, it seems possible that cases temporally related to mumps vaccination are caused by the vaccine virus. However, it is also possible that at least some of the cases of orchitis following administration of mumps vaccine were caused by infection with wild-type virus, because the impetus to immunize males often is exposure to mumps disease. It should be noted that even though millions of doses of mumps vaccine have been administered, very few cases of mumps vaccine-associated orchitis have been reported.

There are no case reports of sterility in the literature or in VAERS (submitted between November 1990 and July 1992). However, these data are difficult to obtain because of the number of years required for follow-up. Because there are case reports of bilateral orchitis following administration of mumps vaccine, there is a possibility of sterility, and thus, a causal relation between mumps vaccine and sterility has not been fully studied.

Conclusion

There is no evidence bearing on a causal relation between measles vaccine and orchitis or sterility.

The available evidence is inadequate to accept or reject a causal relation between mumps vaccine and orchitis.

The available evidence is inadequate to accept or reject a causal relation between mumps vaccine and sterility.

THROMBOCYTOPENIA

Clinical Description

Thrombocytopenia is a decrease in the number of platelets, the cells involved in blood clotting. Thrombocytopenia may stem from the failure of platelet production, a shortened platelet life span, or an abnormal distribution of platelets within the body (Lee et al., 1993). Normal platelet counts are on the order of 150,000 to 450,000/mm^3. Thrombocytopenia occurs in children of all ages, with an incidence of 31.9 cases (defined as a platelet count less than 150,000/mm^3) per 1 million children under age 15 years per year (Cohn, 1976). Approximately 70 percent of cases occur following viral illnesses (Lightsey, 1980). In most cases, thrombocytopenia in children is mild and transient, and it is often discovered only incidentally when a complete blood count is performed. Severe thrombocytopenia associated with spontaneous bleeding, including bleeding into the skin, is called *thrombocytopenic purpura.*

History of Suspected Association

In 1966, Oski and Naiman reported a decrease of greater than 25,000/mm^3 in the platelet counts of 38 of 44 (86 percent) subjects immunized with live, attenuated Edmonston B measles vaccine. The lowest platelet counts were observed 1 week following immunization, and the platelet counts returned to prevaccination levels after 3 weeks in all but two patients. There were no petechiae and no purpura or bleeding problems in any of the patients. Nieminen and colleagues (1993) found acute thrombocytopenic purpura in 23 of approximately 700,000 children after they were immunized with MMR. The mean interval between immunization and purpura was 19 days. There also have been several individual case reports of thrombocytopenia following measles vaccination in the literature and VAERS. These studies are described in detail in a later section.

Evidence for Association

Biologic Plausibility

There is demonstrated biologic plausibility that measles or mumps vaccines could be associated with thrombocytopenia on the basis of experience with wild-type virus infections. Early case reports of purpura and bleeding associated with measles did not provide sufficient data to indicate the cause of bleeding. Specifically, they did not differentiate isolated thrombocytopenia from the thrombocytopenia found in disseminated intravascular coagulation. Severe hemorrhage is a well-documented, but rare, complication of infection with measles virus. It is known as the "black measles" because of hemorrhage into the skin (Hudson et al., 1956) and most likely results from disseminated intravascular coagulation. The first case of fatal purpura associated with measles was reported by Jackson in 1890. Hudson et al. (1956) reported 2 cases of thrombocytopenic purpura in patients with measles and reviewed 20 other cases reported in the literature. They found that the hemorrhagic manifestations began an average of 6 days (range, 2 to 14 days) after the onset of the measles rash. The number of circulating platelets ranged from 5,000 to 90,000 (average, 30,900) in the 12 patients for whom counts were available. In 1934, Perlman reported that there was "a rather constant tendency for the platelet count to drop below normal" (p. 602) in 50 random cases of measles. No data on the degree of thrombocytopenia were provided. Thrombocytopenia has been described as a rare complication of mumps disease (Graham et al., 1974).

Case Reports, Case Series, and Uncontrolled Observational Studies

Even though large numbers of doses of live attenuated measles vaccine have been administered, very few cases of thrombocytopenia have been reported. In 1965, Katz noted that he was aware of two cases of idiopathic thrombocytopenic purpura and one case of hemolytic-uremic syndrome after approximately 5 million doses of live attenuated measles vaccine had been administered over 6 years. The hemolytic-uremic syndrome is characterized by the triad of hemolytic anemia, thrombocytopenia, and acute renal insufficiency (Kaplan et al., 1987; Levin et al., 1989; Srivastava and Bagga, 1992). Rare cases of this syndrome have been documented following immunization (Srivastava and Bagga, 1992). In addition to the case noted above following administration of live attenuated measles vaccine (Katz, 1965), there have been other cases following administration of mumps vaccine (Dosik and Tricarico, 1970) and MMR (Taranger and Wiholm, 1987).

There are several individual case reports in the literature of thrombocytopenia following administration of live attenuated measles vaccine alone (Alter et al., 1968; Bach and Allard, 1974; DeRitis and Pecorari, 1990; Giroud et al., 1983; Kiefaber, 1981; Medical Journal of Australia, 1980) or concomitantly with immune globulin (Bachand et al., 1967; Saxton, 1967; Wilhelm and Paegle, 1967). Cases of thrombocytopenia also have been reported following administration of measles-mumps vaccine (von Muhlendahl, 1989) and MMR (Azeemuddin, 1987; Neiderud, 1983), but not after administration of mumps vaccine alone (other than that associated with hemolytic-uremic syndrome discussed above). The vast majority of cases of thrombocytopenia occur following the first dose of measles vaccine, but thrombocytopenia has been documented following administration of a second dose as well (Wiersbitzky et al., 1992). It should be noted that comparatively few individuals have received more than one dose of measles vaccine to date.

Case series and uncontrolled observational studies provide the bulk of the information regarding measles and measles-containing vaccines and thrombocytopenia. Taranger and Wiholm (1987) and Bottiger and colleagues (1987) found that 16 cases of thrombocytopenia following administration of MMR were reported to the Swedish health authorities over a 3-year period from 1982 through 1984, when an estimated 700,000 doses of MMR (using the same strains that are used in the United States) were sold and approximately 590,000 children were immunized. One other child had hemolytic-uremic syndrome (as noted above), but the child's platelet count was not reported. Fourteen cases of thrombocytopenia occurred in 18-month-old children. Eight of 13 patients with thrombocytopenia considered to have been vaccine related recovered without therapy. One patient had a second episode, and two patients responded to prednisone therapy within 2 months. Only one patient remained thrombocytopenic at 2 years of follow-up, but that patient had no clinical symptoms. Three other patients had a transient petechial rash, but platelet counts were not determined at the time of the rash.

In 1987, a new passive surveillance system for adverse reactions to vaccines was implemented in Canada (Koch et al., 1989). Five cases of thrombocytopenia were reported to this new system, for a cumulative incidence of 1 case per 100,000 doses of MMR distributed.

Fescharek and colleagues (1990) reported 11 cases of thrombocytopenia following administration of measles vaccine between 1976 and December 1989, over which period an estimated 5.5 million doses of measles and measles-mumps vaccines and MMR were sold in the former West Germany. All cases of thrombocytopenia occurred following immunization with vaccines containing the measles virus antigen (the same strain that is used in the United States). The lowest platelet count was 9,000. All 11 patients recovered either spontaneously or after steroid therapy.

Data suggesting that MMR can cause thrombocytopenic purpura have recently been reported by Nieminen and colleagues (1993). They found that 23 of about 700,000 children immunized with MMR in Finland (which uses the same vaccine strains as those used in the United States) developed thrombocytopenic purpura a mean of 19 days (median, 17 days; range, 7 to 59 days) following vaccination. The patients' ages ranged from 1.2 to 7.3 years. The median platelet nadir was $4,000/mm^3$, with a range of 1,000 to $45,000/mm^3$. Fifteen of the patients' platelet counts returned to greater than 100,000 within 1 month, 20 within 2 months, and 22 within 6 months. Thirty months later, one patient had a second episode associated with an infection.

Bone marrow aspirates were performed in 13 patients, and all revealed "at least normal" (p. 268) numbers of megakaryocytes. Platelet survival was decreased in both of the two patients studied, and platelet-associated immunoglobulin was detected in 10 of 15 patients tested. Five of six lost antibodies on follow-up 62 to 206 days after immunization, but one remained weakly positive at 132 days. Five of 15 patients had glycoprotein-specific platelet antibody.

There have been 12 reports in VAERS (submitted between November 1990 and July 1992) of thrombocytopenia following administration of measles vaccine (1 report) or MMR (11 reports). One case occurred after receipt of measles vaccine alone, six after receipt of MMR alone, and five cases after receipt of MMR plus one or more other vaccines (DPT, OPV, or Hib vaccine). The ages of the patients ranged from 12 months to 18 years. Seven of the 10 patients whose ages were given were 2 years old or younger. The interval between immunization and the onset of symptoms for the nine patients for whom these data were provided ranged from 6 to 27 days, and for six patients it was less than 14 days. Platelet counts were provided for 10 patients, and the lowest count for each was 4,000, 9,000, <10,000, 11,800, 17,000, 38,000, 43,000, 43,000, 55,000, and 65,000/mm^3. Five patients were reported to have recovered. The outcomes in the other seven patients were not specified.

Controlled Observational Studies

Data suggesting that the live measles vaccine can cause thrombocytopenia were provided by Oski and Naiman (1966), who found decreases in platelet counts in most subjects following administration of live attenuated measles vaccine (this vaccine is no longer used in the United States). They determined platelet counts of 59 individuals on a weekly basis until 21 days after administration of either live measles vaccine, live measles vaccine plus gamma globulin, gamma globulin alone, or killed measles vaccine. Twenty-five of 28 patients who received immune globulin along with measles vaccine and 13 of 16 patients who received measles vaccine alone had transient decreases in their platelet counts (mean maximum decrease of 92,000/mm^3 [representing a 37 percent decrease from the original platelet count] for those who received immune globulin versus 108,000/mm^3 [36 percent decrease from the original platelet count] for those who received measles vaccine alone). The median decrease in the 38 patients whose platelets fell by more than 25,000/mm^3 was in the range of 76,000 to 100,000/mm^3. In contrast, only 1 of the 10 patients who received gamma globulin alone and none of the 5 patients who received killed measles vaccine experienced a decline in platelet count.

In over 50 percent of patients vaccinated with live attenuated measles vaccine, the platelet count fell more than 75,000/mm^3 below its original level. The most dramatic decline was 317,000/mm^3 in an iron-deficient infant, whose original platelet count had been 570,000/mm^3. The lowest documented platelet count was 64,000/mm^3. The maximum depression was noted at 1 week, and postimmunization platelet counts returned to preimmunization levels in all but two vaccinees by 3 weeks postimmunization. In those patients whose platelet counts were determined more frequently, decreases were seen by 3 days postimmunization. A decrease in the platelet count of one infant was documented after each of three challenges with live attenuated measles vaccine.

The decrease in platelet counts was greater in children less than 2 years of age than in those over 12 years of age (126,000 versus 51,000/mm^3). It is not known whether maternal antibody plays a role in the accentuated platelet count decrease in infants less than 1 year of age. However, it seems unlikely since there was little difference between the degree of thrombocytopenia seen in patients who received measles vaccine alone and that seen in patients who received immune globulin along with the measles vaccine. It should be noted that measles vaccine is rarely given to infants who have the highest levels of maternal antibody (those less than 6 months of age).

Serial bone marrow aspirates from three patients were examined, and a decrease in the number of megakaryocytes was demonstrated by the third day postimmunization. The megakaryocytes also demonstrated morphologic alterations characterized by vacuolization of the cytoplasm and nucleus. In addition to the bone marrow findings, stable or decreasing plasma acid phosphatase determinations also suggested that the decrease in platelet count was more likely the result of decreased platelet production rather than increased destruction. This is in contrast to data of Hudson and colleagues (1956) suggesting that the thrombocytopenia following wild-type measles virus infection is caused by increased destruction of platelets.

Although Oski and colleagues (1966) speculated that the vaccine virus may replicate in the bone marrow since the onset of the vaccine-induced thrombocytopenia occurred during the incubation period of the live attenuated measles virus infection following immunization, they were unable to isolate the virus from the bone marrow on either of two occasions. It has been noted that the thrombocytopenia following wild-type virus infection occurs later, usually about 1 week following the onset of rash, not during the incubation period. Data suggesting that the measles vaccine virus can suppress the bone marrow are provided in a study by Olivares et al. (1989), who found a significant decrease in hemoglobin concentration by days 9 and 14 following administration of live attenuated measles vaccine (Schwarz strain) in infants studied prospectively at 0, 4, 9, 14, 21, and 30 days postimmunization. Platelet counts were not determined in that study.

Controlled Clinical Trials

None.

Causality Argument

Evidence that wild-type measles virus is associated with thrombocytopenia provides biologic plausibility that measles vaccine could also be associated with thrombocytopenia. Evidence from the study by Oski et al. (1966), individual reports in the literature, and VAERS suggests a causal relation between measles vaccine and thrombocytopenia. However, the measles vaccine strain (the live attenuated Edmonston B strain) studied by Oski is no longer used in the United States. The evidence concerning the live, more attenuated measles vaccine strain currently used in the United States is scarce. Although transient decreases in platelet counts following measles vaccination or from other nonvaccine causes may be common, clinically significant thrombocytopenia is extremely rare, especially considering the very large number of doses of measles vaccine that have been administered.

The reports of thrombocytopenia following mumps diseases provide biologic plausibility that mumps vaccine could be associated with thrombocytopenia. The evidence bearing on a causal relation between mumps vaccine and thrombocytopenia consists of one report of a child who had thrombocytopenia as part of hemolytic-uremic syndrome following receipt of mumps vaccine (Dosik and Tricarico, 1970).

Published reports of passive surveillance systems from several countries provide evidence that MMR is associated with clinically significant thrombocytopenia within two months of vaccination. On the basis of data from Finland and Sweden, the incidence appears to be on the order of 1 per 30,000 to 40,000 vaccinated children. This is a six-fold higher incidence than that reported in the only study of background incidence of thrombocytopenia identified by the committee (Cohn, 1976). The committee could not identify the component of MMR responsible for the thrombocytopenia, but the data from Oski and from the experience with wild-type measles virus suggest that the measles vaccine component of MMR might be responsible for the thrombocytopenia that occurs after MMR.

Conclusion

The evidence establishes a causal relation between MMR and thrombocytopenia. On the basis of data from Finland and Sweden, the incidence appears to be on the order of 1 per 30,000 to 40,000 vaccinated children.

The evidence is inadequate to accept or reject a causal relation between monovalent measles and mumps vaccines and thrombocytopenia.

Risk-Modifying Factors

Because so little information is available, the committee does not have the means to recommend any precautions to prevent clinically significant thrombocytopenia from occurring after administration of live attenuated measles vaccine or MMR. One child in the series by Nieminen and colleagues (1993) had had acute idiopathic thrombocytopenic purpura 9 months prior to the episode following MMR administration. Children with a prior history of thrombocytopenia may be at increased risk for developing thrombocytopenia following MMR.

ANAPHYLAXIS

Clinical Description

Anaphylaxis and anaphylactic shock refer to an acute, severe, and potentially lethal systemic allergic reaction. Most cases resolve without sequelae. Signs and symptoms begin within minutes to a few hours after exposure. Death, if it occurs, usually results from airway obstruction caused by laryngeal edema or bronchospasm and may be associated with cardiovascular collapse. Chapter 4 contains a detailed discussion of anaphylaxis.

History of Suspected Association

The suspected relation between measles and mumps vaccines and anaphylaxis is based on several reports of anaphylactic reactions following administration of measles or measles-mumps vaccines or MMR in the literature and VAERS (Aukrust et al., 1980; Fescharek et al., 1990; Herman et al., 1983; McEwen, 1983; Pollock and Morris, 1983; Taranger and Wiholm, 1987; Thurston, 1987; Van Asperen et al., 1981). No reports of anaphylaxis following administration of monovalent mumps vaccine have been published, but the 1991 *Red Book* states that since 1967 there have been rare, isolated reports of allergic reactions (American Academy of Pediatrics, Committee on Infectious Diseases, 1991).

Anaphylaxis to egg proteins has been considered to be a relative contraindication to immunization with live attenuated virus vaccines grown in eggs or in tissue culture cells of chicken embryo origin (American Academy of Pediatrics, Committee on Infectious Diseases, 1991). In 1983, Herman et al. reported generalized urticaria, angioedema, and respiratory difficulty after immunization with MMR in two children who had allergy to egg white protein (ovalbumin). Both had serum immunoglobulin E (IgE) reactive with the ovalbumin-related antigens in measles vaccine and MMR.

Evidence for Association

Biologic Plausibility

Concern has been raised regarding the safety of egg-derived vaccines in individuals who are sensitive to egg protein, since some individuals are exquisitely sensitive. Measles and mumps viruses in currently available monovalent and combination (measles-mumps and MMR) vaccines are grown in cell cultures of chicken embryo fibroblasts (rubella virus is grown in human diploid cell culture). Egg-related antigens can be detected in measles and mumps vaccines, but in extremely small quantities (much less than in the egg-derived vaccines).

Herman and colleagues (1983) reported that two children with systemic allergic reactions to egg white protein (ovalbumin) had anaphylactic reactions to MMR. Both children had serum IgE reactive with ovalbumin-related antigens in the vaccine. They had no detectable IgE directed against the measles vaccine, although IgE directed at ovalbumin was present.

Vaccine components other than egg protein have been implicated in triggering severe allergic reactions to live attenuated virus vaccines. Previously available live attenuated virus vaccines contained small amounts of antibiotics such as penicillin and streptomycin, but currently they have only trace amounts (25 µg/ml) of neomycin sulfate. They also have trace amounts of proteins such as chick embryo tissue culture protein and human serum albumin.

Case Reports, Case Series, and Uncontrolled Observational Studies

In 1981, Van Asperen et al. reported immediate reactions following administration of live attenuated measles vaccine (Rimevax) in three children in Australia. The reactions began within 30 minutes of immunization and consisted of vomiting, fever, and a rash; two of the patients also had cyanosis.

Pollock and Morris (1983) reported that nine reactions in the 170,000 children who received measles vaccine fell into their category of "anaphylaxis and collapse" during a 7-year period (January 1975 through December 1981) of intensified voluntary reporting of vaccine reactions in the North West Thames region of England. Some were felt to be vasovagal reactions, and some included slight facial swelling or pallor. It was unclear whether any of these reactions were anaphylactic.

Fifteen reports of reactions occurring within 30 minutes of vaccination with live attenuated measles virus (Rimevax) were received by the Adverse Drug Reactions Advisory Committee in Australia for the period February 1980 to March 1982 (McEwen, 1983). The most common findings were vomiting, changes in skin coloring, and disturbances of breathing. The mechanism of the reactions was unknown. Insufficient detail was provided to determine whether any of these reactions represented anaphylaxis. All individuals survived, and in 10 individuals the symptoms resolved without active treatment. The authors noted that the role that therapy played in the recovery of the other five children could not be assessed.

In a report from India (Sokhey, 1991), measles vaccine was involved in five incidents of adverse reactions in children. In three incidents, symptoms were felt to be typical of toxic shock. In one incident, 6 of the 12 children who received measles vaccine died. The six children who survived were said to have been saved by timely hospitalization and appropriate (but unspecified) treatment. Most of the incidents were felt to have been caused by contamination of the vaccines with pathogens, because the quality of the sterilization procedures was unsatisfactory. These incidents, however, were not described in sufficient detail to eliminate the possibility of anaphylactic shock.

In 1980, Aukrust et al. reported severe hypersensitivity or intolerance reactions to measles vaccine in six children. No description of the reactions was provided, although the authors felt that the children had immediate hypersensitivity reactions "most probably due to allergy." This measles vaccine was grown in monkey kidney cells (Aukrust et al., 1980). Trace amounts of calf serum proteins, but not egg antigens, were demonstrated in measles vaccine by crossed immunoelectrophoresis, but the exact cause of the untoward reactions was not identified. Four of the cases received the same lot of vaccine, suggesting the presence of an allergenic contaminant. The possibility of lot contamination also was suggested by the higher incidence of severe hypersensitivity reactions in Norway than in other countries (1 case per 15,000 to 20,000 doses versus 1 to 2 cases per 1 million doses, respectively) provided with the same vaccine by the same manufacturer.

Thurston (1987) reported two cases of anaphylaxis in his private practice. The first was an 18-month-old boy who developed bradycardia, cyanosis, periorbital edema, widespread erythema, and hypotonia 5 minutes after receiving MMR. He responded immediately to epinephrine. The second was a 16-month-old girl who started crying and who developed widespread erythema, cyanosis, decreased respiration, and wheezing 5 minutes after receiving MMR. She also responded to epinephrine.

The Swedish health authorities reported that no case with a clear picture of anaphylactic shock following administration of MMR was reported from 1982 to 1984, during which time 700,000 doses of MMR were sold in Sweden (Taranger and Wiholm, 1987). Five children had reactions that were described as anaphylactic or hypersensitivity reactions. These included a 12-year-old boy who developed urticaria with dyspnea and suspected laryngeal edema a couple of hours after immunization. He was treated with epinephrine and cortisone. Two 12-year-olds received epinephrine because of local redness and general symptoms of paleness and itching. An 18-month-old child was reported to have a diagnosis of mucocutaneous syndrome, but no further information was provided. A 5.5-year-old boy received cortisone and antihistamine orally for small urticaria.

In Germany, five reports of so-called immediate reactions were received after distribution of approximately 5.5 million doses of measles, mumps, and measles-mumps vaccines and MMR (Fescharek et al., 1990). Three reports were of siblings who all collapsed after having been vaccinated shortly after one another. These were considered to be probable psychosomatic reactions. Another was the possible aspiration of a piece of candy, and the last case was called an "anaphylactic reaction" but was not described further.

In the new passive surveillance system for adverse reactions to vaccines in Canada, 30 of the 511 reports of adverse events following administration of MMR in 1987 were of allergic reaction, for an estimated incidence of 6.6 reports per 100,000 doses distributed (Koch et al., 1989). No details of these reactions were given.

Nine cases of possible anaphylactic reactions following administration of measles or mumps vaccines have been reported to VAERS (submitted between November 1990 and July 1992). All of these reactions followed receipt of MMR. The ages of the patients ranged from 4 to 31 years, with a median age of 11 years. None of the reactions were described in sufficient detail to verify the diagnosis of anaphylaxis. Also, prompt treatment may have prevented some of the individuals from developing full-blown anaphylaxis. Reactions in six of the patients had at least one component of an anaphylactic reaction. Three cases probably did not represent anaphylaxis. One child began to cry 2 to 4 hours after vaccination, and she complained that she could not hear; then she became pale and sweaty. Her symptoms resolved after she was given a drink of 7-Up. Another had a probable vasovagal reaction. Another case listed complaints of weakness, dizziness, nausea, blurred vision, and decreased hearing in the right ear immediately after the vaccine was administered, but the patient went home with no residual effects.

Egg allergy refers to an IgE-mediated immediate reaction to ovalbumin, the most severe manifestation being anaphylactic shock. Most patients who react to the ovalbumin skin test can ingest ovalbumin without any difficulties. Genuine anaphylactic reactions are very rare. Most physicians feel that patients with severe systemic reactions to egg proteins should be considered to be at some increased risk for a severe systemic reaction to measles and mumps vaccines. Most also agree that patients who are skin test positive to egg protein but who do not have clinical symptoms are not at any higher risk of an adverse reaction than the general population. There is disagreement, however, on the usefulness of vaccine skin testing in predicting those children who should receive the vaccines in graded (desensitizing) doses in order to avert life-threatening reactions.

Several reports in the literature describe safe measles and MMR immunization of patients with varying degrees of allergic symptoms to egg protein, including severe immediate reactions (Brown and Wolfe, 1967; Bruno et al., 1990; Di Cristofano, 1989; Greenberg and Birx, 1988; Kamin et al., 1963, 1965; Kemp et al., 1990).

Herman and colleagues (1983) advocate intracutaneous testing with diluted vaccine prior to immunization with measles vaccine in children with systemic reactions to egg protein. They employed graded doses of measles vaccine to safely immunize six patients who had severe allergic hypersensitivity reactions to ovalbumin and IgE anti-measles vaccine antibody and positive reactions after intracutaneous or intradermal testing with the vaccine.

Lavi and colleagues (1990) gave MMR to 90 egg-allergic children after performing skin tests with diluted MMR. They confirmed the reliability of negative reactions to skin tests with diluted MMR in predicting that the vaccine can safely be administered to such children. However, they stressed the importance of skin testing with diluted MMR because three patients who had positive reactions to MMR skin tests developed generalized urticaria, despite graded challenges, suggesting that they may have developed more pronounced reactions if MMR had been given in a routine fashion. Indeed, Puvvada and colleagues (1993) reported systemic reactions after just intradermal skin testing with MMR in two patients with severe systemic reactions to egg.

Fasano and colleagues (1992) reported a case series of 140 children with egg hypersensitivity in whom the safety of MMR was evaluated. Sixty-nine of the 140 children already had received MMR and were not tested. Two of the remaining 71 children had positive skin prick reactions to MMR. Three of six egg-allergic children, as well as three of six normal adult control subjects, had positive responses to MMR intradermal testing. All 71 children were given MMR in the standard dose under close observation, and the only child with an immediate reaction had four small hives 15 to 25 minutes after immunization. However, systemic reactions to MMR were documented in two nonallergic children. Both were skin test negative to egg and neomycin. One had a positive skin prick test to MMR and its individual components (antigens). The other was skin prick test negative, but intradermal test positive to the same components (antigens). The authors concluded that MMR skin testing was not helpful in predicting an adverse reaction.

Skin prick testing with MMR was performed on subjects with documented or suspected systemic allergies to antigens other than egg before they were immunized with MMR (Juntunen-Backman et al., 1987). Of 135 individuals, 126 had negative skin prick tests to MMR. Mild generalized urticaria or fever was noted in 2 of the 122 vaccinees who eventually were vaccinated with MMR. The authors concluded that children with common forms of systemic allergy can safely be vaccinated with MMR.

MMR contains neomycin sulfate, which may be responsible for some immediate reactions to the vaccine (Kwitten et al., 1993). Elliman and Dhanraj (1991) reported safe MMR vaccination in one child, despite neomycin allergy documented by a positive reaction to skin patch testing with 20 percent neomycin sulfate.

Controlled Observational Studies

None.

Controlled Clinical Trials

None.

Causality Argument

Evidence from individual reports in VAERS and the literature is consistent with a causal relation between measles vaccine and MMR and anaphylaxis. The most compelling evidence consists of the cases reported by Herman and colleagues (1983) and by Thurston (1987). All four patients received MMR. In most cases of MMR-associated anaphylaxis, the precise component of the vaccine responsible for the severe reaction was not identified. In addition to the measles and mumps antigens, egg proteins, antibiotics, and other contaminants have been implicated. Reported cases of anaphylaxis following administration of these vaccines are extremely rare, and several reports suggest that anaphylaxis to measles vaccine is overreported and that not all of the cases are substantiated (Fescharek et al., 1990; McEwen, 1983; Pollock and Morris, 1983; Sokhey, 1991; Taranger and Wiholm, 1987; Thurston, 1987; Van Asperen et al., 1981). In 1983, Pollock and Morris estimated that anaphylaxis or collapse within 24 hours of vaccination occurred with a frequency of about 9 cases per 170,000 doses of measles vaccine administered in a large region of England over 7 years. In children with a history of anaphylactic reactions to egg, only five cases of immediate allergic reaction had been reported after distribution of more than 174 million doses of measles vaccine in the United States (American Academy of Pediatrics, Committee on Infectious Diseases, 1991).

Conclusion

The evidence establishes a causal relation between MMR and anaphylaxis.

The evidence favors acceptance of a causal relation between measles vaccine and anaphylaxis.

Because these conclusions are not based on controlled studies, the criteria for the diagnosis of anaphylaxis are variable, and pharmacologic intervention complicates the diagnosis, no reliable estimate of incidence or relative risk is available. Estimates from the studies described above range from 1 per 20,000 to 1 per 1 million doses distributed.

The evidence is inadequate to accept or reject a causal relation between mumps vaccine and anaphylaxis.

Risk-Modifying Factors

Most anaphylactic reactions occur in individuals who have no known risk factors for severe reactions to these vaccines; thus, no special precautions can be taken. Patients who have demonstrated severe systemic reactions to egg protein or neomycin may be at increased risk of anaphylaxis following receipt of measles or mumps vaccines, and guidelines for immunizing such patients have been provided by the Committee on Infectious Diseases of the American Academy of Pediatrics (1991). Patients with allergies to other antigens, including chickens and feathers, are not at increased risk of severe allergic reactions to these vaccines.

DEATH

A detailed discussion of the evidence regarding death following immunization can be found in Chapter 10. Only the causality argument and conclusions follow. See Chapter 10 for details.

Causality Argument

The data relating death and measles or mumps vaccine are from case reports and case series. The largest series comes from India, but toxic shock syndrome caused by the unhygienic conditions involved in the immunization program was the apparent cause of death reported for eight of nine patients. Evidence based on RNA sequencing techniques has linked measles vaccine and measles infection to subsequent death in some severely immunocompromised children. In contrast, studies of the immunogenic response to measles vaccine in children infected with human immunodeficiency virus, which causes acquired immune deficiency syndrome, have not recorded any deaths from measles infection.

The evidence favors the acceptance of a causal relation between measles vaccine and anaphylaxis. The evidence establishes a causal relation between MMR and thrombocytopenia and anaphylaxis. Anaphylaxis and thrombocytopenia can be fatal. Although there is *no direct evidence* of death as a consequence of measles vaccine-related anaphylaxis or of MMR-related thrombocytopenia or anaphylaxis, in the committee's judgment measles vaccine could cause fatal anaphylaxis and MMR could cause fatal thrombocytopenia or fatal anaphylaxis. There is no evidence or reason to believe that the case fatality rate of vaccine-related thrombocytopenia or anaphylaxis would differ from the case fatality rates for these adverse events associated with any other cause.

Conclusion

The evidence establishes a causal relation between vaccine-strain measles virus infection and death. The conclusion is based on case reports in immunocompromised individuals and not on controlled studies. No relative risk can be calculated. However, the risk of death from measles vaccine-strain infection would seem to be extraordinarily low.

The evidence establishes a causal relation between MMR and death from anaphylaxis or complications of severe thrombocytopenia. There is no direct evidence for this; the conclusion is based on the potential of thrombocytopenia and anaphylaxis to be fatal. The risk would seem to be extraordinarily low.

The evidence favors acceptance of a causal relation between measles vaccine and death from anaphylaxis. There is no direct evidence for this; the conclusion is based on the potential of anaphylaxis to be fatal. The risk would seem to be extraordinarily low.

The evidence is inadequate to accept or reject a causal relation between measles and mumps vaccines and death from causes other than those listed above.

REFERENCES

Abe T, Nonaka C, Hiraiwa M, Ushijima H, Fujii R. Acute and delayed neurologic reaction to inoculation with attenuated live measles virus. Brain and Development 1985;7:421-423.

Afzal MA, Pickford AR, Forsey T, Minor PD. Heterogeneous mumps vaccine. Lancet 1992;340:980-981.

Alderslade R, Bellman MH, Rawson NS, Ross EM, Miller DL. The National Childhood Encephalopathy Study: a report on 1,000 cases of serious neurological disorders in infants and young children from the NCES research team. In: Department of Health and Social Security. Whooping Cough: Reports from the Committee on the Safety of Medicines and the Joint Committee on Vaccination and Immunisation. Lond: Her Majesty's Stationery Office; 1981.

Alter HJ, Scanlon RT, Schechter GP. Thrombocytopenic purpura following vaccination with attenuated measles virus. American Journal of Diseases of Children 1968;115:111-113.

Alves RS, Barbosa ER, Scaff M. Postvaccinal parkinsonism. Movement Disorders 1992;7:178-180.

American Academy of Pediatrics, Committee on Infectious Diseases. The Red Book. Report of the Committee on Infectious Diseases, 22nd edition. Elk Grove, IL: American Academy of Pediatrics; 1991.

Asbury AK, Gibbs CJ Jr, eds. Autoimmune neuropathies: Guillain-Barré syndrome. Annals of Neurology 1990;27(Suppl.):S1-S79.

Association for the Study of Infectious Disease. A retrospective survey of the complications of mumps. Journal of the Royal College of General Practitioners 1974;24:552-556.

Aukrust L, Almeland TL, Refsum D, Aas K. Severe hypersensitivity or intolerance reactions to measles vaccine in six children: clinical and immunological studies. Allergy 1980;35:581-587.

Azeemuddin S. Thrombocytopenia purpura after combined vaccine against measles, mumps, and rubella (letter). Clinical Pediatrics 1987;26:318.

Azimi PH, Cramblett HG, Haynes RE. Mumps meningoencephalitis in children. Journal of the American Medical Association 1969;207:509-512.

Babbott FL Jr., Gordon JE. Modern measles. American Journal of Medical Science 1954;228:334-361.

Bach C, Allard M. Purpura thrombopenique aigu apres vaccination antirougeoleuse. A propos d'une observation. [Acute thrombocytopenic purpura after measles vaccination. Report of a case.] Semaine des Hopitaux de Paris 1974;50:589-593.

Bachand AJ, Rubenstein J, Morrison AN. Thrombocytopenic purpura following live measles vaccine. American Journal of Diseases of Children 1967;113:283-285.

Banatvala JE et al. Insulin-dependent (juvenile-onset, type I) diabetes mellitus: Coxsackie B viruses revisited. Progress in Medical Virology 1987;34:33-54.

Barbor PR, Grant DB. Encephalitis after measles vaccination. Lancet 1969;2:55-56.

Beale AJ. Measles vaccines. Proceedings of the Royal Society of Medicine 1974;67:1116-1119.

Beard CM, Benson RC, Kelalis PP, Elveback LR, Kurland LT. The incidence and outcome of mumps orchitis in Rochester, Minnesota, 1935-1974. Mayo Clinic Proceedings 1977;52:3-7.

Beersma MFC, Kapsenberg, JG, Renier WO, Galama JMD, Van Druten EN, Lucas, CJ. Subacute sclerosing panencephalitis in the Netherlands (1976-1986). Nederlands Tijdschrift voor Geneeskunde 1988;132:1194-1199.

Beghi E, Kurland LT, Mulder DW. Incidence of acute transverse myelitis in Rochester, Minnesota, 1970-1980, and implications with respect to influenza vaccine. Neuroepidemiology 1982;1:176-188.

Beghi E, Nicolosi A, Kurland LT, Mulder DW, Hauser WA, Shuster L. Encephalitis and aseptic meningitis, Olmsted County, Minnesota, 1950-1981. I. Epidemiology. Annals of Neurology 1984;16:283-294.

Bellanti JA, Sanga RL, Klutinis B et al. Antibody responses in serum and nasal secretions of children immunized with inactivated and attenuated measles-virus vaccines. New England Journal of Medicine 1969;260:628-633.

Bendersky-Malbec N. Les oreillons en 1982: mise au point sur le vaccin anti-ourlien. [Mumps in 1982: current situation concerning anti-mumps vaccine.] Concours Medecin 1982;104:167-177.

Blom L, Nystrom L, Dahlquist G. The Swedish childhood diabetes study: vaccinations and infections as risk determinants for diabetes in childhood. Diabetologia 1991;34:176-181.

Borsche A. Wie gefahrlich sind Impfungen im Kindesalter? [What are the hazards of vaccinations in childhood?] Zietschrift für Allemeinmedizin 1976;52:666-674.

Bottiger M, Christenson B, Romanus V, Taranger J, Strandell A. Swedish experience of two dose vaccination programme aiming at eliminating measles, mumps, and rubella. British Medical Journal 1987;295:1264-1267.

British Medical Journal. Prevention of mumps (editorial). British Medical Journal 1980;281:1231-1232.

Brodsky L, Stanievich J. Sensorineural hearing loss following live measles virus vaccination. International Journal of Pediatric Otorhinolaryngology 1985;10:159-163.

Brown EG, Furesz J, Dimock K, Yarosh W, Contreras G. Nucleotide sequence analysis of

Urabe mumps vaccine strain that caused meningitis in vaccine recipients. Vaccine 1991;9:840-842.

Brown FR, Wolfe HI. Chick embryo grown measles vaccine in an egg-sensitive child. Journal of Pediatrics 1967;71:868-869.

Bruno G, Giampietro PG, Grandolfo ME, Milita O, Businco L. Safety of measles immunisation in children with IgE-mediated egg allergy (letter). Lancet 1990;335:739.

Bunnell CE, Monif GR. Interstitial pancreatitis in the congenital rubella syndrome. Journal of Pediatrics 1972;80:465-466.

Buynak EB, Hilleman MR. Live attenuated mumps virus vaccine. I. Vaccine development. Proceedings of the Society for Experimental Biology and Medicine 1966;123:768-775.

Centers for Disease Control. Recommendations of the Public Health Service Advisory Committee on Immunization Practices: measles vaccines. Morbidity and Mortality Weekly Report 1967;16:169-271.

Cernescu C, Popescu-Tismana G, Alaicescu M, Popescu L, Cajal N. The continuous decrease in the number of SSPE annual cases ten years after compulsory anti-measles immunization. Revue Roumaine de Virologie 1990;41:13-18.

Champsaur HF, Bottazzo GF, Bertrams J, Assan R, Bach C. Virologic, immunologic, and genetic factors in insulin-dependent diabetes mellitus. Journal of Pediatrics 1982;100:15-20.

Cho CT, Lansky LJ, D'Souza BJ. Panencephalitis following measles vaccination. Journal of the American Medical Association 1973;224:1299.

Cizman M, Mozetic M, Radescek-Rakar R, Pleterski-Rigler D, Susec-Michieli M. Aseptic meningitis after vaccination against measles and mumps. Pediatric Infectious Disease Journal 1989;8:302-308.

Clark C, Hashim G, Rosenberg R. Transverse myelitis following rubeola vaccination. Neurology 1977;27:360.

Cohn J. Thrombocytopenia in childhood: an evaluation of 433 patients. Scandinavian Journal of Hematology 1976;16:226-240.

Coll JR. The incidence and complications of mumps. General Practitioner 1974;24:545-551.

Colville A, Pugh S. Mumps meningitis and measles, mumps, and rubella vaccine. Lancet 1992;340:786.

Craighead JE. The role of viruses in the pathogenesis of pancreatic disease and diabetes mellitus. Progress in Medical Virology 1975;19:161-214.

Dacou-Voutetakis C, Constantinidis M, Moschos S, Vlachou C, Matsaniotis MD. Diabetes mellitus following mumps: insulin reserve. American Journal of Diseases of Children 1974;127:890-891.

Dahlquist G, Blom L, Lonnberg G. The Swedish childhood diabetes study: a multivariate analysis of risk determinants for diabetes in different age groups. Diabetologia 1991;34:757-762.

De Prins F, Van Assche FA, Desmyter J, DeGroote J, Gepts W. Congenital rubella and diabetes mellitus. Lancet 1978;1:439-440.

De Ritis L, Pecorari R. Porpora trombocitopenica in seguito a vaccinazione antimorbillosa. [Thrombocytopenic purpura following measles vaccination.] Pediatria Medica e Chirurgica 1990;12:161-163.

Di Cristofano A. La vaccinazione contro il morbillo in bambini allergici all'uovo. [Measles vaccination in children allergic to eggs.] Professioni Infermieristiche (Roma) 1989;42:24-30.

Dietzsch HJ, Kiehl W. Zentralnervose Komplikationen nach Mmasern-Schutzimpfung. [Central nervous complications after measles vaccination.] Deutsche Gesundheit-Wesen 1976;31:2489-2491.

Dodson WE, Pasternak J, Trotter JL. Rapid deterioration in subacute sclerosing panencephalitis after measles immunisation (letter). Lancet 1978;1:767-768.

Dosik H, Tricarico F. Haemolytic-uraemic syndrome following mumps vaccination. Lancet 1970;1:247.

Dyken PR, Cunningham SC, Ward LC. Changing character of subacute sclerosing panencephalitis in the United States. Pediatric Neurology 1989;5:339-341.

Dyrberg T, Schwimmbeck PL, Oldstone MBA. Inhibition of diabetes in BB rats by virus infection. Journal of Clinical Investigation 1988;81:928-931.

Ehrengut W, Zastrow K. Komplikationen "nach" Mumpsschutzimpfungen in der Bundesrepublik Deutschland (einschliesslich Mehrfachschutzimpfungen). [Complications "following" mumps vaccinations in the Federal Republic of Germany (including combined vaccine immunizations).] Monatsschrift Kinderheilkunde 1989;137:398-402.

Elliman D, Dhanraj B. Safe MMR vaccination despite neomycin allergy (letter). Lancet 1991;337:365.

Enders JF. Techniques of laboratory diagnosis, tests for susceptibility, and experiments on specific prophylaxis. Journal of Pediatrics 1946;29:129-142.

Enders JF, Peebles TC. Propagation in tissue culture of cytopathic agents from patients with measles. Proceedings of the Society for Experimental Biology and Medicine 1954;86:277-286.

Enders-Ruckle G. Frequency, serodiagnosis and epidemiological features of subacute sclerosing panencephalitis (SSPE) and epidemiology and vaccination policy for measles in the Federal Republic of Germany (FRG). Developments in Biological Standardization 1978;41:195-207.

Fajans SS. Diabetes Mellitus. In: DeGroot LJ et al., ed. Endocrinology. Philadelphia: W.B. Saunders; 1989.

Fasano MB, Wood RA, Cooke SK, Sampson HA. Egg hypersensitivity and adverse reactions to measles, mumps, and rubella vaccine. Journal of Pediatrics 1992;120:878-881.

Fescharek R, Quast U, Maass G, Merkle W, Schwarz S. Measles-mumps vaccination in the FRG: an empirical analysis after 14 years of use. II. Tolerability and analysis of spontaneously reported side effects. Vaccine 1990;8:446-456.

Fujinaga T, Motegi Y, Tamura H, Kuroume T. A prefecture-wide survey of mumps meningitis associated with measles, mumps and rubella vaccine. Pediatric Infectious Disease Journal 1991;10:204-209.

Gale JL, Thapa PB, Bobo JK, Wassilak SGF, Mendelman PM, Foy HM. Acute neurological illness and DTP: report of a case-control study in Washington and Oregon. Sixth International Symposium on Pertussis Abstracts. DHHS Publication No. (FDA) 90-1162. Bethesda, MD: U.S. Public Health Service, U.S. Department of Health and Human Services; 1990.

Gamble DR. Relation of antecedent illness to development of diabetes in children. British Medical Journal 1980;281:99-101.

Gerson K, Haslam RH. Subtle immunologic abnormalities in four boys with subacute sclerosing panencephalitis. New England Journal of Medicine 1971;285:78-82.

Giroud M, Page G, Genelle B, Lacroix X. Les thrombopenies post vaccinales avec purpura [Post-vaccinal thrombopenia with purpura]. Journal de Medecine de Lyon 1983;64:97-100.

Gladisch R, Hofmann W, Waldherr R. Myokarditis und Insulitis nach Coxsackie virus Infektion. Zeitsch rift fur Kardiologie 1976;65:837-849.

Gluck R, Hoskins JM, Wegmann A, Just M, Germanier R. Rubini, a new live attenuated mumps vaccine virus strain for human diploid cells. Developments in Biological Standardization 1986;65:29-35.

Graham DY, Brown CH, Benrey J, Butel JS. Thrombocytopenia. Journal of the American Medical Association 1974;227:1161-1164.

Gray JA, Burns SM. Mumps meningitis following measles, mumps, and rubella immunisation (letter). Lancet 1989a;2:98.

Gray JA, Burns SM. Mumps vaccine meningitis (letter). Lancet 1989b;2:927.

Greenberg MA, Birx DL. Safe administration of mumps-measles-rubella vaccine in egg-allergic children. Journal of Pediatrics 1988;113:504-506.

Griffin MR, Ray WA, Mortimer EA, Fenichel GM, Schaffner W. Risk of seizures after measles-mumps-rubella immunization. Pediatrics 1991;88:881-885.

Grose C, Spigland I. Guillain-Barré syndrome following administration of live measles vaccine. American Journal of Medicine 1976;60:441-443.

Gunderson E. Is diabetes of infectious origin? Journal of Infectious Diseases 1927;41:197-202.

Gutierrez-Lopez MD, Bertera S, Chantres MT, Vavassori C, Dorman JS, Trucco M et al. Susceptibility to Type 1 (insulin-dependent) diabetes mellitus in Spanish patients correlates quantitatively with expression of HLA-DQ(alpha) ARG 52 and HLA-DQ(beta) non-Asp 57 alleles. Diabetologia 1992;35:583-588.

Halsey N. Risk of subacute sclerosing panencephalitis from measles vaccination. Pediatric Infectious Disease Journal 1990;9:857-858.

Halsey NA, Schubert W, Jabbour JT, Preblud SR. Measles vaccine and the course of subacute sclerosing panencephalitis (letter). Lancet 1978;2:783.

Halsey NA, Modlin JF, Jabbour JT, Dubey L, Eddins DL, Ludwig DD. Risk factors in subacute sclerosing panencephalitis: a case-control study. American Journal of Epidemiology 1980;111:415-424.

Harris HF. A case of diabetes mellitus quickly following mumps. Boston Medical and Surgical Journal 1899;140:465-469.

Haun U, Ehrhardt G. Zur problematik postvakzinaler Komplikationen nach Masernschutzimpfung. [Postvaccinal complications following protective vaccination against measles.] Deutsche Gesundheit-Wesen 1973;28:1306-1308.

Helmke K, Otten A, Willems WR, Brockhaus R, Mueller-Eckhardt G, Stief T et al. Islet cell antibodies and the development of diabetes mellitus in relation to mumps infection and mumps vaccination. Diabetologia 1986;29:30-33.

Herman JJ, Radin R, Schneiderman R. Allergic reactions to measles (rubeola) vaccine in patients hypersensitive to egg protein. Journal of Pediatrics 1983;102:196-199.

Hilleman MR, Buynak EB, Weibel RE, Stokes JJ, Whitman JE Jr, Leagus MB. Development and evaluation of the Moraten measles virus vaccine. Journal of the American Medical Association 1968a;206:587-590.

Hilleman MR, Buynak EB, Weibel RE et al. Live attenuated mumps-virus vaccine. New England Journal of Medicine 1968b;278:227-232.

Hinden E. Mumps followed by diabetes. Lancet 1962;1:1381.

Hirayama M. Measles vaccines used in Japan. Reviews of Infectious Diseases 1983;5:495-503.

Hirtz DG, Nelson KB, Ellenberg JH. Seizures following childhood immunizations. Journal of Pediatrics 1983;102:14-18.

Hudson JB, Weinstein L, Chang T et al. Thrombocytopenic purpura in measles. Journal of Pediatrics 1956;48:48-56.

Isomura S. Measles and measles vaccine in Japan. Acta Paediatrica Japonica 1988;30:154-162.

Jabbour JT, Duenas DA, Sever JL, Krebs HM, Horta-Barbosa L. Epidemiology of subacute sclerosing panencephalitis (SSPE). Journal of the American Medical Association 1972;220:959-962.

Jackson H. A fatal case of purpura with a few notes on the recent literature of this disease. Archives of Pediatrics 1890;7:951.

Jagdis F, Langston C, Gurwith M. Encephalitis after administration of live measles vaccine. Canadian Medical Association Journal 1975;112:972-975.

Jenson AB, Rosenberg HS, Notkins AL. Pancreatic islet cell damage in children with fatal viral infections. Lancet 1980;2:354-358.

Juntunen-Backman K, Peltola H, Backman A, Salo OP. Safe immunization of allergic children against measles, mumps, and rubella. American Journal of Diseases of Children 1987;141:1103-1105.

Kamin PB, Fein BT, Britton HA. Live, attenuated measles vaccine. Journal of the American Medical Association 1963;185:99-102.

Kamin PB, Fein BT, Britton HA. Use of live, attenuated measles virus vaccine in children allergic to egg protein. Journal of the American Medical Association 1965;193:1125-1126.

Kaplan BS, Proesmans W et al. The hemolytic uremic syndrome of childhood. Seminars in Hematology 1987;24:148-160.

Kaplan SA. Clinical Pediatric Endocrinology. Philadelphia: W.B. Saunders; 1990.

Katz SL. Immunization with live attenuated measles virus vaccine: five years' experience. Archiv für die Gesamte Virusforschung 1965;16:222-230.

Kazarian EL, Gager WE. Optic neuritis complicating measles, mumps, and rubella vaccination. American Journal of Ophthalmology 1978;86:544-547.

Kemp A, Van Asperen P, Mukhi A. Measles immunization in children with clinical reactions to egg protein. American Journal of Diseases of Children 1990;144:33-35.

Kiefaber RW. Thrombocytopenic purpura after measles vaccination (letter). New England Journal of Medicine 1981;305:225.

Klajman A, Sternbach M, Ranon L, Drucker M, Geminder D, Sadan N. Impaired delayed hypersensitivity in subacute sclerosing panencephalitis. Acta Paediatrica Scandinavica 1973;62:523-526.

Koch J, Leet C, McCarthy R, Carter A, Cuff W. Adverse events temporally associated with immunizing agents—1987 report/Manifestations facheuses associees dans le temps a des agents immunisants—rapport de 1987. Canada Diseases Weekly Report/Rapport Hebdomadaire des Maladies au Canada 1989;15:151-158.

Kremer HU. Juvenile diabetes as a sequel to mumps. American Journal of Medicine 1947;3:257-258.

Krugman S. Further-attenuated measles vaccine: characteristics and use. Reviews of Infectious Diseases 1983;5:477-481.

Krugman S, Giles JP, Jacobs AM, Friedman H. Studies with live attenuated measles-virus vaccine. American Journal of Diseases of Children 1962;103:353-363.

Kumar R, Chandra R, Bhushan V, Srivastava BC. Adverse reaction after measles immunization in a rural population. Indian Pediatrics 1982;19:605-610.

Kwitten PL, Rosen S, Sweinberg SK. MMR vaccine and neomycin allergy (letter). American Journal of Diseases of Children 1993;147:128-129.

Landrigan PJ, Witte JJ. Neurologic disorders following live measles-virus vaccination. Journal of the American Medical Association 1973;223:1459-1462.

Lavi S, Zimmerman B, Koren G, Gold R. Administration of measles, mumps, and rubella virus vaccine (live) to egg-allergic children. Journal of the American Medical Association 1990;263:269-271.

Lee GR, Foerster J, Athens JW, Lukens JN, eds. Wintrobe's Clinical Hematology, 9th edition. London: Lea & Febiger; 1993.

Levin M, Walter MD S., Barratt TM. Hemolytic uremic syndrome. Advances in Pediatric Infectious Disease 1989;4:51-81.

Lidin-Janson G, Strannegard O. Two cases of Guillain-Barré syndrome and encephalitis after measles. British Medical Journal 1972;2:572.

Lightsey AL. Thrombocytopenia in children. Pediatric Clinics of North America 1980;27:293-308.

Lipton RB, Kocova M, LaPorte RE, Dorman JS, Orchard TJ, Riley WJ, Drash Al, Becker Dɪ

Trucco. M. Autoimmunity and genetics contribute to the risk of insulin-dependent diabetes mellitus in families: islet cell antibodies and HLA DQ heterodimers. American Journal of Epidemiology 1992;136:503-512.

Maclaren N, Atkinson M. Is insulin-dependent diabetes mellitus environmentally induced? New England Journal of Medicine 1992;327:348-349.

Marshall GS, Wright PF, Fenichel GM, Karzon DT. Diffuse retinopathy following measles, mumps, and rubella vaccination. Pediatrics 1985;76:989-991.

Maspero A, Cancellieri V, Della Rosa C. Reazioni secondarie alla vaccinazione contro il morbillo. [Adverse reactions to measles vaccine.] Giornale di Malattie Infettive e Parassitarie 1991;43:499-503.

McCrae WM. Diabetes mellitus following mumps. Lancet 1963;1:1300-1301.

McDonald JC, Moore DL, Quennec P. Clinical and epidemiologic features of mumps meningoencephalitis and possible vaccine-related disease. Pediatric Infectious Disease Journal 1989;8:751-755.

McEwen J. Early-onset reaction after measles vaccination: further Australian reports. Medical Journal of Australia 1983;2:503-505.

McKendrick GDW, Nishtar T. Mumps orchitis and sterility. Public Health 1966;80:277-278.

Medical Journal of Australia. Measles vaccination: thrombocytopenia. Medical Journal of Australia 1980;1:561.

Medical Research Council. Vaccination against measles: clinical trial of live measles vaccine given alone and live vaccine preceded by killed virus. The Practitioner 1971;206:458-466.

Menser MA, Forrest JM, Bransby RD. Rubella infection and diabetes mellitus. Lancet 1978;1:57-60.

Messaritakis J. Diabetes following mumps in sibs. Archives of Disease in Childhood 1971;46:561.

Meyer MB. An epidemiologic study of mumps: its spread in school and families. American Journal of Hygiene 1962;75:259.

Mirchamsy H. Measles immunization in Iran. Reviews of Infectious Diseases 1983;5:491-494.

Mitus A, Holloway A, Evans AE, Enders JF. Attenuated measles vaccine in children with acute leukemia. American Journal of Diseases of Children 1962;103:243-248.

Modlin JF, Jabbour JT, Witte JJ, Halsey NA. Epidemiologic studies of measles, measles vaccine, and subacute sclerosing panencephalitis. Pediatrics 1977;59:505-512.

Monif GR. Rubella virus and the pancreas. Medecine et Chirurgie Digestives 1974;3:195-197.

Mori I, Torii S, Hamamoto Y, Kanda A, Tabata Y, Nagafuji H. [Virological evaluation of mumps meningitis following vaccination against mumps.] Kansenshogaku Zasshi [Journal of the Japanese Association for Infectious Diseases] 1991;65:226-283.

Morley DC. Measles in the developing world. Proceedings of the Royal Society of Medicine 1974;67:1112-1115.

Morrow JI, Dowey KE, Swallow MW. Subacute sclerosing panencephalitis in Northern Ireland: twenty years' experience. Ulster Medical Journal 1986;55:124-130.

Nabe-Nielsen J, Walter B. Unilateral total deafness as a complication of the measles-mumps-rubella vaccination. Scandinavian Audiology, Supplementum 1988a;30:69-70.

Nabe-Nielsen J, Walter B. Unilateral deafness as a complication of the mumps, measles, and rubella vaccination. British Medical Journal 1988b;297:489.

Nader PR, Warren RJ. Reported neurologic disorders following live measles vaccine. Pediatrics 1968;41:997-1001.

Neiderud J. Thrombocytopenic purpura after a combined vaccine against morbilli, parotitis and rubella. Acta Paediatrica Scandinavica 1983;72:613-614.

Nicolosi A, Hauser WA, Beghi E, Kurland LT. Epidemiology of central nervous system infections in Olmsted County, Minnesota, 1950-1981. Journal of Infectious Diseases 1986;154:399-408.

Nieminen U, Peltola H, Syrjala MT, Makipernaa A, Kekomaki R. Acute thrombocytopenic purpura following measles, mumps and rubella vaccination: a report on 23 patients. Acta Paediatrica 1993;82:267-270.

Norrby R. Polyradiculitis in connection with vaccination against morbilli, parotitis and rubella. Lakartidningen 1984;81:1636-1637.

Okuno Y, Nakao T, Ishida N, Konno T, Mizutani H, Fukuyama Y, et al. Incidence of subacute sclerosing panencephalitis following measles and measles vaccination in Japan. International Journal of Epidemiology 1989;18:684-689.

Oldstone MBA. Prevention of Type I diabetes in nonobese diabetic mice by virus infection. Science 1988;239:500-502.

Oldstone MBA. Viruses can cause disease in the absence of morphological evidence of cell injury: implication for uncovering new diseases in the future. The Journal of Infectious Diseases 1989;159:384-389.

Oldstone MBA, Ahmed R, Salvato M. Viruses as therapeutic agents II. Viral reassortants map prevention of insulin-dependent diabetes mellitus to the small RNA of lymphocytic choriomeningitis virus. Journal of Experimental Medicine 1990a;171:2091-2100.

Oldstone MBA, Tishon A, Schwimmbeck PL, Shyp S, Lewicki H, Dyrberg T. Cytotoxic T lymphocytes do not control lymphocytic choriomeningitis virus infection of BB diabetes-prone rats. Journal of General Virology 1990b;71(Pt. 4):785-791.

Olivares M, Walter T, Osorio M, Chadud P, Schlesinger L. Anemia of a mild viral infection: the measles vaccine as a model. Pediatrics 1989;84:851-855.

Oski FA, Naiman JL. Effect of live measles vaccine on the platelet count. New England Journal of Medicine 1966;275:352-356.

Otten A, Helmke K, Stief T, Mueller-Eckhard G, Willems WR, Federlin K. Mumps, mumps vaccination, islet cell antibodies and the first manifestation of diabetes mellitus type I. Behring Institute Mitteilungen 1984;75:83-88.

Ozeretskovskii NA, Gurvich EB. Pobochnoe deistvie vaktsin kalendaria profilakticheskikh privivok. [The side effects of vaccines used in prophylactic inoculation schedules.] Zhurnal Mikrobiologii, Epidemiologii, i Immunobiologii 1991;5:59-63.

Parker JC, Klintworth GK, Graham DG, Griffith JF. Uncommon morphologic features in sub-acute sclerosing panencephalities (SSPE). American Journal of Pathology 1970;61:275-291.

Parkkonen P, Hyoty H, Koskinen L, Leinikki P. Mumps virus infects beta cells in human fetal islet cell cultures upregulating the expression of HLA class I molecules. Diabetologia 1992;35:63-69.

Patrick A. Acute diabetes following mumps. British Medical Journal 1924;2:802.

Patterson K, Chandra RS, Jenson AB. Congenital rubella, insulitis, and diabetes mellitus in an infant. Lancet 1981;1:1048-1049.

Pawlowski B, Gries FA. Mumpsimpfung und Typ-I-Diabetes. [Mumps vaccination and type-I diabetes.] Deutsche Medizinische Wochenschrift 1991;116:635.

Payne FE, Baublis JV, Itabashi HH. Isolation of measles virus from cell cultures of brain from a patient with subacute sclerosing panencephalitis. New England Journal of Medicine 1969;281:585-589.

Peig M, Ercilla G, Millan M, Gomis R. Post-mumps diabetes mellitus (letter). Lancet 1981;1:1007.

Penttinen K, Cantell K, Somer P, Poikolainen A. Mumps vaccination in the Finnish defense forces. American Journal of Epidemiology 1968;88:234-244.

Perlman EC. Purpuric and cerebral manifestations following measles. Archives of Pediatrics 1934;51:596-604.

Philip RN, Reinhard KR, Lackman DB. Observations on a mumps epidemic in a "virgin" population. American Journal of Hygiene 1959;69:91-111.

Plotkin SA, Mortimer EA. Vaccines. Philadelphia: W.B. Saunders Co., 1988.

Pollock TM, Morris J. A 7-year survey of disorders attributed to vaccination in North West Thames region. Lancet 1983;1:753-757.

Prince GA, Jenson AB, Billups LC, Notkins AL. Infection of human pancreatic beta cell cultures with mumps virus. Nature 1978;271:158-161.

Puvvada L, Silverman B, Bassett C, Chiaramonte LT. Systemic reactions to measles-mumps-rubella vaccine skin testing. Pediatrics 1993;91:835-836.

Quast U, Hennessen W, Widmark RM. Vaccine induced mumps-like diseases. Developments in Biological Standardization 1979;43:269-272.

Rayfield EJ, Kelly KJ, Yoon JW. Rubella virus-induced diabetes in the hamster. Diabetes 1986;35:1278-1281.

Reed D, Brown G, Merrick R et al. A mumps epidemic on St. George Island, Alaska. Journal of the American Medical Association 1967;199:113-117.

Riikonen R. The role of infection and vaccination in the genesis of optic neuritis and multiple sclerosis in children. Acta Neurologica Scandinavica 1989;80:425-431.

Robbins FC. Measles: clinical features, pathogenesis, pathology, and complications. American Journal of Diseases of Children 1962;103:266-273.

Rubinstein P, Walker ME, Fedun B, Witt ME, Cooper LZ, Ginsberg-Fellner F. The HLA system in congenital rubella patients with and without diabetes. Diabetes 1982;31:1088-1091.

Sandler B. Recovery from sterility after mumps orchitis. British Medical Journal 1954;11:795.

Saxton NL. Thrombocytopenic purpura following the administration of attenuated live measles vaccine. Journal of the Iowa Medical Society 1967;57:1017-1018.

Schacher SA. An epidemiological approach to subacute sclerosing panencephalitis. Neurology 1968;18(1 Pt 2):76-77.

Schneck SA. Vaccination with measles and central nervous system disease. Neurology 1968;18(Pt 2):79-82.

Schwarz AJ. Immunization against measles: development and evaluation of a highly attenuated live measles vaccine. Annales de Paediatrie 1964;202:241-252.

Schwarz AJ, Anderson JT. Immunization with a further attenuated live measles virus vaccine. Archiv für Gesamte Virusforschung 1965;16:273-278.

Schwarz AJ, Jackson JE, Ehrenkranz NJ, Ventura A, Schiff GM, Walters VW. Clinical evaluation of a new measles-mumps-rubella trivalent vaccine. American Journal of Diseases of Children 1975;129:1408-1412.

Sinaniotis CA, Daskalopoulou E, Lapatsanis P, Doxiadis S. Diabetes mellitus after mumps vaccination (letter). Archives of Disease in Childhood 1975;50:749-750.

Sokhey J. Adverse events following immunization: 1990. Indian Pediatrics 1991;28:593-607.

Srivastava RN, Bagga A. Hemolytic uremic syndrome: recent developments. Indian Pediatrics 1992;29:11-24.

Starke G, Hlinak P, Nobel B, Winkler C, Kaesler G. Maserneradikation—eine Moglichkeit? Ergebnisse und Erfahrungen mit der Masernschutzimpfung 1967 bis 1969 in der DDR [Measles control—a possibility? Results and experiences with measles vaccination from 1967 to 1969 in the German Democratic Republic.] Deutsche Gesundheit-Wesen 1970;25:2384-2390.

Stokes JJ, Maris EP, Gelles SS. Chemical, clinical, and immunologic studies on the products of human plasma fractionation. XI. The use of concentrated normal human serum gamma globulin (human immune serum globulin) in the prevention and attenuation of measles. Journal of Clinical Investigations 1944;23:531-540.

Sugiura A, Yamada A. Aseptic meningitis as a complication of mumps vaccination. Pediatric Infectious Disease Journal 1991;10:209-213.

Sultz HA, Hart BA, Zielezny M, Schlesinger ER. Is mumps virus an etiologic factor in juvenile diabetes mellitus? Journal of Pediatrics 1975;86:654-656.

Taranger J, Wiholm BE. Litet antal biverkningar rapporterade efter vaccination mot massling-passjuka-roda hund. [The low number of reported adverse effects after vaccination against measles, mumps, rubella.] Lakartidningen 1987;84:948-950.

Thurston A. Anaphylactic shock reaction to measles vaccine (letter). Journal of the Royal College of General Practice 1987;37:41.

Tishon A, Oldstone MBA. Persistent virus infection associated with chemical manifestations of diabetes. American Journal of Pathology 1987;126:61-72.

Trump RC, White TR. Cerebellar ataxia presumed due to live, attenuated measles virus vaccine. Journal of the American Medical Association 1967;199:129-130.

U.S. Department of Health and Human Services. U.S. Public Health Service, National Vaccine Injury Compensation Program; Revision of the Vaccine Injury Table; Proposed Rule. Federal Register, 42 CFR Part 100, August 14, 1992;57(158):36877-36885.

Valmari P, Lanning M, Tuokko H, Kouvalainen K. Measles virus in the cerebrospinal fluid in postvaccination immunosuppressive measles encephalopathy. Pediatric Infectious Disease Journal 1987;6:59-63.

Van Asperen PP, McEniery J, Kemp AS. Immediate reactions following live attenuated measles vaccine. Medical Journal of Australia 1981;2:330-331.

von Muhlendahl KE. Nebenwirkungen und Komplikationen der Masern-Mumps-Impfung. [Side effects and complications of measles-mumps vaccination.] Monatsschrift Kinderheilkunde 1989;137:440-446.

Walker AM, Jick H, Perera DR, Knauss TA, Thompson RS. Neurologic events following diphtheria-tetanus-pertussis immunization. Pediatrics 1988;81:345-349.

Werner CA. Mumps orchitis and testicular atrophy. I. Occurrence. Annals of Internal Medicine 1950a; 32:1066-1074.

Werner CA. Mumps orchitis and testicular atrophy. II. A factor in male sterility. Annals of Internal Medicine 1950b;32:1075-1086.

White F. Measles vaccine associated encephalitis in Canada (letter). Lancet 1983;2:683-684.

Wiersbitzky S, Bruns R, Schroder C, Warmuth M. Thrombozytopenische Purpura nach Impfung mit Lebendvakzine (Mumps-Masern-Roteln-Schutzimpfung)? [Thrombocytopenic purpura following immunization with a live vaccine (mumps-measles-rubella vaccination)?] Kinderarztliche Praxis 1992;60:28-29.

Wilhelm DJ, Paegle RD. Thrombocytopenic purpura and pneumonia following measles vaccination. American Journal of Diseases of Children 1967;113:534-537.

Yamada A, Takeuchi K, Tanabayashi K, Hishiyama M, Takahashi Y, Sugiura A. Differentiation of the mumps vaccine strains from the wild viruses by the nucleotide sequences of the P gene. Vaccine 1990;8:553-557.

Yoon JW, Ray UR. Perspectives on the role of viruses in insulin-dependent diabetes. Diabetes Care 1985;8(Suppl 1):39-44.

Yoon JW, Onodera T, Notkins AL. Virus-induced diabetes mellitus: XV. Beta cell damage and insulin-dependent hyperglycemia in mice infected with Coxsackie virus B-4. Journal of Experimental Medicine 1978;148:1068-1080.

Yoon JW, Austin M, Onodera T, Notkins AL. Virus-induced diabetes mellitus. New England Journal of Medicine 1979;300:1173-1179.

Yoon JW, Eun HM, Essani K, Roncari DA, Bryan LE. Possible mechanisms in the pathogenesis of virus-induced diabetes mellitus. Medecine Clinique et Experimentale [Clinical and Investigative Medicine] 1987a;10:450-456.

Yoon JW, Kim CJ, Pak CY, McArthur RG et al. Effects of environmental factors on the development of insulin-dependent diabetes mellitus. Medecine Clinique et Experimentale [Clinical and Investigative Medicine] 1987b;10:457-469.

7

Polio Vaccines

BACKGROUND AND HISTORY

Poliomyelitis is an acute infectious disease caused by an enterovirus. There are three types of this virus: types 1, 2, and 3. Each type is capable of infecting humans; there is no cross-immunity and only those individuals immune to each of the three types are protected against all three types. The virus enters the body by the oral or respiratory route and multiplies in the pharynx and small intestine. Within 24 hours it invades the regional lymph nodes, and after an additional 24 to 48 hours it enters the bloodstream, which carries it to the secondary sites of replication in many organs, and thus, viremia develops and is maintained and enhanced. During the period of viremia, the virus can reach the central nervous system and initiate infection there. Antibodies appear within 1 week to 10 days after the initial infection, and viremia then ceases, probably as a consequence of neutralization by the antibodies. Only 1 to 2 percent of infected individuals develop disease in the central nervous system, and fewer still have residual paralysis. Nevertheless, the portent of these rare consequences is great, because they result in death or lifelong disability.

Although there are currently effective vaccines against poliovirus, even before they became available, Hammon et al. (1953) demonstrated the effectiveness of passive immunization by injections of pooled gamma globulin. Various attempts at developing a vaccine had been thwarted by the absence of an effective in vitro system of virus replication. The establishment in 1949 of the tissue culture technique for supporting virus growth made development of a vaccine possible (Enders et al., 1949). It was for these findings that J.F. Enders, F.C. Robbins, and T.H. Weller received the Nobel Prize in 1954. This development was followed by efforts to generate sufficient quantities of the virus to inactivate it and use it as an inert antigen. An alternative approach was to attenuate the wild-type virus and render it safe as a replicating antigen. Both were successful and today there are two forms of the vaccine: the inactivated polio vaccine (IPV), which is administered by the parenteral route, and the live attenuated vaccine, which is administered orally and hence is known as the oral polio vaccine (OPV).

IPV was developed in 1953 by Jonas Salk (Salk, 1953; Salk et al., 1953); OPV was developed by Koprowski and colleagues (1952), who were the first to use it, and Albert Sabin (1956). An enhanced-potency IPV was developed in the late 1970s and is used today. Currently, IPV and the Sabin strains of OPV are available for use in the United States; however, OPV is the vaccine recommended for general use and is the most prevalent (American Academy of Pediatrics, Committee on Infectious Diseases, 1991).

Shortly after the licensure of IPV in 1955, the vaccine manufactured by Cutter was found to cause paralytic disease. It contained residual infectious virus. The reason was traced to the method of inactivation. At that time the dynamics of the inactivation process were not fully understood, and the U.S. government's requirements for vaccine production were ambiguous. All of these problems have since been corrected.

The first OPV was licensed in 1960 after an extensive trial in the former Soviet Union (Benison, 1982). By then, over 100 million people in the former Soviet Union and Eastern Bloc countries—except Poland—had received the Sabin vaccine (LaForce, 1990). Trials of OPV in the United States followed, and monovalent OPVs were quickly licensed. The trivalent OPV used today was licensed in 1963. In the 1962 recommendations of the U.S. Public Health Service, no preference for one or the other form of the vaccine was expressed (U.S. Public Health Service, 1962), but in 1964 the Committee on Infectious Diseases of the American Academy of Pediatrics recommended the use of OPV.

Polio has been eliminated as an endemic disease in the United States and many developing countries. Outbreaks have occasionally occurred in subsets of unvaccinated susceptible individuals. A persistent concern has been the possibility of the rare complication of paralytic poliomyelitis in vaccinees and their contacts, particularly those with impaired immunity. This is discussed in detail later in this chapter. Some countries, for example, Denmark, use a mixed schedule of IPV followed by OPV. Other nations, such as Finland and Holland, continue to rely on IPV. The debate over the relative efficacy of OPV versus that of IPV continues in the literature, as does debate regarding the use of combined schedules of IPV and OPV (Institute of Medicine, 1977, 1988).

The American Academy of Pediatrics and the Advisory Committee on Immunization Practices recommend that OPV be administered at ages 2, 4, and 15 months and again at ages 4 to 6 years. If IPV is used, it should be given according to the same schedule as OPV.

BIOLOGIC EVENTS FOLLOWING IMMUNIZATION

Each of the three immunologically distinct types of poliovirus—types 1, 2, and 3—can cause paralytic disease. Both IPV and OPV stimulate immune responses against all three types of virus. OPV induces gastrointestinal mucosal immunity to a greater degree than IPV. The enhanced-potency IPV used today in the United States produces a humoral antibody response superior to that of OPV (Onorato et al., 1991). It is not clear whether either OPV or IPV confers lifelong immunity (Nishio et al., 1984). The mechanism of attenuation of the neurovirulence and that of occasional reversion to neurovirulence have been described in detail in a recent review (Racaniello, 1992). Recipients of OPV shed the virus in their feces, and contacts exposed to the virus can become infected.

POLIOMYELITIS

Clinical Description

Infection with poliovirus can take several forms: inapparent infection, mild illness, aseptic meningitis (nonparalytic poliomyelitis), and paralytic poliomyelitis. Approximately 4 to 8 percent of all wild-type poliovirus infections result in nonparalytic polio disease. This manifests as fever, malaise, headache, nausea, stiffness of the neck and back, and meningeal signs. Approximately 1 percent of infections results in paralytic disease. In paralytic poliomyelitis, the virus invades the central nervous system, replicating in motor neurons within the anterior horn of the spinal cord, in the brainstem, and in the motor cortex. When viral replication destroys sufficient numbers of neurons, paralysis occurs (Racaniello, 1992). The illness begins with a headache, fever, and stiff neck; this is followed by paralysis of the voluntary muscles previously controlled by the destroyed neurons of either the spinal cord or the brainstem. The muscle paralysis is usually asymmetrical. The spinal fluid contains an increased number of lymphocytes, the protein concentration is elevated, and the glucose concentration is normal.

History of Suspected Association

The association between live attenuated polio vaccine and cases of paralytic poliomyelitis dates back to the time of administration of the first live attenuated polio vaccine tried by Kolmer in the 1930s (Kolmer, 1936). Leake (1935) described nine cases of poliomyelitis that occurred following vaccination with the Kolmer vaccine and that seemed to be caused by the vaccine. The concept that live attenuated polio vaccine causes a small number of poliomyelitis cases thus has a history of at least six decades.

Shortly after licensing of Sabin's OPV, the United States Communicable Diseases Center (CDC; later named the Center for Disease Control, the Centers for Disease Control, and, more recently, the Centers for Disease Control and Prevention) reported its monitoring of vaccine-associated cases of paralytic polio. Henderson et al. (1964) summarized data for the United States collected by the CDC in 1962, 1963, and 1964. They evaluated 123 cases of paralytic polio that had occurred within 30 days of OPV administration and decided that 57 cases were compatible with vaccine-induced disease. Fifteen of the cases occurred after receiving the type 1 vaccine, with an estimated incidence of 0.17 case per 1 million doses. Thirty-six cases occurred following vaccination with the type 3 vaccine, with an incidence of 0.40 case per 1 million doses. Two cases occurred following vaccination with the type 2 vaccine, and four cases occurred following vaccination with the trivalent vaccine. The authors also described three cases of poliomyelitis that occurred in contacts of a recipient of the type 3 vaccine, but it is not clear whether the contact cases were included in the overall counts of vaccine-associated cases. Following publication of the paper by Henderson et al. (1964), case reports documenting vaccine-associated paralytic polio in recipients and contacts of recipients continued to appear. Table 7-1 summarizes the early case reports that described vaccine-associated poliomyelitis. By 1966, Chang et al. described a case of poliomyelitis in a 7-year-old recipient who was then found to have hypogammaglobulinemia. In 1966, Morse et al. documented a case of poliomyelitis in an unimmunized mother of a vaccinated infant. This was similar to the case of polio in an unimmunized father of a recently vaccinated infant reported by Swanson et al. (1967). Two reports provided evidence that contacts other than the parents or household members were also at risk of contracting polio. Balduzzi and Glasgow (1967) and Stolley et al. (1968) described unimmunized children who developed poliomyelitis after contact with recently vaccinated playmates or classmates.

TABLE 7-1 Early Reports of Vaccine-Associated Poliomyelitis, Published Before 1970

Reference	Recipients	Contacts
Chang et al., 1966	One 7-yr-old with hypogammaglobulinemia	
Morse et al., 1966		One adult (mother of infant)
Stolley et al., 1968		One 16-mo-old boy
Swanson et al., 1967		One 29-yr-old father of 2-yr-old recipient
Henderson et al., 1964	57 vaccine-associated cases (1962-1964; may include 3 contact cases)	Three cases
Balduzzi and Glasgow, 1967		One 5-yr-old boy
Cesario et al., 1969		One 5-yr-old

Evidence for Association

Biologic Plausibility

OPV consists of live attenuated viruses that multiply in the intestinal tract and that can revert to a more virulent form, causing disease. A vaccine recipient excretes live virus for several weeks, and recipients or contacts may become infected with the virus.

Case Reports, Case Series, and Uncontrolled Observational Studies

Since the 1960s there have been about 100 studies reporting individual cases, case series, and national surveillances of vaccine-associated cases of paralytic poliomyelitis. Case definitions have been well developed by the CDC and the World Health Organization (WHO); a case of vaccine-associated paralytic poliomyelitis is said to occur in recipients if the onset of the disease begins 7-30 days postvaccination and is said to occur in contacts of vaccine recipients if the onset of the disease begins 7-60 days after a recipient's vaccination. Laboratory tests can identify the strain of the infecting virus as a wild-type or vaccine strain of poliovirus. The cases described above in the section History of Suspected Association are typical of those that followed in the 1970s and 1980s.

WHO and CDC have used standard definitions of cases of paralytic poliomyelitis for almost 30 years, and many nations have implemented polio surveillance systems to monitor their polio immunization programs. Table 7-2 summarizes national data from the United States, England and Wales, Belgium, Spain, Romania, Hungary, Italy, and northern Greece. Despite

TABLE 7-2 National Surveillance Studies of Polio

Reference	Country	Years	Case Description
Andre, 1979	Belgium	1964-1978	25 cases
Bernal et al., 1987	Spain	1982-1984	9 recipients, 10 contacts, 2 immune-deficient
Biberi-Moroeanu and Muntiu, 1978	Romania	1970-1977	58 recipients, 27 contacts, 58 unclear
World Health Organization Consultative Group, 1982	Six unspecified countries	1970-1979	52 recipients, 70 contacts
Centers for Disease Control, 1984	United States	1982-1983	8 recipients, 9 contacts, 3 immune-deficient
Centers for Disease Control, 1986	United States	1975-1984	30 recipients, 41 contacts, 11 immune-deficient
Domok, 1984	Hungary	1961-1981	32 recipients, 13 contacts
Smith and Wherry, 1978	England and Wales	1969-1975	3 recipients, 7 contacts
Novello et al., 1987	Italy	1981-1985	3 cases temporally associated with vaccine
Centers for Disease Control, 1987	United States	1975-1986	37 recipients, 48 contacts, 13 immune-deficient
Frantzidou-Adamopoulou, 1992	Northern Greece	1976-1990	2 recipients

differences in the ways that data are categorized and reported and the changes in the incidence of polio from 1959 to the present, all the national data show a low incidence of vaccine-associated paralytic polio, on the order of a few cases per 1 million doses given or a few cases per 1 million vaccine recipients. The CDC data for the years 1975 to 1984 show an incidence of 1 case of vaccine-associated paralytic polio per 3.22 million doses of OPV distributed (Centers for Disease Control, 1986; Nkowane et al., 1987). When cases among immunodeficient recipients and contacts and patients with vaccine-like virus are included, the incidence is 1 case per 2.64 million doses of OPV distributed (Centers for Disease Control, 1986; Nkowane et al., 1987). The incidence is greater with the first dose of vaccine. The CDC has estimated that the overall dose-related incidence is 1 case per 520,000 first doses distributed versus 1 case per 12.3 million subsequent doses distributed (Nkowane et al., 1987).

The Monitoring System for Adverse Effects Following Immunization (MSAEFI) does not list poliomyelitis as a separate adverse event, although it may be included under categories such as "other neurologic symptoms," "other reactions," and "serious events." The Vaccine Adverse Event Reporting System (VAERS) contains several reports (submitted between November 1990 and July 1992) that may be cases of poliomyelitis, but the data are generally insufficient to state whether a case of vaccine-associated polio has occurred. Of the eight VAERS reports suggestive of vaccine-associated poliomyelitis, six provided insufficient information, one provided enough information to rule out vaccine-associated poliomyelitis (the time interval exceeded WHO guidelines), and one report provided information sufficient to be a well-documented case of vaccine-associated poliomyelitis. The report, which was filled out by a physician, stated, "Vaccine associated paralytic poliomyelitis confirmed by box 12 oligonucleotide sequencing of type III viral isolate. Occurred in an unvaccinated contact of a recently vaccinated eight-month old."

The data regarding OPV-related nonparalytic polio are more scarce than those for paralytic disease. A report of poliomyelitis surveillance in England and Wales from 1969 to 1975 documented 44 cases of nonparalytic poliomyelitis (Smith and Wherry, 1978). (Included in this definition were patients with a clinical diagnosis of nonparalytic poliomyelitis, as well as those with encephalitis or aseptic meningitis who also had cultural or serologic evidence of poliovirus infection.) Twelve of those cases were believed to have been associated with administration of OPV (11 in recipients, 1 in a contact). Poliovirus was isolated from 8 of the 11 recipient cases. All of the viruses were typed as the vaccine strain on the basis of reproductive capacity temperature (RCT) tests. Virus isolated from the one contact case was also typed as the vaccine strain. The authors calculated incidence rates of 0.1 per 1 million population at risk per year for both the paralytic and nonparalytic forms of disease. The authors noted that the definition of nonparalytic disease was, perhaps, broad, and thus, this represents an estimate of the highest possible number of nonparalytic cases. Poliovirus was isolated from recently vaccinated patients in the former West Germany between 1965 and 1970 (Thraenhart and Kuwert, 1972). Of the 34 patients with aseptic meningitis, virus isolated from 17 patients was typed by the RCT test as vaccine strain, from 13 patients as wild-type, and from 4 patients as intermediate. A study of the incidence of aseptic meningitis in Olmsted County, Minnesota, from 1950 to 1981 reported that 2 of the 283 patients with aseptic meningitis had received polio vaccine within 4 weeks prior to the onset of symptoms (Beghi et al., 1984). However, no mention of virus isolation was made, and the disease cannot be ascribed to the vaccine.

Controlled Observational Studies

    None.

Controlled Clinical Trials

    None.

Causality Argument

Vaccination with live virus mimics a natural process of exposure to virus that results in immunity to the disease. Although the vaccine virus is attenuated, approximately 1 in 1 million vaccinations with attenuated virus leads to paralytic disease. Infection in the intestinal tract with the vaccine strain of poliovirus results in virus shedding in the feces and the risk that the contacts of a recipient might become infected. The vaccine virus can revert to a virulent form, and this lends demonstrated biologic plausibility to the finding that occasional contacts of vaccine recipients contract polio.

Paralytic poliomyelitis, as an adverse event associated with OPV vaccination, occurs among OPV recipients and contacts of OPV recipients. The presence of vaccine virus in patients suspected of having vaccine-associated polio is often confirmed by laboratory tests that permit specific identification of the virus as the vaccine or wild-type virus. In countries where wild-type poliovirus has almost been eradicated, there is usually no other means of exposure to poliovirus that could explain a case of polio. The confirmation by laboratory tests, the absence of circulating wild-type virus, and the temporal association of paralytic polio with receipt of OPV (onset of illness within 30 days postvaccination in recipients and 60 days in contacts of vaccine recipients), all of which have been seen in the well-documented cases of vaccine-associated polio, fulfill the criteria of infectious disease causality. Surveillance of nonparalytic polio following OPV administration has been much less rigorous and thus, less well-documented in the literature. The arguments in support of accepting a causal relation between OPV and paralytic poliomyelitis apply, most certainly, to the relation between OPV and nonparalytic polio. The quantitative evidence, however, is less complete.

Conclusion

The evidence establishes a causal relation between OPV and paralytic and nonparalytic polio. The incidence of paralytic polio in OPV recipients has been well documented and is greater with the first dose of vaccine. The CDC has estimated that the overall dose-related incidence of paralytic disease is 1 case per 520,000 first doses administered versus 1 case per 12.3 million subsequent doses administered (Nkowane et al., 1987). It is clear that OPV can lead to vaccine-strain infection in contacts as well. There are no data with which to calculate an incidence, but on the basis of data on wild-type poliovirus infection, the incidence of vaccine-related nonparalytic disease would be expected to be slightly greater than the incidence of paralytic disease.

Risk-Modifying Factors

The immune status of a vaccine recipient or a contact of a vaccine recipient modifies the risk of polio as an adverse event associated with OPV vaccination. Among OPV recipients, various types of immunodeficiency are often diagnosed after a patient develops polio after immunization with OPV. These cases are described in Table 7-3. Nonimmune contacts are at increased risk of developing polio after exposure to a person immunized with OPV. These cases are described in Table 7-4. Most of the case reports describe unimmunized contacts who contracted polio, but two case reports describe immunodeficient contacts who contracted polio. For both vaccine recipients and their contacts, case reports may or may not be representative of the vaccine-associated cases of polio that occur in immunodeficient people. The CDC reports its cases of polio among immunodeficient people without categorizing the case as contacts or recipients (Centers for Disease Control, 1984, 1986). Unimmunized siblings and playmates of recipients continue to be at risk of contracting polio and may constitute a special risk group. With the increasingly younger age of entry into day care, there is a growing group of nonimmunized infants who may be exposed to infants recently immunized with OPV. The committee's review uncovered case reports of two infants, ages 20 days and 4 months (Bergeisen et al., 1986; Wilson and Robinson, 1974), who were unimmunized and who contracted polio from contact with a care giver and other infants.

TABLE 7-3 Cases of Polio Among Immune-Deficient Recipients

Reference	Type of Immune Deficiency
Chang et al., 1966	Hypogammaglobulinemia
Davis et al., 1977	Same case described by Saulsbury et al. (1975)
Loffel et al., 1982	68-yr-old man on chemotherapy for non-Hodgkin's lymphoma
Mathias and Routley, 1985	Chronic lymphatic leukemia in a 63-yr-old man treated with immunosuppressive medication (chlorambucil, prednisone) before and 10 days after vaccination
Sakano et al., 1980	Agammaglobulinemia
Saulsbury et al., 1975	Short-limbed dwarfism, cartilage-hair hypoplasia, small thymus, deficient antibody-mediated immunity as well as cell-mediated immunity
Wright et al., 1977	Agammaglobulinemia

TRANSVERSE MYELITIS

Clinical Description

Transverse myelitis is characterized by the acute onset of signs of spinal cord disease, usually involving the descending motor tracts and the ascending sensory fibers, suggesting a lesion at one level of the spinal cord. The annual incidence of transverse myelitis in Rochester, Minnesota, from 1970 to 1981 was 0.83 per 100,000 people (Beghi et al., 1982). Chapter 3 contains a more complete discussion of transverse myelitis.

History of Suspected Association

There is no particular history of an association between transverse myelitis and polio vaccines.

Evidence for Association

Biologic Plausibility

Chapter 3 contains a discussion of the biologic plausibility for a causal relation between demyelinating disorders and vaccines in general.

TABLE 7-4 Cases of Polio Among Nonimmune Contacts of Polio
Recipients

Reference	Relationship to Recipient	Immune Deficiency or History of Polio Immunization in Contact
Derenne et al., 1989	26-yr-old mother of infant	Remembered receiving polio vaccine as a child
Wiechers, 1988	19-yr-old mother of infant	No information
Arlazoroff et al., 1987	34-yr-old father of infant and 10-yr-old relative of infant	No information
Bateman et al., 1987	16-yr-old uncle of infant, 23-yr-old father of infant	Unimmunized
Canadian Medical Association Journal, 1987	25-yr-old father of infant	Unclear
	19-yr-old mother of infant	Unclear
Gross et al., 1987	40-yr-old father of infant	Patient on long-term steroid therapy for Netherton's syndrome
Maass and Quast, 1987	26-yr-old father of infant	Previous vaccination against type 1 and type 3 polioviruses
	32-yr-old father of infant/ husband of recipients	Unknown
	31-yr-old mother of infant	Previous vaccination against type 1 poliovirus
	48-yr-old grandmother of infant	Unknown
	6-wk-old sibling/son of recipients	Unknown
	21-yr-old male in contact with immunized infant	Unknown
Bell et al., 1986	19-yr-old male—contact not known	Received one dose of OPV as a child
	39-yr-old man—contact not known	Received one dose of Salk vaccine as a child
	24-yr-old woman, neighbor of children	Unvaccinated
Bergeisen et al., 1986	20-day-old contact of baby-sitter and sitter's infant	Unimmunized
British Medical Journal, 1986	23-yr-old father of infant	No information
Daneault et al., 1986	25-yr-old father of infant	Received Salk vaccine as a child
Ishizaki and Noda, 1986	No information	No information
Kruppenbacher et al., 1983	Mother of infant	No information
Openshaw and Lieberman, 1983	43-yr-old grandfather of infant	Unimmunized
Basillico and Bernat, 1978	30 yr-old father of infant	No information
Collingham et al., 1978	5-yr-old sibling of recipient	Unimmunized
	Young adult father of infant	Unknown

continued

TABLE 7-4 *(continued)*

Reference	Relationship to Recipient	Immune Deficiency or History of Polio Immunization in Contact
Adams et al., 1977	31-yr-old mother of infant	Depressed T-cell function
Orzechowska-Wolczyk et al., 1976	25-yr-old mother of child	No information
Wilson and Robinson, 1974	4-mo-old contact of infant	Unimmunized
Kostrzewski, 1973	Six children in group care	No information
Haneberg and Orstavik, 1972	1-yr-old younger brother of 10-yr-old recipient	Unimmunized
Kuwert et al., 1971	48-yr-old grandmother	No information
Riker et al., 1971	8-mo-old sibling of a recipient	Probable hereditary thymic dysplasia
Stolley et al., 1968	16-mo-old cousin of recipient	Probable hypogamma-globulinemia, unimmunized
Balduzzi and Glasgow, 1967	5-yr-old classmate of recipient	Had received four doses of Salk vaccine and one dose of type 2 Sabin vaccine
Swanson et al., 1967	29-yr-old father of 2-yr-old	Unimmunized
Morse et al., 1966	43-yr-old mother of infant	Unimmunized

Case Reports, Case Series, and Uncontrolled Observational Studies

Table 7-5 summarizes the three cases of transverse myelitis that have been reported in the literature to occur following vaccination with OPV. Two cases occurred in infants. A seven-month old girl developed symptoms 6 days after receiving OPV and diphtheria and tetanus toxoids (DT) (Whittle and Roberton, 1977). A 20-month girl developed symptoms 1 month after receiving OPV and diphtheria and tetanus toxoids and pertussis vaccine (DPT). She was found to be hypogammaglobulinemic (Douglas and Anolik, 1981). The third case occurred in a 24-year-old woman who was simultaneously vaccinated with OPV and typhoid and cholera vaccines (D'Costa et al., 1990). The woman had a fever at the time of vaccination and had an upper respiratory tract infection and pharyngitis for the 5 weeks preceding vaccination. The committee is aware of a case of transverse myelitis in a child with severe combined immunodeficiency syndrome (Richard B. Johnston, Yale University, New Haven, personal communication, 1993). Vaccine-strain poliovirus was isolated from the myocardium. VAERS listed two cases (submitted between November 1990 and July 1992) of transverse myelitis that occurred in patients after receiving a combination

TABLE 7-5 Reports Associating Transverse Myelitis with Polio Vaccine

Reference	No. of Cases	Age of Patients	Time of Onset After Vaccination	Vaccine Given
Whittle and Roberton, 1977	1	7 mo	6 days	OPV; DT
Douglas and Anolik, 1981	1	20 mo	1 mo	OPV; DPT
D'Costa et al., 1990	1	24 yr	36 h	OPV; cholera; typhoid

of DPT, OPV, and *Haemophilus influenzae* type b (Hib) vaccine and a combination of DPT, OPV, measles-mumps-rubella vaccine (MMR), and Hib vaccine, but the temporal and clinical details are insufficient for proper evaluation. Another VAERS report of transverse myelitis was a duplicate of the case report published in 1990 and discussed above (the 24-year-old woman). In addition, at a public meeting held in January 1993, the committee heard about a 4-month-old girl who developed transverse myelitis, diagnosed by neurologists, a few days after her second DPT and OPV immunizations. This was thought by the physicians treating the girl to be related to her immunizations (see Appendix B).

Controlled Observational Studies

None.

Controlled Clinical Trials

None.

Causality Argument

There is biologic plausibility that viral vaccines can cause demyelinating disorders. Vaccine-strain poliovirus can enter the central nervous system and has been associated with a peripheral nerve demyelinating disorder, Guillain-Barré syndrome (see next section). The three cases of transverse myelitis following receipt of OPV reported in the literature, the two cases reported in VAERS, and the case identified by the committee in a personal communication are inadequate to indicate an association between OPV and transverse myelitis beyond that due to chance alone. At least five of the cases occurred following multiple immunizations, which complicates an assessment of a causal relation between OPV and transverse myelitis. No cases of transverse myelitis following receipt of IPV have been reported.

Conclusion

The evidence is inadequate to accept or reject a causal relation between OPV and transverse myelitis.

There is no evidence bearing on a causal relation between IPV and transverse myelitis.

GUILLAIN-BARRÉ SYNDROME

Clinical Description

Guillain-Barré syndrome (GBS) is characterized by the rapid onset of flaccid motor weakness with depression of tendon reflexes and inflammatory demyelination of peripheral nerves. The annual incidence of GBS appears to be approximately 1 per 100,000 for adults. The data are not definitive, but the annual incidence of GBS in children under age 5 years appears to be approximately the same. The annual incidence of GBS in children over age 5 years and teenagers appears to be lower. Chapter 3 contains a detailed discussion of GBS.

History of Suspected Association

A relation between attenuated viral vaccines and demyelinating disease has been investigated for many years, as described in Chapter 3. Specific interest in the relation between GBS and polio vaccine was triggered by a report in 1976 of 10 cases of GBS in patients who had received IPV (Andersen and Eeg-Olofsson, 1976).

Evidence for Association

Biologic Plausibility

Chapter 3 contains a detailed discussion of the arguments that vaccines can cause demyelination, including GBS. There are no additional data demonstrating the biologic plausibility of a specific relation between polio vaccines and GBS.

Case Reports, Case Series, and Uncontrolled Observational Studies

Grose and Spigland (1976) describe a 10-month-old girl who developed GBS 4 to 7 days after receiving measles vaccine, DPT, and OPV. Poliovirus type 1 was isolated from a throat swab. The authors attributed the disease to the measles vaccine.

Leneman (1966) reviewed the literature prior to 1966 and described 1,100 case reports of GBS published between 1949 and 1966. In five cases, vaccination with IPV was mentioned, although the time interval between vaccination and the onset of GBS was not described. Changes in diagnostic procedures since 1949 might also disqualify some of the cases included in that summary. This secondhand summary of case reports does not supply sufficient information to determine whether IPV is associated with GBS.

In a study in Sweden, which utilized IPV exclusively, Andersen and Eeg-Olofsson (1976) discussed 10 cases of GBS that occurred in 1971 in individuals less than 60 years of age. In nine of the individuals, the onset of GBS occurred more than 1 year after a vaccination with IPV. The authors concluded that there was no association between IPV and GBS.

Data from the MSAEFI noted 14 cases of GBS following OPV administration from 1979 to 1990. In most cases OPV was given in combination with DPT, or MMR, or both. VAERS listed two cases of GBS (submitted between November 1990 and July 1992) following administration of OPV in combination with DPT and either MMR or Hib vaccine.

Controlled Observational Studies

Two controlled studies examined the association between GBS and polio vaccine (Table 7-6).

The first study took place in a southern province of Finland (Uusimaa), where continuing surveillance of GBS from 1981 to 1986 uncovered an increase in the incidence of GBS following a nationwide program of immu-

TABLE 7-6 Reports Associating Guillain-Barré Syndrome with Polio Vaccines

Reference (location)	No. of Cases	Age of Patients (yr)	Time of Onset After Vaccination	Vaccines Given
Andersen and Eeg-Olofsson, 1976 (Sweden)	10	2-53	>1 yr for all except one case	IPV; others not discussed
Kinnunen et al., 1989 (Finland)	10	15-73	<10 wk	OPV alone (nine patients); IPV + OPV (one patient)
Uhari et al., 1989 (Finland)	27	0.4-14.3	<10 wk	Five patients were immunized with OPV

nizing children and adults against polio (Kinnunen et al., 1989). At that time, Finland generally used IPV, but an outbreak of 10 cases of poliomyelitis between August 1984 and January 1985 led to the decision to carry out a mass immunization with OPV. Ninety-four percent of the Finnish population was vaccinated with OPV during a 5-week period between February 10 and March 15, 1985. During and shortly after the immunization campaign, hospitals in the southern province, Uusimaa (population, approximately 1.17 million), received an unexpectedly high number of patients with GBS. The first and second quarters of 1985 showed a statistically significant higher number of cases of GBS than were found in the other quarters of the observational period. Over the 6-year period from 1981 to 1986 (including the period of OPV immunization), the mean number of cases of GBS per quarter was 3, and Kinnunen estimated a crude annual incidence of 1 case per 100,000 population. This is significantly higher than the mean for the 6-year period. Ten cases occurred in the first quarter and 6 cases occurred in the second quarter of 1985, the times corresponding to the immunization campaign. Ten patients were diagnosed with GBS within 10 weeks after vaccination with OPV, with the mean time of onset occurring at 31 days postvaccination. Six of the cases occurred within 6 weeks of vaccination. All patients with suspected GBS were evaluated separately by two neurologists, and consensus on the diagnosis was reached in every case. The patients' ages ranged from 15 to 73 years.

The study in Finland took advantage of two unique phenomena: a continuing surveillance of GBS that identified cases in the population over a 6-year period and a national program of immunizing adults in a 5-week period. The data showed an increase in the number of cases of GBS temporally associated with the immunization program, and the increase was statistically significant. The diagnosis of GBS was made by using consistent criteria throughout the observation period because of the prospective study on GBS that was in place well before the polio epidemic and immunization against polio occurred.

The study in Finland presents evidence that OPV may be associated with GBS and raises the question of why there have not been other reports of GBS associated with OPV. One explanation may be that the rarity of GBS, the usual predominance of GBS in adults, and the rarity of administration of OPV to adults have not produced any recognized cases of OPV-associated GBS. Kinnunen et al. (1989) estimated a crude annual incidence of 1 case of GBS per 100,000 population. The 10 cases that were considered vaccine associated occurred in patients ages 15 to 73 years. Six of the patients were in their 50s and two were in their 30s. If GBS mainly occurs in adults and relatively few adults receive OPV, the probability of uncovering a case of OPV-associated GBS without a surveillance system is low.

At the same time that Kinnunen et al. (1989) published the results of their study, Uhari et al. (1989) published a letter describing a cluster of GBS cases in children in Finland. They identified 27 cases of GBS in children ages 0.4 to 14.3 years over the 7-year period from 1980 to 1986, with an average incidence of 3.9 cases per year. They also noted a peak of 10 cases in 1985, which was different from the number of cases noted in other years, and the difference was statistically significant ($P = 0.0042$). Unlike Kinnunen et al. (1989), Uhari and colleagues did not confirm that the children with GBS had actually received OPV within the 6 weeks prior to the onset of GBS. They demonstrated an ecologic and temporal association between the OPV campaign and the cluster of GBS cases.

Controlled Clinical Trials

None.

Causality Argument

Other viruses and vaccines have been found to be associated with GBS (see Chapter 3), and it is biologically plausible that OPV may also be associated with GBS. Of the two controlled studies examining the relation between OPV and GBS, one study provided evidence that there may be an effect in adults, and the second study suggested that there may be an effect in children (Table 7-6). The absence of other reports is consistent with the low incidence of GBS (roughly estimated to have an annual incidence rate of 1 case per 100,000 people). The observation of an increased incidence of GBS in Finland temporally associated with a mass immunization with OPV provided a special opportunity to study the association between GBS and OPV. The consistency of diagnostic criteria and statistically significant differences in the incidence of GBS suggest that the increase was not due to chance variation or biased case reporting.

The committee estimated relative risks and risk differences for GBS following OPV based on the studies of Kinnunen et al. (1989) and Uhari et al. (1989). The expected number of cases was calculated by eliminating from the background incidence data the period in which OPV was given (which the authors did not do in their calculations). This led to relative risk (RR) estimates of 3.8 for the study by Kinnunen et al. (1989) and 3.6 for the study by Uhari et al. (1989). The risk difference (calculated as [RR − 1] × background incidence) for GBS in adults on the basis of the relative risk and background incidence derived from Kinnunen et al. is 2.5 per 100,000 per year. Since OPV-induced GBS occurs within 6 weeks of vaccination, the 6-week excess risk is 0.3 per 100,000. By using the background rates and relative risks from Uhari et al., the risk difference for GBS within 6 weeks of OPV in children under 15 years of age is about 0.1 per 100,000.

However, data provided by Winner and Evans (1990) and Hankey (1987) suggest the background incidence rate for children varies by age interval. Based on the latter data, the risk difference in young children could be significantly greater than that based on the background incidence described by Uhari et al. and could approach that in adults. Relatively few adults in the United States receive OPV; thus, the proportion of GBS cases in adults attributable to OPV would be small.

Conclusion

The evidence favors acceptance of a causal relation between OPV and GBS. The relative risk on the basis of studies done in Finland is on the order of 3.5 for adults, and the risk difference is approximately 2.5 per 100,000 people. Estimates of background incidence rates for GBS in children vary. It is not clear what the relative risk and risk difference are for children in the United States (see Chapter 3).

The evidence is inadequate to accept or reject a causal relation between IPV and GBS.

Risk-Modifying Factors

GBS, as a separate discrete attack, recurs in a small percentage of those previously afflicted, perhaps 2 to 3 percent, and some individuals have been known to have three or four separate episodes. Other than the patient described by Pollard and Selby (1978), who experienced three attacks, each within 10-21 days of receipt of tetanus toxoid, cases of recurrence after vaccination are not documented. Nevertheless, if GBS occurs within 5 days to 6 weeks of a vaccination, subsequent vaccinations with either OPV or different immunogens could be associated with a greater risk of GBS than if the person had never had GBS. A previous history of GBS unrelated to vaccination as an antecedent event is even more uncertain as a risk factor.

ANAPHYLAXIS AND THROMBOCYTOPENIA

Clinical Description

Anaphylaxis is a sudden, potentially life-threatening systemic condition mediated by highly reactive molecules from mast cells and basophils. The clinical manifestations of anaphylaxis include pallor and then diffuse erythema, urticaria and itching, subcutaneous edema, edema and spasm of the larynx, wheezing, tachycardia, hypotension, and hypovolemic shock, usually occurring within minutes of intramuscular or subcutaneous exposure to antigen. See Chapter 4 for a more detailed discussion of anaphylaxis.

Thrombocytopenia is a decrease in the number of platelets that are involved in blood clotting. Thrombocytopenia can stem from the failure of platelet production, a shortened platelet life span, or an abnormal distribution of platelets within the body. In most cases, thrombocytopenia in children is mild and transient, and it is often discovered only incidentally when a complete blood count is performed. Severe thrombocytopenia associated with spontaneous bleeding, including bleeding into the skin, is called *thrombocytopenic purpura*. No population-based incidence rates for either condition were identified.

The committee was asked to evaluate the data regarding a possible causal relation between IPV only and anaphylaxis and thrombocytopenia.

Evidence for Association

There are no published reports of anaphylaxis or thrombocytopenic purpura associated with IPV.

Conclusion

There is no evidence bearing on a causal relation between IPV and anaphylaxis.

There is no evidence bearing on a causal relation between IPV and thrombocytopenia.

DEATH

A detailed discussion of the evidence regarding death following immunization can be found in Chapter 10. Only the causality argument and conclusion follow. See Chapter 10 for details.

Causality Argument

The evidence favors acceptance of a causal relation between OPV and GBS. The evidence establishes a causal relation between OPV and paralytic poliomyelitis in recipients or contacts. GBS and paralytic poliomyelitis can be fatal. Although there is no direct evidence of death as a consequence of OPV-induced GBS, in the committee's judgment OPV could cause fatal GBS. There are data regarding death from vaccine-strain poliovirus infection; the data derive primarily from immunocompromised individuals. There is no evidence or reason to believe that the case fatality rate for GBS or vaccine-associated poliovirus infection (including that resulting in paralytic poliomyelitis) is greater than that for these adverse events associated with any other cause.

The possible causal relation between polio vaccines and sudden infant death syndrome (SIDS) has rarely been studied. The evidence is inadequate to accept or reject a causal relation between polio vaccines and SIDS.

Conclusion

The evidence establishes a causal relation between OPV and death from vaccine-strain poliovirus infection, including infection that results in paralytic poliomyelitis. The conclusion is based on case reports and not on controlled studies. No relative risk can be calculated. However, the risk of death from OPV-related polio infection would seem to be extraordinarily low.

The evidence favors acceptance of a causal relation between OPV and death from GBS. There is no direct evidence for this; the conclusion is based on the potential of GBS to be fatal. The risk appears to be extraordinarily low.

The evidence is inadequate to accept or reject a causal relation between polio vaccines and SIDS.

The evidence is inadequate to accept or reject a causal relation between OPV and death from causes other than those listed above.

REFERENCES

Adams, J, Francke, E, Lillestol, M. Poliomyelitis vaccination (letter). New England Journal of Medicine 1977;297:1290-1291.

American Academy of Pediatrics, Committee on Infectious Diseases. Report of the Committee on Infectious Diseases. Elk Grove Village, IL: American Academy of Pediatrics; 1964.

American Academy of Pediatrics, Committee on Infectious Diseases. Report of the Committee on Infectious Diseases: 22nd edition. Elk Grove Village, IL: American Academy of Pediatrics; 1991.

Andersen O, Eeg-Olofsson E. A prospective study of parapareses in western Sweden. Acta Neurologica Scandinavica 1976;54:312-320.

Andre FE. Poliomyelitis vaccines in Belgium: 20 years of experience. Developments in Biological Standardization 1979;43:187-193.

Arlazoroff A, Bleicher Z, Klein C, Vure E, Lahat E, Gross B, et al. Vaccine-associated contact paralytic poliomyelitis with atypical neurological presentation. Acta Neurologica Scandinavica 1987;76:210-214.

Balduzzi P, Glasgow LA. Paralytic poliomyelitis in a contact of a vaccinated child. New England Journal of Medicine 1967;276:796-797.

Basillico FC, Bernat JL. Vaccine-associated poliomyelitis in a contact. Journal of the American Medical Association 1978;239:2275.

Bateman DE, Elrington G, Kennedy P, Saunders M. Vaccine related poliomyelitis in non-immunised relatives and household contacts. British Medical Journal 1987;294:170-171.

Beghi E, Kurland LT, Mulder DW. Incidence of acute transverse myelitis in Rochester, Minnesota, 1970-1980, and implications with respect to influenza vaccine. Neuroepidemiology 1982;1:176-188.

Beghi E, Nicolosi A, Kurland LT, Mulder DW, Hauser WA, Shuster L. Encephalitis and aseptic meningitis, Olmsted County, Minnesota, 1950-1981. I. Epidemiology. Annals of Neurology 1984;16:283-294.

Bell EJ, Riding MH, Grist NR. Paralytic poliomyelitis: a forgotten diagnosis? British Medical Journal 1986;293:193-194.

Benison S. International medical cooperation: Dr. Albert Sabin, live poliovirus vaccine and the Soviets. Bulletin of the History of Medicine 1982;56:460-483.

Bergeisen GH, Bauman RJ, Gilmore RL. Neonatal paralytic poliomyelitis: a case report. Archives of Neurology 1986;43:192-194.

Bernal A, Garcia-Saiz A, Liacer A, De Ory F, Tello O, Najera R. Poliomyelitis in Spain, 1982-1984: virologic and epidemiologic studies. American Journal of Epidemiology 1987;126:69-76.

Biberi-Moroeanu S, Muntiu A. Commentary on the oral poliomyelitis vaccine (Sabin):associated cases of acute persisting spinal paralysis. Archives Roumaines de Pathologie Experimentale et de Microbiologie 1978;37:355-368.

British Medical Journal. Report from the PHLS Communicable Disease Surveillance Centre. British Medical Journal 1986;293:195-196.

Canadian Medical Association Journal. Vaccine-associated poliomyelitis in Quebec. Canadian Medical Association Journal 1987;137:418-419.

Centers for Disease Control. Paralytic poliomyelitis—United States, 1982 and 1983. Morbidity and Mortality Weekly Report 1984;33:635-638.

Centers for Disease Control. Poliomyelitis—United States, 1975-1984. Morbidity and Mortality Weekly Report 1986;35:180-182.

Centers for Disease Control. Epidemiologic classification of reported cases of paralytic poliomyelitis, U.S.A., 1975-1986. Unpublished. Atlanta: Centers for Disease Control; 1987.

Cesario TC, Nakano JH, Caldwell GG, Youmans RA. Paralytic poliomyelitis in an unimmunized child: apparent result of a vaccine-derived poliovirus. American Journal of Diseases of Children 1969;118:895-898.

Chang TW, Weinstein L, MacMahon HE. Paralytic poliomyelitis in a child with hypogammaglobulinemia: probable implication of type I vaccine strain. Pediatrics 1966;37:630-636.

Collingham KE, Pollock TM, Roebuck MO. Paralytic poliomyelitis in England and Wales, 1976-1977. Lancet 1978;1:976-977.

Daneault N, Albert G, Girouard Y, Remillard G, Furesz J. Postvaccinal poliomyelitis: a case report. Canadian Journal of Neurological Science 1986;12:202.

Davis LE, Bodian D, Price D, Butler IJ, Vickers JH. Chronic progressive poliomyelitis secondary to vaccination of an immunodeficient child. New England Journal of Medicine 1977;297:241-245.

D'Costa DF, Cooper A, Pye IF. Transverse myelitis following cholera, typhoid and polio vaccination. Journal of the Royal Society of Medicine 1990;83:653.

Derenne F, Vanderheyden JE, Bain H, Jocquet P, Jacquy J, Yane F, et al. Poliomyelite anterieure aigue maternelle en zone non endemique. [Acute maternal anterior poliomyelitis in a non-endemic zone.] Acta Neurologica Belgica 1989;89:358-365.

Domok I. Experiences associated with the use of live poliovirus vaccine in Hungary, 1959-1982. Reviews of Infectious Diseases 1984;6(Suppl. 2):S413-S418.

Douglas SD, Anolik R. Postvaccination paralysis in a 20-month-old child. Hospital Practice 1981;16:40A.

Enders JF, Weller TH, Robbins, FC. Cultivation of the Lansing strain of poliomyelitis virus in cultures of various human embryonic tissues. Science 1949;109:85-87.

Frantzidou-Adamopoulou F. Poliomyelitis cases in northern Greece during 1976-1990. European Journal of Epidemiology 1992;8:112-113.

Grose C, Spigland I. Guillain-Barré syndrome following administration of live measles vaccine. American Journal of Medicine 1976;60:441-443.

Gross TP, Khurana RK, Higgins T, Nkowane BS, Hirsch RL. Vaccine-associated poliomyelitis in a household contact with Netherton's syndrome receiving long-term steroid therapy. American Journal of Medicine 1987;83:797-800.

Hammon WM, Coriell LL, Wehrle PF, Stokes J. Evaluation of Red Cross gamma globulin as a prophylactic agent for poliomyelitis. 4. Final report of results based on clinical diagnoses. Journal of the American Medical Association 1953;151:1272-1285.

Haneberg B, Orstavik I. Poliomyelitis associated with oral poliovaccine: report on two cases. Acta Paediatrica Scandinavica 1972;61:105-108.

Hankey GJ. Guillain-Barré syndrome in Western Australia, 1980-1985. Medical Journal of Australia 1987;146:130-133.

Henderson DA, Witte JJ, Morris L, Langmuir AD. Paralytic disease associated with oral polio vaccines. Journal of the American Medical Association 1964;190:41-48.

Institute of Medicine. Evaluation of Poliomyelitis Vaccines. Washington, DC: National Academy of Sciences; 1977.

Institute of Medicine. An Evaluation of Poliomyelitis Vaccine Policy Options. Washington, DC: National Academy Press; 1988.

Ishizaki A, Noda Y. [Neurological complications of immunization]. No To Hattatsu 1986;18:105-113.

Kinnunen E, Farkkila M, Hovi T, Juntunen J, Weckstrom P. Incidence of Guillain-Barré syndrome during a nationwide oral poliovirus vaccine campaign. Neurology 1989;39:1034-1036.

Kolmer JA. Vaccination against acute anterior poliomyelitis. American Journal of Public Health and the Nations Health 1936;26:126-135.

Koprowski H, Jervis GA, Norton TW. Immune responses in human volunteers upon oral administration of a rodent-adapted strain of poliomyelitis virus. American Journal of Hygiene 1952;55:108-126.

Kostrzewski JM. Zachorowania na poliomyelitis w otoczeniu szczepionych wirusem atenuowanym. [Case of poliomyelitis in unvaccinated children in contact with persons vaccinated with attenuated virus.] Przeglad Epidemiologiczny 1973;27:259-265.

Kruppenbacher JP, Mertens T, Adrian M, Smolenski S, Leidel J, Eggers HJ. Die Impfpoliomyelitis als Komplikation der Oralvakzination. [Vaccine poliomyelitis as a complication of oral vaccination.] Offentliche Gesundheitswesen 1983;45:528-531.

Kuwert E, Thraenhart O, Hoher PG, Dorndorf W, Voit D, Blumenthal W. Spinale Kinderlahmung nach Kontakt mit Polioimpfvirus. [Spinal poliomyelitis due to contact with polio vaccine virus.] Deutsche Medizinische Wochenschrift 1971;96:1562-1568.

LaForce FM. Poliomyelitis vaccines: success and controversy. Infectious Disease Clinics of North America 1990;4:75-83.

Leake JP. Poliomyelitis following vaccination against this disease. Journal of the American Medical Association 1935;105:2152.

Leneman F. The Guillain-Barré syndrome. Archives of Internal Medicine 1966;118:139-144.

Loffel M, Meienberg O, Diem P, Mombelli G. Impfpoliomyelitis bei einem Erwachsenen unter Chemotherapie wegen Non-Hodgkin-Lymphoms. [Vaccine poliomyelitis in an adult undergoing chemotherapy for non-Hodgkin lymphoma.] Schweiz Medizinische Wochenschrift 1982;112:419-421.

Maass G, Quast U. Acute spinal paralysis after the administration of oral poliomyelitis vaccine in the Federal Republic of Germany (1963-1984). Journal of Biological Standardization 1987;15:185-191.

Mathias RG, Routley JV. Paralysis in an immunocompromised adult following oral polio vaccination (letter). Canadian Medical Association Journal 1985;132:738-739.

Morse LJ, Rubin HE, Blount RE Jr. Vaccine-acquired paralytic poliomyelitis in an unvaccinated mother. Journal of the American Medical Association 1966;197:1034-1035.

Nishio O, Ishihara Y, Sakae K, Nonomura Y, Kuno A, Yasukawa W, et al. The trend of acquired immunity with live poliovirus vaccine and the effect of revaccination: follow-up of vaccinees for ten years. Journal of Biological Standardization 1984;12:1-10.

Nkowane BM, Wassilak SG, Orenstein WA, Bart KJ, Schonberger LB, Hinman AR, et al. Vaccine-associated paralytic poliomyelitis, United States: 1973 through 1984. Journal of the American Medical Association 1987;257:1335-1340.

Novello F, Lombardi F, Amato C, Santoro R, Fiore L, Grandolfo ME, Pasquini, P. Paralytic poliomyelitis in Italy (1981-85). European Journal of Epidemiology 1987;3:54-60.

Onorato IM, Modlin JF, McBean AM, Thoms ML, Losonsky GA, Bernier RH. Mucosal immunity induced by enhanced-potency inactivated and oral polio vaccines. Journal of Infectious Diseases 1991;163:1-6.

Openshaw H, Lieberman JS. Vaccine-related poliomyelitis: serum IgM and cerebrospinal fluid antibodies. Western Journal of Medicine 1983;138:420-422.

Orzechowska-Wolczyk M, Szulc-Kuberska J, Zawadzki Z. Przypadek zapalenia rogow przednich rdzenia kregowego u matki dziecka szczepionego przeciw polio. [Case of poliomyelitis in the mother of a child vaccinated against poliomyelitis.] Wiadomosci Lekarskie 1976;29:1007-1010.

Pollard JD, Selby G. Relapsing neuropathy due to tetanus toxoid: report of a case. Journal of Neurological Science 1978;37:113-125.

Racaniello VR. Poliovirus vaccines. Biotechnology 1992;20:205-222.

Riker JB, Brandt CD, Chandra R, Arrobio JO, Nakano JH. Vaccine-associated poliomyelitis in a child with thymic abnormality. Pediatrics 1971;48:923-929.

Sabin AB. Immunization of chimpanzees and human beings with avirulent strains of poliomyelitis virus. Annals of the New York Academy Sciences 1956;61:1050-1056.

Sakano T, Kittaka E, Tanaka Y, Yamaoka H, Kobayashi Y, Usui T. Vaccine-associated poliomyelitis in an infant with agammaglobulinemia. Acta Paediatrica Scandinavica 1980;69:549-551.

Salk JE. Recent studies in immunization against poliomyelitis. Pediatrics 1953;12: 471-482.

Salk JE, Bennett BL, Lewis LJ, Ward EN, Youngner JS. Studies in human subjects on active immunization against poliomyelitis. 1. A preliminary report of experiments in progress. Journal of the American Medical Association 1953;151:1081-1098.

Saulsbury FT, Winkelstein JA, Davis LE, Hsu SH, D'Souza BJ, Gutcher GR, Butler, IJ. Combined immunodeficiency and vaccine-related poliomyelitis in a child with cartilage-hair hypoplasia. Journal of Pediatrics 1975;86:868-872.

Smith JW, Wherry PJ. Poliomyelitis surveillance in England and Wales, 1969-1975. Journal of Hygiene 1978;80:155-167.

Stolley PD, Joseph JM, Allen JC, Deane G, Janney JH. Poliomyelitis associated with type-2 poliovirus vaccine strain: possible transmission from an immunised child to a non-immunised child. Lancet 1968;1:661-663.

Swanson PD, McAlister R, Peterson DR. Poliomyelitis associated with type 2 virus: paralytic disease in the father of a recently immunized child. Journal of the American Medical Association 1967;201:771-773.

Thraenhart O, Kuwert E. Intratypische charakterisierung von poliovirussammen unter besonderer Berucksichtigung der impfreaktion nach schluckimpfung. [Intratypic differentiation of poliovirus strains with special regard to complication after oral vaccination in West-Germany.] Sentralblatt fur Bakteriologic, Parasitunkunde, Infektionskrankheiten und Hygiene. 1972;221:143-156.

Uhari M, Rantala H, Niemela M. Cluster of childhood Guillain-Barré cases after an oral poliovaccine campaign (letter). Lancet 1989;2:440-441.

U.S. Public Health Service. Interim document gives advice on use of Salk and Sabin vaccines. Journal of the American Medical Association 1962;180:23-26.

Whittle E, Roberton NR. Transverse myelitis after diphtheria, tetanus, and polio immunisation. British Medical Journal 1977;1:1450.

Wiechers DO. New concepts of the reinnervated motor unit revealed by vaccine-associated poliomyelitis. Muscle Nerve 1988;11:356-364.

Wilson J, Robinson R. Poliomyelitis after contact with recently vaccinated infant (letter). British Medical Journal 1974;2:53.

Winner SJ, Evans G. Age-specific incidence of Guillain-Barré syndrome in Oxfordshire. Quarterly Journal of Medicine (New Series) 1990;77:1297-1304.

World Health Organization Consultative Group. The relation between acute persisting spinal paralysis and poliomyelitis vaccine: results of a ten-year enquiry. Bulletin of the World Health Organization 1982;60:231-242.

Wright PF, Hatch MH, Kasselberg AG, Lowry SP, Wadlington WB, Karzon DT. Vaccine-associated poliomyelitis in a child with sex-linked agammaglobulinemia. Journal of Pediatrics 1977;91:408-412.

8

Hepatitis B Vaccines

BACKGROUND AND HISTORY

Hepatitis B virus infection may result in a wide variety of acute or chronic hepatic and extrahepatic manifestations as well as a chronic carrier state. Following an incubation period of 4 weeks to 6 months, the patient develops anorexia, low-grade fever, and, in more severe cases, tender enlargement of the liver associated with jaundice. At least 80 percent of otherwise healthy adult patients and a larger percentage of children with acute hepatitis B virus infection recover completely from the infection with no sequelae. Fewer than 1 percent develop massive hepatic necrosis and then death. Of those who recover from acute hepatitis, up to 15 percent become chronic carriers, that is, have chronic hepatitis B virus infection. There are major differences between children and adults regarding the development of the chronic carrier state. Ninety percent of newborn infants infected with hepatitis B virus become chronic carriers; however, the risk of becoming a chronic carrier following primary infection decreases during early childhood, so that by the age of 4 years, only 10 percent of those infected become chronic carriers. An even smaller percentage of adults (1-4 percent) become chronic carriers. As a result, the infection of children at birth or soon thereafter results in a higher prevalence of chronic carriers, with the consequent higher risk of hepatocellular carcinoma and chronic liver disease and perpetuation of the risk through maternal-fetal transmission.

The public health importance of hepatitis B infection in susceptible populations spurred the search for a vaccine against this virus. While studying serologic polymorphisms, Blumberg discovered an antibody that reacted with the blood from an Australian aborigine (Blumberg et al., 1969). The reactant became known as the Australia antigen (Au) and was the basis of the test used to screen blood for the presence of hepatitis B virus. This work earned B. S. Blumberg the Nobel Prize in 1976. This basic research also led to the development of a vaccine. Krugman and colleagues, in a classic series of studies in the early 1970s, further laid the groundwork for development of the vaccine. They worked with two strains of hepatitis B virus in human volunteer studies. One was labeled MS-1 and was later identified as hepatitis A virus. The other was labeled MS-2 and was later confirmed to be hepatitis B virus. Those investigators found that a 1:10 dilution of serum infected with hepatitis B virus boiled for 1 minute lost its infectivity but retained its antigenicity and prevented or modified hepatitis B virus infection in approximately 70 percent of vaccinated subjects later challenged with infective MS-2 serum (Krugman and Giles, 1973; Krugman et al., 1970, 1971).

Krugman's principle was developed into a more sophisticated vaccine by several groups (Coutinho et al., 1983; Crosnier et al., 1981; McLean et al., 1983; Purcell and Gerin, 1975). The vaccines consisted of inactivated, alum-adsorbed, 22-nm hepatitis B virus surface antigen (HBsAg) particles that had been purified from the plasma of human chronic hepatitis B virus carriers. The method of purification was by a combination of biophysical (ultracentrifugation) and biochemical procedures. Inactivation was a three-fold process with 8 M urea, pepsin at pH 2, and formalin at a 1:4,000 dilution. The plasma-derived hepatitis B vaccine was licensed by the U.S. Food and Drug Administration in late 1981. A belief among some prospective vaccinees that the plasma-derived vaccine might be contaminated with human blood pathogens (particularly human immunodeficiency virus [HIV]) was an important deterrent to the optimal utilization of the hepatitis B vaccine in high-risk individuals. The treatment steps described above were shown to inactivate representatives of various viruses found in human blood, including HIV (Francis et al., 1986).

Hepatitis B vaccines derived from human plasma were subsequently developed in countries other than the United States, including countries in Europe and Asia. All of the plasma-derived vaccines were given safety tests in tissue culture systems, in animals, and then in humans. Trials of efficacy were done among infants born to carrier mothers, children, and various groups of adults, including homosexual men. Those trials demonstrated adequate antibody production after a three-dose schedule and a high rate of protection following immunization in populations with higher levels of exposure to the antigen than those populations currently receiving the vaccine in the United States (Beasley et al., 1983; McLean et al., 1983; Szmuness et al., 1980, 1982; Wong et al., 1984). The vaccines were used very widely, especially in Asia.

Recombinant vaccines are produced by *Saccharomyces cerevisiae* (common baker's yeast), into which a plasmid containing the gene for HBsAg has been inserted. These were developed and licensed in the 1980s (Emini et al., 1986; Stephenne, 1990). Purified HBsAg is obtained by lysing the yeast cells and separating HBsAg from the yeast components by biochemical and biophysical techniques. These vaccines contain more than 95 percent HBsAg protein. Yeast-derived protein constitutes no more than 5 percent of the final product. Hepatitis B vaccines are packaged to contain 10-40 µg of HBsAg protein per ml and are absorbed with aluminum hydroxide (0.5 mg/ml). Thimerosal (1:20,000 concentration) is added as a preservative. In 1986, the first recombinant hepatitis B vaccine was licensed in the United States. Two recombinant vaccines, both produced in yeasts, are currently licensed in the United States (by Merck Sharp & Dohme and SmithKline Biologicals). These recombinant vaccines are also used in many countries worldwide. An additional recombinant vaccine that is produced in mammalian cells (Pasteur-Merieux) is available in some countries in Europe (Hadler and Margolis, 1992). Recombinant vaccines are also produced in Japan and may become widely available in the future. Additional second-generation recombinant vaccines are currently under development.

Plasma-derived vaccine is no longer being produced in the United States, although it is being produced inexpensively in other countries and has become the predominant form of vaccine in much of Asia, where it is being used in national programs to attempt to interrupt maternal-neonatal transmission. In 1991, hepatitis B vaccine was recommended by both the Centers for Disease Control and the American Academy of Pediatrics for universal administration to infants.

The Advisory Committee on Immunization Practices and the American Academy of Pediatrics recommend that hepatitis B vaccine be given at birth and then again at ages 1 to 2 months and 6 to 18 months. The Advisory Committee on Immunization Practices also recommends an alternative to that schedule of administration, that is, at ages 1 to 2 months, 4 months, and 6 to 18 months.

BIOLOGIC EVENTS FOLLOWING IMMUNIZATION

The antibodies produced after infection with hepatitis B virus or after administration of plasma-derived vaccine or recombinant vaccine are alike in terms of their ability to elicit protective determinants that are active against all subtypes of the virus (Hauser et al., 1987). In the United States, hepatitis B recombinant vaccines are given as a three-dose series. This consists of two priming doses given 1 month apart; this is followed by a third dose given 6 months after the first one (Centers for Disease Control, 1990). An alternative schedule, consisting of three priming doses at 1-month intervals and then a fourth dose 12 months after the first one, is approved for one vaccine (SK-RIT). The priming doses induce detectable antibody to HBsAg in 70-85 percent of healthy adults and children, but they are of relatively low titer. The final dose induces adequate high-titer antibody in more than 90 percent of healthy adults under the age of 50 and 95 percent of children and infants (100-3,000 IU/liter in adults and >5,000 IU/liter in children). The immunogenicity and safety of hepatitis B vaccine in premature infants are less well defined (Lau et al., 1992). Studies show seroconversion rates similar to those observed with the plasma-derived vaccine licensed for use in the United States (Andre and Safary, 1989; McLean et al., 1983; Zajac et al., 1986).

Factors affecting the antibody response to recombinant vaccine include vaccine type and handling, timing of doses, and site of injection. Freezing of the vaccine during shipment or excessive heat may reduce its potency. The deltoid muscle is the preferred site for vaccination, and it is now clear that gluteal injection may decrease the response to the vaccine by as much as 50 percent (Shaw et al., 1989). The anterolateral thigh is the preferred site of vaccine injection in infants. Recombinant vaccine has decreased immunogenicity compared with that of plasma-derived vaccine when the vaccine is administered by the intradermal route, so this route of administration is not recommended by the Centers for Disease Control and Prevention. Factors that do not affect the response include simultaneous administration with hepatitis B immune globulin and with other vaccines, including diphtheria and tetanus toxoids and pertussis vaccine (DPT) (Coursaget et al., 1986).

Age is an important factor affecting the immune response (Andre, 1989; Shaw et al., 1989). The maximal response is in children (ages 2-19 years); this is followed by equivalent responses in young adults and infants (West et al., 1990). The poorest response is in older adults, beginning in the sixth decade of life, and only 50 to 70 percent of adults over age 60 have satisfactory antibody responses. The age-related decrease in immune response is significantly greater in men than in women. The response is diminished in persons with immunosuppressive illnesses, including renal failure and HIV infection. Both higher-titer vaccine and increased numbers of doses are required to achieve a 70 percent response in patients who are on hemodialysis (Centers for Disease Control, 1990).

More than 50 trials of plasma-derived vaccine are reported in the literature. These trials were conducted in nearly half that number of countries and have included the vaccination of more than 100,000 individuals (Beasley et al., 1983; Chung et al., 1985; Francis et al., 1982; McLean et al., 1983; Szmuness et al., 1980). All trials dealt with plasma-derived vaccines that were very similar in composition. Although there were some differences in potency and effectiveness, the results were uniform in reporting a vaccine with minimal local side effects. In a double-blind, randomized controlled study, Szmuness and colleagues (1980) reported no significant differences in any response to the vaccine compared with that to placebo except for local pain. The minimal reactions reported in other studies have been local pain, myalgia, and low-grade and transient fever, usually within the first 24 hours. The frequency of such side effects is not cited in reports of many trials, and statements like "reported untoward reactions to immunization were negligible" are often made. When the frequency of side effects is cited, however, particularly in the initial trials, the estimates range from 0 to 45 percent, but in most studies, about 30 percent of adults have local reactions of sore arms and local induration. Fewer children have these side effects (less than 10 percent). Most of the trials have studied vaccination by the standard route, but some studies have evaluated the intradermal route, including the jet injection technique used in mass immunization campaigns such as in the military. Studies have been conducted in infants, children, adult health care workers, health profession students, patients on dialysis and with renal disease, homosexual or bisexual men, and mentally retarded individuals in institutions. The greatest number of studies have been conducted in infants. Most of these are of hepatitis B vaccine alone, but others have examined different combinations of the vaccine and hepatitis B immune globulin. From these studies, the optimal current recommendation for immunization of newborns of HBsAg-positive mothers was developed. The current recommendations incorporate administration of a combination of vaccine and immune globulin with the initial dose shortly after birth; this is followed by administration of vaccine alone at 1- and 6-month intervals.

Trials of more than 12 separate recombinant vaccines have been conducted in more than 25 countries and have involved more than 100,000 recipients. As is the case for plasma-derived vaccines, however, it is important to note that individual trials usually involved a few hundred subjects per study (Andre, 1989). When larger vaccination programs were monitored, observations of adverse events were necessarily less detailed and less accurately reported.

The results of the trials of recombinant vaccine are much the same as those of trials of plasma-derived vaccines (Andre, 1989). Local reactions of soreness were found in approximately one-third of recipients; generalized reactions of fatigue, headache, or fever were found in 10-15 percent of recipients. The frequencies of these side effects were less in infants and children. The trials are notable for the absence of any serious adverse reactions. The studies were not designed to assess serious, rare adverse events; the total number of recipients is too small and the follow-up generally too short to detect rare or delayed serious adverse reactions.

Studies of the immunogenicity of the recombinant vaccine show that, by the third dose, over 95 percent of healthy children and adults have responded by producing antibody. Infants and older individuals produce less antibody than young children and adults, which is the usual case for many vaccines.

GUILLAIN-BARRÉ SYNDROME

Clinical Description

Guillain-Barré syndrome (GBS) is characterized by the rapid onset of flaccid motor weakness with depression of tendon reflexes and inflammatory demyelination of peripheral nerves. The diagnostic criteria for GBS spelled out in Chapter 3 are those used in this chapter, although the data available from case reports in the literature or in reports of adverse events are often sparse and do not fulfill all diagnostic criteria. The annual incidence of GBS appears to be approximately 1 per 100,000 for adults. The data are not definitive, but the annual incidence of GBS in children under age 5 years appears to be approximately the same. The annual incidence of GBS in children over age 5 years and teenagers appears to be lower. Chapter 3 contains a detailed discussion of GBS.

History of Suspected Association

The association of GBS and swine influenza vaccine has been an impetus for scrutinizing all new vaccines for neurologic sequelae. This was, no doubt, the impetus for the postmarketing surveillance study of Shaw et al. (1988). In addition, hepatitis B virus infection itself may have, on occasion, triggered GBS (Berger et al., 1981; Marti-Masso et al., 1979; Ng et al., 1975; Niermeijer et al., 1975; Penner et al., 1982; Tabor, 1987; Tsukada et al., 1987).

Evidence for Association

Biologic Plausibility

Chapter 3 presents background information on the biologic plausibility of a causal relation between vaccines and demyelinating disease. The association with GBS has been reported from various countries and with various versions of both plasma-derived and recombinant hepatitis B vaccines. As already mentioned, GBS has on occasion been reported to occur following hepatitis B viral infection.

Case Reports, Case Series, and Uncontrolled Observational Studies

Following the introduction of plasma-derived hepatitis B vaccine in 1982, a passive surveillance effort was initiated by the Centers for Disease Control (CDC) to monitor for all serious adverse events. A study of the neurologic adverse events reported in approximately 850,000 vaccinees during the first 3 years of surveillance was published in 1988 (Shaw et al., 1988). Nine cases of putative GBS occurring after administration of hepatitis B vaccine came to attention, all in adults. The clinical information for eight cases was reviewed independently by four academic neurologists. They expressed a wide range of opinions as to whether these cases represented GBS. Two of the nine cases were judged to be definite GBS by three of the four reviewers, two cases received two of four votes as definite GBS, one case was thought to be definite GBS by one of the four reviewers, and three cases were not thought to be definite GBS by any of the reviewers.

Although the neurologists did not all agree that each of the nine cases was GBS, the authors used all nine cases in the analysis. Because no concurrent control populations were available, two population-based studies were used to calculate expected numbers of GBS cases for comparison purposes. One set of background incidence data came from a CDC study designed to evaluate the relation between GBS and swine flu vaccination, which presumably used case definition methods similar to those that led to the nine GBS cases in the study of Shaw et al. (1988). The second set of background incidence rates came from a linked medical records system conducted by the Mayo Clinic in Rochester, Minnesota, for Olmsted County, Minnesota. Relative risks for GBS following hepatitis B vaccination were calculated under a variety of assumptions, specifically, a 6- or 8-week at-risk interval and risk evenly distributed among three doses versus all risk associated with the first dose. Statistically significant increases in risk were found under all assumptions when the CDC data were used for comparison purposes, but only with a 6-week at-risk interval after the first vaccine dose when the Olmsted County data were used. Adjustments for age in the CDC data and age and sex in the Olmsted County data did not substantially change the results. The authors stated that "no conclusive epidemiologic association could be made between any neurologic adverse event and the vaccine" (Shaw et al., 1988, p. 337), presumably because their data derived from spontaneous reporting, they had no concurrent control information, and the diagnosis of GBS was sometimes suspect.

A recent uncontrolled observational study of 43,618 Alaskan native vaccinees used a different strategy to investigate the relation between plasma-derived hepatitis B vaccine and GBS (McMahon et al., 1992). A computer search for all GBS cases in hospitals to which these individuals could be admitted disclosed 10 patients with GBS during the period in which hepatitis B vaccine was administered. Of the 10 cases, 5 had been vaccinated with hepatitis B vaccine and 5 had not. Three of the vaccinees had experienced GBS prior to receiving hepatitis B vaccine, and two of the vaccinees had developed GBS long after vaccination (3 and 9 months, respectively). No relation between hepatitis B vaccination and GBS was demonstrated in that study.

Five case reports could be culled from the literature (Lin et al., 1989; Morris and Butler, 1992; Ribera and Dutka, 1983; Tuohy, 1989). Of these, a single case report related to the plasma-derived vaccine licensed for use in the United States (Ribera and Dutka, 1983), and the others were from Taiwan (plasma-derived), New Zealand (two cases, both plasma-derived), and Australia (recombinant). The cases of GBS in Taiwan, New Zealand, and Australia were in children ages 3-7 years, whereas the case of GBS in the United States was in an adult. These age differences probably reflect the predominant ages of the vaccinees in the respective countries. The case from the United States did not qualify clinically as GBS, because no weakness was demonstrated and the only symptoms were fatigue and paresthesias.

In the Monitoring System for Adverse Events Following Vaccination, three cases of GBS were reported as adverse events following hepatitis B vaccination from the time of the introduction of the vaccine until 1990. The Vaccine Adverse Event Reporting System (VAERS) contains 14 adverse reaction reports (submitted between November 1990 and July 1992) in which GBS is mentioned. Two of the reports are for the same patient; consequently, only 13 patients were reported. Of the 13 patients, 4 patients were described as having clinical syndromes that are incompatible with the diagnosis of GBS, and in 2 of these patients the latencies were 2 and 3 months, respectively. These four cases were considered to be other than GBS. An additional four reports contained virtually no information other than a listing of the diagnosis. For these cases, no conclusion regarding the diagnosis can be reached. Five cases appeared to be plausibly diagnosed as GBS, and the patients developed symptoms within 1 month of hepatitis B vaccination. All cases of GBS were in adults and all followed receipt of the recombinant vaccine.

Controlled Observational Studies

None.

Controlled Clinical Trials

None of the clinical trials reviewed by the committee contained information regarding hepatitis B vaccine and GBS.

Causality Argument

There are reports of GBS following vaccination, but it is difficult to determine whether the frequency is greater than expected. There is some biologic plausibility for this association in terms of the occurrence of GBS following hepatitis B infection, the occurrence of demyelinating disease following vaccination in general (see Chapter 3), and the fact that cases have been reported in various countries and with various versions of both plasma-derived and recombinant vaccines. The episodes of GBS that occurred outside the United States are too rare to make any calculation of the incidence of GBS, and no value for the denominator is available. For New Zealand, a calculation of the incidence of GBS was made by using data from Olmsted County, Minnesota, for comparison. This seems inappropriate for geographic and demographic reasons. For the postmarketing surveillance data (Shaw et al., 1988), the authors assumed that the denominator was at least 850,000, which gives a crude rate of slightly greater than 1 case per 100,000 people receiving the vaccine. Shaw and colleagues examined the incidence rate of GBS in hepatitis B vaccine recipients in more depth using background rates from both Olmsted County and a national Centers for Disease Control study, and they also adjusted the data for age and sex. Some of the analyses of Shaw and colleagues, primarily those comparisons using the CDC data, reported a significant increase in the risk of GBS. However, the committee thought that the evidence was not conclusive for many of the same reasons Shaw and colleagues discussed in their report.

Conclusion

The evidence is inadequate to accept or reject a causal relation between hepatitis B vaccine and GBS.

OTHER DEMYELINATING DISEASES

Clinical Description

Three central nervous system demyelinating diseases have been reported to occur following hepatitis B vaccination: a chronic demyelinating disease, multiple sclerosis, and two focal demyelinating lesions, optic neuritis and transverse myelitis. In patients with multiple sclerosis, demyelinating lesions occur in multiple locations and at different times. Transverse myelitis is characterized by the acute onset of signs of spinal cord disease, usually involving the descending motor tracts and the ascending sensory fibers, suggesting a lesion at one level of the spinal cord. On several occasions, it has been described as occurring after vaccination. The annual incidence of transverse myelitis in Rochester, Minnesota, from 1970 to 1981 was 0.83 per 100,000 people (Beghi et al., 1982). Optic neuritis represents a lesion in the optic nerve behind the orbit but anterior to the optic chiasm. Well-documented cases of optic neuritis that occur following vaccination are even rarer than cases of transverse myelitis. No population-based incidence rates were identified. Chapter 3 contains a discussion of demyelinating diseases.

Evidence for Association

Biologic Plausibility

Chapter 3 contains a discussion of the biologic plausibility of a causal relation between hepatitis B vaccine and demyelinating disease. The reports suggesting a relation between vaccination and multiple sclerosis have largely been associated with hepatitis B vaccine. It has been suggested that hepatitis B vaccine might have an inherent propensity to cause demyelinating disease, and a possible mechanism has been offered (Waisbren, 1992). There is a well-established sequence homology between a short sequence of the P antigen of the hepatitis B virus and the encephalitogenic portion of rabbit myelin basic protein. Using a synthesized amino acid sequence with adjuvant, Fujinami and Oldstone (1989) induced inflammatory encephalomyelitis in rabbits. Although molecular mimicry might induce disease in humans given some vaccines or in humans with certain infections, the relevance of this specific study to the hepatitis B vaccine is questionable, since the recombinant vaccine reported to be associated with the majority of the cases does not contain the P protein. In addition, the sequence of the myelin basic protein that is encephalitogenic for rabbits is not the same as the sequence that is encephalitogenic for primates, and the region implicated in monkeys is thought to be similar to the region implicated in humans.

The initial or recurrent attacks of multiple sclerosis following a dose of hepatitis B vaccine may be a chance occurrence. This would be supported by the frequency of the disease, its onset in young adult life at the same time that the hepatitis B vaccine is often administered, the observation that the episodes have occurred at variable times (some as short as 24 hours and some as long as 6 weeks postvaccination), which would stretch the feasibility of a delayed-type hypersensitivity reaction, and the inconsistency of occurrence after any particular sequence of vaccinations. On the other hand, multiple sclerosis is thought to be an autoimmune disease that occurs in genetically susceptible individuals. Antigenic stimulation of any type in such people might precipitate either an exacerbation or even the first clinically evident attack of disease exacerbation.

Case Reports, Case Series, and Uncontrolled Observational Studies

Two cases of multiple sclerosis were reported by Herroelen et al. (1991) in Belgium in two women (ages 26 and 28 years) 6 weeks after receiving recombinant hepatitis B vaccine. One patient had a prior diagnosis of multiple sclerosis and would have been considered to have had a relapse of multiple sclerosis; the onset of the relapse was 6 weeks after receipt of the third dose. The other patient had no history of neurologic disease; the onset of disease occurred 6 weeks after receipt of the first dose of recombinant vaccine. The vaccines administered to both women were licensed in the United States. In both cases, the diagnosis of multiple sclerosis was convincing.

Two more cases of multiple sclerosis were reported to the Institute of Medicine (Waisbren, 1992). One occurred in a 37-year-old pediatric nurse 3 weeks following receipt of her third dose of plasma-derived vaccine. A second case was described in a 32-year-old nurse 2 weeks after receipt of her second dose of recombinant vaccine. Both cases were atypical of multiple sclerosis but were thought to be a form of demyelinating disease. The second patient appeared to have a clear-cut episode of optic neuritis in one eye.

Three cases of transverse myelitis were reported by Shaw et al. (1988) in their postmarketing surveillance study of plasma-derived vaccine. The three cases were in adults, and transverse myelitis occurred 2 to 7 weeks after receipt of doses one to three. (A fourth case reported by Shaw et al. (1988) was not considered because it occurred 16 weeks after vaccination.) Five more cases of transverse myelitis that occurred after administration of recombinant vaccine were reported in VAERS (submitted between November 1990 and July 1992).

Five cases of optic neuritis were reported by Shaw et al. (1988). They were in adults and occurred 1-6 weeks after receipt of doses one to three of plasma-derived vaccine. Fourteen more cases were reported in VAERS (submitted between November 1990 and July 1992). As is usual in VAERS reports, there was variable documentation of the cases.

Controlled Observational Studies

None.

Controlled Clinical Trials

None of the clinical trials reviewed by the committee contained information regarding hepatitis B vaccine and transverse myelitis, optic neuritis, multiple sclerosis, or other central demyelinating diseases.

Causality Argument

The syndromes transverse myelitis, optic neuritis, multiple sclerosis, or other central demyelinating diseases in adults, when examined individually in relation to hepatitis B vaccine, do not appear to have occurred at a greater than expected frequency, and the age distribution reflects the ages of hepatitis B vaccinees in the United States up to this point. The recent recommendation that infants and children receive hepatitis B vaccine will cause a change in the age distribution of vaccinees to younger ages. The possible relation between hepatitis B vaccine and central demyelinating diseases has not been investigated in controlled studies, however. The background incidence rate of these disorders is not particularly well established, nor is the true number of instances of these adverse events following hepatitis B immunization with the recombinant vaccines in use today. These problems preclude a reliable estimate of relative risk. Overall, however, the numbers of examples of adverse neurologic outcomes following receipt of hepatitis B vaccine are of concern, particularly those resulting in demyelinating neurologic disease. There is a need to look for these outcomes in prospective postmarketing surveillance studies, using large computerized data bases, that include appropriate control groups. A number of such prospective studies are under way, and they should be pursued for the occurrence of demyelinating diseases following receipt of hepatitis B vaccine.

Conclusion

The evidence is inadequate to accept or reject a causal relation between hepatitis B vaccine and optic neuritis, multiple sclerosis, or transverse myelitis.

ARTHRITIS

Clinical Description

The general term for joint symptoms, *arthropathy,* refers to any abnormality of the joint. Arthropathy encompasses arthralgia (subjective pain in a joint or joints), stiffness (with arthralgia, commonly referred to as *rheumatism*), and arthritis (objective findings of swelling, redness, heat, and limitation of motion). According to the 1988 National Health Interview Survey, approximately 13 percent of respondents surveyed reported currently having "arthritis or any kind of rheumatism." Prevalence rates increased with age, with approximately 0.2 percent of persons under age 18 years reporting arthritis of any kind or arthralgia.

History of Suspected Association

An association between hepatitis B vaccine and acute arthralgia, arthritis, or both has been suggested since the initial use of plasma-derived hepatitis B vaccines. Joint symptoms have also been reported following receipt of recombinant hepatitis B vaccines (Cockwell et al., 1990; McMahon et al., 1992). The reported instances of arthropathy have occurred more frequently in adults than in infants and children. These data may, however, be misleading, because hepatitis B vaccines have primarily been used in high-risk adult populations in the United States (Committee on Infectious Diseases, 1985).

Evidence for Association

Biologic Plausibility

Biologic plausibility for a relation between hepatitis B vaccine and arthritis derives from the knowledge that experimental acute serum sickness is accompanied by arthritis and that hepatitis B infection is associated with arthropathies and a serum sickness-like syndrome. Experimental acute serum sickness with arthritis can be produced by one or several closely spaced injections of heterologous serum protein. With the initial exposure, the disease usually develops 1 to 2 weeks after antigen injection. On repeated exposure, the disease develops more rapidly after antigen injection. In either case the disease appears as antibody formation begins; the essence of serum sickness is the interaction between antigen and antibody in the circulation with the formation of antigen-antibody complexes in an environment of antigen excess.

Chronic serum sickness with persistent arthritis can be produced in animals if antigen is injected daily in small amounts—just sufficient to be in balance with the amount of antibody produced. This model of chronic serum sickness resembles chronic polyarteritis nodosa in humans.

During the 4-week to 6-month incubation period of hepatitis B infection, but prior to the overt clinical manifestations of hepatitis, a serum sickness-like syndrome consisting of fever, rash, urticaria, arthralgias, or acute arthritis occurs in 10-20 percent of adolescents and adults. This syndrome is accompanied by HBsAg-antibody complexes and low levels of serum complement in the synovial fluid of affected joints (Schumacher and Gall, 1974; Wands et al., 1975). In the serum sickness-like illness associated with acute hepatitis B virus infection, the arthritis, fever, and rash are generally of short duration (3-7 days). These manifestations occur during the period of antigen excess, when the quantitative relation between HBsAg and specific antibody allows the formation of immune complexes that are large enough to affix complement but still small enough to remain soluble and to circulate freely. Once the situation of antibody excess occurs, the antigen-antibody complexes become large and insoluble, are rapidly phagocytized, and are of minimal pathogenicity. Presumably, the immune complex formation during the period of antigen excess is responsible for the transient arthritis observed in patients in the course of acute hepatitis B virus infection.

In addition to the serum sickness-like syndrome associated with hepatitis B infection, arthropathies are among the most common manifestations during the prodromal period of acute hepatitis B virus infection. The arthritis associated with acute hepatitis B virus infection typically resolves over a period of days or, at most, several weeks; it does not appear to result in long-term joint abnormalities.

Joint symptoms related to hepatitis B virus infection in cases of known time of exposure (e.g., following the transfusion of contaminated blood) usually begin within 1 to 4 weeks after the infection. All joints may be involved, usually symmetrically. The joints involved, in decreasing order of frequency, are the small joints of the hands, the wrists, and the knees (Gocke, 1975). Symptoms are often of sudden onset and may consist simply of prominent stiffness and pain or of warmth, redness, and painful joint effusions. The latter are especially prominent in the knees. The arthralgia or arthritis that occurs following acute hepatitis B virus infection is presumed to be caused by antigen-antibody-mediated vascular responses (Coombs and Gell type III).

Polyarteritis following hepatitis B virus infection has clearly been observed in humans (McMahon et al., 1989). Furthermore, 30-50 percent of patients with biopsy-proven polyarteritis nodosa have persistent hepatitis B virus infection (Gocke, 1977). Such patients have low serum complement levels and circulating HBsAg-antibody complexes. Immune complexes and complement components have been detected, albeit rarely, in diseased vessels by immunofluorescence staining. The association of polyarteritis nodosa with hepatitis B infection (McMahon et al., 1989) is thought to be related to a situation of continued antigenic stimulation in individuals who develop antibodies to hepatitis B virus.

Case Reports, Case Series, and Uncontrolled Observational Studies

VAERS contains a large number of cases (submitted between November 1990 and July 1992) in which there was a possible association between arthritis and hepatitis B vaccination. There are 57 reasonably well documented cases of individuals who developed arthritis within 2 months after receiving recombinant hepatitis B vaccine. Of the 57 vaccinated individuals, 52 were health care workers; 79 percent were women.

For purposes of analyses, these case reports can be divided into two reasonably distinct groups. One group consists of 17 individuals in whom arthritis involving multiple joints occurred within 3 weeks after vaccination and the arthritis was associated with fever. The second group includes 40 individuals who developed arthritis not associated with documented fever in one or more joints within 2 months after hepatitis B vaccination.

An associated transient rash was observed in 9 of the 17 patients with polyarticular arthritis and fever. Fifteen of these 17 patients recovered from the arthritis rapidly (with resolution within 3 days to 2 months), whereas 2 individuals developed a more chronic arthritis that persisted for at least 1 year. Nine episodes of arthritis occurred after the first vaccine dose, seven after the second, and one after the third. Among these individuals, 16 were women and 1 was a man. The mean age of the 17 individuals was 43 years. The two individuals who developed a more chronic arthritis were both women, aged 38 and 50 years. The associated skin rashes were transient in all patients; detailed descriptions of the rashes were lacking. All individuals in this group had arthritis in more than one joint; however, a symmetrical polyarthritis of the type typical of a serum sickness-like reaction was described in only three individuals.

For completeness, it should be noted that of the 17 patients with acute onset of arthritis and fever, 1 had associated erythema nodosum. At least three other cases of erythema nodosum have been reported following hepatitis B vaccination (DiGuisto and Bernhard, 1986; Goolsby, 1989; Rogerson and Nye, 1990). Although the rashes in the nine individuals in whom they occurred were not defined, there are reports in the literature of erythema multiforme following hepatitis B vaccination (Feldshon and Sampliner, 1984; Milstien and Kuritsky, 1986; Wakeel and White, 1992). Although both erythema multiforme and erythema nodosum may represent hypersensitivity reactions, neither has been observed sufficiently frequently to support a causal relation with the hepatitis B vaccine. The more severe, potentially fatal variant of erythema multiforme (Stevens-Johnson syndrome) has not been reported in association with hepatitis B vaccines.

The larger group of 40 individuals who developed arthritis, without documentation of associated fever, within 2 months after receiving hepatitis B vaccine presented with a more heterogeneous clinical picture. In these individuals, involvement of a single joint was common, and the predominance in women was less striking than that in individuals with the more acute onset of arthritis with fever (11 men, 29 women). In this group, the mean age was 46 years (range, 21-92 years). Six of the 40 individuals in this group had antecedent rheumatoid arthritis, and the acute arthritis following vaccination was described as a flare-up of rheumatoid arthritis. The arthritis in the 40 individuals was of widely varying duration, persisting for up to 2 years in one instance.

Two large uncontrolled population-based studies provide relevant information on hepatitis B vaccination and arthritis. The largest is the summary of results of a vaccination program involving 166,757 children in New Zealand; each child received at least one injection of plasma-derived hepatitis B vaccine prepared by a U.S. pharmaceutical firm (Morris and Butler, 1992). In this large group of vaccinees, arthralgias or arthritis occurred on 12 occasions in 10 individuals, giving an incidence of less than 1 episode of arthralgia or arthritis in 10,000 vaccinees. Of these 12 episodes, five were reported after receipt of the first vaccine injection, six after the second, and one after the third. One of these patients was hospitalized for 1 day. In none of these individuals were there any chronic sequelae of the arthralgia or arthritis.

The second large observational study described the frequency of adverse reactions to hepatitis B vaccine in 43,618 Alaskan natives who received 101,360 doses of hepatitis B vaccine (McMahon et al., 1989). In that study myalgias or arthralgias lasting for more than 3 days occurred in 12 individuals, an incidence of less than 1 episode in 3,000 vaccinees. The authors felt that the arthralgias were coincidental to the hepatitis B vaccines, since 5 of the 12 patients had negative skin tests to the vaccine. These five patients as well as four others who did not undergo skin testing received additional doses of hepatitis B vaccine without an adverse event. One of the 12 patients did have an Arthus-type reaction, with transient polyarthritis and a positive skin test to the hepatitis B vaccine.

Controlled Observational Studies

None.

Controlled Clinical Trials

No controlled clinical trials reviewed by the committee contained information regarding hepatitis B vaccine and arthritis.

Causality Argument

On the basis of the two largest available observational studies, arthropathy appears to be unusual following vaccination against hepatitis B virus. On the basis of VAERS reports, the possibility exists that a hypersensitivity arthritis occurred in the 17 individuals who developed acute arthritis associated with fever with or without an associated rash. In the absence of a denominator, however, it is not clear that these episodes represented more than coincidental occurrences.

The 1988 National Health Survey indicated that approximately 13 percent of adults surveyed reported having "arthritis or any kind of rheumatism" at the time of the survey (National Center for Health Statistics, 1989). This provides background data against which the VAERS reports of arthritis without fever can be considered.

Since the arthritis that occurs in patients with acute hepatitis B virus infection appears to occur only during the period of antigen excess, it is almost invariably self-limited and appears to subside as the level of antibody increases. It is therefore difficult to relate arthropathy following receipt of the hepatitis B vaccine to the same sort of serum sickness-like antigen-antibody reaction. The quantity of HBsAg (10-40 μg) in recombinant hepatitis B vaccine preparations is very small relative to the amount of HBsAg produced in the acute phase of hepatitis B virus infection; it is therefore unlikely that enough free antigen would be available to produce a serum sickness-like reaction several days or weeks after the vaccine injection.

Therefore, the biologic plausibility of such a reaction occurring after receipt of hepatitis B vaccine appears slim. It seems unlikely that arthritis occurred more commonly in those individuals who developed arthritis without fever than in unvaccinated individuals in the same age group. The incidence of acute arthritis following vaccination appears small relative to the prevalence of arthritis in the population from which the vaccinees were drawn (National Center for Health Statistics, 1989). Again, the lack of a denominator precludes a definite conclusion in this regard.

Polyarteritis nodosa with associated acute arthritis has been observed following hepatitis B vaccination (Le Goff et al., 1988, 1991; McMahon et al., 1989). Yet, the vascular lesions observed in patients with chronic arthritis associated with polyarteritis nodosa appear to demand the continued presence of HBsAg over periods of months to years. It does not seem biologically plausible that chronic antigenic stimulation of this nature would occur after receipt of the relatively small amount of HBsAg contained in each dose of recombinant hepatitis B vaccine. Therefore, the likelihood of a causal relation between hepatitis B vaccination and chronic arthropathy secondary to vasculitis appears small.

The reported flare-up of rheumatoid arthritis within 2 months after receiving hepatitis B vaccine raises the possibility that the vaccine may have precipitated an acute exacerbation of rheumatoid arthritis. However, the prevalence of rheumatoid arthritis in the age group that received the vaccines (0.1 to 1.0 percent) and the lack of a denominator make it impossible to assess causality.

Conclusion

The evidence is inadequate to accept or reject a causal relation between hepatitis B vaccine and either acute or chronic arthropathy.

ANAPHYLAXIS

Clinical Description

The term *anaphylaxis* refers to the rapid onset (within 4 hours after vaccine administration) of a potentially life-threatening illness in which mortality is related either to cardiovascular collapse or to airway obstruction caused by either bronchospasm or laryngospasm. These life-threatening pathophysiologic events are often associated with cutaneous manifestations (hives, angioedema) and arthritis or arthralgias. Chapter 4 contains in-depth discussions of anaphylaxis and other adverse immunologic reactions, for example, the Arthus reaction and serum sickness, to vaccination.

History of Suspected Association

No infants or adults have been reported to have died of anaphylaxis after vaccination with either plasma-derived or recombinant hepatitis B vaccine. However, several cases of anaphylaxis following receipt of recombinant hepatitis B vaccines have been reported in adults. Of the groups of adults in industrialized countries for whom hepatitis B vaccine has been recommended, health care workers make up the great majority of vaccinees (Alter et al., 1988). As a consequence, most anaphylactic reactions have been observed in adult health care workers, of whom over 2 million have now been vaccinated against hepatitis B virus. Most of the documented cases of anaphylaxis occurred in women. This does not, however, justify a conclusion that women are more susceptible than men to anaphylaxis caused by hepatitis B vaccine, because women represent the majority of health care professionals for whom hepatitis B vaccine has been recommended.

Evidence for Association

Biologic Plausibility

The possibility of a causal relation between hepatitis B vaccination and anaphylaxis is supported by biologic plausibility, by the temporal sequence of observed events following vaccination, and by the observation of a spectrum of host responses to the hepatitis B vaccine that follow a logical biologic gradient from true anaphylaxis to milder hypersensitivity reactions. Biologic plausibility derives from the knowledge that injection of foreign protein into humans can be expected to elicit, in some percentage of recipients, immunoglobulin E (IgE)-mediated responses that present as anaphylaxis.

No specific inciting antigen has been demonstrated, and it is not known whether specific antibody of the IgE class is required for such events to occur after hepatitis B immunization. No data from experiments in animals clarify the immunologic events leading to anaphylaxis after hepatitis B vaccination.

Case Reports, Case Series, and Uncontrolled Observational Studies

The largest number of documented cases of anaphylaxis have been reported in VAERS (submitted between November 1990 and July 1992). Those reports include five well-documented cases of anaphylaxis in response to recombinant hepatitis B vaccine, none of which were fatal. Three of the cases of anaphylaxis occurred after the first dose of vaccine, whereas two occurred after the second dose. One of the five cases has been published as a case report (Hudson et al., 1991). There were five additional VAERS reports of apparent anaphylaxis following hepatitis B vaccination that did not meet the strict criteria applied in this report since a low blood pressure was not recorded. In each of these cases the patient received either intramuscular epinephrine (four cases) or diphenhydramine hydrochloride (Benadryl; one case), with excellent clinical responses. An additional eight cases of anaphylactic-type reactions (cardiovascular collapse associated with wheezing) are described in the VAERS reports, but the time interval following vaccination either was greater than 4 hours or was not defined in the VAERS report.

Less severe manifestations of immediate hypersensitivity that do not fulfill the definition of anaphylaxis occur more commonly (Hudson et al., 1991; Lohiya, 1987; numerous VAERS reports). These are usually characterized by urticaria, wheezing, and sometimes, facial edema. Cardiovascular collapse does not occur, however, either because the reactions are inherently less severe or because they are aborted by intervention, usually with epinephrine.

A possible explanation for the occurrence of anaphylaxis after the first vaccine injection is that the patients were sensitized to thimerosal or yeast protein, both of which are components of recombinant vaccines (Kirkland, 1990). An equally tenable hypothesis is that the three patients had previously been exposed to antigens similar to those present in the recombinant hepatitis B vaccine.

Anaphylaxis was not observed in the 166,757 children vaccinated with a plasma-derived vaccine in New Zealand (Morris and Butler, 1992), nor was it observed in 43,618 Alaskan natives who received plasma-derived vaccine (McMahon et al., 1992). The postmarketing surveillance study discussed above (Shaw et al., 1988) investigated only specific adverse neurologic outcomes following receipt of hepatitis B vaccine and provided no data regarding anaphylaxis.

Controlled Observational Studies

None.

Controlled Clinical Trials

None of the clinical trials reviewed by the committee contained information regarding hepatitis B vaccine and anaphylaxis.

Causality Argument

The possibility of a causal relation between hepatitis B vaccination and anaphylaxis is supported by biologic plausibility, by the temporal sequence of observed events following vaccination, and by the observation of a spectrum of host responses to the hepatitis B vaccine that follow a logical biologic gradient from true anaphylaxis to milder hypersensitivity reactions. Biologic plausibility derives from the knowledge that injection of foreign protein into humans can be expected to elicit, in some percentage of recipients, IgE-mediated responses that present as anaphylaxis. Chapter 4 provides the criteria for accepting the diagnosis of anaphylaxis, including cardiovascular collapse and documented hypotension occurring within 4 hours after injection of the vaccine. Only cases meeting these criteria were included as cases of hepatitis B virus-associated anaphylaxis in this report.

In the VAERS reports of suspected anaphylactic reactions, however, a logical biologic gradient can be observed, in that, in addition to the five well-documented reports of anaphylaxis following administration of hepatitis B vaccine, five additional cases of apparent anaphylaxis following hepatitis B vaccination that did not meet the strict criteria applied in this report and an additional eight cases of anaphylactic-type reactions (cardiovascular collapse associated with wheezing) were described.

The evidence concerning a possible relation between hepatitis B vaccination and anaphylaxis is based on VAERS reports. On the basis of these reports, the evidence indicates that anaphylaxis can occur after vaccination against hepatitis B virus and that such an occurrence is an exceedingly rare event. Nonetheless the timing and the unmistakable classic presentation of anaphylaxis, together with the spectrum of host responses that follow a logical biologic gradient from mild to severe following hepatitis B vaccination, indicate that hepatitis B vaccines can cause anaphylaxis.

Conclusion

The evidence establishes a causal relation between hepatitis B vaccine and anaphylaxis. Because the conclusion is not based on controlled studies, no estimate of incidence or relative risk is available. It would seem to be low.

Risk-Modifying Factors

Anaphylaxis may occur, albeit rarely, following hepatitis B vaccination, and there are no known risk factors that predict the likelihood of anaphylaxis after hepatitis B vaccination. Although prior sensitization to thimerosal or yeast protein may predict greater local swelling at the site of vaccination, such sensitization has not been documented to predict anaphylaxis.

DEATH

A detailed discussion of the evidence regarding death following immunization can be found in Chapter 10. Only the causality argument and conclusions follow. See Chapter 10 for details.

Causality Argument

The evidence establishes a causal relation between hepatitis B vaccine and anaphylaxis. Anaphylaxis can be fatal. Although there is no direct evidence of fatal anaphylaxis following hepatitis B vaccination, in the committee's judgment hepatitis B vaccine could cause fatal anaphylaxis. There is no evidence or reason to believe that the case fatality rate for vaccine-associated anaphylaxis would differ from the case fatality rate for anaphylaxis associated with any other cause.

Hepatitis B vaccine has only recently begun to be administered to the age group that is affected by sudden infant death syndrome (SIDS). There are no published studies of a possible causal relation between hepatitis B vaccine and SIDS. There are reports in VAERS of SIDS following immunization with hepatitis B vaccine given in conjunction with other vaccines.

Conclusion

The evidence establishes a causal relation between hepatitis B vaccine and fatal anaphylaxis. There is no direct evidence for this; the conclusion is based on the potential for anaphylaxis to be fatal. The risk would appear to be extraordinarily low.

The evidence is inadequate to accept or reject a causal relation between hepatitis B vaccine and SIDS.

The evidence is inadequate to accept or reject a causal relation between hepatitis B vaccine and death from any cause other than those listed above.

REFERENCES

Alter MJ, Hadler SC, Margolis HS. The changing epidemiology of hepatitis B in the United States: need for alternative vaccination strategies. Journal of the American Medical Association 1988;263:1218-1222.

Andre FE. Summary of safety and efficacy data on a yeast-derived hepatitis B vaccine. American Journal of Medicine 1989;87(3a):14S-20S.

Andre FE, Safary A. Clinical experience with a yeast derived hepatitis B vaccine. In: Zuckerman AJ, ed. Viral Hepatitis and Viral Disease. New York: Alan R. Liss; 1989.

Beasley RP, Hwang LY, Lee GC. Prevention of perinatally transmitted hepatitis B virus infections with hepatitis B immune globulin and hepatitis B vaccine. Lancet 1983;2:1099-1102.

Beghi E, Kurland LT, Mulder DW. Incidence of acute transverse myelitis in Rochester, Minnesota, 1970-1980, and implications with respect to influenza vaccine. Neuroepidemiology 1982;1:176-188.

Berger JR, Ayyar DR, Sheremata WA. Guillain-Barré syndrome complicating acute hepatitis B: a case with detailed electrophysiological and immunological studies. Archives of Neurology 1981;38:366-368.

Blumberg BS, Sutnick AI, London, WT. Australia antigen and hepatitis. Journal of the American Medical Association 1969;207:1895-1896.

Centers for Disease Control. Protection against viral hepatitis. Recommendations of the Immunization Practices Advisory Committee (ACIP). Morbidity and Mortality Weekly Report 1990;39(RR-2):1-26.

Chung WK, Yoo JY, Sun HS, et al. Prevention of perinatal transmission of hepatitis B virus: a comparison between the efficacy of passive and passive-active immunization in Korea. Journal of Infectious Diseases 1985;151:280-286.

Cockwell P, Allen MB, Page R. Vasculitis related to hepatitis B vaccine (letter). British Medical Journal 1990;301:1281.

Committee on Infectious Diseases. Prevention of hepatitis B virus infections. Pediatrics 1985;75:362-364.

Coursaget P, Yvonnet B, Relyveld EH, Barres JL, Diop-Mar I, Chiron JP. Simultaneous administration of diphtheria-tetanus-pertussis-polio and hepatitis B vaccines in a simplified immunization program: immune response to diphtheria toxoid, tetanus toxoid, pertussis, and hepatitis B surface antigen. Infection and Immunity 1986;51:784-787.

Coutinho RA, Lelie N, Albrecht Van Lent P. Efficacy of a heat inactivated hepatitis B vaccine in male homosexuals: outcome of a placebo controlled double blind trial. British Medical Journal 1983;286:1305-1308.

Crosnier J, Jungers P, Courouce AM. Randomised controlled trial of hepatitis B surface antigen vaccine in French haemophilus units. II. Haemodialysis patients. Lancet 1981;2:797-800.

DiGuisto CA, Bernhard JD. Erythema nodosum provoked by hepatitis B vaccine (letter). Lancet 1986;2:1042.

Emini EA, Ellis RW, Miller WJ. Production and immunological analysis of recombinant hepatitis B vaccine. Journal of Infection 1986;13(Suppl. A):3-9.

Feldshon SD, Sampliner RE. Reaction to hepatitis B virus vaccine (letter). Annals of Internal Medicine 1984;100:156-157.

Francis DP, Hadler SC, Thompson SE. The prevention of hepatitis B with vaccine: report of the Centers for Disease Control multi-center efficacy trial among homosexual men. Annals of Internal Medicine 1982;97:362-366.

Francis DP, Feorino PM, McDougal S, Warfield D, Getchell J, Cabradilla C, et al. The safety of the hepatitis B vaccine: inactivation of the AIDS virus during routine vaccine manufacture. Journal of the American Medical Association 1986;256:869-872.

Fujinami RS, Oldstone MB. Molecular mimicry as a mechanism for virus-induced autoimmunity. Immunologic Research 1989;8:3-15.

Gocke DJ. Extrahepatic manifestations of viral hepatitis. American Journal of Medical Science 1975;270:49-52.

Gocke JD. Immune complex phenomena associated with hepatitis. In: Vyas GN, Cohen SN, Schmid R, eds. Viral Hepatitis: A Contemporary Assessment of Etiology, Epidemiology, Pathogenesis and Prevention. Philadelphia: Franklin Institute Press; 1977.

Goolsby PL. Erythema nodosum after recombinant hepatitis B vaccine. New England Journal of Medicine 1989;321:1198-1199.

Hadler SC, Margolis HS. Hepatitis B immunization: vaccine types, efficacy, and indications for immunization. Current Clinical Topics in Infectious Diseases 1992;12:282-308.

Hauser P, Voet P, Simoen E. Immunological properties of recombinant HBsAg produced in yeast. Postgraduate Medical Journal 1987;63(Suppl. 2):83-91.

Herroelen L, De Keyser J, Ebinger G. Central-nervous-system demyelination after immunisation with recombinant hepatitis B vaccine. Lancet 1991;338:1174-1175.

Hudson TJ, Newkirk M, Gervais F, Shuster J. Adverse response to acute hepatitis B vaccine. Journal of Allergy and Clinical Immunology 1991;85:821-822.

Kirkland LR. Occular sensitivity to thiomerosol: a problem with hepatitis B vaccine? Southern Medical Journal 1990;83:497-499.

Krugman S, Giles JP. Viral hepatitis type B (MS-2 strain): further observations on natural history and prevention. New England Journal of Medicine 1973;288:755-760.

Krugman S, Giles JP, Hammond J. Hepatitis virus: effect of heat on the infectivity and antigenicity of the MS-1 and MS-2 strains. Journal of Infectious Diseases 1970;122:432-436.

Krugman S, Giles JP, Hammond J. Viral hepatitis, type B (MS-2 strain): studies on active immunization. Journal of the American Medical Association 1971;217:41-45.

Lau YL, Tam AY, Ng KW, Tsoi NS, Lam B, Yeung CY. Response of preterm infants to hepatitis B vaccine. Journal of Pediatrics 1992;121:962-965.

Le Goff P, Fauquert P, Youinou P, Hoang S. Periarterite noueuse apres vaccination contre l'hepatite B. [Periarteritis nodosa following vaccination against hepatitis B (letter).] Presse Medicale 1988;17:1763.

Le Goff P, Fauquert P, Youinou P, Hoang S. [Periarteritis nodosa (PAN) following vaccine against B hepatitis]. Rhumatologie 1991;43:79.

Lin JJ, Cheng MK, Hsu CT, Tang HS. A rare association between hepatitis B virus vaccination and Guillain-Barré syndrome—a case report. Chinese Journal of Gastroenterology, 1989;6:229-232.

Lohiya G. Asthma and urticaria after hepatitis B vaccination (letter). Western Journal of Medicine 1987;147:341.

Marti-Masso JF, Obeso JA, Cosme A. Guillain-Barré syndrome associated with a type B acute hepatitis. Medicina Clinica (Barcelona) 1979;73:447.

McLean AA, Hilleman MR, McAleer WJ, Buynak EB. Summary of world wide experience with HB-Vax. Journal of Infectious Diseases 1983;7(Suppl.):95-104.

McMahon B et al. Hepatitis B associated polyarteritis in Alaskan eskimos: clinical and epidemiologic features and long-term follow-up. Hepatology 1989;9:97-101.

McMahon BJ, Helminiak C, Wainwright RB, Bulkow L, Trimble BA, Wainwright K. Frequency of adverse reactions to hepatitis B vaccine in 43,618 persons. American Journal of Medicine 1992;92:254-256.

Milstien JB, Kuritsky JN. Erythema multiforme and hepatitis B immunization (letter). Archives of Dermatology 1986;122:511-512.

Morris JA, Butler H. Nature and frequency of adverse reactions following hepatitis B vaccine injection in children in New Zealand, 1985-1988. Submitted to the Vaccine Safety Committee, Institute of Medicine, Washington, DC, May 4, 1992.

National Center for Health Statistics. Current Estimates from the National Health Interview Survey, United States, 1988. Vital and Health Statistics, Series 10, No. 173. Washington, DC: U.S. Government Printing Office; 1989.

Ng PL, Powell LW, Campbell CP. Guillain-Barré syndrome during the preicteric phase of acute type B viral hepatitis. Australia and New Zealand Journal of Medicine 1975;5:367.

Niermeijer P, Gips CH. Guillain-Barré syndrome in acute HBS Ag-positive hepatitis. British Medical Journal 1975;4:732.

Penner E, Maida E, Mamoli B, Gangl A. Serum and cerebrospinal fluid immune complexes containing hepatitis B surface antigen in Guillain-Barré syndrome. Gastroenterology 1982;82:576-580.

Purcell RH, Gerin JL. Hepatitis B subunit vaccine: a preliminary report of safety and efficacy tests in chimpanzees. American Journal of Medical Science 1975;270:395-399.

Ribera EF, Dutka AJ. Polyneuropathy associated with administration of hepatitis B vaccine (letter). New England Journal of Medicine 1983;309:614-615.

Rogerson SJ, Nye FJ. Hepatitis B vaccine associated with erythema nodosum and polyarthritis. British Medical Journal 1990;301:345.

Schumacher HR, Gall EP. Arthritis in acute hepatitis and chronic active hepatitis: pathology of the synovial membranes with evidence of Australian antigen in synovial membranes. American Journal of Medicine 1974;57:655-664.

Shaw FE Jr, Graham DJ, Guess HA, Milstien JB, Johnson JM, Schatz GC, et al. Postmarketing surveillance for neurologic adverse events reported after hepatitis B vaccination: experience of the first three years. American Journal of Epidemiology 1988;127:337-352.

Shaw FE, Guess HA, Roets JM. The effect of anatomic injection site, age and smoking on the immune response to hepatitis B vaccination. Vaccine 1989;7:425-430.

Stephenne J. Development and production aspects of a recombinant yeast derived hepatitis vaccine. Vaccine 1990;8(Suppl.):S69-S73.

Szmuness W, Stevens CE, Harley EJ, Zang EA, Oleszko WR, William DC, et al. Hepatitis B vaccine: demonstration of efficacy in a controlled clinical trial in a high-risk population in the United States. New England Journal of Medicine 1980;303:833-841.

Szmuness W, Stevens CE, Harley EJ, Zang EA, Alter HJ, Taylor PE, et al. Hepatitis B vaccine in medical staff of hemodialysis units: efficacy and subtype cross protection. New England Journal of Medicine 1982;307:1481-1486.

Tabor E. Guillain-Barré syndrome and other neurologic syndromes in hepatitis A, B, and non-A, non-B. Journal of Medical Virology 1987;21:207-216.

Tsukada N, Koh CS, Inoue A, Yanigasawa N. Demyelinating neuropathy associated with hepatitis B virus infection. Journal of Neurological Science 1987;77:203-216.

Tuohy PG. Guillain-Barré syndrome following immunisation with synthetic hepatitis B vaccine (letter). New Zealand Medical Journal 1989;102:114-115.

Waisbren BA. A commentary regarding personal observations of demyelinizing disease caused by viral vaccines, borrelia infections, and proteolytic enzymes. Paper submitted to the Vaccine Safety Committee, Institute of Medicine, Washington, DC, August 11, 1992.

Wakeel RA, White MI. Erythema multiforme associated with hepatitis B vaccine (letter). British Journal of Dermatology 1992;126:94-95.

Wands JR, Mann E, Alpert E. The pathogenesis of arthritis associated with acute hepatitis B surface antigen-positive hepatitis: complement activation and characterization of circulating immune complexes. Journal of Clinical Investigation 1975;55:930-939.

West DH, Calandra GB, Ellis RW. Vaccination of infants and children against hepatitis B. Pediatric Clinics of North America 1990;37:585-601.

Wong VCW, Ip HMP, Reesink HW. Prevention of the HBsAg carrier state in newborn infants of mothers who are chronic carriers of HBsAg and HBeAg by administration of hepatitis B vaccine and hepatitis B immunoglobulin. Lancet 1984;1:921-926.

Zajac BA, West DJ, McAleer WJ, Scolnick EM. Overview of clinical studies with hepatitis B vaccine made by recombinant DNA. Journal of Infection 1986;13(Suppl. A):39-45.

9

Haemophilus influenzae Type b Vaccines

BACKGROUND AND HISTORY

Prior to the introduction of *Haemophilus influenzae* type b (Hib) vaccines, Hib was the leading cause of bacterial meningitis in the United States among children younger than 4 years of age. Each year, an estimated 10,000 cases of Hib meningitis and 5,000 cases of other severe Hib infections occurred, including pneumonia, septic arthritis, epiglottitis, periorbital cellulitis, and facial cellulitis (Schlech et al., 1985; Todd and Bruhn, 1975). The cumulative incidence of invasive Hib disease in the first 5 years of life in the United States was estimated to be approximately 1 case per 200 children. The mortality rate for children with meningitis was 3 to 6 percent, and 20 to 30 percent of survivors had permanent sequelae, including hearing loss, mental retardation, and seizure disorders (Cochi et al., 1985). Nearly 75 percent of cases of Hib disease occurred in children younger than 2 years of age, and the susceptibility of young children to infection with Hib correlated with their lack of antibody to the type b capsular polysaccharide, polyribosylribitol phosphate (PRP) (Ward and Cochi, 1988).

In the 1970s, a vaccine composed of purified PRP, the plain polysaccharide vaccine, was prepared and was found to be immunogenic in adults and older children. However, responsiveness to PRP was highly age dependent. The vaccine was without protective efficacy in children less than 18 months of age and was of variable efficacy even when given at 2 years of age (Black et al., 1988; Harrison et al., 1988; Osterholm et al., 1988; Peltola et al., 1984; Shapiro et al., 1988). In addition to variable estimates of vaccine efficacy, several investigators noted a possible increased incidence of disease in the immediate postimmunization period (less than 7 days) (Black et al., 1988; Harrison et al., 1988; Osterholm et al., 1988; Shapiro et al., 1988).

In the 1980s, several groups of investigators developed the first Hib polysaccharide-protein conjugate vaccines. Enhancement of the immunogenicity of carbohydrate antigens by chemical conjugation with proteins had been reported in 1929 by Avery and Goebel, but the idea had not been previously applied to the development of vaccines for human use. The Hib conjugate vaccines prepared by Schneerson et al. (1980), Gordon (1984), and Anderson (1983) showed enhanced immunogenicity and T-cell-dependent characteristics, that is, responses in immature animals, booster responses, predominance of immunoglobulin G (IgG) antibodies, and priming by prior carrier immunization.

A series of Hib conjugate vaccines was developed, tested, and licensed in the late 1980s. These vaccines differ in the molecular size of the Hib polysaccharide, the protein used as the carrier, and the methods used to link the polysaccharide to the protein (Table 9-1). Thus, in consideration of the side effects of Hib conjugate vaccines, it is plausible that variations in the type or frequency of adverse effects may occur because of differences in the polysaccharide or protein components of the vaccines.

Routine immunization of infants with Hib conjugate vaccine in a multiple-dose schedule is now recommended in the United States (American Academy of Pediatrics, Committee on Infectious Diseases, 1991b; Centers for Disease Control, 1991a). Because of the need to provide protective immunity during the high-risk period of infancy and for parental convenience, Hib conjugate vaccines are given simultaneously with diphtheria and tetanus toxoids and pertussis vaccine (DPT) and polio vaccines. The efficacies of these schedules on the basis of the results of prelicensure trials were estimated to be greater than 90 percent for PRP-outer membrane protein vaccine (PRP-OMP) in Navajo infants when given at 2 and 4 months of age (Santosham et al., 1992) and 100 percent after three doses of oligosaccharide conjugate Hib (HbOC) vaccine given at 2, 4, and 6 months of age (Black et al., 1992a). A new Hib conjugate vaccine, PRP conjugated to tetanus toxoid (PRP-T), was licensed on March 30, 1993 (Centers for Disease Control and Prevention, 1993). The immunogenicity of this vaccine in infants immunized at ages 2, 4, and 6 months is similar to that of previously licensed Hib conjugate vaccines (Decker et al., 1992). Although controlled trials of the efficacy of PRP-T in the United States had to be terminated because of licensure of other conjugate vaccines, no cases of invasive disease were detected in approximately 100,000 infants given two or more doses in these and other studies (Fritzell and Plotkin, 1992; Greenberg et al., 1991), and a controlled trial in the Oxford region of the United King-

TABLE 9-1 Characteristics of Hib Vaccines

Vaccine, (producer, trade name)	Polysaccharide	Protein Carrier	Age of Administration (date of licensure)
PRP (Praxis, b Capsa 1; Lederle, HibImmune; Connaught, HibVAX)	"Native"	None	>24 mo (4/85)[a] (>18 mo if high risk)
PRP-D (Connaught, ProHiBit)	Medium	Diphtheria toxoid	18 mo (12/22/87)[b] 15 mo (12/89)[c]
HbOC (Lederle-Praxis, Hib-TITER)	Small	CRM_{197} mutant of *Corynebacterium diphtheriae* protein	18 mo (12/22/88)[d] 15 mo (12/89)[c] 2 mo (10/4/90)[e]
PRP-OMP (Merck Sharp & Dohme, PedvaxHIB)	Medium	*Neisseria meningiditis* outer membrane protein complex	15 mo (12/89)[c] 2 mo (12/13/90)[f]
PRP-T, (Pasteur Merieux-Connaught Vaccins, ActHIB)	Large	Tetanus toxoid	2 mo (3/30/93)[g]

[a]Centers for Disease Control (1985).
[b]Centers for Disease Control (1988).
[c]Centers for Disease Control (1990a).
[d]Centers for Disease Control (1989).
[e]Centers for Disease Control (1990b).
[f]Centers for Disease Control (1990d).
[g]Centers for Disease Control and Prevention (1993).

dom demonstrated efficacy of the vaccine when given at ages 2, 3, and 4 months (Booy et al., 1992). Following the widespread distribution and administration of Hib conjugate vaccines, few cases of vaccine failure (a case of Hib disease occurring more than 14 days after the second or third doses) have been reported (Black et al., 1992a; Holmes et al., 1991; Santosham et al., 1992), and postlicensure studies have shown a marked decrease in the incidence of Hib disease in the United States (Adams et al., 1993; Black et al., 1992b; Broadhurst et al., 1993; Centers for Disease Control, 1990c; Murphy et al., 1993b).

The American Academy of Pediatrics and the Advisory Committee on Immunization Practices recommend that conjugate Hib vaccines be administered as two to three doses beginning at age 2 months and then a booster at 12 to 15 months.

BIOLOGIC EVENTS FOLLOWING IMMUNIZATION

The Hib vaccines themselves contain no infective agents, just the organism's capsular polysaccharide; thus, there is no risk of developing Hib infection or clinical manifestations of Hib disease from any of the Hib vaccine components themselves (Granoff and Osterholm, 1987; Weinberg and Granoff, 1988). Occasionally, however, Hib disease is falsely diagnosed following immunization with both plain PRP and conjugated Hib vaccines, on the basis of the results of urine PRP antigen detection tests, because children excrete PRP in their urine for several days following immunization (Goepp et al., 1992; Jones et al., 1991; Spinola et al., 1986). The risk of developing a Hib infection within the first 7 days following immunization with Hib vaccines is discussed later in this chapter.

Rates of local reactions to Hib vaccines, such as pain, tenderness, swelling, and erythema at the site of injection, have varied from study to study, but the overall reaction rates to plain PRP vaccines are lower than those to conjugate vaccines. Approximately 20 to 25 percent of children develop local pain or tenderness, and 5 to 15 percent have redness or swelling at the injection sites in the 24 to 72 hours following immunization. These reactions are almost always mild and transient. Low-grade fever has been reported in the first 24 to 72 hours postimmunization in from 1 to 20 percent of Hib vaccine recipients. Temperatures of 39°C (102.2°F) or greater have been reported in less than 2 percent of Hib vaccine recipients. Most investigators have reported irritability in 10 percent or fewer of plain PRP vaccine recipients and about 10 to 25 percent of conjugate vaccine recipients. These systemic reactions are short-lived and are not felt to be serious by parents or physicians (Ahonkhai et al., 1990, 1991; Barkin et al., 1987; Black et al., 1987, 1991b; Campbell et al., 1990; Claesson et al., 1988, 1989, 1991; Clements et al., 1990; Dashefsky et al., 1990; Decker et al., 1992; Eskola et al., 1990a; Ferreccio et al., 1991; Frayha et al., 1991; Fritzell and Plotkin, 1992; Granoff and Cates, 1985; Granoff and Osterholm, 1987; Greenberg et al., 1987; Hendley et al., 1987; Kayhty et al., 1988, 1989; Kovel et al., 1992; Lenoir et al., 1987; Lepow et al., 1984a, 1985, 1986, 1987; Milstien et al., 1987; Parke et al., 1991; Peltola et al., 1977; Popejoy et al., 1989; Rowe et al., 1990; Santosham et al., 1991a; Vadheim et al., 1990; Watemberg et al., 1991; Weinberg and Granoff, 1988).

Rates of local and systemic reactions to Hib vaccines have usually been similar to or lower than those to injections with placebo or DPT, inactivated polio vaccine, or measles-mumps-rubella vaccine (MMR) alone or to those vaccines plus Hib vaccines (Ahonkhai et al., 1991; Black et al., 1991b; Campbell et al., 1990; Clements et al., 1990; Eskola et al., 1987; Lepow et al., 1984a, 1987; Vadheim et al., 1990; Watemberg et al., 1991). Exceptions include a study by Dashefsky et al. (1990), in which 71 percent of infants receiving the PRP-OMP vaccine plus MMR were reported to develop irritability compared with 35 percent for groups receiving either vaccine alone, and a study by Ferreccio et al. (1991), which found a 7 to 20 percent increase in fever in children who received PRP-T with DPT than in those who received DPT alone.

Immunization with the first-generation Hib polysaccharide, or purified PRP, vaccine stimulates production of anti-PRP antibody in the same manner as natural infection (Granoff and Cates, 1985; Norden et al., 1976; Trollfors et al., 1992). This immune response is felt to be T-cell independent. In contrast, the immune responses to PRP conjugate vaccines appear to use T cells as well as B cells (Robbins and Schneerson, 1990; Steinhoff et al., 1991; Weinberg and Granoff, 1988). Antibodies produced in response to the intact organism, plain PRP vaccines, and conjugate vaccines have subtle differences, but all have been demonstrated to have in vitro opsonic and bactericidal activities and to be protective in animal models of Hib disease as well as in human trials (Adams, 1992; Anderson et al., 1972; Black, 1992; Black et al., 1988, 1991a,b; Cates, 1985; Cates et al., 1985; Eskola et al., 1987, 1990a,b, 1992; Fothergill and Wright, 1933; Fritzell and Plotkin, 1992; Gray, 1990; Kulhanjian, 1992; Loughlin et al., 1992; Musher et al., 1988; Newman et al., 1973; Peltola, 1992; Peltola et al., 1984; Robbins et al., 1973; Santosham et al., 1991b; Schneerson et al., 1971; Schreiber et al., 1986; Smith et al., 1989; Vadheim, 1992).

The difference in reliance on T cells for antibody production results in differences in the age at which the antibody response occurs, the amount of antibody produced, and the ability to boost antibody production by revaccination or exposure to the organism. The conjugate vaccines stimulate anti-PRP antibody responses in young infants, whereas the plain PRP vaccines do not provide protective amounts of antibody in most individuals until after the age of 2 years. The conjugate vaccines also induce larger amounts of anti-PRP antibodies in vaccinees of all ages, and they induce an anti-PRP antibody response in many individuals who do not respond well to natural infection with Hib or to the plain PRP vaccine, including patients with Hib disease before the age of 2 years and those with splenectomy; sickle cell disease; malignancy; IgG_2 deficiency; Navajo, Apache, and Alaskan natives; and allogeneic bone marrow recipients (Barra et al., 1992; Edwards et al., 1989; Feldman et al., 1990; Frank et al., 1988; Gigliotti et al., 1989, 1991; Granoff et al., 1989; Kafidi and Rotschafer, 1988; Kaplan et al., 1988; Marcinak et al., 1991; Rubin et al., 1989, 1992; Santosham et al., 1992; Siber et al., 1990; Steinhoff et al., 1991; Walter et al., 1990; Weinberg and Granoff, 1990; Weisman et al., 1987).

It is evident that the different Hib vaccines produce not only different quantities of anti-PRP antibody but also that this antibody differs in such characteristics as IgG subclass, avidity, and affinity (Ambrosino et al., 1992;

Decker et al., 1992; Granoff et al., 1988; Hetherington and Lepow, 1992; Holmes et al., 1991; Insel and Anderson, 1986; Parke et al., 1991; Schlesinger and Granoff, 1992; Shackelford and Granoff, 1988). These differences produce subtle functional differences in vitro, but the implications for protective activity in vivo are unknown (Amir et al., 1990a,b).

Individuals who produce protective levels of antibody to Hib vaccines generally do so within 1 month of immunization (Kayhty et al., 1989; Peltola et al., 1977). Good immune responses to the conjugate vaccines have been demonstrated as soon as 1 week after immunization in older children and adults (Daum et al., 1989; Marchant et al., 1989).

Unlike plain PRP vaccines, PRP conjugate vaccines stimulate memory B cells capable of generating booster responses to immunization with either plain PRP or PRP conjugate vaccines and, thus, presumably, to the intact Hib organism (Weinberg et al., 1987). PRP conjugate vaccines reduce the Hib oropharyngeal carrier state (Barbour, 1992; Mohle-Boetani, 1992; Murphy, 1991; Takala et al., 1991).

TRANSVERSE MYELITIS

Clinical Description

Myelitis is inflammation of the spinal cord. Transverse myelitis is myelitis in which the inflammatory process principally involves one or more spinal cord segments, showing the manifestations of a transverse cord lesion that usually develops acutely. Initially, many cases of transverse myelitis are not complete. Early symptoms in some patients include sphincter paralysis associated with a total or partial loss of sensation below the level of the lesion. As the acute spinal shock resolves, the paraplegia becomes spastic. Acute multiple sclerosis and postinfective myelitis are among the commonest causes of this syndrome. The annual incidence of transverse myelitis in Rochester, Minnesota, from 1970 to 1980 was 0.83 per 100,000 people (Beghi et al., 1982).

History of Suspected Association

The history of a suspected association between Hib vaccines and transverse myelitis is based solely on three case reports in the Vaccine Adverse Event Reporting System (VAERS). There are no reports in the literature of an association between Hib vaccines and transverse myelitis.

Evidence for Association

Biologic Plausibility

A general discussion of transverse myelitis and vaccination can be found in Chapter 3. There are no data specifically bearing on the biologic plausibility of a causal relation between Hib vaccines and transverse myelitis.

Case Reports, Case Series, and Uncontrolled Observational Studies

There have been three cases reported in VAERS (submitted between November 1990 and July 1992) labeled as "transverse myelitis" following Hib vaccination. HbOC vaccine was the Hib vaccine used in all three cases. In one patient (there appeared to be two reports of this one case), the HbOC vaccine was administered alone, in the second the HbOC vaccine was administered with DPT and oral polio vaccine (OPV), and in the third HbOC vaccine was administered with DPT, OPV, and MMR. Only the third case provided sufficient evidence to establish a diagnosis of transverse myelitis. This child developed transverse myelitis 14 days after immunization with the HbOC, DPT, OPV, and MMR. She had a diffuse rash, diarrhea, and a fever 10 days after vaccination and 4 days prior to the onset of transverse myelitis. This case report was the only one to provide information on follow-up. At 4.5 months following vaccination, a magnetic resonance image (MRI) of the thoracic spine showed extensive atrophic change of the thoracic cord, extending from the seventh thoracic vertebra (T-7) through T-12. At 10 months postvaccination there was "persistent transverse myelitis" at the T-8 through T-10 level.

Insufficient data were provided for the other two cases to determine whether the children actually had transverse myelitis. One of these children developed a temperature of 40.6°C (105°F) and "extreme floppiness and toxic appearance" 24 to 36 hours after immunization with the HbOC vaccine alone. He had a "multitude of lab tests and MRI" and was hospitalized for 30 days. The other baby was noted to be unable to crawl 12 days after immunization with the HbOC vaccine, DPT, and OPV. The mother reported that a neurologist felt that this child had possible transverse myelitis from polio vaccine. She reported that the lumbar puncture and brain scan were normal. The child was hospitalized for 2 days, and no further follow-up information was provided.

There have been no cases of transverse myelitis reported in any case series or uncontrolled observational studies of Hib vaccines (Ahonkhai et al., 1990, 1991; Black et al., 1987; Claesson et al., 1991; Fritzell and Plotkin, 1992; Milstien et al., 1987; Parke et al., 1991; Popejoy et al., 1989; Rowe et al., 1990; Santosham et al., 1991a; Vadheim et al., 1990).

Controlled Observational Studies

There have been no controlled observational studies investigating an association between Hib vaccines and transverse myelitis.

Controlled Clinical Trials

Transverse myelitis has not been reported in any of the controlled clinical trials of plain PRP or PRP conjugate vaccines that have been performed (Barkin et al., 1987; Black et al., 1991b; Campbell et al., 1990; Claesson et al., 1988, 1989; Clements et al., 1990; Dashefsky et al., 1990; Decker et al., 1992; Eskola et al., 1987, 1990a,b; Ferreccio et al., 1991; Frayha et al., 1991; Granoff and Osterholm, 1987; Greenberg et al., 1987; Hendley et al., 1987; Kayhty et al., 1988, 1989; Kovel et al., 1992; Lenoir et al., 1987; Lepow et al., 1984a,b, 1985, 1986, 1987; Peltola et al., 1977; Santosham et al., 1992; Watemberg et al., 1991).

Causality Argument

There is no animal model or other data supporting the association between Hib vaccines and transverse myelitis. There are three cases reported in VAERS labeled "transverse myelitis" in children aged 6, 9, and 15 months occurring following the administration of HbOC vaccine during a period when an estimated several million doses of HbOC vaccine were administered. One of these children received HbOC vaccine alone, and the interval between immunization and the development of neurologic symptoms in this child was brief (less than 48 hours). A second child also received DPT and OPV. The patient for whom sufficient documentation of transverse myelitis was provided also had received DPT, OPV, and MMR. No cases of transverse myelitis have been reported following administration of the other Hib vaccines, nor have any cases been reported in the literature.

Conclusion

The evidence is inadequate to accept or reject a causal relation between Hib vaccines and transverse myelitis.

GUILLAIN-BARRÉ SYNDROME

Clinical Description

The Guillain-Barré syndrome (GBS) is an acute polyneuropathy that gives rise to muscular weakness, paralysis, and areflexia usually in an ascending pattern. About one-third of patients with GBS require assisted ventilation, but rarely is the condition fatal. In most patients there is spontaneous improvement after weeks or months, usually leading to complete recovery. The annual incidence of GBS appears to be approximately 1 per 100,000 for adults. The data are not definitive, but the annual incidence of GBS in children under age 5 years appears to be approximately the same. The annual incidence of GBS in children over age 5 years and teenagers appears to be lower. Chapter 3 contains a detailed discussion of GBS.

History of Suspected Association

In 1989, D'Cruz and coworkers reported three cases of GBS following immunization with the Hib conjugate vaccine PRP-diphtheria toxoid (PRP-D). Two children received the PRP-D vaccine alone, but the third child received DPT and OPV as well. The onset of symptoms in this child occurred 1 day following immunization. One day is too short a period of time, as described in Chapter 3, to support the notion that the GBS attack was plausibly related to the vaccination.

Evidence for Association

Biologic Plausibility

A general discussion of GBS and vaccination can be found in Chapter 3. There are no data specifically bearing on the biologic plausibility of a causal relation between Hib vaccines and GBS.

Case Reports, Case Series, and Uncontrolled Observational Studies

A total of seven cases labeled GBS have been described following immunization with the three Hib conjugate vaccines that are currently licensed for use in the United States. The three cases following administration of the PRP-D vaccine noted above occurred during a period when approximately 6.2 million doses of PRP-D vaccine were distributed (D'Cruz et al., 1989). None of these children were noted to have an antecedent infection. A different lot of PRP-D vaccine was used in each child.

A fourth case of GBS following vaccination with PRP-D vaccine was reported recently by Gervaix and colleagues (1993). A 4-year-old girl developed signs of GBS (progressive weakness in legs with hypotonia and complete loss of tendon reflexes, difficulty in swallowing, and bilateral facial weakness) 10 days after receiving PRP-D Hib vaccine. The report documented decreased nerve conduction velocities and prolonged distal latencies. Serological tests were negative for cytomegalovirus, herpesvirus, Epstein-Barr virus, *Borrelia burgdorferi,* and *Campylobacter* species. IgM antibodies to PRP in plasma were high 15 days after immunization. The child responded to intravenous immunoglobulin therapy.

The other three reports of GBS following the administration of Hib conjugate vaccines were detected by VAERS (submitted between November 1990 and July 1992). Two of the three children developed an infection between the time of immunization and the onset of the neurologic symptoms. These two children developed GBS (within the time frame described by the committee as plausible) following immunization with HbOC vaccine. One of these children also had received MMR, and the other child had received DPT and OPV at the time of the HbOC immunization. The former developed GBS 12 days following immunization and 6 days following the onset of otitis media and bronchospasm. The latter developed GBS 6 days after immunization and was noted to be on amoxicillin, but the indication for antibiotic therapy was not specified.

The third VAERS report described a child who was immunized as part of a PRP-OMP vaccine safety trial and was not noted to have received any other vaccine. This child developed an unsteady gait and decreased deep tendon reflexes 44 days after immunization and had otitis media, an upper respiratory tract infection, and a rash about 1 month following receipt of Hib vaccine and 2 weeks prior to the onset of neurologic symptoms. The child's discharge diagnosis was GBS. Although the latency is close to the window specified by the committee as reasonable (see Chapter 2), the other antecedent events (infection and rash) also suggest that if this child had GBS, it was far more likely related to these antecedent events.

In one of the PRP-D vaccine recipients (D'Cruz et al., 1989) and one of the HbOC vaccine recipients reported by VAERS, OPV was given concurrently. An increased incidence of GBS was reported to have coincided with a national OPV immunization campaign in Finland, as discussed in Chapter 8 (Farkkila et al., 1991; Kinnunen et al., 1989; Uhari et al., 1989).

The time of onset of symptoms following Hib vaccine administration ranged from 1 day (D'Cruz et al., 1989) to 44 days (a report from VAERS) in seven patients, with the onset of symptoms in five of the patients beginning 6 to 12 days after vaccination. The cases beginning 1 and 44 days after vaccination are not considered likely to be related to vaccination (see Chapter 3). The ages of the patients whose GBS began 6 to 12 days after vaccination were 15, 19, 20, and 33 months and 4 years. The symptoms of GBS resolved in three of these patients, and the outcomes for the others were not reported.

There have been no cases of GBS reported in any case series or uncontrolled observational studies of Hib vaccines (Ahonkhai et al., 1990, 1991; Black et al., 1987; Claesson et al., 1991; Fritzell and Plotkin, 1992; Milstien et al., 1987; Parke et al., 1991; Popejoy et al., 1989; Rowe et al., 1990; Santosham et al., 1991a; Vadheim et al., 1990).

Controlled Observational Studies

There have been no controlled observational studies investigating an association between Hib vaccines and GBS.

Controlled Clinical Trials

GBS has not been reported in any of the controlled clinical trials of plain PRP or PRP conjugate vaccines that have been performed (Barkin et al., 1987; Black et al., 1991b; Campbell et al., 1990; Claesson et al., 1988, 1989; Clements et al., 1990; Dashefsky et al., 1990; Decker et al., 1992; Eskola et al., 1987, 1990a,b; Ferreccio et al., 1991; Frayha et al., 1991; Granoff and Osterholm, 1987; Greenberg et al., 1987; Hendley et al., 1987; Kayhty et al., 1988, 1989; Kovel et al., 1992; Lenoir et al., 1987; Lepow et al., 1984a,b, 1985, 1986, 1987; Peltola et al., 1977; Santosham et al., 1992; Watemberg et al., 1991).

Causality Argument

There are no animal models of GBS following immunization for Hib; however, Chapter 3 presents evidence that GBS is biologically plausible as a consequence of vaccines in general. Data bearing on causality are limited to case reports. Seven cases labeled as GBS were reported to occur following immunization with three different Hib conjugate vaccines over a period when an estimated several million doses of Hib conjugate vaccines were distributed. Five of these cases fit the criteria for possible vaccine-related GBS discussed in Chapter 3. Hib conjugate vaccine administration was the only potential predisposing factor cited for the development of GBS in three of the five children who fit the case definition of GBS following immunization for Hib. Gervaix and colleagues (1993) speculated that the anti-PRP IgM antibodies detected in the plasma of the patient they described might have cross-reacted with glycoproteins of peripheral nerve myelin, leading to GBS. Two of the five children who developed GBS following immunization with Hib vaccine had possible predisposing factors (infections, OPV immunization) other than Hib immunization.

Conclusion

The evidence is inadequate to accept or reject a causal relation between Hib vaccines and GBS.

THROMBOCYTOPENIA

Clinical Description

Thrombocytopenia is a decrease in the number of platelets, the cells involved in blood clotting. Thrombocytopenia may stem from the failure of platelet production, a shortened platelet life span, or an abnormal distribution of platelets within the body (Lee et al., 1993). Thrombocytopenia occurs in children of all ages, with an incidence of 31.9 cases per 1 million children per year (Cohn, 1976). Approximately 70 percent of cases occur following viral illnesses (Lightsey, 1980). In most cases, thrombocytopenia in children is mild and transient, and it is often discovered only incidentally when a complete blood count is performed. Severe thrombocytopenia associated with spontaneous bleeding, including bleeding into the skin, is called *thrombocytopenic purpura*.

History of Suspected Association

A possible association of Hib vaccine with thrombocytopenia was noted by Granoff et al. (1984) in a trial of the PRP-D vaccine in adults. Thirty subjects were randomly assigned to receive two doses of either the PRP or the PRP-D vaccine. Because this was one of the first trials of Hib conjugate vaccine in human subjects, multiple hematologic, renal, and hepatic tests were performed after the administration of each dose. One subject developed transient, asymptomatic thrombocytopenia after receiving the second injection of PRP-D vaccine. His platelet count fell from $173,000/mm^3$ before the second injection to $80,000/mm^3$ 7 days after the injection. There was no associated evidence of bleeding, and the platelet count was $153,000/mm^3$ 12 days later (normal range, 150,000 to $350,000/mm^3$). The causal relation between PRP-D vaccine and thrombocytopenia in this subject was not clear because he had received tetanus toxoid 4 weeks earlier and also was taking a number of medications for migraine headaches. None of the other subjects in that study experienced a decrease in platelet count, including the remaining 14 subjects who received PRP-D vaccine and the 15 subjects who received PRP vaccine. A second study of the effect of two doses of PRP and PRP-D vaccines on hematologic indices was conducted in 61 adults (Lepow et al., 1984b). No effect of either vaccine on platelet count was observed.

Evidence for Association

Biologic Plausibility

There are no studies in experimental animals or human subjects to suggest a possible mechanism by which Hib polysaccharide or its protein conjugates might produce thrombocytopenia. Natural infections with live viruses may induce thrombocytopenia by damage to megakaryocytes, destruction of circulating platelets, or induction of viral antigen-antibody complexes that sensitize platelets to increased destruction or sequestration (Kaplan et al., 1992; Lee et al., 1993). In patients with severe bacterial infections, including Hib infections, thrombocytopenia frequently occurs as a manifestation of disseminated intravascular coagulation (DIC). Thrombocytopenia also has been reported in adult patients with gram-negative and gram-positive septicemia but without evidence of DIC (Keltow et al., 1979). The thrombocytopenia in these patients was thought to result from the interaction of platelets with immune complexes.

Thrombocytopenia without evidence of DIC also has been observed in children with bacterial septicemia, including systemic Hib infections (Corrigan, 1974; Thomas and O'Brien, 1986). The mechanism by which the decreased platelet count occurs in these children is unknown, but it should be noted that intact Hib organisms contain many components not present in Hib vaccines. Some of these components, such as lipooligosaccharide, can induce an inflammatory response, including activation of platelet-activating factor and the coagulation cascade. These events can induce platelet aggregation and thus decrease the intravascular platelet count. There is no evidence that the capsular polysaccharide of Hib causes a similar inflammatory response (Quagliarello and Scheld, 1992; Saez-Llorens et al., 1990; Syrogiannopoulos et al., 1988). No published data from studies in animals were found, but Lepow et al. (1984b) referred to hematologic studies in rats, including serial bone marrow evaluations, that failed to demonstrate any effect of PRP-D vaccine on platelet counts.

Case Reports, Case Series, and Uncontrolled Observational Studies

Five cases of thrombocytopenia following immunization for Hib were reported through VAERS between November 1990 and July 1992, a period during which approximately 29.5 million doses of Hib vaccine were distributed in the United States (a rough estimate based on 1991 data provided by the Centers for Disease Control). In one case, the thrombocytopenia occurred 7 days after receipt of DPT, OPV, and HbOC vaccine and was associated with high fever, diarrhea, weight loss, seizures, and renal failure, a symptom complex resembling hemolytic-uremic syndrome. The report stated that there was a "possibility of permanent renal dysfunction and possible brain damage," but no follow-up information was available. The other four cases occurred in children who had received MMR in addition to the Hib vaccines (two children received HbOC vaccine, one child received PRP-D vaccine, and one child received an unspecified Hib vaccine). Thrombocytopenia developed 5 to 13 days after immunization, and all four patients recovered. Two of the children had only petechiae and purpura in association with the thrombocytopenia, one child had a high fever and maculopapular rash in addition to petechiae, and one child had fever, a maculopapular rash, erythema multiforme, petechiae, and purpura.

Milstien and coworkers (1987) published a summary of the adverse reactions reported to the U.S. Food and Drug Administration (FDA) during the first year after marketing of the PRP vaccine (1985-1986). During that time, 4.5 million doses of vaccine were sold. Included in that summary was one report of petechiae (platelet count not given), one case of idiopathic thrombocytopenic purpura (ITP) (platelet count, 15,000/mm^3) diagnosed 18 days after immunization, and one child who developed a low platelet count associated with hemolytic-uremic syndrome that began 2 days after receiving PRP vaccine.

Controlled Observational Studies

A study of the effect of two doses of PRP and PRP-D vaccines on hematologic indices was conducted in 61 adults (Lepow et al., 1984b). No effect of either vaccine on platelet count was observed.

Controlled Clinical Trials

In several large prospective trials of PRP and Hib conjugate vaccine efficacy and safety (Black et al., 1987, 1991b; Eskola et al., 1990a; Peltola et al., 1977; Santosham et al., 1991b; Vadheim et al., 1990), no subjects developed petechiae or purpura. Platelet counts were not measured, so the incidence of asymptomatic thrombocytopenia after immunization with Hib vaccines is unknown.

Causality Argument

The information concerning thrombocytopenia and Hib vaccines is limited. There is no biologic plausibility (data from animal models or experimental studies) to suggest a mechanism for thrombocytopenia following immunization for Hib. One case of thrombocytopenia without clinical illness occurred in a clinical trial study subject who had other possible risk factors that could have been responsible for the decline in platelet count

(Granoff et al., 1984). Four cases of thrombocytopenia have been reported through VAERS, and all subjects received other vaccines including a live viral vaccine, MMR. MMR is associated with thrombocytopenia (see Chapter 6). An additional report in VAERS described an event resembling hemolytic-uremic syndrome following immunization for Hib, diphtheria, tetanus, and pertussis (DPT), and polio (OPV). One case of ITP and one case of hemolytic-uremic syndrome were reported to the FDA following immunization with PRP vaccine (Milstien et al., 1987). No information regarding other medications or illnesses in the child with ITP was provided in the summary report. Most cases of hemolytic-uremic syndrome are now known to follow enteritis caused by intestinal pathogens that produce verotoxins (shigella-like toxins) (Centers for Disease Control, 1991b; Rowe et al., 1991). Both patients with hemolytic-uremic syndrome associated with Hib vaccine administration (noted above) presented with diarrhea. Thus, it is most likely that these were related to enteritis caused by verotoxin-producing *Escherichia coli* or *Shigella dysenteriae* rather than the Hib vaccines, which contain no toxins.

Conclusion

The evidence is inadequate to accept or reject a causal relation between Hib vaccines and thrombocytopenia.

EARLY SUSCEPTIBILITY TO *H. INFLUENZAE* TYPE b

Clinical Description

Early-onset Hib disease following immunization is defined as a case of serious systemic infection caused by Hib that occurs within the 7-day interval following immunization for Hib. The annual incidence of Hib has decreased dramatically with the introduction of Hib vaccines.

History of Suspected Association

In conducting vaccine efficacy trials for Hib vaccines, investigators expected to observe a number of vaccine "failures" (i.e., none of the Hib vaccines was likely to be 100 percent effective in the prevention of disease, particularly after administration of a single dose to young infants). For calculation of efficacy, "immunization" was usually defined as receipt of vaccine more than 14 days prior to the onset of disease; 14 days was considered a reasonable time period for development of a protective antibody response. In studies of vaccine efficacy for the unconjugated PRP vaccine, a wide range of estimates of vaccine efficacy was observed in various locations in the United States (Black et al., 1988; Harrison et al., 1988; Osterholm et al., 1988; Shapiro et al., 1988). This observation was not easily explained by differences in study design or vaccine potency or by genetic differences among study populations. Furthermore, in several case-control studies there appeared to be an increased incidence of disease in the immediate postimmunization period (7 days or less) (Black et al., 1988; Harrison et al., 1988; Osterholm et al., 1988; Shapiro et al., 1988).

Evidence for Association

Biologic Plausibility

PRP vaccine contained only purified capsular polysaccharide, so the early-onset cases of Hib infection could not have been caused by infectious material in the vaccine itself. Several investigators postulated that the apparent increased susceptibility to infection in the immediate postimmunization period might be related to a transient decrease in preexisting antibody caused by the formation of complexes of antigen with antibody or by transient suppression of antibody synthesis (Marchant et al., 1989; Sood and Daum, 1990). Black and coworkers (1988) postulated that the clustering of early cases in the first week after immunization and the absence of cases in the second and third weeks after immunization observed in their study suggest that immunization may shorten the incubation period of Hib in children already destined to become ill. This mechanism implies that there is a redistribution of cases of disease to earlier in the time postimmunization rather than an actual increase in the rate of disease.

Observations of decreased immunity in the immediate postimmunization period were recorded as early as 1893 by Brieger and Ehrlich in a study of immunity in goat's milk after immunization with tetanus cultures. In 1896, Salomonsen and Madsen noted a decreased anti-diphtheria antibody content in the serum of horses early after immunization with diphtheria toxin, and those workers pointed out three phases of antitoxin response: (1) a fall, later called the "negative" phase, (2) a rise, and, after phase 2 reaches a maximum, (3) a fall. Madsen and coworkers (1937) studied the "negative" phase of the antitoxin curve in detail using rabbits immunized with diphtheria toxin. They were able to demonstrate that the negative phase in their experiments resulted from fixation between antigen and antitoxin in the bloodstream. Studies of individuals immunized for typhoid fever have suggested that immunization may transiently enhance susceptibility to infection both in epidemics of typhoid fever and in experimental murine infections (Raettig, 1959; Topley, 1938).

Using an infant rat model of Hib infection, Sood and colleagues (Sood and Daum, 1990; Sood et al., 1988) showed that the passive protection of animals provided by human immunoglobulin containing 5 μg of anti-PRP antibody per ml was diminished by administration of a wide range of doses of PRP vaccine (25-250 ng). These doses of antibody and antigen were chosen to simulate clinically relevant amounts in children who receive a 25-μg dose of PRP in the vaccine. The magnitude but not the incidence of bacteremia varied with the dose of vaccine. Interestingly, small doses of vaccine that significantly affected the incidence and degree of bacteremia did not measurably affect antibody concentrations in the serum of rats, and thus, the relation between the decrease in the level of antibody and the occurrence of bacteremia in this model remains unclear. The conjugate vaccines varied in their ability to reverse passive immunity in rats, a phenomenon that may be related to variations in the binding of anti-capsular antibody to the different vaccine antigens (Sood and Daum, 1990).

The demonstration of detectable antigenuria in many children for as long as 7 days following immunization with PRP vaccine (Spinola et al., 1986) or with Hib conjugate vaccines (Jones et al., 1991; Sood and Daum, 1990) implies that children are antigenemic after immunization and, thus, that binding of free antibody and depression of the levels of free antibody can occur.

Anti-PRP antibody concentrations were sequentially measured in the serum of human subjects for 7 days following immunization with PRP (adults and children) or PRP-D (adults) vaccine. A decline was observed in most 2-year-old children immunized with PRP vaccine and in adults immunized with either vaccine (Daum et al., 1989). The nadir occurred on days 1 to 3, and the decrease averaged 25 percent for adults and 15 percent for children. Thus, it is theoretically possible that some Hib infections that occur early after immunization with vaccine are the result of this transient decrease in free antibody levels. However, in the same study, antibody levels were shown to rise rapidly after immunization and were greater than preimmunization levels in adults by day 7. In children, the distribution of antibody levels in sera obtained at 4 or 5 days postimmunization (with PRP vaccine) did not differ from that in preimmunization serum. In another study (Marchant et al., 1989), among 30 infants aged 18 to 21 months immunized with PRP-D vaccine, 9 had detectable preimmunization anti-PRP antibody concentrations (greater than 0.025 μg/ml). Although all nine of these children had depression of antibody on the second day after immunization, all achieved anti-PRP concentrations of greater than 0.15 μg/ml (a level thought to be protective against Hib challenge) by day 7. In that same study, 21 children were found to have undetectable antibody concentrations before immunization. All but 2 of these 21 children developed detectable antibody by day 7, and 67 percent of these children achieved protective levels by that time. The investigators concluded that although the small proportion of infants among previously unimmunized infants with preexisting antibody may develop a transient depression of antibody following immunization with Hib vaccine, the more important determinant of susceptibility to early Hib disease in this age group is acquisition of protective antibody rather than depression of preexisting antibody levels. A recent study (Granoff et al., in press) demonstrated that PRP vaccine induces high antibody responses within 6 to 9 days after vaccination when given to 12-month-old infants who were previously vaccinated with Hib conjugate vaccine beginning at 2 months of age. Proof that transient suppression of preexisting antibody may be associated with increased susceptibility to Hib disease can come only from epidemiologic studies of recently immunized versus unimmunized populations.

Another possible mechanism of enhanced susceptibility to Hib disease in the early postimmunization period is the transient suppression of antibody synthesis. This alternative is unlikely on the basis of the observation that children with "early" cases of Hib disease after vaccination have excellent antibody responses to their disease (Murphy, 1987).

Case Reports, Case Series, and Uncontrolled Observational Studies (PRP)

LeMay (1986) presented the first report of a case of Hib infection occurring early after immunization. This case was in a 2.5-year-old child who developed epiglottitis with a blood culture positive for Hib within 24 hours after immunization with PRP vaccine. The child attended a day-care center but had not been in contact with individuals known to have Hib disease. The author emphasized the implication of using rifampin prophylaxis rather than reliance upon postexposure immunization for the prevention of disease following identification of an index case in a day-care center or household.

Hiner and Frasch (1988) examined the spectrum of Hib disease occurring in children immunized with PRP vaccine on the basis of reports received by the Food and Drug Administration between May 1985 and September 1987. At least some of these cases overlap with the cases described in the case-control studies outlined below. The purposes of the study were (1) to examine the types of Hib disease in vaccinated children compared with the types in unvaccinated children and (2) to determine whether there was any interval after immunization in which invasive disease was more likely to occur. Reports of 216 cases were analyzed. Vaccination did not alter the frequencies of the different clinical entities associated with invasive Hib disease except in the children who developed disease within 72 hours after immunization, when meningitis was less frequent and epiglottitis and cellulitis were relatively more frequent. In the 6-month interval after immunization, more cases (53 percent) occurred in the first 2 months than at later intervals. Of the 13 cases that occurred in the first 10-day interval, 10 occurred within 72 hours of vaccination. However, the authors noted that the "data do not provide evidence for increased susceptibility immediately after immunization, because the frequency of cases by days to onset occurring within the first 60 days was random" (Hiner and Frasch, 1988, p. 346).

Controlled Observational Studies (PRP)

Four case-control studies, all of which were published in 1988 (Black et al., 1988; Harrison et al., 1988; Osterholm et al., 1988; Shapiro et al., 1988) and all of which used similar designs and methods of surveillance, bear on the question of the increased risk of early disease after receipt of PRP vaccine. The four studies are summarized in Table 9-2. The first, by Black et al. (1988), is from the Northern California Kaiser Permanente Medical Care Program. The studies by Harrison et al. (1988), Shapiro et al. (1988), and Osterholm et al. (1988) all appeared in a single issue of the *Journal of the American Medical Association* and were based on study populations throughout the United States. Although the studies of Harrison et al. (1988), Shapiro et al. (1988), and Osterholm et al. (1988) used a matched design in the primary analyses, the data on early disease were reported in an unmatched fashion.

All four of the case-control studies provided data bearing on the risk of early Hib disease within the first 7 days following vaccination. For the study by Black et al. (1988), the committee used only three of the four vaccinated (exposed) cases in the analysis, since one of the patients had requested vaccine because of contact with an individual with Hib disease (see below for the possibility of increased risk in this situation). Based on the method of Mantel and Haenszel (1959), the meta-analysis of all four studies yielded an odds ratio of 2.6 (95 percent confidence interval [CI], 1.1-7.50) for the association between PRP vaccine and the development of Hib disease within 7 days of vaccination.

Controlled Clinical Trials (PRP)

A large, randomized trial to test the efficacy of the PRP (unconjugated) vaccine was carried out by Peltola and coworkers, and the results of long-term follow-up were reported in 1984 (Peltola et al., 1984). In that study, protective efficacy was observed only in those children immunized at 18 months of age or older. Among children immunized at 18-71 months of age, no cases of Hib disease were observed within the 7-day interval following immunization. Among 37,393 children immunized with Hib vaccine, 2 developed bacteremic Hib infection (20 and 21 months after receiving vaccine, respectively). Among 38,431 controls of the same age who

TABLE 9-2 Epidemiologic Studies of Early Hib Disease with Unconjugated (PRP only) Hib Vaccine

References	Location	Design	No. Exposed[a]/ No. of Hib Cases	No. Exposed[a]/ No. of Controls	OR (95% CI)[b]
Black et al., 1988	Northern California	Case-control	3/30	61/2,774	4.9 (1.2-17.7)
Harrison et al., 1988	Los Angeles, Missouri, New Jersey, Oklahoma, Tennessee, Washington	Case-control	3/104	5/207	1.2 (0.2-5.9)
Shapiro et al., 1988	Pennsylvania, Texas, Connecticut	Case-control	1/76	1/152	2.0 (0-74.8)
Osterholm et al., 1988	Minnesota	Case-control	3/88	1/176	6.2 (0.6-156.4)
Pooled (Mantel-Haenszel) estimate					2.6 (1.1-7.5)

[a]Exposed to vaccine within preceding 7 days.
[b]OR, odds ratio; CI, confidence interval.

were immunized with group A meningococcal capsular polysaccharide vaccine, 20 developed Hib infections (1 to 42 months after receiving vaccine).

Case Reports (Hib Conjugate Vaccines)

Ten cases of early Hib disease following immunization were reported through VAERS between November 1990 and July 1992. Nine cases occurred in children who received HbOC vaccine and one in a child who received PRP-D vaccine, presumably reflecting the distribution of Hib vaccine types during that period. Five of the nine cases occurred after the administration of one dose each to infants ages 2, 2, 3, and 4.5 months and 2 years. Two infants aged 4 months developed disease after receiving two doses of vaccine, one infant aged 8 months developed disease after receiving the third dose, and one infant aged 6 months developed disease after an unspecified number of doses. The child who received PRP-D vaccine was 2 years of age. Information regarding his previous vaccine history was not available. All cases occurred within 5 days of immunization. There were eight cases of meningitis, one case of periorbital cellulitis, and one case of septicemia with disseminated intravascular coagulation and shock that occurred less than 24 hours after receiving Hib vaccine. All cases were documented by a positive culture of blood or cerebrospinal fluid, but the serotype was specified as type b in only four instances. Serotype data are crucial, because in the post-Hib vaccine era, the proportion of cases of invasive disease caused by non-type b strains may increase, reflecting the dramatic decline in type b isolates (Adams et al., 1993; Black et al., 1992b; Broadhurst et al., 1993; Centers for Disease Control, 1990c; Murphy et al., 1993).

Uncontrolled Observational Studies, Controlled Observational Studies, and Controlled Clinical Trials (Hib conjugate vaccines)

Studies that bear on the risk of early Hib disease in recipients of the more recently developed Hib conjugate vaccines (first dose only) are summarized in Table 9-3. All are based on cohort designs. Two studies (Eskola et al., 1990a; Santosham et al., 1991b) were randomized trials, one was a controlled observational cohort study (Black et al., 1991b), and the others were all based on follow-up of vaccine recipients only. Several differences among the studies are worthy of note. The studies by Black et al. (1991b, 1992b) were based on HbOC vaccine, that of Santosham et al. (1991b) was based on PRP-OMP vaccine, and those of Eskola et al. (1990a), Vadheim et al. (1990), and Scheifele (1989) used PRP-D vaccine. The studies of Eskola et al. (1990a), Black et al. (1991b), and Santosham et al. (1991b) were based on the first dose administered to young infants (6 weeks to 6 months of age), who are currently the largest group of recipients of the conjugate vaccine. The studies of both Vadheim et al. (1990) and Scheifele (1989) were based on a single dose administered to children 18 months to 60 months of age, that is, those who were formerly immunized with the unconjugated vaccine (PRP) (see studies above). In the study of Eskola et al. (1990a), the control children received one dose of PRP-D vaccine at 24 months of age.

The randomized, prospective field trial of PRP-D vaccine in 114,000 infants in Finland (Eskola et al., 1990a) showed a vaccine efficacy of 94 percent (95 percent CI, 83-98 percent) when given at 3, 4, 6, and 14-18 months of age. Eight cases of Hib disease occurred in 58,000 vaccinated children, but no cases of early Hib disease occurred following immunization. Four cases occurred after one to two doses (interval after immunization, 25 days-2.5 years) (J. Eskola, National Public Health Institute, Helsinki, Finland, personal communication, 1993), and four cases occurred after three doses (days 55-173 after immunization) (Eskola et al., 1990a). The control children received PRP-D vaccine at 24 months of age, and one child in this group developed epiglottitis with Hib bacteremia at 24 months of age on the same day that she received PRP-D vaccine and DPT.

Although control groups were studied by Eskola et al. (1990a), Black et al. (1991b), and Santosham et al. (1991b), no relative risk estimate for early disease can be calculated, since no cases of Hib were observed within 7 days of vaccination in either the vaccinated or unvaccinated groups in any of those studies.

Because the studies of Vadheim et al. (1990) and Scheifele (1989) and the small immunogenicity studies did not include control groups, meta-analysis could not be used to estimate the relative risk of early Hib disease following receipt of the conjugate vaccines. Nonetheless, a pooled relative risk can be estimated from the ratio of the total number of observed cases among vaccine recipients in all of the studies combined (i.e., ignoring the control groups of Black et al. [1991b] and Santosham et al. [1991b]) to the total number of expected cases. The number of cases of early Hib disease in each study can be treated as having a Poisson distribution. The expected number of cases for each study is estimated from the age-specific annual incidence rates reported from the prevaccine era, that is, an external comparison group (Ward and Cochi, 1988), and was considered to be a constant. The results are shown in Table 9-3. No statistically significant increase in the risk of early disease is apparent with the conjugate vaccines. It should be noted that recent studies have demonstrated that immunization with Hib conjugate vaccines decreases colonization rates in immunized subjects and may decrease the level of transmission of Hib to their contacts (Murphy et al., 1993; Takala et al., 1991), thus potentially decreasing the risk of disease both in unimmunized and in recently immunized children. This argues for

TABLE 9-3 Epidemiologic Studies of Early Hib Disease After First Dose of Hib Conjugate Vaccines (Vaccine Recipients Only)

Reference	Location	Vaccine	Ages	No.	Cases of Hib Disease Within 7 Days of Vaccination	
					Observed	Expected[a]
Scheifele, 1989	British Columbia	PRP-D	18-60 mo	5,263	1	0.04
Eskola, 1990a, and personal communication	Finland	PRP-D	3 mo	58,000	0	1.65
	Finland	PRP-D	24 mo	56,000	1	0.77
Vadheim et al., 1990	Southern California	PRP-D	18-60 mo	29,309	1	0.23
Black et al., 1991b	Northern California	HbOC	6 wk-6 mo	30,400	0	0.85
Santosham et al., 1991b	Arizona	PRC-OMP	6 wk-4 mo	2,588	0	0.07
b		HbOC	1-6 mo	664	0	.02
			15-23 mo	268	0	.01
c		PRP-D	7-14 mo	678	0	.03
			15-24 mo	300	0	.01
d		PRP-OMP	1-6 mo	918	0	.03
			7-11 mo	300	0	.02
			12-17 mo	476	0	.02
			18-23 mo	249	0	.00
			24-71 mo	361	0	.00
e		PRP-T	2-3 mo	269	0	.01
			18-23 mo	55	0	.00
Black et al., 1992b, and personal communication	Northern California	HbOC	6 wk-6 mo	53,000	0	1.48
	California		15-18 mo	22,000	1	0.68
				Total	4	5.92
				95% CI[f]	(1.09-10.24)	
				RR[g] (95% CI)	0.68 (0.18-1.73)	

[a]Expected based on age-specific annual incidence figures in Ward and Cocchi (1988).

[b]HbOC studies: Madore et al., 1990a,b; Rowe et al., 1990; Tudor-Williams et al., 1989; Anderson et al., 1987.

[c]PRP-D studies: Berkowitz et al., 1987; Lepow et al., 1987.

[d]PRP-OMP studies: Ahonkai et al., 1990; Campbell et al., 1990.

[e]PRP-T studies: Claesson et al., 1988, 1989; Parke et al., 1991; Booy et al., 1992.

[f]CI, confidence interval.

[g]RR, relative risk.

caution in comparing observed rates among recent vaccinees with historical (expected) rates in children from the prevaccine era.

Causality Argument

The biologic plausibility of a causal relation is provided by studies in human subjects and experimental animals that demonstrate a transient decrease in protective antibody levels following immunization with the unconjugated PRP vaccine. Both individually and by meta-analysis, data from four case-control trials suggest that immunization of children over 18 months of age who receive their first Hib immunization with unconjugated PRP vaccine is associated with an increased risk of disease in the 7-day interval following immunization. Because these were not controlled clinical trials, it is theoretically possible that the results are confounded (biased) by indication for receipt of the vaccine. For example, children in the immunized group may have been at greater risk for early-onset disease if they were immunized because of day-care center attendance or exposure to an individual with Hib disease.

The epidemiologic evidence from prospective observational studies favors rejection of a causal relation between immunization with Hib conjugate vaccines and an increased risk of disease in the early postvaccination interval. Although these vaccines also appear to be capable of causing a transient decline in serum antibody levels following immunization, conjugate vaccines produce a rapid and more predictable rise in protective antibody levels, and thus, the interval of increased risk, if any, is very short. In addition, conjugate vaccines are given to young infants, who generally have little preexisting protective antibody to be decreased, and thus, it is highly likely that the vaccine will provide protection rather than suppression of antibody (and increased risk of disease).

There are no epidemiologic data regarding the risk of Hib disease in the early period following immunization with PRP vaccine in individuals who have previously received one or more doses of Hib conjugate vaccine. However, the immunologic data showing rapid development of high antibody levels in previously immunized children given PRP vaccine at 12 months of age suggest that these children, like unimmunized children receiving Hib conjugate vaccine, would not be at increased risk of Hib disease in the early postvaccination interval.

Conclusion

The evidence favors acceptance of a causal relation between unconjugated PRP vaccine and early-onset Hib disease in children over 18 months of age who receive their first Hib immunization with unconjugated PRP vaccine.

On the basis of the incidence in the prevaccine era (Ward and Cochi, 1988) for the 24- to 35-month age group (presumably, the main age group previously immunized with PRP vaccine) of 1.0 per 100,000 per week (i.e., the annual rate divided by 52) and the Mantel-Haenszel odds ratio for the meta-analysis of 2.62, the attributable incidence is $2.62 - 1.0 = 1.62$ cases of early-onset (within 7 days of vaccination) Hib disease per 100,000 vaccinees. It should be stated, however, that the above figures may not be valid, since today the 7-day incidence of disease is probably less than the 1.0 per 100,000 from the prevaccine era owing to decreased colonization and transmission of disease.

The evidence favors rejection of a causal relation between immunization with Hib conjugate vaccines and early-onset Hib disease.

The evidence is inadequate to accept or reject a causal relation between PRP vaccine and early-onset disease in individuals who previously received one or more doses of Hib conjugate vaccine.

Risk-Modifying Factors

Because immunization with Hib vaccines may lead to a transient decrease in protective antibody levels, unimmunized children at increased risk of colonization (household or day-care contact with individuals with recent cases of Hib infection) may require special measures (see the recommendations of the American Academy of Pediatrics, Committee on Infectious Diseases [1991a]). A number of studies have demonstrated the safety and efficacy of Hib conjugate vaccines in high-risk groups such as adults with human immunodeficiency virus infection (Steinhoff et al., 1991) and children with sickle cell anemia (Frank et al., 1988; Rubin et al., 1992), cancer (Feldman et al., 1990), and asplenia (Jakacki et al., 1990), although in the latter two groups the antibody responses to vaccine were lower than normal.

ANAPHYLAXIS

Clinical Description

Anaphylaxis and anaphylactic shock refer to an acute, severe, and potentially lethal systemic allergic reaction. Signs and symptoms begin within minutes to a few hours after exposure. Death, if it occurs, usually results from airway obstruction caused by laryngeal edema or bronchospasm and may be associated with cardiovascular collapse. Most cases resolve without sequelae, and early treatment with alpha-adrenergic drugs can abort the full expression of the syndrome. A general discussion of anaphylaxis can be found in Chapter 4.

Evidence for Association

Biologic Plausibility

The biologic plausibility for a causal relation between Hib vaccines and anaphylaxis derives from the knowledge that injection of foreign protein into humans can be expected to elicit, in some percentage of recipients, IgE-mediated responses that present as anaphylaxis.

Case Reports, Case Series, and Uncontrolled Observational Studies

A study of efficacy and reactions to vaccination against either Hib or *Neisseria meningitidis* reported two cases of apparent anaphylactic reactions (Mäkelä et al., 1977). One child had received unconjugated Hib vaccine. There had been a total of 48,977 people vaccinated against Hib. Both children responded to epinephrine. No other details were provided. A summary of adverse reaction reports submitted to FDA for a 1-year period beginning in April 1985 lists two cases of what the authors termed *anaphylactoid-like reactions* (Milstien et al., 1987). A 3-year-old boy became pale, started wheezing, and exhibited hypotension 5 minutes after vaccination. A 4-year-old boy became nauseated, pale, bradycardic, and cyanotic 20 minutes after vaccination. Both children responded to epinephrine.

There are no published case reports. The reports in VAERS (submitted between November 1990 and July 1992) include one case of an immediate reaction to Hib vaccine alone and three cases of a response to a combination of vaccines that included a Hib conjugate vaccine. The first of these probably does not represent true anaphylaxis and may have been a severe breath-holding spell. The last three all received a combination of Hib vaccine, DPT, and OPV. One of these, in which a 6-month-old child developed acute flushing and edema 10 minutes after immunization, may have represented an anaphylactic reaction that was aborted by the early use of epinephrine.

Controlled Observational Studies and Controlled Clinical Trials

None of the controlled studies identified by the committee contained reports of anaphylaxis in association with the administration of any Hib vaccine.

Causality Argument

There is biologic plausibility that Hib vaccines, like all foreign proteins, could cause anaphylaxis. There are no data to suggest that Hib vaccines would be more likely than any other foreign protein, including other vaccines, to cause anaphylaxis. There are few cases of anaphylaxis following Hib vaccination in the literature. Insufficient details are provided by Mäkelä and colleagues (1977) to determine whether the responses represented anaphylaxis. The symptoms described in the paper by Milstien et al. (1987) are suggestive but not conclusive of anaphylaxis, but the administration of epinephrine might have aborted development of enough signs of anaphylaxis to be convincing.

Conclusion

The evidence is inadequate to accept or reject a causal relation between Hib vaccines and anaphylaxis.

DEATH

A detailed discussion of the evidence regarding death following immunization can be found in Chapter 10.

Conclusion

The evidence favors acceptance of a causal relation between PRP vaccine and death from early-onset Hib disease in children 18 months of age or older who receive their first Hib immunization with unconjugated PRP vaccine. There is no direct evidence for this; the conclusion is based on the potential for Hib disease to be fatal. The risk would appear to be extraordinarily low.

The evidence favors rejection of a causal relation between conjugated Hib vaccines and death from early-onset Hib disease.

The evidence is inadequate to accept or reject a causal relation between Hib vaccines and sudden infant death syndrome.

The evidence is inadequate to accept or reject a causal relation between Hib vaccine and death from causes other than those listed above.

REFERENCES

Adams J. Program Abstracts of the 32nd Interscience Conference on Antimicrobial Agents and Chemotherapy. Abstract 974, p. 273. Washington, DC: American Society for Microbiology; 1992.

Adams WG, Deaver KA, Cochi SL. Decline of childhood *Haemophilus influenzae* type b (Hib) disease in the Hib vaccine era. Journal of the American Medical Association 1993;269:221-226.

Ahonkhai VI, Lukacs LJ, Jonas LC, Matthews H, Vella PP, Ellis RW, et al. *Haemophilus influenzae* type b conjugate vaccine (meningococcal protein conjugate) (PedvaxHIB): clinical evaluation. Pediatrics 1990;85(4 Pt 2):676-681.

Ahonkhai VI, Lukacs LJ, Jonas LC, Calandra GB. Clinical experience with PedvaxHIB, a conjugate vaccine of *Haemophilus influenzae* type b polysaccharide-Neisseria meningitidis outer membrane protein. Vaccine 1991;9(Suppl.):S38-S41, S42-S43.

Ambrosino DM, Sood SK, Lee MC, Chen D, Collard HR, Bolon DL, et al. IgG1, IgG2 and IgM responses to two *Haemophilus influenzae* type b conjugate vaccines in young infants. Pediatric Infectious Disease Journal 1992;11:855-859.

American Academy of Pediatrics, Committee on Infectious Diseases. The Red Book. Report of the Committee on Infectious Diseases, 22nd edition. Peter G, ed. Elk Grove, IL: American Academy of Pediatrics; 1991a.

American Academy of Pediatrics, Committee on Infectious Diseases. *Haemophilus influenzae* vaccines: recommendations for immunization of infants and children 2 months of age and older: update. Pediatrics 1991b;88:169-172.

Amir J, Liang X, Granoff DM. Variability in the functional activity of vaccine-induced antibody to *Haemophilus influenzae* type b. Pediatric Research 1990a;27:358-364.

Amir J, Scott MG, Nahm MH, Granoff DM. Bactericidal and opsonic activity of IgG$_1$ and IgG$_2$ anticapsular antibodies to *Haemophilus influenzae* type b. Journal of Infectious Diseases 1990b;162:163-171.

Anderson P. Antibody responses to *Haemophilus influenzae* type b and diphtheria toxin induced by conjugates of oligosaccharides of the type b capsule with the nontoxic protein CRM197. Infection and Immunity 1983;39:233-238.

Anderson P, Johnston RB Jr, Smith DH. Human serum activities against *Hemophilus influenzae*, type b. Journal of Clinical Investigation 1972;51:31-38.

Anderson P, Pichichero M, Edwards K, Porch CR, Insel R. Priming and induction of *Haemophilus influenzae* type b capsular antibodies in early infancy by Dpo20, an oligosaccharide-protein conjugate vaccine. Journal of Pediatrics 1987;111:644-650.

Avery OT, Goebel WF. Chemo-immunological studies on conjugated carbohydrate-proteins. II. Immunological specificity of synthetic sugar-protein antigens. Journal of Experimental Medicine 1929;50:533-550.

Barbour ML, Booy R, Crook DW, Griffiths H. *Haemophilus influenzae* type b: carriage and immunity four years after conjugate vaccination. Program Abstracts of the 32nd Interscience Conference on Antimicrobial Agents and Chemotherapy. Abstract 978, p. 273. Washington, DC: American Society for Microbiology; 1992.

Barkin RM, Hendley JO, Zahradnik J. Capsular polysaccharide *Haemophilus influenzae* type b vaccine: clinical and immunologic responses to two vaccines. Pediatric Infectious Disease Journal 1987;6:20-23.

Barra A, Cordonnier C, Preziosi MP, Intrator L, Hessel L, Fritzell B, et al. Immunogenicity of *Haemophilus influenzae* type b conjugate vaccine in allogeneic bone marrow recipients. Journal of Infectious Diseases 1992;166:1021-1028.

Beghi E, Kurland LT, Mulder DW. Incidence of acute transverse myelitis in Rochester, Minnesota, 1970-1980, and implications with respect to influenza vaccine. Neuroepidemiology 1982;1:176-188.

Berkowitz CD, Ward JI, Meier K et al. Safety and immunogenicity of *Haemophilus influenzae* type b polysaccharide and polysaccharide diphtheria toxoid conjugate vaccines in children 15 to 24 months of age. Journal of Pediatrics 1987;110:509-514.

Black SB. Dramatic reduction in invasive Hib disease in a large California population following HbOC conjugate vaccine in infancy. Program Abstracts of the 32nd Interscience Conference on Antimicrobial Agents and Chemotherapy. Abstract 309, p. 162. Washington, DC: American Society for Microbiology; 1992.

Black SB, Shinefield HR, Northern California Permanente Medical Care Program Departments of Pediatrics Vaccine Study Group. b-CAPSA I *Haemophilus influenzae*, type b, capsular polysaccharide vaccine safety. Pediatrics 1987;79:321-325.

Black SB, Shinefield HR, Hiatt RA, Fireman BH, Beekly M, Callas ER, et al. Efficacy of

Haemophilus influenzae type b capsular polysaccharide vaccine. Pediatric Infectious Disease Journal 1988;7:149-156.

Black SB, Shinefield HR, Fireman B, Hiatt R, Polen M, Vittinghoff E, et al. Efficacy in infancy of oligosaccharide conjugate *Haemophilus influenzae* type b (HbOC) vaccine in a United States population of 61,080 children. Pediatric Infectious Disease Journal 1991a;10:97-104.

Black SB, Shinefield HR, Lampert D, Fireman B, Hiatt RA, Polen M, et al. Safety and immunogenicity of oligosaccharide conjugate *Haemophilus influenzae* type b (HbOC) vaccine in infancy. Pediatric Infectious Disease Journal 1991b;10:92-96.

Black SB, Shinefield HR, Fireman B, Hiatt R. Safety, immunogenicity, and efficacy in infancy of oligosaccharide conjugate *Haemophilus influenzae* type b vaccine in a United States population: possible implications for optimal use. Journal of Infectious Diseases 1992a;165(Suppl. 1):S139-S143.

Black SB, Shinefield HR, Kaiser Permanente Pediatric Vaccine Study Group. Immunization with oligosaccharide conjugate *Haemophilus influenzae* type b (HbOC) vaccine in a large health maintenance organization population: extended follow-up and impact on *Haemophilus influenzae* disease epidemiology. Pediatric Infectious Disease Journal 1992b;11:610-613.

Booy R, Moxon ER, MacFarlane JA, Mayon-White RT, Slack MPE. Efficacy of *Haemophilus influenzae* type b conjugate vaccine in the Oxford region (letter). Lancet 1992;340:47.

Brieger P, Ehrlich P. Beiträge zur Kenntniss der Milch immunisirter Thiere. Zeitschrift für Hygiene und Infektionskrankheiten 1893;13:336-346.

Broadhurst LE, Erickson RL, Kelley PW. Decreases in invasive *Haemophilus influenzae* diseases in US Army children, 1984 through 1991. Journal of the American Medical Association 1993;269:227-231.

Campbell H, Byass P, Ahonkhai VI, Vella PP, Greenwood BM. Serologic responses to an *Haemophilus influenzae* type b polysaccharide-Neisseria meningitidis outer membrane protein conjugate vaccine in very young Gambian infants. Pediatrics 1990;86:102-107.

Cates KL. Serum opsonic activity for *Haemophilus influenzae* type b in infants immunized with polysaccharide-protein vaccines. Journal of Infectious Diseases 1985;152:1076-1079.

Cates KL, Marsh KH, Granoff DM. Serum opsonic activity after immunization of adults with *Haemophilus influenzae* type b-diphtheria toxoid conjugate vaccine. Infection and Immunity 1985;48:183-189.

Centers for Disease Control, Immunization Practices Advisory Committee. Polysaccharide vaccine for prevention of *Haemophilus influenzae* type b disease. Morbidity and Mortality Weekly Report 1985;34:201-205.

Centers for Disease Control. Update: prevention of *Haemophilus influenzae* type b disease. Morbidity and Mortality Weekly Report 1988;37:13-16.

Centers for Disease Control. Update: *Haemophilus influenzae* type b vaccine. Morbidity and Mortality Weekly Report 1989;38:14.

Centers for Disease Control. Recommendations of the Immunization Practices Advisory Committee, Supplementary Statement: change in administration schedule for *Haemophilus b* conjugate vaccines. Morbidity and Mortality Weekly Report 1990a;39:232-233.

Centers for Disease Control. Food and Drug Administration approval of a *Haemophilus b* conjugate vaccine for infants. Morbidity and Mortality Weekly Report 1990b;39:698-699.

Centers for Disease Control. Decline in *Haemophilus influenzae* type b meningitis—Seattle-King County, Washington, 1984-1989. Morbidity and Mortality Weekly Report 1990c;39:924-925.

Centers for Disease Control. Food and Drug Administration approval of use of *Haemophilus b* conjugate vaccine for infants. Morbidity and Mortality Weekly Report 1990d;39:925-926.

Centers for Disease Control. *Haemophilus b* conjugate vaccines for prevention of *Haemophilus influenzae* type b disease among infants and children two months of age and older.

Recommendations of the Immunization Practices Advisory Committee (ACIP). Morbidity and Mortality Weekly Report 1991a;40(RR 1):1-7.

Centers for Disease Control. Surveillance of Escherichia coli O157 isolation and confirmation, United States, 1988. Morbidity and Mortality Weekly Report 1991b;40(SS-1):1-6.

Centers for Disease Control and Prevention. Food and Drug Administration approval of use of a new *Haemophilus* b conjugate vaccine and a combined diphtheria-tetanus-pertussis and *Haemophilus* b conjugate vaccine for infants and children. Morbidity and Mortality Weekly Report 1993;42:296-298.

Claesson BA, Trollfors B, Lagergard T, Taranger J, Bryla D, Otterman G, et al. Clinical and immunologic responses to the capsular polysaccharide of *Haemophilus influenzae* type b alone or conjugated to tetanus toxoid in 18- to 23-month-old children. Journal of Pediatrics 1988;112:695-702.

Claesson BA, Schneerson R, Robbins JB, Johansson J, Lagergard T, Taranger J, et al. Protective levels of serum antibodies stimulated in infants by two injections of *Haemophilus influenzae* type b capsular polysaccharide-tetanus toxoid conjugate. Journal of Pediatrics 1989;114:97-100.

Claesson BA, Schneerson R, Lagergard T, Trollfors B, Taranger J, Johansson J, et al. Persistence of serum antibodies elicited by *Haemophilus influenzae* type b-tetanus toxoid conjugate vaccine in infants vaccinated at 3, 5 and 12 months of age. Pediatric Infectious Disease Journal 1991;10:560-564.

Clements DA, Rouse JB, London WL, Yancy WS, Moggio MV, Wilfert CM. Antibody response of 18 month old children 1 month and 18 months following *Haemophilus influenzae* type b vaccine administered singly or with DTP vaccine. Journal of Paediatrics and Child Health 1990;26:46-49.

Cochi SL, Broome CV, Hightower AW. Immunization of U.S. children with *H. influenzae* vaccine: a cost-effectiveness model of strategy assessment. Journal of the American Medical Association 1985;253:521-529.

Cohn J. Thrombocytopenia in childhood: an evaluation of 433 patients. Scandinavian Journal of Hematology 1976;16:226-240.

Corrigan JJ Jr. Thrombocytopenia: a laboratory sign of septicemia in infants and children. Journal of Pediatrics 1974;83:219-221.

Dashefsky B, Wald E, Guerra N, Byers C. Safety, tolerability, and immunogenicity of concurrent administration of *Haemophilus influenzae* type b conjugate vaccine (meningococcal protein conjugate) with either measles-mumps-rubella vaccine or diphtheria-tetanus-pertussis and oral poliovirus vaccines in 14- to 23-month-old infants. Pediatrics 1990;85(4 Pt 2):682-689.

Daum RS, Sood SK, Osterholm MT, Pramberg JC, Granoff PD, White KE, et al. Decline in serum antibody to the capsule of *Haemophilus influenzae* type b in the immediate postimmunization period. Journal of Pediatrics 1989;114:742-747.

D'Cruz OF, Shapiro ED, Spiegelman KN, Leicher CR, Breningstall GN, Khatri BO, et al. Acute inflammatory demyelinating polyradiculoneuropathy (Guillain-Barré syndrome) after immunization with *Haemophilus influenzae* type b conjugate vaccine. Journal of Pediatrics 1989;115:743-746.

Decker MD, Edwards KM, Bradley R, Palmer P. Comparative trial in infants of four conjugate *Haemophilus influenzae* type b vaccines. Journal of Pediatrics 1992;120(2 Pt 1):184-189.

Edwards KM, Decker MD, Porch CR, Palmer P, Bradley R. Immunization after invasive *Haemophilus influenzae* type b disease: serologic response to a conjugate vaccine. American Journal of Diseases of Children 1989;143:31-33.

Einhorn MS, Weinberg GA, Anderson EL. Immunogenicity in infants of *Haemophilus influenzae* type b polysaccharide in a conjugate vaccine with Neisseria meningitidis outer-membrane protein. Lancet 1986;2:299-302.

Eskola J, Peltola H, Takala AK, Kayhty H, Hakulinen M. Efficacy of *Haemophilus influenzae* type b polysaccharide-diphtheria toxoid conjugate vaccine in infancy. New England Journal of Medicine 1987;317:717-722.

Eskola J, Kayhty H, Takala AK, Peltola H, Ronnberg PR, Kela E, et al. A randomized, prospective field trial of a conjugate vaccine in the protection of infants and young children against invasive *Haemophilus influenzae* type b disease. New England Journal of Medicine 1990a;323:1381-1387.

Eskola J, Kayhty H, Takala A, Ronnberg PR, Kela E, Peltola H. Reactogenicity and immunogenicity of combined vaccines for bacteraemic diseases caused by *Haemophilus influenzae* type b, meningococci and pneumococci in 24-month-old children. Vaccine 1990b;8:107-110.

Eskola J, Takala AK, Kayhty H, Peltola H, Makela PH. *Haemophilus influenzae* type b (Hib) conjugate vaccine is better than expected on the basis of efficacy trials. Program Abstracts of the 32nd Interscience Conference on Antimicrobial Agents and Chemotherapy. Abstract 979, p. 273. Washington, DC: American Society for Microbiology; 1992.

Farkkila M, Kinnunen E, Weckstron P. Survey of Guillain-Barré syndrome in southern Finland. Neuroepidemiology 1991;10:236-241.

Feldman S, Gigliotti F, Shenep JL, Roberson PK, Lott L. Risk of *Haemophilus influenzae* type b disease in children with cancer and response of immunocompromised leukemic children to a conjugate vaccine. Journal of Infectious Diseases 1990;161:926-931.

Ferreccio C, Clemens J, Avendano A, Horwitz I, Flores C, Avila L, et al. The clinical and immunologic response of Chilean infants to *Haemophilus influenzae* type b polysaccharide-tetanus protein conjugate vaccine coadministered in the same syringe with diphtheria-tetanus toxoids-pertussis vaccine at two, four and six months of age. Pediatric Infectious Disease Journal 1991;10:764-771.

Fothergill LD, Wright J. Influenzal meningitis: the relation of age incidence to the bactericidal power of blood against the causal organism. Journal of Immunology 1933;24:273-284.

Frank AL, Labotka RJ, Rao S, Frisone LR, McVerry PH, Samuelson JS, et al. *Haemophilus influenzae* type b immunization of children with sickle cell diseases. Pediatrics 1988;82:571-575.

Frayha HH, Dent P, Shannon HS, Johnson SE, Gordon L. Safety and immunogenicity of subcutaneous *H. influenzae* vaccines in 15-17 month-old children. Medicine Clinique et Experimentale [Clinical and Investigative Medicine] 1991;14:379-387.

Fritzell B, Plotkin S. Efficacy and safety of a *Haemophilus influenzae* type b capsular polysaccharide-tetanus protein conjugate vaccine. Journal of Pediatrics 1992;121:355-362.

Gervaix A, Caflisch M, Suter S, Haenggeli CA. Guillain-Barré syndrome following immunization with *Haemophilus influenzae* type b conjugate vaccine. European Journal of Pediatrics 1993;152:613-614.

Gigliotti F, Feldman S, Wang WC, Day SW, Brunson G. Immunization of young infants with sickle cell disease with a *Haemophilus influenzae* type b saccharide-diphtheria CRM 197 protein conjugate vaccine. Journal of Pediatrics 1989;114:1006-1010.

Gigliotti F, Feldman S, Wang WC, Day SW, Brunson G. Serologic follow-up of children with sickle cell disease immunized with a *Haemophilus influenzae* type b conjugate vaccine during early infancy. Journal of Pediatrics 1991;118:917-919.

Goepp JG, Hohenboken M, Almeidohill J, Santosham M. Persistent urinary antigen excretion in infants vaccinated with *Haemophilus influenzae* type b capsular polysaccharide conjugated with outer membrane protein from Neisseria meningitidis. Pediatric Infectious Disease Journal 1992;11:2-5.

Gordon LK. Characterization of a hapten-carrier conjugate vaccine: *H. influenzae*-diphtheria conjugate vaccine. In: Chanock RM, Lerner RA, eds. Modern Approaches to Vaccines. Cold Spring Harbor, NY: Cold Spring Harbor Laboratory; 1984.

Granoff DM, Cates KL. *Haemophilus influenzae* type b polysaccharide vaccines. Journal of Pediatrics 1985;107:330-336.

Granoff DM, Osterholm MT. Safety and efficacy of *Haemophilus influenzae* type b polysaccharide vaccine. Pediatrics 1987;80:590-592.

Granoff DM, Boies EG, Munson RS. Immunogenicity of *Haemophilus influenzae* type b polysaccharide-diphtheria toxoid conjugate vaccine in adults. Journal of Pediatrics 1984;105:22-27.

Granoff DM, Weinberg GA, Shackelford PE. IgG subclass response to immunization with *Haemophilus influenzae* type b polysaccharide-outer membrane protein conjugate vaccine. Pediatric Research 1988;24:180-185.

Granoff DM, Chacko A, Lottenbach KR, Sheetz KE. Immunogenicity of *Haemophilus influenzae* type b polysaccharide-outer membrane protein conjugate vaccine in patients who acquired *Haemophilus* disease despite previous vaccination with type b polysaccharide vaccine. Journal of Pediatrics 1989;114:925-933.

Granoff DM, Holmes SJ, Osterholm MT. Induction of immunologic memory in infants primed with *Haemophilus influenzae* type b conjugate vaccines. Journal of Infectious Diseases, In press.

Gray BM. Opsonophagocidal activity in sera from infants and children immunized with *Haemophilus influenzae* type b conjugate vaccine (meningococcal protein conjugate). Pediatrics 1990;85(4 Pt 2):694-697.

Greenberg DP, Ward JI, Burkart K. Factors influencing immunogenicity and safety of two *Haemophilus influenzae* type b polysaccharide vaccines in children 18 and 24 months of age. Pediatric Infectious Disease Journal 1987;6:660-665.

Greenberg DP, Vadheim CM, March SM, Ward JI, Kaiser-UCLA Hib Vaccine Study Group. Evaluation of the safety, immunogenicity, and efficacy of *Haemophilus* b (Hib) PRP-T conjugate vaccine in a prospective, randomized, and placebo-controlled trial in young infants. Program Abstracts of the 32nd Interscience Conference on Antimicrobial Agents and Chemotherapy. Abstract 65, p. 109. Washington, DC: American Society for Microbiology; 1991.

Harrison LH, Broome CV, Hightower AW, Hoppe CC, Makintubee S, Sitze SL, et al. A day care-based study of the efficacy of *Haemophilus* b polysaccharide vaccine. Journal of the American Medical Association 1988;260:1413-1418.

Hendley JO, Wenzel JG, Ashe KM, Samuelson JS. Immunogenicity of *Haemophilus influenzae* type b capsular polysaccharide vaccines in 18-month-old infants. Pediatrics 1987;80:351-354.

Hetherington SB, Lepow ML. Correlation between antibody affinity and serum bactericidal activity in infants. Journal of Infectious Diseases 1992;165:753-756.

Hiner EE, Frasch CE. Spectrum of disease due to *Haemophilus influenzae* type b occurring in vaccinated children. Journal of Infectious Diseases 1988;158:343-348.

Holmes SJ, Murphy TV, Anderson RS, Kaplan SL, Rothstein EP, Gan VN, et al. Immunogenicity of four *Haemophilus influenzae* type b conjugate vaccines in 17- to 19-month old children. Journal of Pediatrics 1991;118:364-371.

Insel RA, Anderson PW. Response to oligosaccharide-protein conjugate vaccine against *Haemophilus influenzae* b in two patients with IgG_2 deficiency unresponsive to capsular polysaccharide vaccine. New England Journal of Medicine 1986;315:499-503.

Jakacki R, Luery N, McVerry P, Lange B. *Haemophilus influenzae* diphtheria protein conjugate immunization after therapy in splenectomized patients with Hodgkin disease. Annals of Internal Medicine 1990;112:143-144.

Jones RG, Bass JW, Weisse ME, Vincent JM. Antigenuria after immunization with *Haemophilus influenzae* oligosaccharide crm197 conjugate (HbOC) vaccine. Pediatric Infectious Disease Journal 1991;10:557-559.

Kafidi KT, Rotschafer JC. Bacterial vaccines for splenectomized patients. Drug Intelligence and Clinical Pharmacy 1988;22:192-197.

Kaplan C, Morinet F, Cartron J. Virus-induced autoimmune thrombocytopenia and neutropenia. Seminars in Hematology 1992;29:34-44.

Kaplan SL, Zahradnik JM, Mason EO Jr, Dukes CM. Immunogenicity of the *Haemophilus influenzae* type b capsular polysaccharide conjugate vaccine in children after systemic *Haemophilus influenzae* type b infections. Journal of Pediatrics 1988;113:272-277.

Kayhty H, Peltola H, Eskola J. Immunogenicity and reactogenicity for four *Haemophilus influenzae* type b capsular polysaccharide vaccines in Finnish 24-month-old children. Pediatric Infectious Disease Journal 1988;7:574-577.

Kayhty H, Peltola H, Eskola J, Ronnberg PR, Kela E, Karanko V, et al. Immunogenicity of *Haemophilus influenzae* oligosaccharide-protein and polysaccharide-protein conjugate vaccination of children at 4, 6, and 14 months of age. Pediatrics 1989;84:995-999.

Keltow JG, Neame PB, Gauldie J, Hirsch J. Elevated platelet-associated IgG in the thrombocytopenia of septicemia. New England Journal of Medicine 1979;300:760-764.

Kinnunen E, Farkkila M, Hovi T, Juntunen J, Weckstrom P. Incidence of Guillain-Barré syndrome during a nationwide oral poliovirus vaccine campaign. Neurology 1989;39:1034-1036.

Kovel A, Wald ER, Guerra N, Serdy C, Meschievitz CK. Safety and immunogenicity of acellular diphtheria-tetanus-pertussis and *Haemophilus* conjugate vaccines given in combination or at separate injection sites. Journal of Pediatrics 1992;120:84-87.

Kulhanjian J. The decline in invasive *Haemophilus influenzae* type b (Hib) disease in a large pediatric referral hospital following introduction to Hib conjugate vaccines. Program Abstracts of the 32nd Interscience Conference on Antimicrobial Agents and Chemotherapy. Abstract 1727, p. 398. Washington, DC: American Society for Microbiology; 1992.

Lee GR, Foerster J, Athens JW, Lukens JN, eds. Wintrobe's Clinical Hematology, 9th edition, London: Lea & Febiger; 1993.

LeMay M. Infection after *Haemophilus* vaccine (letter). Pediatric Infectious Disease Journal 1986;5:387.

Lenoir AA, Granoff PD, Granoff DM. Immunogenicity of *Haemophilus influenzae* type b polysaccharide-Neisseria meningitidis outer membrane protein conjugate vaccine in 2- to 6-month-old infants. Pediatrics 1987;80:283-287.

Lepow ML, Peter G, Glode MP. Response of infants to *Haemophilus influenzae* type b polysaccharide and diphtheria-tetanus-pertussis vaccines in combination. Journal of Infectious Diseases 1984a;149:950-955.

Lepow ML, Samuelson JS, Gordon LK. Safety and immunogenicity of *Haemophilus influenzae* type b polysaccharide-diphtheria toxoid conjugate vaccine in adults. Journal of Infectious Diseases 1984b;150:402-406.

Lepow ML, Samuelson JS, Gordon LK. Safety and immunogenicity of *Haemophilus influenzae* type b-polysaccharide diphtheria toxoid conjugate vaccine in infants 9 to 15 months of age. Journal of Pediatrics 1985;106:185-189.

Lepow M, Randolph M, Cimma R. Persistence of antibody and response to booster dose of *Haemophilus influenzae* type b polysaccharide diphtheria toxoid conjugate vaccine in infants immunized at 9 to 15 months of age. Journal of Pediatrics 1986;108:882-886.

Lepow ML, Barkin RM, Berkowitz CD, Brunell PA, James D, Meier K, et al. Safety and immunogenicity of *Haemophilus influenzae* type b polysaccharide-diphtheria toxoid conjugate vaccine (PRP-D) in infants. Journal of Infectious Diseases 1987;156:591-596.

Lightsey AL. Thrombocytopenia in children. Pediatric Clinics of North America 1980;27:293-308.

Loughlin AM, Marchant CD, Lett S, Shapiro ED. Efficacy of *Haemophilus influenzae* type b vaccines in Massachusetts children 18 to 59 months of age. Pediatric Infectious Disease Journal 1992;11:374-379.

Madore DV, Johnson CL, Phipps DC, Pennridge Pediatric Associates, Popejoy LA, Eby R, et al. Safety and immunologic response to *Haemophilus influenzae* type b oligosaccharide-CRM197 conjugate vaccine in 1- to 6-month-old infants. Pediatrics 1990a;85:331-337.

Madore DV, Johnson CL, Phipps DC, Pennridge Pediatric Associates, Myers MG, Eby R, et al. Safety and immunogenicity of *Haemophilus influenzae* type b oligosaccharide-CRM197 conjugate vaccine in infants aged 15 to 23 months. Pediatrics 1990b;86:527-534.

Madsen T, Jensen C, Ipsen J. Problems in active and passive immunity. Bulletin of the Johns Hopkins Hospital 1937;61:221-245.

Mäkelä PH, Peltola H, Käyhty H, Jousimies H, Pettay O, Ruoslahti E, Sivonen A, Renkonen OV. Polysaccharide vaccines in group A Neisseria meningitidis and *Haemophilus influenzae* type b: a field trial in Finland. Journal of Infectious Diseases 1977;136(Supplement);S43-S50.

Mantel N, Haenszel W. Statistical aspects of the analysis of data from retrospective studies of disease. Journal of the National Cancer Institute 1959;22:719-748.

Marchant CD, Band E, Froeschle JE, McVerry PH. Depression of anticapsular antibody after immunization with *Haemophilus influenzae* type b polysaccharide-diphtheria conjugate vaccine. Pediatric Infectious Disease Journal 1989;8:508-511.

Marcinak JF, Frank AL, Labotka RL, Fao S, Frisone LR, Yogev R, et al. *Haemophilus influenzae* after vaccination at age one and one-half to six years. Pediatric Infectious Disease Journal 1991;10:157-159.

Milstien JB, Gross TP, Kuritsky JN. Adverse reactions reported following receipt of *Haemophilus influenzae* type b vaccine: an analysis after 1 year of marketing. Pediatrics 1987;80:270-274.

Mohle-Boetani J. Oropharyngeal carriage of *Haemophilus influenzae* type b (Hib) in a heavily vaccinated population of 2-5 year olds. Program Abstracts of the 32nd Interscience Conference on Antimicrobial Agents and Chemotherapy. Abstract 1729, p. 399. Washington, DC: American Society for Microbiology; 1992.

Murphy TV. *Haemophilus* b polysaccharide vaccine: need for continuing assessment. Pediatric Infectious Disease Journal 1987;6:701-703.

Murphy TV. Is *Haemophilus influenzae* type b colonization of children in day care reduced by Hib conjugate (Conj) and plain polysaccharide (PRP) vaccine (Vac)? Program Abstracts of the 31st Interscience Conference on Antimicrobial Agents and Chemotherapy. Abstract 66, p. 121. Washington, DC: American Society for Microbiology; 1991.

Murphy TV, Pastor P, Medley F, Osterholm MT, Granoff DM. Decreased *Haemophilus* colonization in children vaccinated with *Haemophilus influenzae* type b conjugate vaccine. Journal of Pediatrics 1993a;122:517-523.

Murphy TV, White KE, Pastor P. Declining incidence of *Haemophilus influenzae* type b disease since introduction of vaccination. Journal of the American Medical Association 1993b;269:246-248.

Musher DM, Watson DA, Lepow ML, McVerry P, Hamill R, Baughn RE. Vaccination of 18-month-old children with conjugated polyribosyl ribitol phosphate stimulates production of functional antibody to *Haemophilus influenzae* type b. Pediatric Infectious Disease Journal 1988;7:156-159.

Newman SL, Waldo B, Johnston RB Jr. Separation of serum bactericidal and opsonizing activities for *Haemophilus influenzae* type b. Infection and Immunity 1973;8:488-490.

Norden CW, Michaels RH, Melish M. Serologic responses of children with meningitis due to *Haemophilus influenzae* type b. Journal of Infectious Diseases 1976;134:495-499.

Osterholm MT, Rambeck JH, White KE, Jacobs JL, Pierson LM, Neaton JD, et al. Lack of efficacy of *Haemophilus* b polysaccharide vaccine in Minnesota. Journal of the American Medical Association 1988;260:1423-1428.

Parke JC Jr, Schneerson R, Reimer C, Black C, Welfare S, Bryla D, et al. Clinical and immunologic responses to *Haemophilus influenzae* type b-tetanus toxoid conjugate vaccine in infants injected at 3, 5, 7, and 18 months of age. Journal of Pediatrics 1991;118:184-190.

Peltola H. Clinical efficacy of the PRP-D versus HbOC conjugate vaccine *Haemophilus influenzae* type b (Hib). Program Abstracts of the 32nd Interscience Conference on Antimicrobial Agents and Chemotherapy. Abstract 975, p. 273. Washington, DC: American Society for Microbiology; 1992.

Peltola H, Kayhty H, Sivonen A, Makela PH. *Haemophilus influenzae* type b capsular polysaccharide vaccine in children: a double-blind field study of 100,000 vaccinees 3 months to 5 years of age in Finland. Pediatrics 1977;60:730-737.

Peltola H, Kayhty H, Virtanen M, Makela PH. Prevention of *Hemophilus influenzae* type b bacteremic infections with the capsular polysaccharide vaccine. New England Journal of Medicine 1984;310:1561-1566.

Popejoy LA, Rivera AI, Gonzales-Torres I. Side-effects and immunogenicity of *Haemophilus influenzae* type b polysaccharide vaccine in a multi-ethnic pediatric population. Military Medicine 1989;154:25-29.

Quagliarello V, Scheld WM. Bacterial meningitis: pathogenesis, pathophysiology, and progress. New England Journal of Medicine 1992;327:864-872.

Raettig H. Provokation einer infektion durch Schutzimpfung. Zentralblatt für Bakteriologie, Parasitendunde, Infektionskrankheiten und Hygiene 1959;174:192-217.

Robbins JB, Schneerson R. Polysaccharide-protein conjugates: a new generation of vaccines. Journal of Infectious Diseases 1990;161:821-832.

Robbins JB, Parke JC Jr, Schneerson R, Whisnant JK. Quantitative measurement of "natural" and immunization-induced *Haemophilus influenzae* type b capsular polysaccharide antibodies. Pediatric Research 1973;7:103-110.

Rowe JE, Messinger IK, Schwendeman CA, Popejoy LA. Three-dose vaccination of infants under 8 months of age with a conjugate *Haemophilus influenzae* type b vaccine. Military Medicine 1990;155:483-486.

Rowe PC, Orrbine E, Wells GA, McLaine PN. Epidemiology of hemolytic-uremic syndrome in Canadian children from 1986 to 1988. Journal of Pediatrics 1991;119:218-224.

Rubin LG, Voulalas D, Carmody L. Immunization of children with sickle cell disease with *Haemophilus influenzae* type b polysaccharide vaccine. Pediatrics 1989;84:509-513.

Rubin LG, Voulalas D, Carmody L. Immunogenicity of *Haemophilus influenzae* type b conjugate vaccine in children with sickle cell disease. American Journal of Diseases of Children 1992;146:340-342.

Saez-Llorens X, Ramilo O, Mustafa MM, Mertsola J. Molecular pathophysiology of bacterial meningitis: current concepts and therapeutic implications. Journal of Pediatrics 1990;116:671-684.

Salomonsen CJ, Madsen TH. Bulletin de l'Academie Royale des Sciences et des Lettres de Danemark. 1896.

Santosham M, Hill J, Wolff M, Reid R, Lukacs L, Ahonkhai V. Safety and immunogenicity of a *Haemophilus influenzae* type b conjugate vaccine in a high risk American Indian population. Pediatric Infectious Disease Journal 1991a;10:113-117.

Santosham M, Wolff M, Reid R, Hohenboken M, Bateman M, Goepp J, et al. The efficacy in Navajo infants of a conjugate vaccine consisting of *Haemophilus influenzae* type b polysaccharide and Neisseria meningitidis outer-membrane protein complex. New England Journal of Medicine 1991b;324:1767-1772.

Santosham M, Rivin B, Wolff M, Reid R, Newcomer W, Letson GW, et al. Prevention of *Haemophilus influenzae* type b infections in Apache and Navajo children. Journal of Infectious Diseases 1992;165(Suppl. 1):S144-S151.

Scheifele DW. Postmarketing surveillance of adverse reactions to ProHIBit vaccine in British Columbia. Canadian Medical Association Journal 1989;141:927-929.

Schlech WF, Ward JI, Bard JD. Bacterial meningitis in the United States, 1978-81: the National Bacterial Meningitis Surveillance Study. Journal of the American Medical Association 1985;253:1749-1754.

Schlesinger Y, Granoff DM. Avidity and bactericidal activity of antibody elicited by different *Haemophilus influenzae* type b conjugate vaccines. Journal of the American Medical Association 1992;267:1489-1494.

Schneerson R, Rodrigues LP, Parke JC Jr, Robbins JB. Immunity to disease caused by *Hemophilus influenzae* type b. II. Specificity and some biologic characteristics of "natural," infection-acquired, and immunization-induced antibodies to the capsular polysaccharide of *Hemophilus influenzae* type b. Journal of Immunology 1971;107:1081-1089.

Schneerson R, Barrera O, Sutton A, Robbins JB. Preparation, characterization, and immunogenicity of *H. influenzae* type b polysaccharide-protein conjugates. Journal of Experimental Medicine 1980;152:361-376.

Schreiber JR, Barrus V, Cates KL, Siber GR. Functional characterization of human IgG, IgM, and IgA antibody directed to the capsule of *Haemophilus influenzae* type b. Journal of Infectious Diseases 1986;153:8-16.

Shackelford PG, Granoff DM. IgG subclass composition of the antibody response of healthy adults, and normal or IgG2-deficient children to immunization with *H. influenzae* type b polysaccharide vaccine or Hib PS-protein conjugate vaccines. Monographs in Allergy 1988;23:269-281.

Shapiro ED, Murphy TV, Wald ER, Brady CA. The protective efficacy of *Haemophilus* b polysaccharide vaccine. Journal of the American Medical Association 1988;260:1419-1422.

Siber GR, Santosham M, Reid GR, Thompson C, Almeido-Hill J, Morell A, et al. Impaired antibody response to *Haemophilus influenzae* type b polysaccharide and low IgG2 and IgG4 concentrations in Apache children. New England Journal of Medicine 1990;323:1387-1392.

Smith DH, Madore DV, Eby RJ, Anderson PW, Insel RA, Johnson CL. *Haemophilus* b oligosaccharide-CRM197 and other *Haemophilus* b conjugate vaccines: a status report. Advances in Experimental and Medical Biology 1989;251:65-82.

Sood SK, Daum RS. Disease caused by *Haemophilus influenzae* type b in the immediate period after homologous immunization: immunologic investigation. Pediatrics 1990;85(4 Pt 2):698-704.

Sood SK, Schreiber JR, Siber GR, Daum RS. Postvaccination susceptibility to invasive *Haemophilus influenzae* type b disease in infant rats. Journal of Pediatrics 1988;113:814-819.

Spinola SM, Sheaffer CI, Philbrick KB, Gilligan PH. Antigenuria after *Haemophilus influenzae* type b polysaccharide immunization: a prospective study. Journal of Pediatrics 1986;109:835-838.

Steinhoff MC, Auerbach BS, Nelson KE, Vlahov D, Becker RL, Graham NMH, et al. Antibody responses to *Haemophilus influenzae* type b vaccines in men with human immunodeficiency virus infection. New England Journal of Medicine 1991;325:1837-1842.

Syrogiannopoulos GA, Hansen EJ, Erwin AL, et al. *Haemophilus influenzae* type b lipooligosaccharide induced meningeal inflammation. Journal of Infectious Diseases 1988;157:237-244.

Takala AK, Eskola J, Leinonen M, Kayhty H, Nissinen A, Pekkanen E, et al. Reduction of oropharyngeal carriage of *Haemophilus influenzae* type b (Hib) in children immunized with an Hib conjugate vaccine. Journal of Infectious Diseases 1991;164:982-986.

Thomas GA, O'Brien RT. Thrombocytosis in children with *Haemophilus influenzae* meningitis. Clinical Pediatrics 1986;25:610-611.

Todd JK, Bruhn FW. Severe *Haemophilus influenzae* infections: spectrum of disease. American Journal of Diseases in Children 1975;129:607-611.

Topley WW. The role of active or passive immunization in the control of enteric infection. Lancet 1938;1:181-186.

Trollfors B, Lagergard T, Claesson BA, Thornberg E, Martinell J, Schneerson R. Characterization of the serum antibody response to the capsular polysaccharide *Haemophilus influenzae* type b in children with invasive infections. Journal of Infectious Disease 1992;166:1335-1339.

Tudor-Williams G, Frankland J, Isaacs D, Mayon-White RT, MacFarlane JA, Rees DG, et al. *Haemophilus influenzae* type b conjugate vaccine trial in Oxford: implications for the United Kingdom. Archives of Disease in Childhood 1989;64:520-524.

Uhari M, Rantala H, Niemela M. Cluster of childhood Guillain-Barré cases after an oral poliovaccine campaign (letter). Lancet 1989;2:440-441.

Vadheim CM. Reduction of Hib disease in Southern California, 1983-1991. Program Abstracts of the 32nd Interscience Conference on Antimicrobial Agents and Chemotherapy. Abstract 1726, p. 398. Washington, DC: American Society for Microbiology; 1992.

Vadheim CM, Greenberg DP, Marcy SM, Froeschle J, Ward JI. Safety evaluation of PRP-D *Haemophilus influenzae* type b conjugate vaccine in children immunized at 18 months of age and older: follow-up study of 30,000 children. Pediatric Infectious Disease Journal 1990;9:555-561.

Walter EB, Moggio MV, Drucker RP, Wilfert CM. Immunogenicity of *Haemophilus* b conjugate vaccine (meningococcal protein conjugate) in children with prior invasive *Haemophilus influenzae* type b disease. Pediatric Infectious Disease Journal 1990;9:632-635.

Ward J, Cochi S. *Haemophilus influenzae* vaccines. In: Plotkin SA, Mortimer EA, eds. Vaccines. Philadelphia: W.B. Saunders; 1988.

Watemberg N, Dagan R, Arbelli Y, Belmaker I, Morag A, Hessel L, et al. Safety and immunogenicity of *Haemophilus* type b-tetanus protein conjugate vaccine, mixed in the same syringe with diphtheria-tetanus-pertussis vaccine in young infants. Pediatric Infectious Disease Journal 1991;10:758-763.

Weinberg GA, Granoff DM. Polysaccharide-protein conjugate vaccines for the prevention of *Haemophilus influenzae* type b disease. Journal of Pediatrics 1988;113:621-631.

Weinberg GA, Granoff DM. Immunogenicity of *Haemophilus influenzae* type polysaccharide-protein conjugate vaccines in children with conditions associated with impaired antibody responses to type b polysaccharide vaccine. Pediatrics 1990;85(4 Pt 2):654-661.

Weinberg GA, Einhorn MS, Lenois AA, Granoff PD, Granoff DM. *Haemophilus influenzae* type b polysaccharide-Neisseria meningitidis outer membrane protein conjugate vaccine. Journal of Pediatrics 1987;111:22-27.

Weisman SJ, Cates KL, Allegretta GJ, Quinn JJ, Altman AJ. Antibody response to immunization with *Haemophilus influenzae* type b polysaccharide vaccine in children with cancer. Journal of Pediatrics 1987;111:727-729.

Yogev R, Arditi M, Chadwick EG, Amer MD, Sroka PA. *Haemophilus influenzae* type b conjugate vaccine (meningococcal protein conjugate): immunogenicity and safety at various doses. Pediatrics 1990;85(4 Pt 2):690-693.

10

Death

The Vaccine Safety Committee was charged with assessing a causal relation between all of the vaccines that it reviewed and death. The myriad possible causes of death made this a difficult task. To facilitate review of this serious adverse event, the committee used a categorization scheme, which is discussed below. Because the vast majority of reports of death following vaccination reside in passive surveillance systems, the committee used the scheme to analyze data from a currently operating one, the Vaccine Adverse Event Reporting System (VAERS). A description of the system is included in this chapter, and the results of this analysis are also discussed. All evidence reviewed by the committee (published literature and reports from the passive surveillance systems of the Centers for Disease Control and Prevention [CDC] and U.S. Food and Drug Administration [FDA]) regarding deaths in association with immunization is discussed later in this chapter.

To answer the question "Can any deaths be attributed to the use of the vaccines discussed in this review?," the committee categorized reports of death following immunization into seven categories:

- deaths for which the available data were insufficient to allow a judgment of cause;
- deaths associated with vaccine administration but attributable to inappropriate handling, contamination, production error, or error of medical care;

- deaths temporally associated with vaccine administration but clearly caused by something other than the vaccine;
- deaths classified as sudden infant death syndrome (SIDS);
- deaths that are a consequence of vaccine-strain viral infection (applies to measles, mumps, or oral polio vaccine [OPV] for this report);
- deaths that are a consequence of an adverse event that itself is causally related to a vaccine reviewed in this report; and
- deaths temporally associated with vaccine administration and the cause of death is other than those listed above.

EXAMPLES

Deaths for Which the Available Data Were Insufficient to Allow a Judgment of Cause

The reports from passive surveillance systems accessed by the committee vary in the quantity and quality of the information that they contain. Many of the reports contained phrases such as "died" or "found dead at baby-sitter's." Reports with more information frequently had no additional documentation submitted with them, so assessment of the diagnosis was not possible. The information in VAERS is discussed below in great detail. The published literature contains reports of deaths following immunization that lack sufficient information for a causality assessment as well. This is most common in uncontrolled observational studies intended to give a broad picture of the results of immunization campaigns.

Deaths Associated with Vaccine Administration but Attributable to Inappropriate Handling, Contamination, Production Error, or Error of Medical Care

This category includes a wide range of contamination or handling problems; vaccines, like any other pharmaceutical agent, are subject to mishandling that might, in extreme cases, lead to death. The Cutter incident is a well-known example of vaccine contamination caused by errors in quality control by the manufacturer and lack of clear guidelines from a regulatory agency; 60 vaccine recipients and 89 contacts of recipients contracted polio as a result of contamination of two production pools of inactivated polio vaccine (IPV) with live virus in 1955 (Nathanson and Langmuir, 1963). Contamination can occur at a more local level. Sokhey (1991) reported several deaths following administration of measles vaccine in India. The report lists the cause of death as "toxic shock syndrome" and notes that contamination was likely because syringes and needles were reused and the sterilization procedures were unsatisfactory. *Staphylococcus aureus* was isolated from a few available implicated vials. That report is discussed later in this chapter.

Deaths Temporally Associated with Vaccine Administration but Clearly Caused by Something Other Than the Vaccine

Passive surveillance systems contain many reports that fall into this category. Reports to the manufacturer or to the government regarding the death of a vaccine recipient in temporal relation to vaccination can be made before a cause of death is established. Once an autopsy is performed, it is sometimes clear that the death was temporally but not causally related to vaccination. An example of such a death is one that was reported to VAERS. This report describes the death of a 5-year-old 10 days after receipt of diphtheria and tetanus toxoids and pertussis vaccine (DPT), OPV, and measles-mumps-rubella vaccine (MMR). The cause of death was *Haemophilus influenzae* type b meningitis, which did not appear to be vaccine related.

Deaths Classified as SIDS

For many years, the standard immunization schedule in the first year of life (the period in which most cases of SIDS occur) included only DPT and polio vaccine. Use of hepatitis B and *H. influenzae* type b vaccines during the first year of life is increasing rapidly. Although the scientific question of interest is, "Does vaccination increase an infant's probability of dying of SIDS," the research has focused on the role of DPT, even though polio vaccine is often given with DPT. The previous Institute of Medicine report on rubella and pertussis vaccines (Institute of Medicine, 1991) concluded that the evidence favors rejection of a causal relation between DPT and SIDS. "Studies showing a temporal relation between these events are consistent with the expected occurrence of SIDS over the age range in which DPT immunization typically occurs" (Institute of Medicine, 1991, p. 141). A few studies that primarily investigated the role of DPT in SIDS also examined the role of polio vaccine (Bouvier-Colle et al., 1989; Hoffman et al., 1987; Taylor and Emery, 1982; Walker et al., 1987). Only Hoffman and colleagues (1987) report odds ratio estimates of the relative risk of a SIDS case infant being immunized with OPV (0.57 for age-matched controls and 0.61 for age-, race-, and low-birth-weight-matched controls). These odds ratios were very similar to those obtained for the relative risk from DPT immunization. The committee's evaluation of the causal relation between diphtheria and tetanus toxoids for pediatric use (DT) and SIDS is discussed later in this chapter.

Passive surveillance systems such as the Monitoring System for Adverse Events Following Immunization (MSAEFI) and VAERS contain many reports of SIDS that occurred within 24 or 48 hours following vaccination, but these case reports often contain inadequate information to substantiate the diagnosis, and they are not necessarily evidence of a causal relation, because cases will occur in the 24- to 48-hour period following vaccination by chance alone. The licensure and recommendations for administration in the first year of life of vaccines to prevent hepatitis B and *H. influenzae* type b infections would suggest that studies of a possible role of vaccines in SIDS will continue. There are no controlled studies of a relation between either of these two newer vaccines and SIDS. MMR is customarily given after the first year of life in the United States; therefore, a relation between MMR and SIDS has not been investigated.

Deaths That Are a Consequence of Vaccine-Strain Viral Infection

Measles and mumps vaccines and OPV are made up of live attenuated viruses. It is plausible that administration of a live viral vaccine could cause a systemic infection in the recipient that could, in certain circumstances, be fatal. The committee identified a few such reports; they are discussed later in this chapter.

Deaths That Are a Consequence of an Adverse Event That Itself Is Causally Related to a Vaccine Reviewed in This Report

Several of the adverse events studied by the committee can lead to death. If the adverse event was caused by the vaccine and led to death, then one may say that the vaccine caused the death. An example would be a patient who suffers fatal anaphylaxis associated with vaccine administration.

If the evidence favors the acceptance of (or establishes) a causal relation between a vaccine and an adverse event and that adverse event can be fatal, then in the committee's judgment the evidence favors the acceptance of (or establishes) a causal relation between the vaccine and death from that adverse event. The case fatality rate for adverse events associated with vaccines (other than, possibly, the live viral vaccines) should not be different from that for adverse events associated with all other causes. For example, anaphylaxis caused by a vaccine should be no more or less likely to result in death than anaphylaxis precipitated by any other antigen. It is plausible, however, that some adverse events caused by an attenuated viral vaccine might be milder than that same adverse event caused by the wild-type virus. In later sections of this chapter, the committee discusses the data regarding death from adverse events that are causally related to vaccines. If the evidence is inadequate to accept or reject a causal relation between a vaccine and an adverse event, then in the committee's judgment the evidence is inadequate to accept or reject a causal relation between the vaccine and death resulting from that adverse event.

Deaths Temporally Associated with Vaccine Administration and the Cause of Death Is Other Than Those Listed Above

The committee explored the possibility that vaccines may cause death by mechanisms other than vaccine-strain viral infection or an adverse event that itself is causally related to vaccine administration. The committee considered whether it might have overlooked possible vaccine-related mechanisms or pathways that could lead to death. The committee was unable to hypothesize such causes. However, had the committee identified reports of death following vaccination that did not fall into any of the other six categories, de facto those reports would have been placed into this category and causality would have been assessed for those reports. The committee found no reports of death that could be placed in this category, either in theory or by exclusion from the other causes listed above.

REPORTS OF DEATH IDENTIFIED FROM VAERS

The preponderance of data concerning death as an adverse consequence of vaccination comes from passive surveillance systems. The committee made a concerted effort to evaluate these data. The number of reports in VAERS of death in temporal association with vaccination has been the topic of presentations to the Advisory Commission on Childhood Vaccines (ACCV), the Advisory Committee on Immunization Practices, an FDA-sponsored workshop on contraindications to vaccination, a public session regarding changes to the Vaccine Injury Table, and the Vaccine Safety Committee of the Institute of Medicine. Because of this interest, because VAERS has a number of advantages over its predecessor data bases (the Spontaneous Reporting System [SRS], which was run by the FDA, and MSAEFI, which was run by the CDC), and because VAERS contains reports of reactions to hepatitis B vaccine (particularly in infants and children) and *H. influenzae* type b vaccine (which would be scarce in MSAEFI and SRS because of the recent licensure of these vaccines), the committee focused its investigations of reports to the U.S. government-run passive surveillance systems of death after vaccination on the information contained in VAERS. A description of VAERS and a discussion of its strengths and weaknesses will help in the analysis of the data that follow.

History and Background

VAERS was established by the National Childhood Vaccine Injury Act of 1986 (P.L. 99-660) to collect reports of adverse reactions following vaccination. The database is managed by a contractor under the aegises of both the CDC and the FDA. Reporting forms are available in drugstores and elsewhere, and anyone may file a report. A blank form appears in Appendix B (Figure B-1). A toll-free phone number (800-822-7967) can be used instead of the form. Physicians and nurses may report an adverse event, as may the parents, relatives, or neighbors of a patient. Health care providers are obligated to report specific adverse reactions to vaccines covered by the National Vaccine Injury Compensation Program (see box entitled The Vaccine Injury Table; see Chapter 1 for more information on the compensation program); however, reports can be made regarding any reaction to any vaccine.

Several people may submit reports about one patient. The person reporting the adverse event may supply additional information, but no supporting information is required. The form asks for the following items: the patient's initials, age, and sex; the time of event onset; description of events; general assessment of condition (dead, hospitalized, disabled, etc.); relevant diagnostic tests or laboratory data; date of vaccination; and the vaccines that were given. Once submitted to the contractor, the data are entered into a computerized database. The narrative regarding the description of the adverse event is used to determine the index terms used to categorize the adverse reaction. Up to eight terms can be assigned to each report. The indexing system used is the Coding Symbol for Thesaurus of Adverse Reaction Terms (COSTART) system.

VAERS began operation in November 1990. By July 31, 1992, there were over 17,000 reports in VAERS, almost 11,000 of which concerned vaccines covered by the National Vaccine Injury Compensation Program. Of the total number of reports, just over 2,500 of them were considered to be "serious," which is defined as the following: the patient died, suffered a life-threatening illness, or suffered a reaction that resulted in, or prolonged, hospitalization or that resulted in permanent disability.

Strengths and Weaknesses

The ease and accessibility of the reporting system might be useful in allowing VAERS to cast a large net, bringing attention to any possible adverse event. The negative aspect of this open system is that data may be inaccurate, poorly documented, or incomplete and that records may be duplicated. Although VAERS may be useful as a monitor for detecting ad-

THE VACCINE INJURY TABLE

Vaccine/Toxoid	Event	Interval from Immunization
DPT, pertussis vaccine DPT/poliovirus combined	A. Anaphylaxis or anaphylactic shock	24 hours
	B. Encephalopathy (encephalitis)[a]	3 days
	C. Shock-collapse or hypotonic-hyporesponsive collapse[b]	3 days
	D. Residual seizure disorder[c]	3 days
	E. Any acute complication or sequela (including death) of above event which arose within the time period prescribed	No limit
Measles, mumps, and rubella; DT, Td, tetanus toxoid	A. Anaphylaxis or anaphylactic shock	24 hours
	B. Encephalopathy (or encephalitis)[a]	15 days for measles, mumps and rubella vaccines; 3 days for DT, Td and tetanus toxoids
	C. Residual seizure disorder[c]	15 days for measles, mumps and rubella vaccines; 3 days for DT, Td and tetanus toxoids
	D. Any acute complication or sequela (including death) of above event which arose within the time period prescribed	No limit
Oral poliovirus vaccine	A. Paralytic poliomyelitis	
	—in a nonimmunodeficient recipient	30 days
	—in an immunodeficient recipient	6 months
	—in a vaccine-associated community case	Not applicable

	B. Any acute complication or sequela (including death) of above event which arose within the time period prescribed	No limit
Inactivated poliovirus vaccine	A. Anaphylaxis or anaphylactic shock	24 hours
	B. Any acute complication or sequela (including death) of above event which arose within the time period prescribed	No limit

NOTE: Events listed are required by law to be reported by health care providers to the U.S. Department of Health and Human Services; however, VAERS will accept *all* reports of suspected adverse events after the administration of *any* vaccine. Aids to interpretation follow as footnotes.

[a]Encephalopathy means any substantial acquired abnormality of, injury to, or impairment of brain function. Among the frequent manifestations of encephalopathy are focal and diffuse neurologic signs, increased intracranial pressure, or changes lasting ≥6 hours in level of consciousness, with or without convulsions. The neurologic signs and symptoms of encephalopathy may be temporary with complete recovery, or they may result in various degrees of permanent impairment. Signs and symptoms such as high-pitched and unusual screaming, persistent uncontrollable crying, and bulging fontanel are compatible with an encephalopathy, but in and of themselves are not conclusive evidence of encephalopathy. Encephalopathy usually can be documented by slow wave activity on an electroencephalogram.

[b]Shock-collapse or hypotonic-hyporesponsive collapse may be evidenced by signs or symptoms such as decrease in or loss of muscle tone, paralysis (partial or complete), hemiplegia, hemiparesis, loss of color or change of color to pale white or blue, unresponsiveness to environmental stimuli, depression of or loss of consciousness, prolonged sleeping with difficulty arousing, or cardiovascular or respiratory arrest.

[c]Residual seizure disorder may be considered to have occurred if no other seizure or convulsion unaccompanied by fever or accompanied by a fever of <102°F occurred before the first seizure or convulsion after the administration of the vaccine involved, AND, if in the case of measles-, mumps-, or rubella-containing vaccines, the first seizure or convulsion occurred within 15 days after vaccination OR in the case of any other vaccine, the first seizure or convulsion occurred within 3 days after the vaccination, AND, if two or more seizures or convulsions unaccompanied by fever or accompanied by a fever of <102°F occurred within 1 year after vaccination. The terms seizure and convulsion include grand mal, petit mal, absence, myoclonic, tonic-clonic, and focal motor seizures and signs.

SOURCE: Adapted from Public Law 99-660.

verse events, it is less useful for scientific analysis and assessments of causality (Chen et al., submitted for publication).

Two issues, data quality and record duplication, limit the usefulness of the VAERS data set for analysis. Under the category of data quality are the concerns of validity, documentation, and completeness of information. Because the forms can be submitted by medical and nonmedical personnel, there is bound to be variability in the quality (and availability) of information. Even among health care providers there can be great variation in the use of diagnostic terms. Although this variation in diagnosis may be random (and not biased by the reporter's concern about the contributory effect of the vaccine), death is such a serious outcome that one would like to have information that confirms or clarifies the VAERS reports. Linkage to hospital records, autopsy reports, laboratory files, and death certificates could help validate the information. Besides accurate data regarding the cause of death, one would wish to confirm the validity of key variables such as the age of the patient at the time of vaccination, type of vaccination, calendar date (and perhaps time of day) of vaccination, date of onset of adverse event, and date of death. These would be minimal data requirements for a preliminary analysis of the overall pattern of deaths following vaccination.

Table 10-1 illustrates some of the problems associated with VAERS reports. The committee assembled a table of 28 samples of VAERS reports of deaths. The sample was not necessarily random or representative, but examples were chosen to illustrate the problem of data quality. In the majority of cases, the cause of death was not stated, and there was no information to indicate whether an autopsy was performed. The VAERS data by themselves frequently do not supply enough information to allow informative data analysis.

Some VAERS reports contain enough reliable information that the report can be evaluated and weighed as one would a published case report. For example, one specific report was filed by a nurse, the cause of death was stated to be *H. influenzae* type b meningitis, and laboratory tests were performed. The death occurred 10 days following immunization with DPT, OPV, and MMR. Such VAERS reports were often very useful to the committee in its assessments of all adverse reactions reviewed, not just the reports of death.

Multiple reports relating to the same adverse event in a given patient are an obvious disadvantage of analyzing the VAERS database. Many duplicates can be found by going through the VAERS reports by hand, but one cannot be certain that all duplicate reports have been identified. Verification of data quality would probably help to eliminate more duplicate records.

There are other problematic aspects of VAERS, most notably, the problem of underreporting. The accessibility of VAERS should encourage reporting, but underreporting of events may still occur. The possible incompleteness of the data hampers any attempt to analyze the data. VAERS is a passive reporting system that could serve as a sentinel for as yet unsuspected adverse events that occur following immunization. If linked to other detailed and accurate information, such a surveillance system could be a database for scientific analysis.

Follow-up of Reports of Death to VAERS

The FDA followed up all reports of death following immunization submitted to VAERS during the time period July 1, 1990, to September 30, 1991 (R. P. Wise, FDA, presentation to the ACCV, December 1992). Of 235 reports, 29 were duplicates, leaving 206 unduplicated reports. The submitted data were considered to be adequate for 78 of those reports. Complete follow-up was achieved for an additional 81 reports. Thus, the number of reports with completed assessments was 159. Follow-up was done by FDA staff. Most queries were by telephone, and a few were by mail. There were 3.5 calls per clarified report and 2.5 completed calls per clarified report. The typical succession of calls was first to the reporting physician's office and then one or more referrals to the hospital medical records department, the coroner or medical examiner's office, and occasionally, the county recorder or state public health vaccination department.

As a result, for 159 VAERS reports the diagnosis was confirmed or clarified by the FDA. Before analyzing the reports, the committee excluded 17 VAERS reports because for 16 reports the deaths followed administration of a vaccine or vaccines not under consideration by the present committee and one report concerned a miscarriage, which the committee classified as an adverse event in temporal relation to vaccination experienced by the woman who was vaccinated.

All of the 90 cases of SIDS reported to VAERS during this 15-month period occurred within 28 days of vaccination, and 78 occurred within 7 days of vaccination. There have been no changes in the incidence of SIDS over recent years; each year, on the order of 5,000 deaths in the United States are classified as SIDS (Little and Peterson, 1990). The committee calculated the number of SIDS deaths that might be expected to occur within 7 days of vaccination if vaccination had no effect on the incidence of SIDS. Assuming that all infants receive three separate immunizations during the first year of life, there are three 7-day periods when a SIDS death would occur within 7 days of vaccination by chance alone. Of the SIDS deaths in a 1-year period, 288 deaths (21/365 of the total 5,000 SIDS deaths in 1 year) would occur within 7 days following a vaccination. If it is assumed that only half of all children receive their immunizations (a low estimate), one might expect 144 SIDS deaths in the 7 days following vaccination.

TABLE 10-1 Quality and Quantity of Data in a Sample of VAERS
Reports of Death Following Immunization

Report No.	Was Vaccine Suspected?	Is Report by an MD or RN?	Is Cause of Death Stated?	Was an Autopsy Performed?
1	No information	No	No information	No information
2	No	No	Yes, meningitis	No
3	No information	Yes—MD	No	No information
4	No information	Yes—RN	No	No information
5	No information	No information	No	No information
6	No information	No information	No	No information
7	No information	Yes—MD	No	No information
8	No information	Yes—RN	No	No information
9	No information	No information	No	No information
10	No	No information	No	Yes
11	No information	Yes—MD	No	No information
12	No information	Yes—MD	No	No information
13	No information	Yes—RN	No	No information
14	No information	No information	No	No information
15	No information	Yes—RN	No	No information
16	No information	Yes—RN	No	No information
17	No information	Yes—MD	No	No information
18	No information	Yes—RN	Yes, *H. influenzae* type b meningitis	No information
19	No information	No information	No	No information
20	No information	Yes—MD	No	Yes
21	No information	No information	No	No information
22	No information	Yes—RN	No	No information
23	No information; drug company summary	Yes	No	No information
24	Not sure; drug company report	No information	No	Yes
25	No; drug company report	No	No	No information
26	No information; drug company report	No	No	No information
27	No information	No information	Yes, meningitis	No information
28	No; drug company duplicate reports	No information	No	No information

Were Lab Tests Done?	Which Vaccines Were Given?	Age at the Time of Death?	Time Since Receipt of Vaccine (days)
No information	DPT, Hib, polio	19 mo	2
Yes	MMR, Hib	16 mo	4
No information	IPV, Hib, hepatitis B	4 mo	30
No	DPT, Hib, OPV	5.5 mo	1
No	DPT, OPV	3 mo	1
No	DPT, OPV, Hib	2.5 mo	8
No	DPT, OPV, Hib	2 mo	3
No	DPT, OPV, Pedivax 129	2.5 mo	17
No	OPV, DPT, Hib	2 mo	1
No information	DPT, OPV, Hib	4 mo	3
No information	DPT, polio, Hib	1.5 mo	2
No information	DPT, OPV, Hib	2.5 mo	1
No information	DPT, OPV, Hib	2.5 mo	1
No information	DPT, OPV, Hib	3 mo	1
No	DPT, OPV, Hib	2 mo	3
No information	DPT, OPV, Hib	4 mo	23
No information	DPT, OPV, Hib	2 mo	1
Yes	DPT, OPV, MMR	5 yr	10
No information	DT, MMR, OPV	5 yr	Same day
No information	DPT, polio, MMR	18 mo	9
No	MMR, OPV, DPT	15 mo	12
No information	Polio, DPT, MMR	5 yr	Same day
No information	MMR	11 yr	15
No information	MMR, DPT, polio	18 mo	Same day
No information	MMR	15 yr	19
No information	Orimune	No information	4 mo
No information	Hib	2 yr	1 yr
No information	Hepatitis B	No information	No information

This may be an underestimate because SIDS is not distributed evenly over the first year of life—it peaks at about 12 weeks and tapers off toward 12 months (Little and Peterson, 1990). Over a 15-month period comparable to the FDA survey period, 180 cases of SIDS would be expected to occur in the 7-day period following vaccination. Only 78 such deaths were reported to VAERS, suggesting not only that VAERS does not contain an excessive number of reports of SIDS following immunization but also that it does not pick up all cases of SIDS that occur within 7 days of vaccination.

The remaining 52 VAERS reports of deaths following vaccinations were reviewed individually by members of the Vaccine Safety Committee and were classified into the categories discussed at the beginning of the chapter. The committee received all supporting documentation (e.g., autopsy reports or letters sent by the attending physician in response to requests for follow-up information) submitted to VAERS for these reports as well as the cause of death determination made by the FDA on the basis of the follow-up described earlier in this section. After the independent reviews, the results were compared and discussed until a consensus was reached for each death.

For 10 reports, details about the cause of death were inadequate, and the review panel could not judge whether the vaccine was causally related to the death. No deaths in this group were caused by manufacturing or handling errors. Forty deaths were considered to be not caused by the vaccine. These included cases in which there were unequivocal explanations of the cause of death such as neuroblastoma of the adrenal, congenital heart disease, viral pneumonia, and asphyxiation from a foreign body, and the review panel determined that the relation between vaccine and death was not causal. One death was considered to be a result of SIDS by the committee's review panel; FDA had left the diagnosis unclear for that case, resulting in a total of 91 SIDS deaths in the data set reviewed by the committee. One death resulted from an adverse event possibly caused by a vaccine. This was a case in which a 28-year-old woman died of common complications of Guillain-Barré syndrome (GBS) that developed after receiving diphtheria and tetanus toxoids for adult use (Td). The committee determined that the evidence favors acceptance of a causal relation between Td and GBS (see Chapter 5). There were no reports for which the committee thought the cause of death was plausibly related to vaccine or that did not clearly fall into one of the other six categories.

The committee's assessment of data in VAERS is similar to those of both the FDA (R. P. Wise, FDA, presentation to ACCV, December 1992) and the CDC (R. T. Chen, presentation to ACCV, March 1993), both of which concluded that the vast majority of deaths reported to VAERS are temporally but not causally related to vaccination.

VACCINE-SPECIFIC DATA CONCERNING DEATH AFTER IMMUNIZATION

The preceding discussion sets the stage for discussion of the evidence regarding the causal relation between the vaccines reviewed in this report and death. The discussion will focus on deaths that are classified as SIDS and deaths that are a consequence of vaccine-strain viral infection. However, reports of death from all other causes (particularly from passive surveillance systems such as MSAEFI and VAERS) will be summarized for completeness. The committee evaluated VAERS reports submitted between November 1990 and July 1992.

Diphtheria and Tetanus Toxoids

Deaths Classified as SIDS

The relation between DPT and SIDS was examined by a previous Institute of Medicine committee in its investigation of the adverse effects of pertussis vaccine (Institute of Medicine, 1991). That committee concluded that the evidence favors rejection of a causal relation between DPT and SIDS. "Studies showing a temporal relation between these events are consistent with the expected occurrence of SIDS over the age range in which DPT immunization typically occurs" (Institute of Medicine, 1991, p. 141). Since both diphtheria and tetanus toxoids are components of DPT, it is likely that these toxoids are not causally associated with SIDS, although it is theoretically possible that pertussis vaccine could protect children from an effect of DT immunization on SIDS. Only one study (Pollock et al., 1984) compared the incidence of SIDS in cohorts of children who were immunized with DPT (13,917 doses) and DT (10,601 doses). Seven cases of SIDS occurred within 6 weeks of immunization, three (2.2 cases per 100,000 doses) in the DPT group and four (3.8 cases per 100,000 doses) in the DT group. The relative risk of SIDS after receipt of DPT versus that after receipt of DT was 0.6, with a 95 percent confidence interval (CI) of 0.1 to 2.3; thus, the relative risk was not significantly different from 1.0 (Institute of Medicine, 1991).

In a 7-year survey of vaccine reactions in the North West Thames region conducted by Pollock and Morris (1983), two deaths attributed to SIDS occurred among 133,500 children who received a primary series of DT (three doses). No deaths occurred among 221,000 children who received booster immunizations with DT.

A small case-control study conducted by Taylor and Emery (1982) concluded that infants who had received DT and polio vaccine were not more likely to have died "unexpectedly" than age-matched controls.

Deaths That Are a Consequence of an Adverse Event That Itself Is Causally Related to a Vaccine Reviewed in This Report

The evidence favors acceptance of a causal relation between Td and GBS. The evidence establishes a causal relation between tetanus toxoid and anaphylaxis (see Chapter 5). A VAERS report described a 28-year-old woman who received a Td booster following laceration of her foot, developed GBS, and required mechanical ventilation. After initial improvement, she developed interstitial pneumonitis and progressive ventilatory failure, and she died 20 days after immunization. Postmortem examination revealed massive interstitial pneumonitis and no inflammatory infiltrates in the nervous system.

A study by Kovalskaya (1967) demonstrated that it is possible to sensitize mice to fatal anaphylactic reactions to DPT. Only two cases of death associated with the administration of tetanus toxoid given as a single antigen have been described, one by Regamey in 1965 and one by Staak and Wirth in 1973. In both cases, anaphylaxis was thought to be the cause of death.

Other Reports of Death Following Immunization

Available Data Were Insufficient to Allow a Judgment of Cause Three deaths associated with DT or Td were reported to VAERS between November 1990 and September 1992. One patient received DT, MMR, and OPV at 60 months of age and died 1 day after immunization; no further clinical details were provided, and a cause of death was not indicated. The other two reports are discussed in other sections in this chapter.

Deaths Associated with Vaccine Administration but Attributable to Inappropriate Handling, Contamination, Production Error, or Error of Medical Care Early reports of death associated with toxin-antitoxin mixtures of diphtheria toxin and diphtheria toxoid were shown to be related to inadequate inactivation of toxin (see Background and History in Chapter 5); modern techniques of toxoid preparation and testing have eliminated this problem.

Deaths Temporally Associated with Vaccine Administration and the Cause of Death Is Other Than Those Listed Above Korger and colleagues (1986) reported data collected over 15 years (1970-1984) in Marburg, Germany, regarding the adverse effects of the tetanus toxoid produced by Behring. Reports were made by practicing physicians, the Drug Commission of the German Medical Association, the Paul-Ehrlich-Institut, druggists, and patients from 1970 to 1984. Data were stored on computer, and the physicians and the manufacturer tried to determine the details of the reactions with a questionnaire. Five deaths were reported during a period when about 100 million doses were administered. When analyzed by those investigators, none of the deaths appeared to be causally related to the administration of tetanus toxoid, although one case was reported as "circulatory collapse in a patient with bronchial asthma." Clinical details of this case were not provided in the report.

In one of the three deaths associated with DT or Td reported to VAERS between November 1990 and September 1992, the cause of death in a 9-month-old child who received DT was reported as "Wilms tumor with nephrotic syndrome." The other two reports are discussed in the sections on deaths that are a consequence of an adverse event that is itself causally related to a vaccine reviewed in this report and on deaths for which the available data were insufficient to allow a judgment of cause.

In the hospital activity analysis of acute neurologic disease in the North West Thames region of England (this study is discussed in detail in Chapter 5), one case of fatal encephalopathy occurred 28 days after DT immunization (Pollock and Morris, 1983).

The National Childhood Encephalopathy Study described in the encephalopathy section of Chapter 6 was a large case-control study carried out between July 1976 and June 1979 to address the relation between vaccine administration and acute neurologic events (Alderslade et al., 1981). As part of that study, outcome data were collected, including any deaths that occurred in the children who experienced neurologic events. Of the 20 children with onset of a neurologic event within 7 days after immunization with DT, 4 died. Two children who had been normal prior to immunization developed encephalopathy or encephalitis. One child died on the same day after receiving the first DT immunization, and the other child died after 20 days. A third, previously normal child who died was originally thought to have Reye syndrome, but endocardial fibroelastosis was found at autopsy. The fourth child who died after DT immunization had a preceding neurologic abnormality, developed acute infantile hemiplegia after immunization, and died at 2.5 years of age. In the committee's judgment the evidence favors rejection of a causal relation between DT and encephalopathy (see Chapter 5).

Causality Argument

The evidence favors rejection of a causal relation between DPT and SIDS (Institute of Medicine, 1991). Pollock et al. (1984) presented data suggesting that the relative risk of SIDS after DPT versus that after DT is not significantly different from 1. In the committee's judgment the evidence favors rejection of a causal relation between DT and SIDS.

The evidence favors acceptance of a causal relation between DT, Td, and tetanus toxoid and GBS. The evidence establishes a causal relation between DT, Td, and tetanus toxoid and anaphylaxis (see Chapter 5). Both GBS and anaphylaxis can be fatal. The only well-documented cases of death causally related to immunization with tetanus toxoid, DT, or Td are attributable to anaphylaxis; the evidence regarding death as a consequence of GBS that temporally followed administration of one of these toxoids is limited (one case report). In the committee's judgment DT, Td, or tetanus toxoid may rarely cause fatal GBS or anaphylaxis. There is no evidence or reason to believe that the case fatality rate from vaccine-associated GBS or anaphylaxis would differ from the case fatality rate for these adverse events associated with any other cause.

Reports of death from all other causes are not clearly linked to the preceding immunization. No cases of death were reported by Christensen (1972) in Denmark between 1952 and 1970, a time during which 2.5 million doses of monovalent tetanus toxoid, 2.67 million doses of DT, and 1.1 million doses of Td were given. No cases of death associated with tetanus toxoid, DT, or Td were reported through MSAEFI between 1979 and 1990. During that time, approximately 1.3 million doses of DT and 29 million doses of Td were distributed.

Conclusion

The evidence establishes a causal relation between DT, Td, and tetanus toxoid and death from anaphylaxis. Although this conclusion is based on direct evidence, it is not based on controlled studies and no relative risk can be calculated. However, the risk of death from anaphylaxis following receipt of DT, Td, or tetanus toxoid would appear to be extraordinarily low.

The evidence favors acceptance of a causal relation between DT, Td, and tetanus toxoid and death from GBS. This conclusion is not based on controlled studies and no relative risk can be calculated. However, the risk of death from GBS following receipt of DT, Td, or tetanus toxoid would seem to be extraordinarily low.

The evidence favors rejection of a causal relation between DT and SIDS.

The evidence is inadequate to accept or reject a causal relation between tetanus toxoid, DT, or Td and death from causes other than those listed above.

Measles and Mumps Vaccines

Deaths Classified as SIDS

Measles and mumps vaccines are not administered in the United States to the age group in which most cases of SIDS occur (under age 6 months). There are scattered reports of sudden death in temporal relation to measles vaccine (Hirayama, 1983; Miller, 1982; Nader and Warren, 1968), but insufficient information was provided to classify these as SIDS.

Deaths That Are a Consequence of Vaccine-Strain Viral Infection

Several articles have reported the death from measles infection of immunocompromised children following administration of live attenuated measles vaccine. Hong and colleagues (1985) reported the death of a 4-month-old boy with Omenn's disease following immunization with an unspecified strain of live attenuated measles vaccine. He was first seen at 4 months of age because of a skin eruption and fever following immunization with live attenuated measles vaccine. Attempts to culture measles virus from throat, skin, lymph node, and stool specimens were not successful. His skin rash persisted for several weeks, and he experienced unexplained high fevers and chronic diarrhea and cough. He was readmitted to the hospital at 15 months of age and died soon thereafter. The autopsy showed lymphoma and measles virus antigen in his bone marrow and lymphoid tissue. There was no evidence of subacute sclerosing panencephalitis. It thus appears that because of the patient's T-cell deficiency, the measles virus was not contained, suggesting a chronic measles infection following vaccination.

Bellini and colleagues reported on two cases of fatal measles following vaccination of two children with severe combined immunodeficiency syndrome (Bellini et al., 1992; Coffin et al., 1993). In both cases, RNA-templated nucleotide sequencing showed that the gene sequences of the RNAs isolated from the children's tissues were identical to the gene sequences of the RNA of the vaccine strain. Two other case reports link measles vaccine and the subsequent development of measles that led to death in immunocompromised children. One child each suffered from dysgammaglobulinemia (Mawhinney et al., 1971) and acute leukemia (Mitus et al., 1962). The technology used by Bellini and colleagues described above was not available at the time of the latter two studies, so the findings do not permit as confident an inference of a causal association.

Deaths That Are a Consequence of an Adverse Event That Itself Is Causally Related to a Vaccine Reviewed in This Report

The evidence favors acceptance of a causal relation between measles vaccine and anaphylaxis. The evidence establishes a causal relation between MMR and thrombocytopenia anaphylaxis (see Chapter 6). The committee identified no reports of death from these adverse events that occurred in temporal relation to vaccination.

Other Reports of Death Following Immunization

The committee does not consider the apparent increased relative risk of death following administration of high-titer Edmonston-Zagreb or Schwarz strain measles vaccine such as has been seen in clinical trials conducted in Senegal (Garenne et al., 1991) to be relevant to the United States because these high-titer vaccines are not licensed for use in the United States. The cause of the increased mortality such as that seen in Senegal is not known.

Available Data Were Insufficient to Allow a Judgment of Cause   Starke and colleagues (1970) described three deaths that occurred during a mass measles immunization campaign in the former East Germany from 1967 to 1969. One child died of toxic circulatory collapse 6 days after immunization. The article stated that virologic examinations showed no proof of a pathogenic agent, but it is not clear how rigorously this was pursued. Another child died 3 days after measles vaccination. Autopsy results report cerebral edema as the cause of death. Another child died approximately 6 weeks after immunization. Autopsy results showed encephalitis as the cause of death. Haun and Ehrhardt (1973) described an 11-month-old child who developed clonic seizures and encephalitis within 12 days of receiving measles vaccine (Leningrad-16 SSW) and who died soon thereafter of probable disseminated intravascular coagulation. The authors were unsure whether vaccine-strain virus was responsible. Nader and Warren (1968) described 23 cases of neurologic disease following measles vaccination reported to the U.S. Communicable Disease Center (now CDC) between 1965 and 1967. Two deaths were reported 7 and 13 days following vaccination. Measles antibody was not detectable in either patient. One of the cases was diagnosed as encephalitis (herpes simplex virus was isolated from brain, but there were no detectable antibodies against this virus in serum) and the other was diagnosed as a sudden death. Landrigan and Witte (1973) reported on 84 cases of neurologic disorders reported to the CDC between 1963 and 1971 and diagnosed within 1 month following administration of measles vaccine. Five of these patients had extensive neurologic disorders that were ultimately fatal. They also reported five fatalities in which the clinical course was consistent with overwhelming bacterial or viral infec-tion. Culturing was inadequate, and no cause of death was established. Hirayama (1983) described complications from measles vaccine reported as part of a compensation system established by the Preventive Vaccination Law in Japan in 1976. During the time period covered by the article (1978 to approximately 1982), 2.15 million individuals were inoculated with the Schwarz measles vaccine and 1.39 million individuals were inoculated with the Biken-CAM live attenuated measles vaccine. The authors estimated that during the 18 days following administration of the vaccine in children younger than 1 year of age, the combined risk of acute neurologic disease and sudden death was 9.8 per 100,000 doses per year. The annual back-ground incidence of acute neurologic disease and sudden deaths was 200 per 100,000 infants younger than 1 year.

The evidence is inadequate to accept or reject a causal relation between measles vaccine and encephalitis, encephalopathy, or residual seizure disor-der (see Chapter 6). In the committee's judgment the evidence is inad-equate to accept or reject a causal relation between measles vaccine and death from encephalitis, encephalopathy, and residual seizure disorder.

Summary statistics from MSAEFI from 1979 to 1990 showed 3 deaths after administration of measles vaccine, 16 deaths after administration of MMR alone, and 8 deaths after administration of MMR in conjunction with DPT and OPV. No other data regarding deaths were obtained from MSAEFI. The committee identified 32 reports in VAERS (submitted between Novem-ber 1990 and July 1992) of death in association with administration of measles and mumps vaccines. One of these was in association with measles vaccine, one with mumps vaccine, one with measles-mumps vaccine, and nine with MMR. Twenty reports were of MMR administered in conjunction with other vaccines. The vaccinees ranged in age from 2 months to 15 years, and the interval from the time of vaccination to death ranged from 1 day to at least 56 days. Missing data from some VAERS reports precludes the listing of more precise information concerning the age of the child or the interval from the time of vaccination to death.

Deaths Associated with Vaccine Administration but Attributable to Inappro-priate Handling, Contamination, Production Error, or Error of Medical Care Sokhey (1991) reported the results of a monitoring effort following immunization in India for the year 1990. The monitoring effort covered a number of childhood vaccines, although only the events possibly associated with measles vaccines are described here. There were apparently five sepa-rate locations where children received the measles vaccine, and 9 of 54 children died after receiving the vaccine. The authors attributed the deaths of eight children to toxic shock syndrome (TSS). In one incident, 6 of the 12 immunized children died within 24 hours of receiving the vaccine (the vaccine strain was unidentified). Apparently, all 12 children had adverse reactions and 6 survived. The ages of those who died ranged from 9 to 18 months. This extraordinary mortality rate was attributed by the author to TSS and, specifically, the use of unhygienic conditions in administering the vaccine. A second incident involved the death of the only child (age 8 months) immunized at a particular location. Death occurred within 24 hours of vaccine administration and was attributed to TSS. In a third incident, 1 of 33 immunized children died following measles vaccination. This child was 23 months old and died of TSS 17 hours after immunization. A fourth incident involved the death of one of seven immunized children. The 16-month-old child became semiconscious within 30 minutes of receiving the vaccine and died approximately 40 hours later. The death was attributed to underlying hemorrhagic diathesis.

Deaths Temporally Associated with Vaccine Administration, and the Cause of Death Is Other Than Those Listed Above Miller (1982) described a case series of 10,035 children who were vaccinated between 1970 and 1980 in Oxford, England, with the Beckenham 31 and Schwarz measles vaccine strains. One 12-month-old child died 36 hours after the vaccination. The report indicated that the coroner's death certificate stated "sudden death in infancy and acute bronchiolitis" (Miller, 1982, p. 535).

Causality Argument

The data relating death and measles or mumps vaccine are from case reports and case series. The largest series comes from India, but TSS caused by the unhygienic conditions involved in the immunization program was the apparent cause of death reported for eight of nine patients. Evidence based on RNA sequencing techniques has linked measles vaccine and measles infection to subsequent death in some severely immunocompromised children. In contrast, studies of the immunogenic response to measles vaccine in children infected with human immunodeficiency virus (HIV), which causes acquired immune deficiency syndrome (AIDS), have not recorded any deaths from measles vaccine-strain viral infection.

The evidence favors the acceptance of a causal relation between measles vaccine and anaphylaxis. The evidence establishes a causal relation between MMR and thrombocytopenia and anaphylaxis (see Chapter 6). Anaphylaxis and thrombocytopenia can be fatal. Although there is no direct evidence of death as a consequence of measles vaccine-related anaphylaxis or of MMR-related thrombocytopenia or anaphylaxis, in the committee's judgment measles vaccine could cause fatal anaphylaxis and MMR could cause fatal thrombocytopenia or anaphylaxis. There is no evidence or reason to believe that the case fatality rate from measles vaccine-related thrombocytopenia or anaphylaxis would differ from the case fatality rates for these adverse events associated with any other cause.

Conclusion

The evidence establishes a causal relation between vaccine-strain measles virus infection and death. The conclusion is based on case reports in immunocompromised individuals and not on controlled studies. No relative risk can be calculated. However, the risk of death from measles vaccine-strain infection would seem to be extraordinarily low.

The evidence establishes a causal relation between MMR and death from complications associated with severe thrombocytopenia. The evidence establishes a causal relation between MMR and death from anaphylaxis. There is no direct evidence for this; the conclusion is based on the potential of severe thrombocytopenia and anaphylaxis to be fatal. The risk would seem to be extraordinarily low.

The evidence favors acceptance of a causal relation between measles vaccine and death from anaphylaxis. There is no direct evidence for this; the conclusion is based on the potential of anaphylaxis to be fatal. The risk would seem to be extraordinarily low.

The evidence is inadequate to accept or reject a causal relation between measles and mumps vaccines and death from causes other than those listed above.

Risk-Modifying Factors

There is evidence that some severely immunocompromised children, such as those with severe combined immunodeficiency syndrome, dysgamma-globulinemia, or leukemia, are susceptible to overwhelming measles infection and subsequent death, even from attenuated measles vaccine. Infection with HIV has not been associated with death from measles vaccine-strain viral infection.

Polio Vaccines

Deaths Classified as SIDS

For many years, the standard immunization schedule in the first year of life (the period in which SIDS occurs) included only DPT and polio vaccine. The research on SIDS has focused on DPT. A few studies that primarily investigated the role of DPT in SIDS also looked at polio vaccine (Bouvier-Colle et al., 1989; Hoffman et al., 1987; Taylor and Emery, 1982; Walker et al., 1987). Only Hoffman and colleagues (1987) report odds ratio estimates of the relative risk of a SIDS case infant being immunized with OPV (0.57 for age-matched controls and 0.61 for age-, race-, and low-birth-weight-matched controls). These odds ratios were very similar to those obtained for the relative risk of SIDS after DPT immunization. A small case-control study conducted by Taylor and Emery (1982) concluded that infants who had received DT and polio vaccine were not more likely to have died "unexpectedly" than age-matched controls. Mobius and colleagues (1972) described 13 deaths that occurred in the 21 days following receipt of polio vaccine over the years 1959 to 1968 in the former East Germany. Three deaths labeled sudden death followed administration of OPV and one labeled fever and sudden death followed administration of IPV.

Passive surveillance systems such as MSAEFI and VAERS contain many reports of SIDS occurring within 24 or 48 hours following vaccination, but these case reports are not necessarily evidence of an association or a causal relation, because cases will occur in the 24- to 48-hour period following vaccination by chance alone.

Deaths That Are a Consequence of Vaccine-Strain Viral Infection

One VAERS report states that molecular biologic techniques were used to identify vaccine-strain poliovirus from the myocardium of a 3.5-month-old baby who died of myocarditis 4 days after receiving his second doses of OPV and DPT. On the basis of details in the VAERS report, the committee believes this report concerns the same baby described to the committee at its May 1992 public meeting (see Appendix B).

Deaths That Are a Consequence of an Adverse Event That Itself Is Causally Related to a Vaccine Reviewed in This Report

The evidence favors acceptance of a causal relation between OPV and GBS. The evidence establishes a causal relation between OPV and paralytic poliomyelitis (see Chapter 7).

The committee identified no reports of death following GBS that occurred in temporal relation to OPV immunization. In the committee's review of over 90 papers reporting cases of vaccine-associated polio, the committee found 6 papers that described deaths among patients with vaccine-associated polio. These deaths are summarized in Table 10-2. Two papers described the same case (Davis et al., 1977; Saulsbury et al., 1975) of a female infant with immunodeficiency associated with cartilage-hair hypoplasia who contracted polio but who died of pneumonia 3 months after the diagnosis of polio. Two other deaths reported in the United States (Chang et al., 1966; Gaebler et al., 1986) also occurred in immunodeficient individuals. The sixth paper describes the first year of Peru's vaccination

TABLE 10-2 Deaths Among Patients with Vaccine-Associated Polio

Reference	Case Description
Davis et al., 1977	Female diagnosed with polio at age 8 mo, diagnosed with dwarfism because of cartilage-hair hypoplasia at 10 mo, died of pneumonia at age 11 mo
Gross et al., 1987	40-yr-old man receiving long-term steroid therapy; he developed polio 51 days after daughter's immunization with OPV and died of cardiac arrest 1 year later
Gaebler et al., 1986	Infant boy received typical course of immunizations and developed polio at age 7.5 mo; he died at age 21 mo; the authors considered boy to be immune deficient, but evidence of vaccine-associated polio was not definitive
Saulsbury et al., 1975	Same as Davis et al., 1977
Roedenbeck and Diaz, 1967	Fourteen deaths among patients with polio occurring in the first year (1966) of Peru's vaccination program
Chang et al., 1966	A 7-yr-old boy diagnosed with "vaccine-like" polio and then discovered to be hypogammaglobulinemic; he died of pneumococcal meningitis more than 1 yr following diagnosis of polio

program (Roedenbeck and Diaz, 1967). The authors described 14 deaths that occurred in children who were recently immunized with OPV. This was at a time when wild-type poliovirus was still circulating; the cases of polio and the deaths may therefore have been associated with wild-type strains. A third case occurred in a person who had been on long-term steroids and might have been immunocompromised (Gross et al., 1987).

The CDC reported five deaths that occurred in people with vaccine-associated polio over the years 1980 to 1991 (Division of Immunization, Centers for Disease Control, personal communication, 1993). Four of the deaths occurred in immunodeficient or immunosuppressed patients. The fifth patient was not considered to be immunosuppressed but was described in the published case report described above (Gross et al., 1987) as possibly being immunocompromised because of long-term steroid use.

There may have been other deaths among people with vaccine-associated polio, but the case reports in the literature do not always follow the patients long enough. It is interesting to note that all the deaths in the United States reported in the literature occurred in immunodeficient or immune-suppressed people. This suggests that immunodeficiency is a risk-modifying factor that increases the case fatality rate of polio. In such immunodeficient patients with polio, other infections contributed to the patients' deaths. The immunodeficient patients may therefore be at increased risk of dying compared with the risk for other people who contract vaccine-associated polio.

Death from Other Causes Following Immunization

Available Data Were Insufficient to Allow a Judgment of Cause Summary statistics from MSAEFI for the years 1979 to 1990 include 1 report of death following administration of OPV only, 1 report following IPV only, 445 reports following OPV plus other vaccines, and 1 report following IPV and other vaccines. VAERS (reports submitted between November 1990 and July 1992) contained 1 report of death following OPV only, 267 following OPV plus other vaccines, and 1 following IPV and other vaccines. Many VAERS reports contain insufficient data to assess a causal relation between polio vaccines and death.

Deaths Temporally Associated with Vaccine Administration and the Cause of Death Is Other Than Those Listed Above Ehrengut and Ehrengut-Lange (1969) reviewed the deaths in which illness started in the 4 weeks following vaccination that occurred in Bavaria, Germany, during the years 1962 to 1964. They found that 26 such deaths occurred among 702,348 children aged 0 to 3 years. In all cases, poliomyelitis or polyradiculitis was ruled out as the cause of death. The main causes of death were respiratory infections (pneumonia, bronchitis, etc.). The authors did not comment on the causes of death, but suggested that mortality following receipt of polio vaccine was similar to that following receipt of smallpox vaccine in the same years.

Mobius and colleagues (1972) described 13 deaths that occurred in the 21 days following receipt of polio vaccine over the years 1959 to 1968 in the former East Germany. Eleven deaths occurred following receipt of OPV and two occurred following receipt of IPV. The causes of death following receipt of OPV were as follows: three were "found dead," three were "sudden death," and there was one each of epiglottitis, aspiration, pneumonia, and "unclear." One of the fatalities was in a child who died of myocarditis. The authors report that the child had been administered oral polio vaccine stains 1 and 3, however polio virus type II was isolated. The causes of death following IPV were convulsions and fever/sudden death.

Causality Argument

The evidence favors acceptance of a causal relation between OPV and GBS. The evidence establishes a causal relation between OPV and paralytic poliomyelitis in recipients or contacts (see Chapter 7). GBS and paralytic poliomyelitis can be fatal. Although there is no direct evidence of death as a consequence of OPV-induced GBS, in the committee's judgment OPV could cause fatal GBS. There are data regarding death from vaccine-strain polio infection; the data derive primarily from immunocompromised individuals. There is no evidence or reason to believe that the case fatality rate for GBS or vaccine-associated poliovirus infection (including that resulting in paralytic poliomyelitis) is less than that for these adverse events associated with any other cause.

The possible causal relation between polio vaccines and SIDS has rarely been studied. The evidence is inadequate to accept or reject a causal relation between polio vaccines and SIDS.

Conclusion

The evidence establishes a causal relation between OPV and death from vaccine-strain poliovirus infection, including infection that results in paralytic poliomyelitis. The conclusion is based on case reports and not on controlled studies. No relative risk can be calculated. However, the risk of death from OPV-related polio infection would seem to be extraordinarily low.

The evidence favors acceptance of a causal relation between OPV and death from GBS. There is no direct evidence for this; the conclusion is based on the potential of GBS to be fatal. The risk would appear to be extraordinarily low.

The evidence is inadequate to accept or reject a causal relation between polio vaccines and SIDS.

The evidence is inadequate to accept or reject a causal relation between OPV and death from causes other than those listed above.

Risk-Modifying Factors

Immunodeficient individuals may be at greater risk of dying than immunocompetent persons if they contract vaccine-associated poliovirus infection.

Hepatitis B Vaccine

Deaths Classified as SIDS

Hepatitis B vaccine has only recently been used in infants under 1 year of age. A possible causal relation between hepatitis B vaccine and SIDS has not been studied. There are reports in VAERS (submitted between November 1990 and July 1992) of SIDS occurring in temporal relation to hepatitis B vaccination.

Deaths That Are a Consequence of an Adverse Event That Itself Is Causally Related to a Vaccine Reviewed in This Report

The committee did not identify any reports of fatal anaphylaxis following hepatitis B vaccination.

Death from Other Causes Following Immunization

Available Data Were Insufficient to Allow a Judgment of Cause Two deaths following hepatitis B vaccination were reported to MSAEFI for the years 1979 to 1990. Both deaths occurred in vaccinees who concurrently received DPT and OPV. No other data regarding deaths were obtained from MSAEFI.

The committee identified nine reports in VAERS (submitted between November 1990 and July 1992) of death that occurred in association with administration of hepatitis B vaccines. Six of these were associated with administration of hepatitis B vaccine only; the other three were associated with administration of hepatitis B vaccine in conjunction with other vaccines. The ages of the vaccinees ranged from 1 month to 70 years, and the interval from vaccination to death ranged from 1 to 30 days.

Causality Argument

The evidence establishes a causal relation between hepatitis B vaccine and anaphylaxis (see Chapter 8). Anaphylaxis can be fatal. Although there is no direct evidence of fatal anaphylaxis following hepatitis B vaccination, in the committee's judgment hepatitis B vaccine could cause fatal anaphylaxis. There is no evidence or reason to believe that the case fatality rate for vaccine-associated anaphylaxis would differ from the case fatality rate for anaphylaxis associated with any other cause.

Hepatitis B vaccine has only recently begun to be administered to the age group that is affected by SIDS. There are no published studies of a possible causal relation between hepatitis B vaccine and SIDS. There are reports in VAERS of SIDS following immunization with hepatitis B vaccine given in conjunction with other vaccines.

Conclusion

The evidence establishes a causal relation between hepatitis B vaccine and fatal anaphylaxis. There is no direct evidence for this; the conclusion is based on the potential for anaphylaxis to be fatal. The risk would appear to be extraordinarily low.

The evidence is inadequate to accept or reject a causal relation between hepatitis B vaccine and SIDS.

The evidence is inadequate to accept or reject a causal relation between hepatitis B vaccine and death from any cause other than those listed above.

Haemophilus influenzae Type b Vaccine

Deaths Classified as SIDS

There are no published studies of the relation between *H. influenzae* type b (Hib) vaccines and SIDS. Hib vaccines are licensed for administration to children under 1 year of age. There are reports in VAERS of SIDS occurring in temporal relation to Hib vaccine administration. As part of an investigation of VAERS reports of death following administration of Hib vaccines, the CDC has preliminary data suggesting that Hib vaccines do not appear to be causally related to SIDS (R. T. Chen, presentation to ACCV, March 1993).

Deaths That Are a Consequence of an Adverse Event That Itself Is Causally Related to a Vaccine Reviewed in This Report

The committee found no reports of death caused by Hib disease that occurred within 7 days of immunization with the unconjugated (polyribosylribitol phosphate [PRP]) Hib vaccine in children over 18 months of age who receive their first Hib immunization with unconjugated PRP vaccine, although in 10 instances outcome information was not provided.

Death from Other Causes Following Immunization

Available Data Were Insufficient to Allow a Judgment of Cause The committee identified 223 reports of death in association with the administration of Hib vaccine from VAERS between November 1990 and August 1992. Of these 223 reports, 17 were of children who received Hib vaccine alone. The ages of the children in the 223 reports ranged from 2 months to at least 36 months. The interval from the time of vaccination to death ranged from 1 to 210 days. Because data were missing from some VAERS reports, more precise information about the age of the child or the time interval from vaccination to death is unavailable.

There were no reports to MSAEFI regarding death in association with Hib vaccination from 1979 to 1984. There were reports to MSAEFI of two deaths following Hib vaccination from 1985 to 1990. The recent licensure of the Hib vaccine makes this finding not surprising.

Causality Argument

The evidence favors rejection of a causal relation between conjugated Hib vaccines and early-onset Hib disease. The evidence favors acceptance of a causal relation between PRP vaccine and early-onset Hib disease in children 18 months of age or older who receive their first Hib immunization with unconjugated PRP vaccine (see Chapter 9). Hib disease can be fatal. Although there is no direct evidence of death as a consequence of early-onset Hib disease in children 18 months of age or older who receive their first Hib immunization with PRP vaccine, in the committee's judgment PRP vaccine could cause fatal Hib disease in children 18 months of age or older who receive their first Hib immunization with PRP vaccine. There is no evidence or reason to believe that the case fatality rate from PRP-associated Hib disease would differ from the case fatality rate from Hib disease not associated with PRP vaccine.

Conclusion

The evidence favors acceptance of a causal relation between PRP vaccine and death from early-onset Hib disease in children 18 months of age or older who receive their first Hib immunization with unconjugated PRP vaccine. There is no direct evidence for this; the conclusion is based on the potential for Hib disease to be fatal. The risk would appear to be extraordinarily low.

The evidence favors rejection of a causal relation between conjugated Hib vaccines and death from early-onset Hib disease.

The evidence is inadquate to accept or reject a causal relation between Hib vaccines and SIDS.

The evidence is inadequate to accept or reject a causal relation between Hib vaccine and death from causes other than those listed above.

REFERENCES

Alderslade R, Bellman MH, Rawson NS, Ross EM, Miller DL. The National Childhood Encephalopathy Study: a report on 1000 cases of serious neurological disorders in infants and young children from the NCES research team. In: Department of Health and Social Security. Whooping Cough: Reports from the Committee on the Safety of Medicines and the Joint Committee on Vaccination and Immunisation. London: Her Majesty's Stationery Office; 1981.

Bellini WJ, Rota JS, Greer FW, Zaki SR. Measles vaccination death in a child with severe combined immunodeficiency: report of a case. Laboratory Investigation 1992;66:19A.

Bouvier-Colle MH, Flahaut A, Messiah A, Jougla E, Hatton F. Sudden infant death and immunization: an extensive epidemiological approach to the problem in France—winter 1986. International Journal of Epidemiology 1989;18:121-126.

Chang TW, Weinstein L, MacMahon HE. Paralytic poliomyelitis in a child with hypogamma-globulinemia: probable implication of type I vaccine strain. Pediatrics 1966;37:630-636.

Chen RT, Rastogi SC, Mullen JR, Hayes SW, Cochi SL, Donlon JA, et al. The Vaccine Adverse Event Reporting System (VAERS). Atlanta: Centers for Disease Control; submitted for publication.

Christensen PE. Side reactions to tetanus toxoid. Scientific Publication, Pan American Health Organization 1972;253:36-43.

Coffin CM, Roberts RL, Monafo WJ, Haslam DB, Bellini WJ, Zaki S, et al. Disseminated measles infection following vaccination in severe combined immune deficiency syndrome. Society for Pediatric Pathology 1993;13:102.

Davis LE, Bodian D, Price D, Butler IJ, Vickers JH. Chronic progressive poliomyelitis secondary to vaccination of an immunodeficient child. New England Journal of Medicine 1977;297:241-245.

Ehrengut W, Ehrengut-Lange J. Interkurrente todliche Erkrankungen nach Polioschluckimpfung und Pockenschutzimpfung. [Intercurrent fatal diseases after oral polio vaccination and smallpox vaccination.] Munchener Medizinische Wochenschrift 1969;111:1092-1099.

Gaebler JW, Kleiman MB, French ML, Chastain G, Barrett C, Griffin C. Neurologic complications in oral polio vaccine recipients. Journal of Pediatrics 1986;108:878-881.

Garenne M, Leroy O, Beau J-P, Sene I. Child mortality after high titre measles vaccines: prospective study in Senegal. Lancet 1991;338:903-907.

Gross TP, Khurana RK, Higgins T, Nkowane BS, Hirsch RL. Vaccine-associated poliomyelitis in a household contact with Netherton's syndrome receiving long-term steroid therapy. American Journal of Medicine 1987;83:797-800.

Haun U, Ehrhardt G. Zur problematik postvakzinaler Komplikationen nach Masernschutzimpfung. [Postvaccinal complications following protective vaccination against measles.] Deutsche Gesundheitswesen 1973;28:1306-1308.

Hirayama M. Measles vaccines used in Japan. Reviews of Infectious Diseases 1983;5:495-503.

Hoffman HJ, Hunter JC, Damus K, Pakter J, Peterson DR, van Belle G, Hasselmeyer EG. Diphtheria-tetanus-pertussis immunization and sudden infant death: results of the National Institute of Child Health and Human Development Cooperative Epidemiological Study of Sudden Infant Death Syndrome Risk Factors. Pediatrics 1987;79:598-611.

Hong R, Gilbert EF, Opitz JM. Omenn disease: termination in lymphoma. Pediatric Pathology 1985;3:143-154.

Institute of Medicine. Adverse Effects of Pertussis and Rubella Vaccines. Washington, DC: National Academy Press; 1991.

Korger G, Quast U, Dechert G. Tetanusimpfung: Vertraglichkeit und Vermeidung von Nebenreaktionen. [Tetanus vaccination: tolerance and avoidance of adverse reactions.] Klininische Wochenschrift 1986;64:767-775.

Kovalskaya SI. Anafilaktogennye svoistva adsorbipovannoi i neadsorbirovannoi kokliusnodifterino-stolbniachnoi vaktsin. [The anaphylactogenic properties of absorbed and non-absorbed pertussis-diphtheria-tetanus vaccines.] Zhurnal Mikrobiologii, Epidemiologii, i Immunobiologii 1967;44:105-109.

Landrigan PJ, Witte JJ. Neurologic disorders following live measles-virus vaccination. Journal of the American Medical Association 1973;223:1459-1462.

Little RE, Peterson DR. Sudden infant death syndrome epidemiology: a review and update. Epidemiologic Reviews 1990;12:241-246.

Mawhinney H, Allen IV, Beare JM, Bridges JM, Connolly HH, Haire M, et al. Dysgamma-globulinaemia complicated by disseminated measles. British Medical Journal 1971;2:380-381.

Miller CL. Surveillance after measles vaccination in children. The Practitioner 1982;226:535-537.

Mitus A, Holloway A, Evans AE, Enders JF. Attenuated measles vaccine in children with acute leukemia. American Journal of Diseases of Children 1962;103:243-248.

Mobius G, Wiedersberg H, Wunscher W, Backer F. Pathologisch-anatomische Befunde bei Todesfallen nach Poliomyelitis- und Dreifach-Schutzimpfung. [Pathological-anatomical findings in cases of death following poliomyelitis and diphtheria-pertussis-tetanus vaccination.] Deutsche Gesundheitswesen 1972;27:1382-1386.

Nader PR, Warren RJ. Reported neurologic disorders following live measles vaccine. Pediatrics 1968;41:997-1001.

Nathanson N, Langmuir AD. The Cutter incident: poliomyelitis following formaldehyde-inactivated poliovirus vaccination in the United States during the spring of 1955. I. Background. American Journal of Hygiene 1963;78:16-28.

Pollock TM, Morris J. A 7-year survey of disorders attributed to vaccination in North West Thames region. Lancet 1983;1:753-757.

Pollock TM, Miller E, Mortimer JY, Smith G. Symptoms after primary immunisation with DTP and with DT vaccine. Lancet 1984;2:146-149.

Regamey RH. Die Tetanus-Schutzimpfung. In: Herrlick A, ed. Handbuch der Schutzimpfungen. Berlin: Springer; 1965.

Roedenbeck SD, Diaz C. Poliomielitis y vacuna oral. [Poliomyelitis and oral vaccine.] Revista de Neuro-Psiquiatria 1967;30:38-56.

Saulsbury FT, Winkelstein JA, Davis LE, Hsu SH, D'Souza BJ, Gutcher GR, Butler, IJ. Combined immunodeficiency and vaccine-related poliomyelitis in a child with cartilage-hair hypoplasia. Journal of Pediatrics 1975;86:868-872.

Sokhey J. Adverse events following immunization: 1990. Indian Pediatrics 1991;28:593-607.

Staak M, Wirth E. Zur problematik anaphylaktischer Reaktionen nach aktiver Tetanus-Immunisierung. [Anaphylactic reactions following active tetanus immunization.] Deutsche Medizinische Wochenschrift 1973;98:110-111.

Starke VG, Hlinak P, Nobel B, Winkler C, Kaesler G. Masernradikation—eine Moglichkeit? Ergebnisse und Erfahrungen mit der Masernschutzimpfung 1967 bis 1969 in der DDR [Measles eradication—a possibility? Results and experiences with the measles inoculation from 1967 to 1969 in the GDR.] Deutsche Gesundheitswesen 1970;25:2384-2390.

Taylor EM, Emery JL. Immunisation and cot deaths (letter). Lancet 1982;2:721.

Walker AM, Jick H, Perera DR, Thompson RJ, Knauss TA. Diphtheria-tetanus-pertussis immunization and sudden infant death syndrome. American Journal of Public Health 1987;77:945-951.

11

Need for Research and Surveillance

The lack of adequate data regarding many of the adverse events under study was of major concern to the committee. Presentations at public meetings indicated that many parents and physicians share this concern. Although the committee was not charged with proposing specific research investigations, in the course of its reviews additional obvious needs for research and surveillance were identified, and those are briefly described here.

DIPHTHERIA AND TETANUS TOXOIDS

Recent advances in molecular analysis of diphtheria and tetanus toxins make it possible to construct mutant toxins that would be potentially safer, more immunogenic, and more readily purified for use as vaccines. A nontoxic variant of diphtheria toxin (CRM_{197}) is already used as a protein carrier molecule in one of the licensed *Haemophilus influenzae* type b polysaccharide-protein conjugate vaccines (see Chapter 9). If mutant toxin vaccines are more immunogenic than the presently used chemically inactivated toxins, successful immunization might be achieved with fewer doses and fewer adverse events.

The possibility of lot-specific reactions to diphtheria and tetanus toxoids, as has been demonstrated for diphtheria and tetanus toxoids and pertussis vaccine preparations, suggests that studies could be more revealing if the vaccines were tracked by lot.

MEASLES AND MUMPS VACCINES

Understanding the molecular basis for the risk of aseptic meningitis after immunization with the Urabe mumps strain (compared to the experience with the Jeryl Lynn strain) might lead to better understanding of the pathogenetic capacity of mumps virus and to principles of viral pathogenesis that would aid in the development of safe attenuated virus vaccines in the future.

Insulin-dependent diabetes mellitus (IDDM) is a serious and relatively common disorder. The large number of reports raising the suspicion that mumps vaccine might induce the onset of IDDM suggests the need for systematic study of the question.

POLIO VACCINES

There is a need to understand the basis for reversion of oral polio vaccine to a more virulent form to prevent its occurrence.

HEPATITIS B VACCINES

Evidence is inadequate to accept or reject a causal relation between hepatitis B vaccine and Guillain-Barré syndrome, transverse myelitis, optic neuritis, multiple sclerosis, or other demyelinating syndromes. The absence of reports of such outcomes in large-scale field trials suggests that if hepatitis B vaccine causes these adverse events, it does so at a very low frequency. Nevertheless, the number of reports questioning the relation between hepatitis B vaccine to one or the other of these disorders of similar character suggests the need for systematic research.

The possibility that hepatitis B vaccine can cause an exacerbation of rheumatoid arthritis should be carefully evaluated in a population-based study.

GUILLAIN BARRÉ SYNDROME

The committee found that the evidence favors acceptance of a causal relation between tetanus toxoid and Guillain-Barré syndrome (GBS) and between oral polio vaccine and GBS. For the other vaccines, the association with GBS is inconclusive, and research is needed to clarify the association. The following information is potentially obtainable through research: (1) the background incidence of GBS in the U.S. by year of life in the pediatric age group, particularly in infants and preschool-age children; (2) the incidence of GBS after the receipt of each vaccine and combination of vaccines administered to children or adults; and (3) more precise knowledge of the mechanisms and sequence of events that result in vaccine-induced GBS.

DEATH

The committee encourages active and aggressive follow-up of the reports to passive surveillance system of death in association with immunization. This follow-up should be timely and might include elements such as medical records, laboratory tests, and autopsy results. See the section on General Surveillance and Epidemiologic Studies for elaboration.

SIMULTANEOUS ADMINISTRATION OF MORE THAN ONE VACCINE

The committee was able to identify little information pertaining to the risk of serious adverse events following administration of multiple vaccines simultaneously. This is an issue of increasing concern as more vaccines and vaccine combinations are developed for routine use. Both pre- and postmarketing research should address the issue.

RISK-MODIFYING FACTORS

The committee was able to identify little information pertaining to why some individuals react adversely to vaccines when most do not. When it is clear that a vaccine can cause a specific adverse event, research should be encouraged to elucidate the factors that put certain people at risk for that adverse reaction.

GENERAL SURVEILLANCE AND EPIDEMIOLOGIC STUDIES

Postmarketing surveillance of licensed vaccines in the United States depends upon voluntary reporting. Large numbers of alleged adverse events are reported to the Vaccine Adverse Event Reporting System (VAERS) of the Centers for Disease Control and Prevention and the U.S. Food and Drug Administration. The committee found, however, that follow-up of serious adverse events was often incomplete, and the reported event was often not confirmed because of insufficient clinical, laboratory, or pathologic data. The committee suggests that, in the least, research should be conducted on the performance of passive reporting systems like VAERS. What is the quality and completeness of the information supplied? Can the reports received be used to estimate the true risk of vaccine-induced adverse events? Perhaps most important, how well does the surveillance system detect new adverse events, events not previously reported in the medical literature or demonstrated in epidemiologic studies?

The committee encourages the consideration of a more active system. Such a system might follow a representative sample of new vaccine recipients rather than the population at large. Alternatively, a randomly selected subgroup of serious adverse events reported to VAERS might be investigated fully. This latter approach suffers the inevitable limitations of retrospective review. It may be necessary to retain some broad-based passive reporting system to serve an early-warning function for unpredicted adverse events.

The committee found that a judgment regarding causality was often limited by the absence of background data for the occurrence of the pathologic condition (the putative adverse event) in apparently normal individuals not recently exposed to the vaccine. Regional or national disease registries could be established for those rare but serious conditions suspected of sometimes being caused by one or more licensed vaccines, for example, GBS, transverse myelitis, optic neuritis, and Stevens-Johnson syndrome. Such disease registries, if reasonably complete, would provide information about the descriptive epidemiology of these conditions, including age-, sex-, and race-specific background incidence rates. This information would facilitate the performance of case-control studies and other attempts to investigate vaccines as potential causes of the disorders.

The committee believes that future clinical trials of vaccines licensed or under development should study the serious adverse events examined by the present committee and its predecessor committee. Although any single trial may be too small to detect an effect of vaccine on rare adverse events, meta-analyses of several large trials may provide useful information. Meta-analysis could also be used to improve the statistical power of case-control studies to detect rare sequelae of vaccine administration.

With the existence of the large databases that have recently been established for defined populations, cohort studies become a feasible and desirable epidemiologic method of detecting the adverse effects of vaccines. Cohort studies would also permit the follow-up of patients exposed to specific vaccine types or batches that are suspected (e.g., on the basis of case reports) of being associated with a pathologic condition. Here, too, meta-analyses of cohort studies from different settings and different databases may permit identification of effects not detectable within individual studies.

Executive Summary from *Adverse Effects of Pertussis and Rubella Vaccines*

Reprinted from Institute of Medicine, *Adverse Effects of Pertussis and Rubella Vaccines*, National Academy Press, 1991.

1

Executive Summary

Next to clean water, no single intervention has had so profound an effect on reducing mortality from childhood diseases as has the widespread introduction of vaccines. Immunization, the process in which the body's own protective mechanisms are primed to thwart the invasion or multiplication of pathogens, is effective and relatively inexpensive, simple, and easy to deliver.

The use of vaccines is not entirely without risk, however. Vaccines, including the whole-cell pertussis (whooping cough) vaccine and the rubella (German measles) vaccine, the subjects of this report, typically contain small quantities of material derived from disease-causing organisms. The pertussis vaccine contains dead bacteria and is termed a *killed* or *inactivated vaccine*; the rubella vaccine contains laboratory-weakened live viruses and is termed a *live, attenuated vaccine*.

This study responds to a request to the Institute of Medicine (IOM) to conduct a thorough review of the evidence pertaining to a set of serious adverse events and immunization with pertussis or rubella vaccine. The request to IOM originated in the 1986 National Childhood Vaccine Injury Act (Public Law 99-660), whose primary purpose was to establish a federal compensation scheme for persons potentially injured by a vaccine. Section 312 of Public Law 99-660 called for IOM review of scientific and other information on specific adverse consequences of pertussis and rubella vaccines. The 11-member interdisciplinary committee, constituted by IOM to conduct this study, recognized that its charge was to focus on questions of causation and not broader topics, such as cost-benefit or risk-benefit analyses of vaccination. These topics are therefore not addressed in the report.

After formation of the committee, additional adverse events were added both by the committee and at the request of the Advisory Commission on Childhood Vaccines. During the 20 months of the study, the committee reviewed altogether *17 adverse events for pertussis vaccine*—infantile spasms; hypsarrhythmia; aseptic meningitis; encephalopathy (including acute encephalopathy and chronic neurologic damage); deaths classified as sudden infant death syndrome (SIDS); anaphylaxis; autism; erythema multiforme or other rashes; Guillain-Barré syndrome (polyneuropathy); peripheral mononeuropathy; hemolytic anemia; juvenile diabetes; learning disabilities and hyperactivity; protracted inconsolable crying or screaming; Reye syndrome; shock and "unusual shock-like state" with hypotonicity, hyporesponsiveness, and short-lived convulsions (usually febrile); and thrombocytopenia—and *3 adverse events for rubella vaccine*—arthritis (acute and chronic); radiculoneuritis and other neuropathies; and thrombocytopenic purpura. Although the committee was not asked expressly to examine febrile seizures, afebrile seizures, or epilepsy in relation to diphtheria-pertussis-tetanus (DPT) vaccine, it did so because these conditions may also be serious and are considered by some to be components of encephalopathy. Conclusions regarding these conditions are given in Chapter 4. The committee's conclusions on acute encephalopathy, also presented in Chapter 4, refer only to conditions diagnosed as encephalopathy, encephalitis, or encephalomyelitis. (For additional information on the committee's charge and the events leading to the enactment of Public Law 99-660, see the Preface and Appendix B, Pertussis and Rubella Vaccines: A Brief Chronology.)

The following three sections of this summary briefly review the methods used by the committee to evaluate the evidence relating the 20 adverse events to pertussis or rubella vaccine, the evidence considered and the conclusions reached for each adverse event, and the research directions recommended by the committee.

METHODOLOGIC CONSIDERATIONS IN EVALUATING THE EVIDENCE

The committee undertook the task of judging whether each of a set of adverse events can occur as a result of exposure to pertussis or rubella vaccine. These judgments have both quantitative and qualitative aspects; they reflect the nature of the exposures, events, and populations at issue; the specific questions to be considered; the characteristics of the evidence examined; and the approach taken to evaluate that evidence. To facilitate the independent assessment of the committee's conclusions, the committee wishes to make the process of its evaluation as explicit as possible.

The adverse events under consideration by the committee are, in most instances, rare in the exposed population. They also are known to occur in the absence of vaccination, are clinically ill-defined, and are generally of unknown causation in the general population. The exposures—pertussis and rubella vaccinations—are very widespread in the population, so that the absence of exposure may itself require an explanation in the interpretation of comparative studies. These and other features raise a number of difficulties both in the investigation and in the evaluation of the resulting evidence.

The committee considered causal questions of three kinds in connection with adverse events that have been reported to occur after administration of pertussis or rubella vaccine. The first of these questions about exposure to pertussis or rubella vaccine is, in general, *can it cause* the specified adverse condition? For example, can rubella vaccine cause chronic arthritis? If the conclusion is affirmative, a second question becomes pertinent: *How frequently does it cause* that condition? Or, how frequently is arthritis a result of rubella vaccination? The third question, which applies to a particular instance or case of an adverse event, is *did it cause* that specific event? Or, did rubella vaccine cause this particular individual to develop arthritis? The committee has undertaken its evaluation from a neutral posture, presuming neither the existence nor the absence of association between these vaccines and the events under consideration.

The identification and acquisition of the relevant evidence were major tasks of the committee throughout the course of its work. The preponderance of this material comprised either reports of controlled, observational epidemiologic studies (case-comparison or cohort studies) or uncontrolled case reports or case series. There was no experimental evidence, whether in humans or animals, that clearly proved or disproved a causal relation. Each study or report reviewed by the committee was first assessed individually and then, as appropriate, incorporated into the collective results that underlie the committee's conclusions.

Both quantitative and qualitative approaches to integration of the evidence were utilized. Formal meta-analysis was applied when it was feasible and appropriate. All of the studies were assessed insofar as possible with respect to the roles of error, bias, confounding, and chance in producing the observed results. Several considerations bearing on the inference that an association may reflect a true causal relation were also included in the committee's evaluation of the overall body of evidence pertaining to each type of adverse event under review. These included the strength of association, temporal relation between exposure and event, consistency of results between studies, specificity of the relation between exposure and event, and biologic plausibility of such a relation.

SUMMARY AND CONCLUSIONS

Table 1-1 summarizes the categories of evidence reviewed for each adverse event and the respective contribution of each to the committee's judgments about causation. The evidence is organized under five headings: (1) human experiments; (2) animal experiments; (3) case-comparison, cohort, and other controlled studies, (4) case reports and case series; and (5) biologic plausibility. Methods for interpreting evidence in the first four categories are discussed in Chapter 3. The fifth category, biologic plausibility, includes background knowledge concerning the pathophysiology of an adverse event, attributes of a particular vaccine, or other biologic information derived from research in such areas as immunology and physiology. The evidence in these five categories, elaborated in the body of the report, forms the basis of the committee's conclusions.

Where evidence was available in a particular category, the committee judged whether that evidence was generally supportive or not supportive of causation or whether it was insufficient for a determination. For example, where there were relevant controlled studies which, overall, found relative risks greater than 1, the evidence was classified as "supportive of causation." Blanks for any given category of evidence indicate that evidence of that type was lacking. It is important to note that any one category of evidence generally was not sufficient in itself to support a conclusion of causality, since other aspects of the evidence, including the details of the results and the number and quality of contributing studies, as well as the assessment of the other categories of evidence, were also considered in the evaluation.

Table 1-2 summarizes the committee's conclusions about the 20 adverse events evaluated in this report. As shown in the table, the committee found it convenient to organize its conclusions about the adverse events into five categories. These categories reflect the strength and direction of the conclusions about the causal relations between DPT or rubella vaccine and the 20 adverse events evaluated in the report. The bases of these conclusions are discussed in Chapters 4 through 7 of the report. Conclusions on rubella vaccine apply to the RA 27/3 rubella strain currently in use. Evidence does not differentiate between DPT vaccine and the pertussis component of DPT vaccine, except in the case of protracted crying (see below). As shown in Table 1-2, the committee found:

• no evidence bearing on a causal relation between DPT vaccine and autism;
• insufficient evidence to indicate a causal relation between DPT vaccine and aseptic meningitis, chronic neurologic damage, erythema multiforme or other rash, Guillain-Barré syndrome, hemolytic anemia, juvenile diabetes, learning disabilities and attention deficit disorder, peripheral mononeurop-

TABLE 1-1 Categories of Evidence Reviewed for Each Adverse Event: Is the Evidence Supportive of Causation?[a]

Vaccine and Adverse Event (Chapter of Report)	Human Experiments			Animal Experiments			Case-Comparison, Cohort, and Other Controlled Studies			Case Reports and Case Series			Biologic Plausibility		
	Yes[b]	?[c]	No[d]	Yes	?	No	Yes	?	No	Yes	?	No	Yes	?	No
DPT															
Infantile spasms (4)									X		X				
Hypsarrhythmia (4)			X								X				
Aseptic meningitis (4)								X			X				
Acute encephalopathy[e] (4)					X		X			X				X	
Chronic neurologic damage (4)					X			X			X			X	
Sudden infant death syndrome (5)									X		X				
Anaphylaxis (6)					X			X		X			X		
Autism (6)															
Erythema multiforme or other rash (6)															
Guillain-Barré syndrome (polyneuropathy) (6)									X		X		X		
Peripheral mononeuropathy (6)											X				
Hemolytic anemia (6)											X		X		
Juvenile diabetes (6)					X			X			X				
Learning disabilities and hyperactivity (6)											X				
Protracted inconsolable crying and screaming (6)							X			X			X		
Reye syndrome (6)								X				X			

TABLE 1-1 *Continued*

Vaccine and Adverse Event (Chapter of Report)	Human Experiments			Animal Experiments			Case-Comparison, Cohort, and Other Controlled Studies			Case Reports and Case Series			Biologic Plausibility		
	Yes[b]	?[c]	No[d]	Yes	?	No	Yes	?	No	Yes	?	No	Yes	?	No
Shock and "unusual shock-like state" (6)								X		X				X	
Thrombocytopenia (6)											X				
RA 27/3 Rubella															
Arthritis (7)															
Acute	X						X			X			X		
Chronic		X								X			X		
Radiculoneuritis and other neuropathies (7)											X		X		
Thrombocytopenic purpura (7)											X		X		

[a]Blanks for any given category of evidence indicate that evidence of this kind is lacking.

[b]Yes, Evidence of this kind is supportive of causation.

[c]?, Evidence of this kind cannot be classified either as supportive or as not supportive of causation.

[d]No, Evidence of this kind is not supportive of causation.

[e]Defined in controlled studies reviewed as encephalopathy, encephalitis, or encephalomyelitis.

TABLE 1-2 Summary of Conclusions by Adverse Event for DPT[a] and RA 27/3 MMR[b] Vaccines

Conclusion	Adverse Events Reviewed	
	DPT Vaccine	RA 27/3 Rubella Vaccine
1. No evidence bearing on a causal relation[c]	Autism	
2. Evidence insufficient to indicate a causal relation[d]	Aseptic meningitis Chronic neurologic damage Erythema multiforme or other rash Guillain-Barré syndrome Hemolytic anemia Juvenile diabetes Learning disabilities and attention-deficit disorder Peripheral mononeuropathy Thrombocytopenia	Radiculoneuritis and other neuropathies Thrombocytopenic purpura
3. Evidence does not indicate a causal relation[e]	Infantile spasms Hypsarrythmia Reye syndrome Sudden infant death syndrome	
4. Evidence is consistent with a causal relation[f]	Acute encephalopathy[g] Shock and "unusual shock-like state"	Chronic arthritis
5. Evidence indicates a causal relation[h]	Anaphylaxis Protracted, inconsolable crying	Acute arthritis

[a]Evidence does not differentiate between DPT vaccine and the pertussis component of DPT vaccine except in the case of protracted, inconsolable crying where the evidence implicates the pertussis component specifically.

[b]RA 27/3 MMR, Trivalent measles-mumps-rubella vaccine containing the RA 27/3 rubella strain.

[c]No category of evidence was found bearing on a judgment about causation (all categories of evidence left blank in Table 1-1).

[d]Relevant evidence in one or more categories was identified but was judged to be insufficient to indicate whether or not a causal relation exists (no category of evidence checked as supporting causation in Table 1-1; exceptions are this designation under biologic plausibility for erythema multiforme and hemolytic anemia).

[e]The available evidence, on balance, does not indicate a causal relation (one or more categories of evidence checked as not supporting causation in Table 1-1, with evidence supporting causation being either absent or outweighed by the other evidence).

[f]The available evidence, on balance, tends to support a causal relation (one or more categories of evidence checked as supporting causation in Table 1-1, with evidence checked as insufficient or not supporting causation being absent or outweighed by the other evidence).

[g]Defined in controlled studies reviewed as encephalopathy, encephalitis, or encephalomyelitis.

[h]The available evidence, on balance, supports a causal relation, and the evidence is more persuasive than that for conclusion 4 above (the categories of evidence are coded similarly to those in conclusion 4, with evidence checked as insufficient or not supporting causation in Table 1-1 being absent or less than for 4).

athy, or thrombocytopenia, and between the currently used rubella vaccine (RA 27/3) and radiculoneuritis and other neuropathies or thrombocytopenic purpura;

• that the evidence does not indicate a causal relation between DPT vaccine and infantile spasms, hypsarrythmia, Reye syndrome, or SIDS;

• that the evidence is consistent with a causal relation between DPT vaccine and acute encephalopathy and shock and "unusual shock-like state," and between RA 27/3 rubella vaccine and chronic arthritis; and

• that the evidence indicates a causal relation between DPT vaccine and anaphylaxis, between the pertussis component of DPT vaccine and pro-tracted, inconsolable crying, and between RA 27/3 rubella vaccine and acute arthritis.[1]

RESEARCH NEEDS

In the course of its review, the committee encountered many gaps and limitations in knowledge bearing directly and indirectly on the safety of vaccines. These include inadequate understanding of the biologic mecha-nisms underlying adverse events following natural infection or immuniza-tion, insufficient or inconsistent information from case reports and case series, inadequate size or length of follow-up of many population-based epidemiologic studies, and limited capacity of existing surveillance systems of vaccine injury to provide persuasive evidence of causation. The commit-tee found few experimental studies published in relation to the number of epidemiologic studies published. Clearly, if research capacity and accom-plishment in these areas are not improved, future reviews of vaccine safety will be similarly handicapped.

With respect to pertussis and rubella vaccines, careful review is needed to identify what sorts of questions might be best answered by further inves-tigations and which kinds of studies could be carried out economically. The availability and introduction of new forms of pertussis vaccine, for ex-ample, could offer valuable opportunities for comparison of vaccine safety as well as efficacy. The committee's experience points to fresh possibilities and to the need for such a review.

---

[1] The available evidence is consistent with a causal relation, but, on balance, is more persua-sive than that in the previous bullet.

B

Strategies for Gathering Information

LITERATURE SEARCHES OF COMPUTERIZED DATABASES

Because the primary purpose of this study was to examine any available information about specific adverse events associated with particular vaccines, the committee undertook an extensive search of relevant electronic databases. The initial searches were conducted by the Institute of Medicine (IOM) librarian in the winter of 1992, with follow-up searches for newly published literature carried out in August 1992, December 1992, and March 1993. Table B-1 lists the vaccine and adverse event combinations that were under consideration by the committee and that formed the basis of the search strategies.

Several database vendors[1] (including Dialog Information Services, Info Pro Technologies, and the National Library of Medicine [NLM]) were used. A total of 31 individual databases were searched. Four of the databases were primarily biomedical; these included NLM's MEDLINE, Excerpta Medica's EMBASE, BIOSIS, and the Life Sciences Collection. Three databases were health sciences related: CINAHL (Cumulative Index to Nursing and Allied Health), Health Planning and Administration, and the Health Periodicals

---

[1]The use of the name of a particular database service or software program is for information only and does not constitute endorsement of any particular product by the Institute of Medicine or the National Academy of Sciences.

TABLE B-1 Vaccines and Adverse Events Studied

Adverse Event	T/D/Td	Measles	Mumps	OPV	IPV	Hib	Hep. B
Encephalopathy (acute and chronic)	X	X	X				
Aseptic meningitis		X	X	X			
Subacute sclerosing panencephalitis		X					
Residual (chronic) seizure disorder	X	X	X				
Guillain-Barré syndrome	X	X		X	X	X	X
Transverse myelitis	X	X		X	X	X	X
Paralytic poliomyelitis (in recipient or contact)				X			
Myelitis							X
Neuropathy	X		X				
Optic neuritis		X					
Sensorineural deafness		X	X				
Sterility via orchitis		X	X				
Death	X	X	X	X	X	X	X
Anaphylaxis	X	X	X		X	X	X
Arthritis	X						X
Erythema multiforme	X						
Insulin-dependent diabetes mellitus		X	X				
Early susceptibility to Hib disease						X	
Thrombocytopenia		X	X		X	X	

NOTE: T/DT/Td, tetanus toxoid/diphtheria and tetanus toxoids for pediatric use/tetanus and diphtheria toxoids for adult use; OPV, oral polio vaccine; IPV, inactivated polio vaccine; Hib, *Haemophilus influenzae* type b vaccine; Hep. B, hepatitis B vaccine.

Database. Two were industry oriented: Pharmaceutical News Index and International Pharmaceutical Abstracts. Two others were primarily agricultural and included international materials: Agricola and Agris International. Seven were either business or general news databases: ABI/INFORM, Trade and Industry Index, Magazine Index, Newspaper and Periodical Abstracts, National Newspaper Index, PTS Prompt, and Newssearch. Four miscellaneous databases included Dissertation Abstracts, the U.S. Government Printing Office database, the National Technical Information Service (NTIS) file, and the Library of Congress' LC-Marc database. Monographs were searched in Books in Print Online, the Online Computer Library Center (OCLC) database, and NLM's Catline file.

Current literature was found in Current Contents Online and through Conference Papers Index. Three databases covered legal and regulatory affairs: Diogenes, Legal Resources Index, and Legi-Slate. In addition, the histories of the reviewed vaccines were searched by using the History of Medicine (Histline) file on the NLM's system and the Legis-Slate database.

Each database was searched in its entirety. Years of coverage vary among databases, beginning no earlier than the mid-1960s, however. Both English- and non-English- language articles were included. When possible, the literature searches were sorted into studies of humans, studies of animals, and review articles.

Much of the retrieved literature came from MEDLINE and EMBASE. The NLM's MEDLINE databases and the Excerpta Medica EMBASE database files have approximately a 40 percent overlap in the journals indexed. MEDLINE's unique content is primarily North American journals published in English, whereas EMBASE's unique content is primarily non-U.S. and non-English-language journals.

Each database has unique indexing structures and thesauri. For example, some databases index *Guillain-Barré syndrome* as such while others use the term *polyradiculoneuritis*. Even such overarching terms as *adverse events* or *adverse effects* are defined as subject headings in some of the databases but not in others. This inconsistency in classification is very common and presents difficulties. To help ensure that relevant articles would not be missed, search strategies were intentionally broad. In addition to lists of synonyms for the particular adverse events being reviewed for each vaccine, more general terms such as *risk*, *danger*, and *contraindication* were used. A unique search strategy was thus created for each vaccine in each database. Further, the terms were searched for in the title, abstract, and descriptor fields of each database. Limiting a search to the descriptor field might have resulted in missing relevant articles if an indexer happened not to list a particular adverse event.

In addition to the initial searches of vaccine and adverse event combinations (Table B-1), the committee requested searches of the following at various points in the study: all vaccines and anaphylaxis, including anaphylactic shock and anaphylactoid reaction; measles vaccine and deafness or hearing loss; measles or mumps disease and deafness or hearing loss; transverse myelitis (including terms such as *myelitis, myelopathy, spinal cord, brachial neuritis, neuropathy, lumbar neuritis, lumbar neuropathy, radiculopathy, radiculitis,* and *neuralgic amyotrophy*) and the reviewed vaccines; sudden infant death syndrome (SIDS) and the reviewed vaccines; a follow-up on the Guillain-Barré syndrome search, including polyradiculitis and the reviewed vaccines; optic neuritis, including retrobulbar neuritis, and the reviewed vaccines; diabetes and all vaccines; and serum sickness and hepatitis B vaccine.

Every effort was undertaken to make the literature searches as thorough as possible. However, the results of any search are subject to the limitations of the particular databases being searched and the selection of search strategies. In addition, as a consequence of the broad search strategy as well as the eccentricities of individual databases, many citations that were not directly relevant to the desired topic were retrieved. Of the more than 8,000 citations retrieved in the course of the various searches, about 1,800 were found to be relevant to the committee's work. The limitations of using computerized databases for literature searches have been explored by Dickersin and others (Dickersin et al., 1985). Later sections of this appendix describe other steps taken by the committee to ensure a thorough review of the literature. The bibliography to this report lists the relevant material reviewed.

After the literature searches were conducted, the retrieved citations were converted (using a software package called Biblio-Links) into a format readable by Pro-Cite (version 1.41), a bibliographic management program. Subject-specific working bibliographies were produced; staff and committee members reviewed the citations (including abstracts when available) and determined whether a particular article might contain information pertinent to the committee's task. Articles were then obtained for each selected citation, and copies were distributed to the appropriate committee members. Many of the articles were obtained through NLM's interlibrary loan system, DOCLINE.

All or part of publications written in languages other than English were translated by professional translation services or read by committee members fluent in those languages. In all, about 150 items were translated from 18 languages.

A bibiliography of references cited in the report and organized both by vaccine and by adverse event entitled "Bibliography of Adverse Consequences Associated with Childhood Vaccines" is available from the National Technical Information Service, 5285 Port Royal Road, Springfield, Virginia 22161 (703-487-4650).

OTHER SOURCES OF INFORMATION

Additional information sources used by the committee included the reference lists of the articles obtained by the committee and staff; this was particularly true with respect to vaccines in existence before about 1966, the date after which computerized reference listings are generally available. Particular attention was paid to citations in review articles and in books and reports with extensive reference lists (e.g., Institute of Medicine, 1977, 1985a,b, 1991; National Library of Medicine, 1988; Office of Technology Assessment, 1980; Plotkin and Mortimer, 1988). The American Academy of Pediatrics *Red Book* (1991) and the Physicians' Desk Reference (1992) were consulted for their information on adverse events and contraindications. In addition, committee members' own libraries of articles and books often provided relevant information.

Committee staff regularly attended meetings of the federal Advisory Commission on Childhood Vaccines and the Centers for Disease Control and Prevention's (CDC's) Advisory Committee on Immunization Practices. In addition, in September 1992 staff members attended a session sponsored by the U.S. Food and Drug Administration (FDA), Workshop to Review Warnings, Use Instructions, and Precautionary Information for Childhood Vaccines. Relevant information, including reference material, from those meetings was provided to committee members.

REVIEW OF INTERIM BIBLIOGRAPHY

Midway through the project (December 1992), an interim bibliography of the more than 1,600 citations being reviewed by the committee was sent to 22 individuals representing a range of views on the topic of adverse events following vaccination. These individuals were asked to identify pertinent sources of information missing from the bibliography to ensure that no important information was overlooked by the committee. A few additional items were suggested by these reviewers, but no significant gaps were identified.

INFORMATION FROM ADVERSE EVENT
SURVEILLANCE SYSTEMS

The committee reviewed case reports from the Vaccine Adverse Event Reporting System (VAERS), the passive surveillance system administered by CDC and FDA. VAERS was established by the National Childhood Vaccine Injury Act (P.L. 99-660) to collect reports of adverse reactions following vaccination; it began operation in November 1990. VAERS combined and replaced the two previous federal surveillance systems, the public-sector Monitoring System for Adverse Events Following Immunization (MSAEFI) and the private-sector Spontaneous Reporting System (SRS). The database is managed by a contractor under the aegises of both CDC and FDA. Health care providers are obligated to report specific adverse events following particular vaccines, as set out in a Vaccine Injury Table also established under the Vaccine Injury Act. Parents, other relatives, or anyone aware of the occurrence of an adverse event may also file a report with VAERS. (A blank VAERS form appears in Figure B-1.)

By July 31, 1992, VAERS had received more than 17,000 reports, of which almost 11,000 concerned vaccines listed in the Vaccine Injury Table (oral and inactivated polio vaccines and the trivalent or monovalent constituents of diphtheria and tetanus toxoids and pertussis vaccine [DPT] and measles, mumps, and rubella vaccine [MMR]). Of the total number of reports, just over 2,500 were considered to be serious, that is, the patient died, suffered a life-threatening illness, suffered a reaction that resulted in or prolonged hospitalization, or resulted in permanent disability.

The committee requested all available VAERS case reports (submitted up to July 31, 1992) for every vaccine-adverse event combination in its charge (see Table B-1). The committee received approximately 575 reports. The individual reports were reviewed by the committee member(s) who had responsibility for the particular vaccine or adverse event described in the report. The staff also purchased computer disks containing data submitted to VAERS for use with the Paradox (version 3.0) database software.

Because of the improvements in VAERS over MSAEFI and SRS, the committee focused its efforts on case reports from VAERS. However, the committee considered summary information from the two earlier surveillance systems. The committee reviewed three publications presenting data from MSAEFI (Centers for Disease Control, 1984, 1986, 1989). It also reviewed summary information on reports to MSAEFI for 1989-1990. In addition, it reviewed information from SRS on deaths reported between July 1, 1989, and June 30, 1990.

Care must be taken in interpreting information from passive surveillance systems. The extent of underreporting cannot be known. Duplicate reports of the same event for the same patient are common and are not always easy to detect, making totals questionable. Medical information provided on reporting forms is often incomplete. In general, passive surveillance systems are useful in flagging potential problems and suggesting hypotheses. See Chapters 2, 10, and 11 for further discussion.

VAERS

VACCINE ADVERSE EVENT REPORTING SYSTEM
24 Hour Toll-free information line 1-800-822-7967
P.O. Box 1100, Rockville, MD 20849-1100
PATIENT IDENTITY KEPT CONFIDENTIAL

For CDC/FDA Use Only

VAERS Number _____

Date Received _____

Patient Name:

Last   First   M.I.

Address

City   State   Zip

Telephone no. (_____)

Vaccine administered by (Name):

Responsible
Physician _____
Facility Name/Address

City   State   Zip

Telephone no. (_____)

Form completed by (Name):

Relation   ☐ Vaccine Provider   ☐ Patient/Parent
to Patient ☐ Manufacturer   ☐ Other
Address (if different from patient or provider)

City   State   Zip

Telephone no. (_____)

1. State	2. County where administered	3. Date of birth mm / dd / yy	4. Patient age	5. Sex ☐ M ☐ F	6. Date form completed mm / dd / yy

7. Describe adverse event(s) (symptoms, signs, time course) and treatment, if any

8. Check all appropriate:
☐ Patient died   (date ___ / ___ / ___)
☐ Life threatening illness mm   dd   yy
☐ Required emergency room/doctor visit
☐ Required hospitalization (_____days)
☐ Resulted in prolongation of hospitalization
☐ Resulted in permanent disability
☐ None of the above

9. Patient recovered ☐ YES ☐ NO ☐ UNKNOWN

10. Date of vaccination ___ / ___ / ___ mm dd yy Time _____ AM PM

11. Adverse event onset ___ / ___ / ___ mm dd yy Time _____ AM PM

12. Relevant diagnostic tests/laboratory data

13. Enter all vaccines given on date listed in no. 10

	Vaccine (type)	Manufacturer	Lot number	Route/Site	No. Previous doses
a.					
b.					
c.					
d.					

14. Any other vaccinations within 4 weeks of date listed in no. 10

	Vaccine (type)	Manufacturer	Lot number	Route/Site	No. Previous doses	Date given
a.						
b.						

15. Vaccinated at:
☐ Private doctor's office/hospital   ☐ Military clinic/hospital
☐ Public health clinic/hospital   ☐ Other/unknown

16. Vaccine purchased with:
☐ Private funds   ☐ Military funds
☐ Public funds   ☐ Other /unknown

17. Other medications

18. Illness at time of vaccination (specify)

19. Pre-existing physician-diagnosed allergies, birth defects, medical conditions (specify)

20. Have you reported this adverse event previously?
☐ No   ☐ To health department
☐ To doctor ☐ To manufacturer

21. Adverse event following prior vaccination (check all applicable, specify)

	Adverse Event	Onset Age	Type Vaccine	Dose no. in series
☐ In patient				
☐ In brother or sister				

Only for children 5 and under

22. Birth weight _____ lb. _____ oz.

23. No. of brothers and sisters

Only for reports submitted by manufacturer/immunization project

24. Mfr. / imm. proj. report no.

25. Date received by mfr. / imm. proj.

26. 15 day report? ☐ Yes ☐ No

27. Report type ☐ Initial ☐ Follow-Up

Health care providers and manufacturers are required by law (42 USC 300aa-25) to report reactions to vaccines listed in the Vaccine Injury Table.
Reports for reactions to other vaccines are voluntary except when required as a condition of immunization grant awards.

Form VAERS -1

FIGURE B-1 Form used to report adverse events to the Vaccine Adverse Event Reporting System.

"Fold in thirds, tape & mail - DO NOT STAPLE FORM"

NO POSTAGE
NECESSARY
IF MAILED
IN THE
UNITED STATES
OR APO/FPO

BUSINESS REPLY MAIL
FIRST CLASS MAIL   PERMIT NO. 1895   ROCKVILLE, MD

POSTAGE WILL BE PAID BY ADDRESSEE

 VAERS
c/o Ogden BioServices Corporation
P.O. Box 1100
Rockville MD 20849-1100

IııIıIIIııIıIıIıIIIıIıııIIııIIIIııIIıııIıIıI

DIRECTIONS FOR COMPLETING FORM
(Additional pages may be attached if more space is needed.)

GENERAL

- Use a separate form for each patient. Complete the form to the best of your abilities. Items 3, 4, 7, 8, 10, 11, and 13 are considered essential and should be completed whenever possible. Parents/Guardians may need to consult the facility where the vaccine was administered for some of the information (such as manufacturer, lot number or laboratory data.)
- Refer to the Vaccine Injury Table (VIT) for events mandated for reporting by law. Reporting for other serious events felt to be related but not on the VIT is encouraged.
- Health care providers other than the vaccine administrator (VA) treating a patient for a suspected adverse event should notify the VA and provide the information about the adverse event to allow the VA to complete the form to meet the VA's legal responsibility.
- These data will be used to increase understanding of adverse events following vaccination and will become part of CDC Privacy Act System 09-20-0136, "Epidemiologic Studies and Surveillance of Disease Problems". Information identifying the person who received the vaccine or that person's legal representative will not be made available to the public, but may be available to the vaccinee or legal representative.
- Postage will be paid by addressee. Forms may be photocopied (must be front & back on same sheet).

SPECIFIC INSTRUCTIONS

Form Completed By: To be used by parents/guardians, vaccine manufacturers/distributors, vaccine administrators, and/or the person completing the form on behalf of the patient or the health professional who administered the vaccine.

Item 7: Describe the suspected adverse event. Such things as temperature, local and general signs and symptoms, time course, duration of symptoms diagnosis, treatment and recovery should be noted.

Item 9: Check "YES" if the patient's health condition is the same as it was prior to the vaccine, "NO" if the patient has not returned to the pre-vaccination state of health, or "UNKNOWN" if the patient's condition is not known.

Item 10: Give dates and times as specifically as you can remember. If you do not know the exact time, please
and 11: indicate "AM" or "PM" when possible if this information is known. If more than one adverse event, give the onset date and time for the most serious event.

Item 12: Include "negative" or "normal" results of any relevant tests performed as well as abnormal findings.

Item 13: List ONLY those vaccines given on the day listed in Item 10.

Item 14: List ANY OTHER vaccines the patient received within four weeks of the date listed in Item 10.

Item 16: This section refers to how the person who gave the vaccine purchased it, not to the patient's insurance.

Item 17: List any prescription or non-prescription medications the patient was taking when the vaccine(s) was given.

Item 18: List any short term illnesses the patient had on the date the vaccine(s) was given (i.e., cold, flu, ear infection).

Item 19: List any pre-existing physician-diagnosed allergies, birth defects, medical conditions (including developmental and/or neurologic disorders) the patient has.

Item 21: List any suspected adverse events the patient, or the patient's brothers or sisters, may have had to previous vaccinations. If more than one brother or sister, or if the patient has reacted to more than one prior vaccine, use additional pages to explain completely. For the onset age of a patient, provide the age in months if less than two years old.

Item 26: This space is for manufacturers' use only.

FIGURE B-1 (*continued*)

PRESENTATIONS

Committee Meetings

At various times in the course of the study, the committee heard presentations from Regina Rabinovich, the study's project officer from the National Institute of Allergy and Infectious Diseases; Geoffrey Evans, Chief Medical Officer of the Division of Vaccine Injury Compensation; John Mullen (CDC), Suresh Rastogi (FDA), and Stephen Gordon (Ogden Bioservices Corp.), representatives of VAERS; and Dirk Teuwen, SmithKline Beecham.

At its November 1992 meeting, the committee heard a presentation from Joanne Hatem, Medical Director of the National Vaccine Information Center. (Because of a scheduling conflict, Dr. Hatem was unable to present this information at the scientific workshop held on the following day.) Dr. Hatem spoke about her concerns in three areas: circumstances under which a vaccine should not be administered (i.e., contraindications), circumstances for delaying the administration of a vaccine, and potential high-risk groups for adverse events following vaccination. She asked the committee to be conscientious about reviewing adverse events that were not a part of its original charge, if the evidence should warrant such a review.

Scientific Workshops

The committee held a scientific workshop on September 11, 1992, in Woods Hole, Massachusetts. Notice of the meeting was sent to more than 1,000 people. Six invited speakers made presentations on the possible mechanisms of neurologic adverse events after vaccination. Approximately 90 people attended the session.

Another scientific workshop took place in Washington, D.C., on November 6, 1992. Six invited speakers made presentations on the contraindications to vaccination and on the possible role of viral vaccines in the etiology of insulin-dependent diabetes mellitus. Approximately 75 people attended the session.

The box entitled Presentations at Scientific Workshops Held by the Vaccine Safety Committee provides lists of the individuals who made presentations at the scientific workshops. (Transcripts of the workshops may be purchased from the National Technical Information Service, 5285 Port Royal Road, Springfield, Virginia 22161; 703-487-4650.)

Public Meetings

The committee held a public meeting on May 11, 1992, in Washington, D.C. Again, notices were mailed to an extensive list of interested individu-

PRESENTATIONS AT SCIENTIFIC WORKSHOPS HELD BY THE VACCINE SAFETY COMMITTEE

September 11, 1992

Robert Fujinami, University of Utah, Salt Lake City. Molecular Mimicry.

Diane Griffin, The Johns Hopkins University School of Medicine, Baltimore. Measles and Rabies Encephalitis.

Dale McFarlin, National Institute of Neurologic Diseases and Stroke, National Institutes of Health. Neural Antigens.

Neal Nathanson, University of Pennsylvania School of Medicine, Philadelphia. The Cutter and Swine Flu Incidents.

Vincent Racaniello, Columbia University, New York, New York. Polio Neurovirulence.

Klaus Toyka, Neurologische Universitätsklinik und Poliklinik im Kopfklinikum, Wurzburg, Germany. Guillain-Barré Syndrome.

November 6, 1992

James Froeschle, Connaught Laboratories, Swiftwater, Pennsylvania. Contra-indications to Vaccination.

Samuel Katz, Advisory Committee on Immunization Practices. Contraindications to Vaccination.

Noel Maclaren, University of Florida, Gainesville. Possible Mechanisms of the Etiology of Insulin-Dependent Diabetes Mellitus.

David Nalin, Merck Sharp & Dohme, West Point, Pennsylvania. Contraindications to Vaccination.

Georges Peter, American Academy of Pediatrics. Contraindications to Vaccination.

Amy Scott, U.S. Food and Drug Administration. Contraindications to Vaccination.

---

als and organizations. Eleven individuals made presentations (in person or by telephone) at the meeting, which was attended by approximately 175 people.

A second public meeting was held on January 16, 1993, in Irvine, California. Thirteen individuals made presentations (in person or by telephone) at the meeting, which was attended by approximately 65 people.

The following is a brief summary of the comments of individuals who made presentations at the public meetings. Committee members were present at the sessions and were provided with full transcripts of the meetings afterward. (Transcripts may be purchased from the National Technical Information Service, 5285 Port Royal Road, Springfield, Virginia, 22161; 703-487-4650.)

Presentations, May 11, 1992, Washington, D.C.

Shannon Dixon, Honolulu, Hawaii Mr. Dixon explained that he developed poliomyelitis in 1962 following receipt of oral poliovirus vaccine. He made a complete recovery and lived an active life until the early 1980s, when he began to develop symptoms that have been diagnosed as post-polio syndrome. He is now severely physically disabled and requires attendant care. Mr. Dixon urged the committee to recognize that recovery from polio is not always the end of medical problems for patients with polio. He noted that the National Vaccine Injury Compensation Program must take into account the possibility of post-polio syndrome when developing compensation plans for those who contract polio from the oral vaccine.

Jesse Ferguson, Milwaukee, Wisconsin Mr. Ferguson described health problems that began shortly after receipt of tetanus toxoid following a work-related injury. These health problems culminated in the loss of use of his right arm and a diagnosis of brachial neuritis. More than a year later, he was still unable to return to construction work and had been told that his medical condition would not improve. Mr. Ferguson urged the committee to ensure that the public is made more aware of the possible side effects of vaccines and to consider new guidelines for the implementation of vaccination programs.

Barbara Loe Fisher, Dissatisfied Parents Together, Vienna, Virginia Mrs. Fisher expressed concern about the concurrent administration of multiple vaccines to children—particularly the possibility that multiple vaccination might result in a greater risk of adverse reactions and/or interference with proper immune response. She maintained that large-scale definitive scientific studies of the effects of simultaneous administration of vaccines have not been carried out and that, in the absence of such studies, it is not possible to make decisions about safety.

James Froeschle, Connaught Laboratories, Swiftwater, Pennsylvania Dr. Froeschle gave information about adverse events following diphtheria and tetanus toxoids (DT) that had been reported to Connaught. From a comparison of spontaneous reports with postmarketing surveillance data, the company estimates about a 50-fold underreporting of adverse events in the passive reporting system. The distribution of types of events, however, was found to be approximately the same; in both cases, the majority of reported events were local reactions or fever. The company has seen a marked decrease in adverse event reports since the inception of VAERS late in 1991, because physicians are now requested to send reports directly to the VAERS contractor.

Joanne Hatem, National Vaccine Information Center, Vienna, Virginia Dr. Hatem stressed the importance of reviewing case reports submitted to FDA, CDC, and VAERS. She reported that her review of measles and mumps vaccines shows inaccurate medical evaluation and a trend toward minimizing reported injuries on the part of manufacturers and FDA. Dr. Hatem also addressed the issue of concurrent administration of multiple vaccines, stating that adequate research has not been carried out to establish its safety.

Walter Kyle, attorney, Franconia, New Hampshire Mr. Kyle maintained that, because of incomplete inactivation, the inactivated polio vaccine (IPV) manufactured in the 1950s caused polio disease in addition to those cases reported as part of the well-known Cutter incident. He suggested that polio following IPV should be an adverse event listed in the Vaccine Injury Table of the National Vaccine Injury Compensation Program. He also asked the committee to look into the possibility of seizures following administration of the oral polio vaccine (OPV) or the simultaneous administration of DPT and OPV.

Susan Maloney, Rowley, Massachusetts Mrs. Maloney told the committee about the death of her 15-week-old son 4 days after receiving his second dose of OPV. The death was initially classified as sudden infant death syndrome. She described the 7-year process that took place before the family received the results of pathology tests. Ultimately, it was revealed that vaccine-strain poliovirus had been isolated from the child's tissue, including the heart. Mrs. Maloney urged the committee to recognize death as a potential adverse outcome after administration of OPV. She also called for improved autopsy protocols following infant deaths.

Ann Millan, National Vaccine Information Center, Vienna, Virginia Mrs. Millan expressed concern that doctors do not always report adverse events after vaccination, as required by law. She criticized the federal government for not following up the case reports presented to the National Vaccine Advisory Committee by her organization. She was also concerned about the simultaneous administration of multiple vaccines. She stated that, with regard to the safety of vaccines, the burden should be to prove or disprove a relationship rather than to assume safety in the absence of data. Mrs. Millan expressed particular concern about the possibility of delayed death or injury caused by live virus vaccines.

John Mullen, Division of Immunization, Centers for Disease Control, Atlanta, Georgia Mr. Mullen, project officer for VAERS, briefly traced the history of adverse event reporting in the U.S. Public Health Service.

Separate surveillance systems for vaccines administered in the private sector and the public sector existed until 1990, when the congressionally mandated VAERS system began operation. Mr. Mullen outlined the limitations of passive surveillance systems. He expressed the belief that VAERS can serve as a useful complement to other mechanisms of postmarketing surveillance for vaccines.

Mary Pearce, Philadelphia, Pennsylvania   Mrs. Pearce spoke about her daughter, who became ill following receipt of the measles-mumps-rubella vaccine (MMR) at age 15 months. The child was diagnosed with febrile seizures and, ultimately, with diabetes. Mrs. Pearce urged the committee to consider the possibility of a link between MMR and diabetes.

Susan Weinberg, Baltimore, Maryland   Mrs. Weinberg detailed the symptoms of her daughter, who was diagnosed with diabetes mellitus several weeks after receiving her first dose of MMR at age 15 months. At age 11 years, the child now leads an outwardly normal life and requires insulin twice a day. Citing research indicating that viral illness may be linked to the onset of diabetes, Mrs. Weinberg expressed concern that MMR can cause diabetes in children with a genetic predisposition for the disorder. She suggested that, when it becomes possible technologically, all infants should be tested for such genetic tendencies before receiving the vaccine.

Presentations, January 16, 1993, Irvine, California

John Brydon, attorney, Long Beach, California   Mr. Brydon expressed concern about whether the inactivated polio vaccine produced in the 1950s adequately inactivated the poliovirus. He believes that the vaccine was capable of producing polio in a small number of children who received the vaccine. Mr. Brydon also spoke about transverse myelitis following receipt of MMR, calling for studies of the possible relationship.

Christine Buhk, Sturgeon Bay, Wisconsin   Mrs. Buhk related the case of her 18-month-old daughter, who became ill 3 days after receiving MMR and *Haemophilus influenzae* type b (Hib) vaccine. The child became progressively ill with a rash, fever, diarrhea, and vomiting and died approximately 2 weeks later. Eight months later, Mrs. Buhk had not yet received an autopsy report.

Kim Chapman, Colorado Springs, Colorado   Mrs. Chapman described the case of her 18-month-old daughter, who developed a high fever 4 days after receiving DPT, Hib vaccine, and OPV and who eventually was hospitalized with dehydration, disseminated intravascular coagulation, encephalitis, and renal failure. The child has severe residual brain damage. Mrs. Chapman questioned the rigid use of the 72-hour guideline for vaccine reactions listed in the Vaccine Injury Table of the National Vaccine Injury Compensation Program. She expressed further concern about the incomplete understanding of contraindications to vaccination among physicians and parents. She also questioned the wisdom of concurrent administration of multiple vaccines without adequate research into their safety when administered in combination.

Mark Geier, medical/legal consultant, Silver Spring, Maryland   Dr. Geier expressed concerns about the National Vaccine Injury Compensation Program: that it is more adversarial than intended by Congress, that plaintiff's expert testimony is too often dismissed as biased, and that decisions made under the program are inconsistent. He criticized the 1991 IOM report (Institute of Medicine, 1991) on pertussis and rubella vaccines for contributing to the problems of the compensation program by not making clear the level of certainty required to make decisions about causal relations between vaccines and adverse events.

Cynthia Goldenberg, Laguna Niguel, California   Mrs. Goldenberg spoke about her son, who was diagnosed as autistic as an infant. She subsequently discovered that he had a very high rubella antibody level and very low immunoglobulin G (IgG) levels. She stated that intravenous IgG treatments have been followed by marked improvement and that, at age 4, her son attends a regular school and no longer meets the criteria for autism. She urged parents of children with autism or similar diagnoses to seek advice from an immunologist.

Marjorie Grant, Determined Parents to Stop Hurting Our Tots, Beaver Dam, Wisconsin   Mrs. Grant expressed strong concern about the safety of administering combination vaccines to infants. She cited the case of her son, who received a combined DPT-polio vaccine (Quadrigen) at the age of 6 months and subsequently suffered seizures, paralysis, and severe mental retardation. She urged the committee to consider the evidence with regard to the safety of combined vaccines in carrying out its work.

Michael Hugo, attorney, Boston, Massachusetts   Mr. Hugo questioned the arbitrary time criteria used by the compensation program for determining the relationship between a vaccine and an adverse event, noting that events that fall outside the guidelines by only a few hours are not compensated, are returned to the jurisdiction of the civil courts, and thus result in more lawsuits. He called for the biologic variability of individuals to be taken into account so that the Vaccine Injury Table guidelines would not be considered as rigid rules.

Marcel Kinsbourne, Winchester, Massachusetts   Dr. Kinsbourne, a neurologist, questioned some of the new criteria being proposed by the federal government for the vaccine compensation program. He further questioned the conclusions of the 1991 IOM report on pertussis and rubella vaccines (Institute of Medicine, 1991), particularly in regard to a differentiation between acute and chronic encephalopathy. He concurred with Dr. Geier (see above) that the confidence level for making decisions about vaccine injury should be more lenient than is usual for strictly scientific decisions.

Andrea Martin, Woodland, California   Mrs. Martin spoke about her daughter, who became ill following receipt of DPT and OPV at ages 2 and 4 months and who was ultimately diagnosed with transverse myelitis. Mrs. Martin was told by her doctors that the child should not be immunized further.

Sandy Mintz, Parents Concerned About the Safety of Vaccines, Anchorage, Alaska   Mrs. Mintz took exception to elements of the 1991 IOM report (Institute of Medicine, 1991) and expressed a wish that the current committee would avoid the same problems, such as acceptance of studies with flawed designs, improper definitions of control groups, and risk estimates based on the number of doses of vaccine rather than on the number of children vaccinated. She expressed concern about measles vaccine and the possibility that widespread vaccination has increased the case fatality rate for those cases of measles that do occur. She made suggestions for the direction and design of future vaccine safety and efficacy research, including taking into account, in risk-benefit analyses, the changing disease epidemiology that results when vaccines are in widespread use, and the need for properly designed long-term (20-30 years) studies of adverse effects.

Robert Moxley, attorney, Cheyenne, Wyoming   Mr. Moxley addressed the issue of the effect of vaccination on children with tuberous sclerosis. He criticized the 1991 IOM report (Institute of Medicine, 1991) for not dealing adequately with the issue. He maintained that both DPT and MMR can trigger seizures or worsen an existing seizure disorder in children with tuberous sclerosis and urged the committee to address the issue specifically and to call for more research on the subject if necessary.

Eugene Robin, Stanford University School of Medicine, Stanford, California   Dr. Robin expressed concern about the balance between the risks and benefits of vaccination and urged that the public be dealt with honestly with respect to such risks and benefits. He noted that, often, randomized controlled clinical trials are not available as evidence about the potential risk of a particular vaccine and that the quality of the available evidence must be considered as part of any discussion of the risks or benefits of vaccination.

Arthur Zahalsky, Southern Illinois University, Edwardsville Dr. Zahalsky addressed the need for new and improved vaccines against diphtheria and tetanus. He cited the low purity and undesired side effects of the vaccines and maintained that the bovine components of the vaccines are responsible for adverse events, particularly in the adult population. He made suggestions for the further purification of diphtheria and tetanus toxins in the manufacture of vaccines.

ADDITIONAL INDIVIDUALS AND ORGANIZATIONS WHO PROVIDED INFORMATION

In addition to the formal presentations, information on adverse events following vaccination was received from the following sources:

Bell of Atri, Inc., College Park, Maryland. Material from J. Anthony Morris and Hillary Butler on adverse events after hepatitis B vaccination.

Colette Cogliandro, Chesapeake, Virginia. Case report regarding MMR vaccination.

Philippe Duclos, Health and Welfare Canada. Information on adverse events following hepatitis B vaccine.

Reinhard Fescharek, Behringwerke AG, Marburg, Germany. Published literature on diabetes and measles/mumps vaccine.

Bonnie Plumeri Franz, Ogdensburg, New York. Letter regarding concerns about the adequacy and accuracy of research relating to adverse events following receipt of vaccines.

Susan Garzonio, Brodhead, Wisconsin. Case report regarding diphtheria-tetanus toxoids.

Cynthia Goldenberg, Laguna Niguel, California. Information on autism and vaccination.

Terry and Kurt Johnson, Mission Viejo, California. Book by Neil Z. Miller, *Vaccines: Are They Really Safe and Effective?*, New Atlantean Press, Santa Fe, New Mexico, 1992.

Gloria Koslofsky, Norwood, New York. Case report regarding DPT and DT.

Kathleen Lane, Spring City, Pennsylvania. Case report regarding inactivated poliovirus vaccine.

Ruth Macrides, Naples, Florida. Case report regarding hepatitis B vaccine.

Robert Moxley, Gage and Moxley, Cheyenne, Wyoming. Information on tuberous sclerosis and vaccination.

National Vaccine Information Center, Vienna, Virginia. Case reports, newsletters, and informational material.

John Pollard, University of Sydney, Sydney, Australia. Case report on Guillain-Barré syndrome following receipt of tetanus toxoid.

Dirk Teuwen, SmithKline Beecham, Rixensart, Belgium. Information on a manufacturers' experience with adverse events following vaccination.

Burton Waisbren, Waisbren Clinic, Milwaukee, Wisconsin. Case reports and published material relating to demyelinating disorders following receipt of hepatitis B vaccine.

Curtis Webb, Webb, Pedersen & Webb, Twin Falls, Idaho. Letter regarding methodology of 1991 IOM report and suggestions for current report.

REFERENCES

American Academy of Pediatrics, Committee on Infectious Diseases. Report of the Committee on Infectious Diseases: 22nd Edition. Elk Grove, IL: American Academy of Pediatrics; 1991.

Centers for Disease Control. Adverse Events Following Immunization: Surveillance Report No. 1, 1979-1982. Atlanta: U.S. Public Health Service, U.S. Department of Health and Human Services; August 1984.

Centers for Disease Control. Adverse Events Following Immunization: Surveillance Report No. 2, 1982-1984. Atlanta: U.S. Public Health Service, U.S. Department of Health and Human Services; December 1986.

Centers for Disease Control. Adverse Events Following Immunization: Surveillance Report No. 3, 1985-1986. Atlanta: U.S. Public Health Service, U.S. Department of Health and Human Services; February 1989.

Dickersin K, Hewitt P, Mutch L, Chalmers I, Chalmers TC. Perusing the literature: comparison of MEDLINE searching with a Perinatal Trials Database. Controlled Clinical Trials 1985;6:306-317.

Institute of Medicine. Evaluation of Poliomyelitis Vaccines. Washington, DC: National Academy of Sciences; 1977.

Institute of Medicine. New Vaccine Development: Establishing Priorities. Volume I. Diseases of Importance in the United States. Washington, DC: National Academy Press; 1985a.

Institute of Medicine. Vaccine Supply and Innovation. Washington, DC: National Academy Press; 1985b.

Institute of Medicine. Adverse Effects of Pertussis and Rubella Vaccines. Washington, DC: National Academy Press; 1991.

National Library of Medicine. Vaccine-Preventable Diseases of Childhood: Current Bibliographies in Medicine, No. 88-12. Washington, DC: U.S. Department of Health and Human Services; 1988.

Office of Technology Assessment. Compensation for Vaccine-Related Injuries: A Technical Memorandum. Washington, DC: U.S. Government Printing Office; 1980.

Physicians' Desk Reference, 46th edition. Montvale, NJ: Medical Economics Company Inc.; 1992.

Plotkin SA, Mortimer EA, eds. Vaccines. Philadelphia: W.B. Saunders; 1988.

Glossary

Acute disseminated encephalomyelitis. A clinical syndrome characterized by acute depression of consciousness and multifocal neurologic findings that usually occur a few days or weeks following vaccine administration or virus-like disease. It is characterized pathologically by diffuse foci of perivenular inflammation and demyelination. See Chapter 3.

ADEM. See *Acute disseminated encephalomyelitis*.

Anaphylaxis. Generalized anaphylaxis is an acute, often explosive, systemic reaction characterized by pruritus, generalized flush, hives, respiratory distress, and vascular collapse and, occasionally, by seizures, vomiting, abdominal cramps, and incontinence. It occurs in a previously sensitized person who again receives the sensitizing antigen. See Chapter 4.

Arthralgia. Pain in a joint or joints.

Arthritis. Inflammation of a joint or joints detectable as swelling, redness, and tenderness.

Arthropathy. Any joint disease.

Arthus reaction. A reaction that follows injection of an antigen into an animal in which hypersensitivity has been previously established and that involves infiltrations, edema, sterile abscesses, and in severe cases, gangrene. See Chapter 4.

Aseptic meningitis. An inflammation of the meninges with typical changes in the cerebrospinal fluid, including increased numbers of leukocytes, normal glucose, and absence of bacteria on examination and culture.

The most common causes include viral infection and noninfectious causes such as lead poisoning.

Attenuated. Having decreased virulence; used especially for live virus vaccines. Attenuation is achieved either through selection of less virulent mutants or through physiologic alteration by exposure to unfavorable conditions.

Attributable risk (exposed). The rate of a disease or other outcome in exposed individuals that can be attributed to the exposure. Synonymous with risk difference and excess risk. This measure is estimated by subtracting the rate of the outcome (usually incidence or mortality) among unexposed individuals from the rate among exposed individuals. It is assumed that causes other than the one under investigation have had equal effects on exposed and unexposed groups and that the effects of different causes are additive. This term is often used, incorrectly, to denote the attributable fraction among exposed individuals in the population.

Bayes theorem. A theorem in probability theory. In epidemiology, it is used to obtain the probability of disease in a group of people with some characteristic on the basis of the overall rate of that disease (the prior probability of disease) and of the likelihoods of that characteristic in healthy and diseased individuals. The most familiar application is in clinical decision analysis where it is used for estimating the probability of a particular diagnosis given the appearance of some symptom or test result.

Bias. Deviation of results or inferences from the truth, or processes leading to such deviation. Any trend in the collection, analysis, interpretation, publication, or review of data that can lead to conclusions that are systematically different from the truth. Not to be confused with *prejudice* or *partisan point of view*, as is the conventional usage.

Brachial neuritis. Also known as brachial plexus neuropathy or as neuralgic amyotrophy. A neuropathy which presents as a deep, steady, often severe aching pain in the shoulder and upper arm. See Chapter 3.

Case-control study (*Syn: case-comparison study*). A controlled observational study that starts with the identification of persons with the disease or condition (adverse event) of interest and a suitable control (comparison) group of persons without the disease. The relation of an attribute (e.g., immunization) to the disease is examined by comparing the diseased and nondiseased groups with regard to how frequently the attribute is present, or if quantitative, the levels of the attribute, in each of the groups.

Cohort study. (*Syn: prospective, follow-up study*). A controlled observational study in which subsets of a defined population can be identified who are, have been, or in the future may be exposed or not exposed, or exposed in different degrees, to a factor or factors hypothesized to influence the probability of occurrence of a given disease (adverse event) or other outcome. The essential feature of the cohort design is observation of the population for a sufficient length of time to generate reliable incidence or mortality rates.

Confidence interval. A range of values estimated for a given variable. The range has a specified probability, e.g., 95 percent, of including the true value of the variable. The specified probability is called the confidence level.

Controlled study. Controlled studies are studies that use a comparison group that differs from the subjects of the study in either disease experience (outcome) or allocation to a regimen (exposure). Allocation to a regimen can be random, as in a randomized clinical trial, or nonrandom, as in an observational cohort study or a case-control study.

EAE. See *Experimental allergic encephalomyelitis.*

EAN. See *Experimental allergic neuritis.*

Ecologic study. A study in which the units of analysis are populations or groups of people, rather than individuals.

Encephalitis. Refers to an encephalopathy caused by an inflammatory response in the brain. This is usually manifested with systemic constitutional symptoms, particularly fever and pleocytosis of the cerebrospinal fluid. However, the terms *encephalopathy* and *encephalitis* have been used imprecisely and even interchangeably in the literature.

Encephalopathy. Refers to a variety of conditions affecting the brain resulting in alterations in the level of consciousness, ranging from stupor to coma. At times, febrile seizures, afebrile seizures, and epilepsy have been considered components of encephalopathy. However, the terms *encephalopathy* and *encephalitis* have been used imprecisely and even interchangeably in the literature. See Chapter 3.

Erythema multiforme. An inflammatory eruption characterized by symmetrical erythematous, or edematous lesions of the skin or mucous membranes. It is usually nonpruritic, lasts several days, and leaves no sequelae. Stevens-Johnson syndrome is a rare, severe, potentially fatal form of erythema multiforme that is associated with bullous lesions.

Experimental allergic encephalomyelitis. Also known as EAE. An experimental model for acute disseminated encephalomyelitis. See Chapter 3.

Experimental allergic neuritis. Also known as EAN. An experimental model of Guillain-Barré syndrome. See Chapter 3.

GBS. See Guillain-Barré syndrome.

Guillain-Barré syndrome. Also known as postinfectious neuritis or acute inflammatory demyelinating polyneuritis, it is a syndrome characterized by rapid onset of flaccid motor weakness with depression of tendon reflexes and inflammatory demyelination of peripheral nerves. Commonly abbreviated as GBS. See Chapter 3.

Haemophilus influenzae. A haemophilus found normally in the human nasopharynx; the influenza bacillus. Strains with polysaccharide capsules, of six types (designated a to f), may cause disease. Type b is the most frequent. The organism was the commonest cause of meningitis in children before introduction of the vaccine against the organism. It also causes sinusitis, otitis media, pneumonia, arthritis, and a fulminating epiglottitis and obstructive laryngitis. The organism was once considered, mistakenly, the cause of pandemic influenza. Also called *Pfeiffer's bacillus*.

Hepatitis B. Inflammation of the liver caused by hepatitis B virus. The infectious agent may circulate in the blood for long periods of time (months or years) and is characteristically transmitted by parenteral, percutaneous, or permucosal inoculation of even minute amounts of blood, blood products, or bodily secretions. The disease may be acute or chronic, symptomatic or asymptomatic. Also called viral hepatitis type B, homologous serum hepatitis, human serum jaundice, and homologous serum jaundice.

Hepatitis B virus. A virus of an unnamed family that is composed of a membrane-bound particle called a *Dane particle* containing double-stranded circular DNA and a DNA polymerase. It is one of the major causes of posttransfusion hepatitis. Human disease can be characterized by acute or chronic hepatitis or an asymptomatic carrier state. Transmission is predominantly via parenteral routes or contact with infected blood. Also called *serum hepatitis virus* (outmoded).

Immunization. The process of rendering a subject immune or of becoming immune. In this report the term has been accepted to be synonymous with *vaccination*. See *Vaccination*.

active i. Inoculation with a specific antigen to induce an immune response.
passive i. The conferral of specific immunity by the administration of sensitized lymphoid cells or serum from immune individuals.

Inactivate. To make biologically inactive, as viruses or bacteria, toxins, or serum complement, by any of various means, such as by physical means (exposure to X rays, ultraviolet irradiation, or heating) or by exposure to chemical agents or to immunologic antagonists.

Inactivated polio vaccine (IPV). A sterile suspension of three types of inactivated polioviruses. The viruses are grown separately in monkey renal tissue cultures and are then inactivated and combined. The vaccine is administered subcutaneously and confers active immunity against poliomyelitis. Also called *Salk vaccine* and *killed poliovirus vaccine*.

Infantile spasms. A condition characterized by sudden flexion of the arms, forward flexion of the trunk, and extension of the legs. The attacks last only a few seconds but may be repeated many times a day. They are restricted to the first 3 years of life, often to be replaced by other forms of seizures.

Insulin-dependent diabetes mellitus. Also known as *juvenile diabetes* or *type I diabetes*. A disease characterized most frequently by low or absent levels of circulating endogenous insulin. See Chapter 7.

IPV. See *Inactivated Polio vaccine*.

Juvenile diabetes. An autoimmune disease characterized most frequently by low or absent levels of circulating endogenous insulin (more properly called *insulin-dependent diabetes mellitus*).

Koch's postulates. Koch stated that these postulates should be met before a causative relationship between a particular bacterial parasite or disease agent and the disease in question can be accepted.

1. The agent must be shown to be present in every case of the disease by isolation in pure culture.
2. The agent must not be found in cases of other diseases.
3. Once isolated, the agent must be capable of reproducing the disease in experimental animals.
4. The agent must be recovered from the experimental disease produced.

Monitoring System for Adverse Events Following Immunization (MSAEFI). A passive surveillance system designed and monitored by the Centers for Disease Control for the purpose of collecting nationwide data on adverse events temporally associated with receipt of vaccines purchased with federal, state, or local government funds. See *Vaccine Adverse Event Reporting System*.

Mononeuropathy. Neuropathic dysfunction limited to the distribution of a single peripheral nerve that is large enough to be named. See Chapter 3.

MSAEFI. See *Monitoring System for Adverse Events Following Immunization*.

Multiple sclerosis. A chronic central nervous system demyelinating disease in which the lesions occur in multiple locations and at different times.

Odds ratio (OR). In studies of adverse events following immunization, the odds ratio generally refers to the exposure-odds ratio, which, for a set of case-control data, is the ratio of the odds of exposure among the cases to the odds of exposure among controls (noncases). When the adverse event under study is rare, the odds ratio is a good estimate of the relative risk.

Optic neuritis. Represents a central demyelinating disease of the optic nerve anterior to the optic chiasm. It can occur as a solitary unexplained monophasic disease or it may be an early sign of multiple sclerosis. See Chapter 3.

Paralytic poliomyelitis. A paralytic disease caused by invasion of the poliovirus into the central nervous system and death of nerve cells in the anterior horn of the spinal cord, the brainstem, and in the motor cortex. The muscle paralysis is usually asymmetrical.

Peripheral mononeuropathy. See *Mononeuropathy.*

Relative risk (RR). The ratio of the risk of disease, death, or other outcome among the exposed to the risk among the unexposed. Generally derived from controlled cohort studies or clinical trials. If used in conjunction with adverse events following immunization, when the adverse event under study is rare, the odds ratio is a good estimate of the RR.

Residual seizure disorder. Recurrent, afebrile seizures; also known as epilepsy.

Reye syndrome. An acute and occasionally fatal childhood syndrome of encephalopathy and fatty degeneration of the liver marked by rapid development of brain swelling and altered levels of consciousness.

Risk difference. See attributable risk.

Sensorineural deafness. A form of hearing loss resulting from pathologic changes in the end organ structures within the cochlea or in the neural connections between the cochlea and the cochlear nuclei. See Chapter 3.

Stevens-Johnson syndrome. See *Erythema multiforme.*

Serum sickness. Caused by interaction between antigen and antibody in the circulation with the formation of antigen-antibody complexes in an environment of antigen excess. Symptoms include urticaria, swelling, arthritis, and fever. See Chapter 4.

Subacute sclerosing panencephalitis (SSPE). A rare form of encephalitis involving both grey and white matter that can affect children and adolescents that is characterized by insidious onset of a progressive cerebral dysfunction occurring over the course of weeks or months. See Chapter 3.

Sudden infant death syndrome (SIDS). The unexpected and unexplained death of an apparently well, or virtually well, infant. SIDS is the most common cause of death of infants between ages 2 weeks and 1 year, accounting for one-third of all deaths in this age group.

Thrombocytopenia. A severe decrease in the number of platelets, the cells involved in clotting. Thrombocytopenia may stem from failure of platelet production, splenic sequestration of platelets, increased platelet destruction, increased platelet utilization, or dilution of platelets.

Thrombocytopenic purpura. Severe thrombocytopenia characterized by mucosal bleeding and bleeding into the skin in the form of multiple petechiae, most often evident on the lower legs, and scattered small ecchymoses (bruises) at sites of minor trauma. In children, idiopathic thrombocytopenic purpura is usually self-limited and follows a viral infection.

Transverse myelitis. A clinical syndrome characterized by the acute onset of signs of spinal cord disease, usually involving the descending motor tracts and the ascending sensory fibers, suggesting a lesion at one level of the spinal cord. It can occur in isolation or as part of a multifocal demyelinating disease such as multiple sclerosis or acute disseminated encephalomyelitis. See Chapter 3.

Vaccination. Inoculation with a vaccine for the purposes of inducing immunity. In this report the term has been accepted to be synonymous with immunization. See *Immunization*.

Vaccine. A material containing live attenuated or killed microorganisms, or constituents of microorganisms, capable of eliciting protection against infection.

Vaccine Adverse Event Reporting System (VAERS). A passive surveillance system intended to collect reports of reactions to vaccines that is under the aegis of the Centers for Disease Control and Prevention and the U.S. Food and Drug Administration. This system replaces the Monitoring System for Adverse Events Following Immunization (MSAEFI) and a similar system formerly run by the Food and Drug Administration. See Chapter 10.

VAERS. See *Vaccine Adverse Event Reporting System*.

D

Committee and Staff Biographies

COMMITTEE

RICHARD B. JOHNSTON, JR. (Chair) is the Senior Vice President for Programs and Medical Director of the March of Dimes Birth Defects Foundation in White Plains, New York, and Adjunct Professor of Pediatrics at the Yale University School of Medicine in New Haven, Connecticut. He received his undergraduate and medical education at Vanderbilt University and his postgraduate training at Children's Hospital, Boston, and Harvard Medical School. He was formerly chairman of the Department of Pediatrics at the National Jewish Center for Immunology and Respiratory Medicine, Denver, and at the University of Pennsylvania. He is board certified in pediatrics and serves as a clinical immunologist for children. His research interests include host defense mechanisms against infection and the biochemical basis for the killing of invading microorganisms by phagocytic cells. He presently chairs the Advisory Committee for Vaccines and Related Biological Products for the U.S. Food and Drug Administration. Dr. Johnston was also a member of the Institute of Medicine Committee to Review the Adverse Consequences of Pertussis and Rubella Vaccines.

E. RUSSELL ALEXANDER is Chief of Epidemiology at the Seattle-King County Department of Public Health and Professor in the Department of Epidemiology at the School of Public Health and Community Medicine of the University of Washington. He received his undergraduate, M.D. degree, and pediatric training at the University of Chicago. He is certified by the American Board of Pediatrics, and his clinical specialty is infectious diseases. He has been a member of the pediatric faculty of the universities of Chicago, Washington and Arizona, and Emory University. He is a former Chairman of the Department of Epidemiology at the University of Washington. He holds membership in a number of professional societies and is a past President of the American Epidemiologic Society. He has been a recipient of several awards and has been a member of a number of committees and advisory panels.

ALAN M. ARON is the Director of Child Neurology and Professor of Neurology at the Mount Sinai School of Medicine in New York City. He received his M.D. degree from Columbia University, New York, and did his undergraduate work at Tufts University in Medford, Massachusetts. Dr. Aron is board certified by the American Board of Pediatrics, the American Board of Psychiatry and Neurology, and the American Board of Psychiatry and Neurology, with special competence in child neurology. This specialization in child neurology led to numerous faculty and hospital appointments, memberships, and consultative positions. He holds membership in a number of professional societies and is a recipient of several awards.

ARTHUR K. ASBURY is the Van Meter Professor of Neurology and Vice Dean for Research at the University of Pennsylvania School of Medicine, Philadelphia. He received his M.D. degree from the University of Cincinnati and did his undergraduate work at the University of Kentucky. Dr. Asbury's specialization in neurology and neuropathology led to numerous faculty and hospital appointments, memberships, and consultative positions. He is a member of the Institute of Medicine and is board certified by the American Board of Psychiatry and Neurology. He has received a number of awards, is past President of the American Neurological Association and the Association of University Professors of Neurology, and was Chief Editor of the *Annals of Neurology*.

CHARLES C. J. CARPENTER is Professor of Medicine at Brown University and Physician-in-Chief at the Miriam Hospital, Providence, Rhode Island. He received his M.D. degree from the Johns Hopkins University School of Medicine and did his undergraduate work at Princeton University. Dr. Carpenter is a member of the Institute of Medicine and numerous other professional societies; he is also a recipient of several academic honors and awards. He has served on numerous Institute of Medicine committees; most recently he chaired the Committee on Malaria Prevention and Control.

K. LYNN CATES is Associate Professor of Pediatrics, Case Western Reserve University School of Medicine, and Chief, Pediatric Infectious Diseases at Rainbow Babies and Children's Hospital in Cleveland, Ohio. She received her M.D. degree from Northwestern University in Chicago and did her undergraduate work at Grinnell College, Grinnell, Iowa. She did her pediatric internship and residency at Children's Memorial Hospital in Chicago and did a pediatric infectious diseases fellowship at the University of Minnesota Hospitals. She is certified by the American Board of Pediatrics and is a member of many professional societies, including the Pediatric Infectious Diseases Society, the Infectious Diseases Society of America, and the Society for Pediatric Research.

KAY DICKERSIN is Assistant Professor in the Department of Epidemiology and Preventive Medicine at the University of Maryland School of Medicine, Baltimore. She received her Ph.D. degree from the Johns Hopkins School of Hygiene and Public Health and did undergraduate work at the University of California in Berkeley. Her major research interests are in clinical trials, meta-analysis, and publication bias. She is particularly interested in the development and utilization of methods for the evaluation of medical care and its effectiveness. Dr. Dickersin has memberships in several professional societies and is a recipient of a number of fellowships and awards. Dr. Dickersin has also served on the Institute of Medicine Committee to Advise the Department of Defense on its FY 1993 Breast Cancer Program and the Forum on Drug Development.

RICHARD T. JOHNSON is Professor and Chair of the Department of Neurology at the Johns Hopkins University School of Medicine, Baltimore, Maryland. He received his M.D. degree from the University of Colorado School of Medicine, Denver. He is certified by the American Board of Neurology and Psychiatry and has held numerous faculty and hospital appointments and fellowships in his neurologic specialty. Dr. Johnson is a member of the Institute of Medicine as well as numerous other honorary and professional societies. He chaired the Institute of Medicine's Committee to Review an Epidemiologic Study of Neurologic Illness and Vaccination in Children. Dr. Johnson is a recipient of many awards and honors, lectures extensively, and is involved in numerous federal, nonfederal, editorial, and voluntary agencies and boards.

MICHAEL KATZ is Vice President for Research at the March of Dimes Birth Defects Foundation in White Plains, New York. He is also Carpentier Professor of Pediatrics, Emeritus, Columbia University, New York. Dr. Katz, a pediatrician, has a clinical specialty of infectious diseases and parasitology, and his research interests have dealt with host defense in malnourished children and mechanisms of latent virus infections. He is an author and coauthor of original scientific papers dealing with these subjects and, with two colleagues, an author of a textbook on parasitic diseases. Dr. Katz is a member of the Institute of Medicine and a number of professional societies, a fellow of the American Association for the Advancement of Science, and a recipient of several awards, among them the Humboldt Award for Senior U.S. Scientists, given by the German government. He has been a visiting professor in universities in the United States and abroad. He has been a consultant to the World Health Organization, the

United Nation's Children's Fund, and various government organizations. Dr. Katz also served on the Institute of Medicine Committee to Review the Adverse Consequences of Pertussis and Rubella Vaccines.

MICHAEL S. KRAMER is a Professor in the Departments of Pediatrics and of Epidemiology and Biostatistics at McGill University Faculty of Medicine, Montreal, Quebec, Canada. He received his M.D. degree from Yale University School of Medicine. He is certified by the National Board of Medical Examiners and the American Board of Pediatrics, and he is a fellow of the American College of Epidemiology. He is a National Health Research Scientist of the National Health Research and Development Program, Health and Welfare, Canada, a member of numerous professional societies, and a recipient of many awards and honors.

KENNETH MCINTOSH is a Professor in the Department of Pediatrics at Harvard Medical School and Chief of the Division of Infectious Diseases at Children's Hospital in Boston, Massachusetts. He received his M.D. degree and did his undergraduate work at Harvard University. He is certified by the American Board of Internal Medicine, is a recipient of several awards and honors, and is a member of many professional societies. His work in infectious diseases has led to numerous faculty and hospital appointments and consultancies.

CATHERINE J. ROSE is a board certified pediatrician in private practice in San Jose, California. She received her M.D. degree from West Virginia University School of Medicine, Morgantown. She did her internship and pediatric residency at the University of California, San Diego. She was a fellow in general academic pediatrics at Stanford University, Palo Alto, California. Following her fellowship, she was an associate in general pediatrics at Duke University. She is a fellow of the American Academy of Pediatrics.

PENELOPE G. SHACKELFORD is Professor of Pediatrics and Associate Professor of Molecular Microbiology at Washington University School of Medicine in St. Louis, Missouri. She received her M.D. degree from Washington University and did undergraduate work at the University of Wisconsin in Madison. She did her pediatric internship at Babies and Children's Hospital, Cleveland, Ohio, and her pediatric residency and fellowship in infectious diseases at St. Louis Children's Hospital, St. Louis, Missouri. She is certified by the American Board of Pediatrics and is a member of several professional societies, including the Infectious Diseases Society of America and the American Association of Immunologists. Her research interest is the development of antibody responses in children.

PAUL D. STOLLEY is Professor and Chairman of the Department of Epidemiology and Preventive Medicine at the University of Maryland School of Medicine, Baltimore. He received his M.D. degree from Cornell University Medical College, New York, and his M.P.H. from the Johns Hopkins

University School of Hygiene and Public Health. He is certified in public health by the American Board of Preventive Medicine and is a fellow of the American College of Physicians. Dr. Stolley is a member of the Institute of Medicine and several other professional societies, as well as a recipient of numerous awards and honors. Dr. Stolley also serves on the Institute of Medicine's Board on Health Sciences Policy.

STAFF

KATHLEEN R. STRATTON is a Senior Program Officer in the Division of Health Promotion and Disease Prevention of the Institute of Medicine. She received a B.A. degree in natural sciences from Johns Hopkins University, Baltimore, Maryland, and received her Ph.D. in pharmacology and toxicology from the University of Maryland at Baltimore. She did a postdoctoral research fellowship in the Department of Neuroscience at Johns Hopkins University School of Medicine. Other projects during her 3 years at the National Research Council and the Institute of Medicine include work with the Committee to Study the Co-Administration of Research and Services at the National Institutes of Health and the Alcohol, Drug Abuse, and Mental Health Administration, Committee on Risk Assessment of Hazardous Air Pollutants, Committee on Risk Assessment Methodology, and the Committee on Neurotoxicology and Models for Assessing Risks.

CYNTHIA JOHNSON HOWE is a Program Officer in the Division of Health Promotion and Disease Prevention of the Institute of Medicine. She received a B.A. degree in psychology from Wittenberg University in Springfield, Ohio, and has done graduate work in experimental psychology at the University of Maryland, College Park. Other projects during 12 years at the Institute of Medicine include a review of the adverse consequences of pertussis and rubella vaccines; an evaluation of poliomyelitis vaccine policy options; and a study of pain, disability, and chronic illness behavior. Ms. Howe, along with four colleagues, is a recipient of the National Research Council's 1992 Group Recognition Award, as well as the 1991 Group Achievement Award of the Institute of Medicine for her work on the report *Adverse Effects of Pertussis and Rubella Vaccines.*

DOROTHY R. MAJEWSKI is a Project Assistant in the Institute of Medicine and has been with the National Academy of Sciences for 5 years. She received a B.A. degree in education from Carlow College in Pittsburgh, Pennsylvania. She served as project assistant on this study, with the review of adverse consequences of pertussis and rubella vaccines, and previously in the same capacity for studies on nuclear energy engineering for the Energy Engineering Board and on diet and health for the Food and Nutrition Board. Ms. Majewski, along with four colleagues, is a recipient of the National Research Council's 1992 Group Recognition Award, as well as the

1991 Group Achievement Award of the Institute of Medicine for her work on the report *Adverse Effects of Pertussis and Rubella Vaccines.*

MICHAEL A. STOTO is the Director of the Division of Health Promotion and Disease Prevention of the Institute of Medicine of the National Academy of Sciences. He received an A.B. in statistics from Princeton University and a Ph.D. in statistics and demography from Harvard University. He was formerly an associate professor of public policy at Harvard's John F. Kennedy School of Government. He recently directed the Institute of Medicine effort in support of the Public Health Service's Healthy People 2000 project, and the Health Effects in Vietnam Veterans of Exposure to Herbicides; he also worked on the study reviewing the adverse consequences of pertussis and rubella vaccines. His current projects address a number of issues in public health, health statistics, health promotion and disease prevention, and AIDS. Dr. Stoto, along with four colleagues, is a recipient of the National Research Council's 1992 Group Recognition Award, as well as the 1991 Group Achievement Award of the Institute of Medicine for his work on the report *Adverse Effects of Pertussis and Rubella Vaccines.*

TAMAR LASKY is Research Assistant to the Chairman, Department of Epidemiology and Preventive Medicine, at the University of Maryland School of Medicine, Baltimore. She received her Ph.D. and M.S.P.H. degrees at the University of North Carolina, Chapel Hill, and did her undergraduate work at Grinnell College, Grinnell, Iowa. Dr. Lasky has extensive research experience and has coauthored many public health publications.

MICHAEL K. HAYES has been an editorial consultant with the National Academy of Sciences, among other organizations, since 1985. He has edited numerous publications for the Institute of Medicine, including *The Children's Vaccine Initiative: Achieving the Vision, Adverse Effects of Pertussis and Rubella Vaccines,* and *Nutrition Labeling.* Mr. Hayes also edits research articles published in the monthly journals *Antimicrobial Agents and Chemotherapy* and the *Journal of Clinical Microbiology.*

Bibliography

Aaby P, Clements CJ. Measles immunization research: a review. Bulletin of the World Health Organization 1989;67:443-448.

Abe T, Nonaka C, Hiraiwa M, Ushijima H, Fujii R. Acute and delayed neurologic reaction to inoculation with attenuated live measles virus. Brain and Development 1985;7:421-423.

Abrahamson HA. Vaccines, poliomyelitis, and the Guillain-Barre syndrome (editorial). Journal of Asthma Research 1976;14:1-4.

Abu Eldan J, Borcic B, Smerdel S. Persistence of immunity against measles in persons immunized with Edmonston-Zagreb vaccine. Acta Medica Croatica 1991;45:297-304.

Adam E, Burian V, Kubatova E, Kratochvilova M, Burianova B, Kyselova M et al. Comparative study of the reactogenicity and efficacy of different combined vaccines against diphtheria, pertussis and tetanus. Progress in Immunobiological Standardization 1969;3:290-291.

Adam E, Burian V, Kubatova E, Kratochvilova M, Burianova B, Kyselova M et al. Comparative study of the reactogenicity and effectiveness of different combined vaccines against diphtheria, pertussis and tetanus. Journal of Hygiene, Epidemiology, Microbiology, and Immunology 1970;14:88-101.

Adam E, Domorazkova E, Kratochvilova M, Burian V, Janotova J, Drevo M et al. [The experience with vaccination against measles in Czech districts] Zkusenosti s ockovanim proti spalnickam v ceskych krajich. Ceskoslovenska Pediatrie 1970;25:438-440.

Adam E, Fosenbauerova E, Domorazkova E, Kratochvilova M, Kubatova E, Mares I et al. [Comparative studies of measles vaccines prepared from further attenuated strains Schwarz and SEVAC] Srovnavaci studie spalnickovych vakcin pripravenych z dale atenuovanych kmenangu Schwarz a SEVAC. Ceskoslovenska Pediatrie 1968;23:581-593.

Adams JM. Persistent or slow viral infections and related diseases. Western Journal of Medicine 1975;122:380-393.

Adams JM. Program Abstracts of the 32nd Interscience Conference on Antimicrobial Agents and Chemotherapy. Abstract 974, p. 273. Washington, DC: American Society for Microbiology; 1992.

Adams JM, Brown WJ, Cremer NE, Eberle ED, Fewster ME, Lennette EH. Atypical demyelinating disease. Journal of Neurology, Neurosurgery and Psychiatry 1974;37:874-878.

Adams JM, Brown WJ, Eberle ED, Verity A. Vaccinia virus implicated in diffuse demyelinating disease. Proceedings of the Society for Experimental Biology and Medicine 1973;143:799-803.

Adams JM, Francke E, Lillestol M. Poliomyelitis vaccination (letter). New England Journal of Medicine 1977;297:1290-1291.

Adams WG, Deaver KA, Cochi SL et al. Decline of childhood *Haemophilus influenzae* type b (Hib) disease in the Hib vaccine era. Journal of the American Medical Association 1993;269:221-226.

Adenyi-Jones SC, Faden H, Ferdon MB, Kwong MS, Ogra PL. Systemic and local immune responses to enhanced-potency inactivated poliovirus vaccine in premature and term infants. Journal of Pediatrics 1992;120:686-689.

Adler JB, Mazzotta SA, Barkin JS. Pancreatitis caused by measles, mumps, and rubella vaccine. Pancreas 1991;6:489-490.

Adler SP. The effects and side effects of vaccines. Virginia Medical Journal 1982;109:410-411.

Advisory Commission on Childhood Vaccines, Martin Smith, Chairman. Vaccine Injury Compensation Program: past, present, and future. June 20, 1991. Unpublished.

Afzal MA, Pickford AR, Forsey T, Minor PD. Heterogeneous mumps vaccine. Lancet 1992;340:980-981.

Agrawal K, Pandit K, Kannan AT. Single dose tetanus toxoid: a review of trials in India with special reference to control of tetanus neonatorum. Indian Journal of Pediatrics 1984;81:285-295.

Aho K, Somer T, Salo OP. Rheumatoid factor and immuno-conglutinin responses following various vaccinations. Proceedings of the Society for Experimental Biology and Medicine 1967;124:229-33.

Ahonkhai VI, Lukacs LJ, Jonas LC, Calandra GB. Clinical experience with PedvaxHIB, a conjugate vaccine of *Haemophilus influenzae* type b polysaccharide—Neisseria meningitidis outer membrane protein. Vaccine 1991;9(Suppl.):S38-41, S42-43.

Ahonkhai VI, Lukacs LJ, Jonas LC, Matthews H, Vella PP, Ellis RW et al. *Haemophilus influenzae* type b conjugate vaccine (meningococcal protein conjugate) (PedvaxHIB): clinical evaluation. Pediatrics 1990;85(4 Pt 2):676-681.

Ahronheim G, Allard M, Forsey T, Rydbeck R, Teuwen D, Yamada A. Mumps associated with trivalent vaccine containing Urabe Am 9 mumps strain (abstract). Program Abstracts of the 30th Interscience Conference on Antimicrobial Agents and Chemotherapy, p. 148. Washington, DC: American Society for Microbiology; 1990.

Ahronheim GA, Allard M, Forsey T, Rydbeck R, Teuwen DE, Yamada A. Mumps associated with trivalent vaccine containing Urabe Am 9 mumps strain (abstract). Pediatric Research 1991;29:166A.

Ajjan N, Bentejac MC. [Anti-mumps vaccination] La vaccination anti-ourlienne. Revue de Pediatrie 1985;21:55-61.

Ajjan N, Biron G, Bentejac MC. [The dangers of vaccination] Les dangers de la vaccination. Revue Medicale 1980;21:739-750.

Ajjan N, Fayet MT, Biron G et al. Combination of attenuated measles vaccine (Schwarz) with meningococcus A and A + C vaccine. Developments in Biological Standardization 1978;41:209-216.

Akama K, Yamamoto A. [Side effects of tetanus toxoid. II. Antigenic materials derived from the constituents of the medium for toxoid preparation]. Nippon Saikingaku Zasshi 1969;24:595-601.

Akosa AB, Ali MH, Khoo CT, Evans DM. Angiolymphoid hyperplasia with eosinophilia associated with tetanus toxoid vaccination. Histopathology 1990;16:589-593.

Al-Qudah AA, Shahar E, Logan WJ, Murphy EG. Neonatal Guillain-Barre syndrome. Pediatric Neurology 1988;4:255-256.

Albert JM, Ott HJ. Calcifying dermatomyositis following antitetanus vaccination. Archives of Internal Medicine 1983;143:1457-1458.

Albrecht P, Lorenz D, Klutch MJ, Vickers JH, Ennis FA. Fatal measles infection in marmosets: pathogenesis and prophylaxis. Infection and Immunity 1980;27:969-978.

Albrecht RM. Poliomyelitis from a vaccinee. Lancet 1968;1:1371.

Alderslade R, Bellman MH, Rawson NS B., Ross EM, Miller DL. The National Childhood Encephalopathy Study: a report on 1000 cases of serious neurological disorders in infants and young children from the NCES research team. In: Department of Health and Social Security. Whooping Cough: Reports from the Committee on the Safety of Medicines and the Joint Committee on Vaccination and Immunisation. London: Her Majesty's Stationery Office; 1981.

Alexander ER. Landmark perspective: Inactivated poliomyelitis vaccination—issues reconsidered. Journal of the American Medical Association 1984;251:2710-2712.

Allen TW. Efficacy of PRP, PRP-D vaccines in children 18 months of age and older. Journal of the American Osteopathic Association 1991;91:323.

Allerdist H. [Epidemiologic problems of measles-mumps vaccination] Epidemische Probleme der Masern-Mumpsimpfung. Offentliche Gesundheitswesen 1979;41(Suppl. 1):51-56.

Allerdist H. Neurological complications following measles vaccination. Developments in Biological Standardization 1979;43:259-264.

Allerdist H. [Neurological complications following measles virus vaccination: Evaluation of the cases seen between 1971-1977] Uber Zentralnervose Komplikationen nach Masernschutzimpfung: eine Analyse des Hamburger Krankengutes von 1971 bis 1977. Monatsschrift fur Kinderheilkunde 1979;127:23-28.

Alter HJ, Scanlon RT, Schechter GP. Thrombocytopenic purpura following vaccination with attenuated measles virus. American Journal of Diseases of Children 1968;115:111-113.

Alter M. The epidemiology of Guillain-Barre syndrome. Annals of Neurology 1990;27(Suppl.):S7-S12.

Alter MJ, Hadler SC, Margolis HS. The changing epidemiology of hepatitis B in the United States: need for alternative vaccination strategies. Journal of the American Medical Association 1988;263:1218-1222.

Alves RS, Barbosa ER, Scaff M. Postvaccinal parkinsonism. Movement Disorders 1992;7:178-180.

Alvord EC Jr. Incubation period and severity of experimental allergic encephalomyelitis: analogy with swine-flu-vaccine-induced Guillain-Barre syndrome (letter). Annals of Neurology 1986;19:100-101.

Alvord EC Jr., Jahnke U, Fischer EH. The causes of the syndromes of Landry (1859) and of Guillain, Barre and Strohl (1916). Revue Neurologique 1987;143:571-579.

Ambrosino DM, Lee MY, Chen D, Shamberger RC. Response to *Haemophilus influenzae* type b conjugate vaccine in children undergoing splenectomy. Journal of Pediatric Surgery 1992;27:1045-1048.

Ambrosino DM, Sood SK, Lee MC, Chen D, Collard HR, Bolon DL et al. IgG1, IgG2 and IgM responses to two *Haemophilus influenzae* type b conjugate vaccines in young infants. Pediatric Infectious Disease Journal 1992;11:855-859.

American Family Physician. Combining DTP vaccine and *H. influenzae* type b vaccine. American Family Physician 1992;45:909-910.

American Family Physician. New poliovirus vaccine. American Family Physician 1991;43:2270.

American Journal of Diseases of Children. Recommendations of the Immunization Practices Advisory Committee (ACIP): mumps prevention. American Journal of Diseases of Children 1989;143:1141-1142.

American Academy of Pediatrics, Committee on Infectious Diseases. *Haemophilus influenzae* type b conjugate vaccine. Pediatrics 1988;81:908-911.

American Academy of Pediatrics, Committee on Infectious Diseases. *Haemophilus influenzae* type b conjugate vaccines: immunization of children at 15 months of age. Pediatrics 1990;86:794-796.

American Academy of Pediatrics, Committee on Infectious Diseases. *Haemophilus influenzae* type b conjugate vaccines: recommendations for immunization of infants and children 2 months of age and older: update. Pediatrics 1991;88:169-172.

American Academy of Pediatrics, Committee on Infectious Diseases. Health guidelines for the attendance in daycare and foster care settings for children infected with human immuno-deficiency virus. Pediatrics 1987;79:466-471.

American Academy of Pediatrics, Committee on Infectious Diseases. Personal and family history of seizures and measles immunization. Pediatrics 1987;80:741-742.

American Academy of Pediatrics, Committee on Infectious Diseases. Report of the Committee on Infectious Diseases. Elk Grove Village, IL: American Academy of Pediatrics; 1964.

American Academy of Pediatrics, Committee on Infectious Diseases. Report of the Committee on Infectious Diseases: 22nd edition. Elk Grove Village, IL: American Academy of Pediatrics; 1991.

American Academy of Neurology, Therapeutics and Technology Assessment Subcommittee. Assessment: DTP vaccination. Neurology 1992;42(3 Pt. 1):471-472.

Aminova MG, Cheredova NG, Novokreshchenova FA, Atakhanov KA, Shakhmuradova VS. [Clinical reactions in children after the administration of the Leningrad-4 live measles vaccine according to data from Kirghizia] Klinicheskie reaktsii u detei na vvedenie zhivoi korevoi vaktsiny iz shtamma Leningrad-4 po dannym Kirgizii. Trudy Leningradskogo Nauchno-issledovatelskogo Instituta Epidemiologii i Mikrobiolgii 1965;28:186-191.

Amir J, Liang X, Granoff DM. Variability in the functional activity of vaccine-induced antibody to *Haemophilus influenzae* type b. Pediatric Research 1990;27(4 Pt 1):358-364.

Amir J, Scott MG, Nahm MH, Granoff DM. Bactericidal and opsonic activity of IgG1 and IgG2 anticapsular antibodies to *Haemophilus influenzae* type b. Journal of Infectious Diseases 1990;162:163-171.

Ammundsen E. [Complications of polio vaccination with Sabin vaccine] Komplikationer ved poliovaccinationen med Sabin-vaccine. Fra Sundhedsstyrelsen 1968;4:337-338.

Amsel SG, Hanukoglu A, Fried D, Wolyvovics M. Myocarditis after triple immunisation. Archives of Disease in Childhood 1986;61:403-405.

Anand JK. Multiple factors in leukaemogenesis. British Medical Journal 1972;4:364.

Andelman MB, Schwarz A, Spiegelblatt H. Field trials with further attenuated live measles vaccine without gamma globulin. American Journal of Public Health / Nations Health 1966;56:1891-1897.

Andersen O, Eeg-Olofsson E. A prospective study of parapareses in western Sweden. Acta Neurologica Scandinavica 1976;54:312-320.

Anderson GR, Gottshall RY, Nelsom E, Angela F. Quadruple vaccines containing pertussis and poliomyelitis vaccines. Health Laboratory Science 1978;15:138-43.

Anderson P. Antibody responses to *H. influenzae* type b and diphtheria toxin induced by conjugates of oligosaccharides of the type b capsule with the nontoxic protein CRM_{197}. Infection and Immunity 1983;39:233-238.

Anderson P, Johnston RB Jr., Smith DH. Human serum activities against *Haemophilus influenzae*, type b. Journal of Clinical Investigation 1972;51:31-38.

Anderson P, Pichichero M, Edwards K, Porch CR, Insel R. Priming and induction of *Haemophilus influenzae* type b capsular antibodies in early infancy by Dpo20, an oligosaccharide-protein conjugate vaccine. Journal of Pediatrics 1987;111:644-650.

Andersson T, Siden A. A clinical study of the Guillain-Barre syndrome. Acta Neurologica Scandinavica 1982;66:316-327.

Andre FE. Control of poliomyelitis by vaccination in Belgium. Reviews of Infectious Diseases 1984;6(Suppl. 2):S419-S423.

Andre FE. Poliomyelitis vaccines in Belgium: 20 years of experience. Developments in Biological Standardization 1979;43:187-193.

Andre FE. Summary of safety and efficacy data on a yeast-derived hepatitis B vaccine. American Journal of Medicine 1989;87(3a):14S-20S.

Andre FE, Peetermans J. Effect of simultaneous administration of live measles vaccine on the "take rate" of live mumps vaccine. Developments in Biological Standardization 1986;65:101-107.

Andre FE, Safary A. Clinical experience with a yeast derived hepatitis B vaccine. In: Zuckerman AJ, ed. Viral Hepatitis and Viral Disease. New York: Alan R Liss; 1988.

Andreoni G, Curatolo D, Cervini E, Provvidenza G, Rocchi G, Velli V. [Isolation of poliovirus in poliomyelitic patients vaccinated with Sabin vaccine] Isolamento di virus polio in poliomiefitici vaccinati con vaccino Sabin. Giornale di Malattie Infettive e Parassitarie 1966;18:662-663.

Andreoni G, Rocchi G. [Etiologic studies in the patients with central nervous system diseases hospitalized in Rome during the period 1964-1970] Indagine eziologica in pazienti con affezioni del sistema nervoso centrale ricoverati a Roma nel periodo 1964-1970. Annali Sclavo 1971;13:291-298.

Andrews NC, Baltimore D. Lack of evidence for VPg priming of poliovirus RNA synthesis in the host factor-dependent in vitro replicase reaction. Journal of Virology 1986;58:212-215.

Annals of Emergency Medicine. Tetanus immunization recommendations for persons seven years of age and older. Annals of Emergency Medicine 1986;15:1111-1112.

Annals of Internal Medicine. Mumps vaccine. Annals of Internal Medicine 1968;68:632-633.

Annals of Internal Medicine. Mumps vaccine: recommendation of the Public Health Service Advisory Committee on Immunization Practices, Centers for Disease Control, U.S. Department of Health, Education, and Welfare, Atlanta, Georgia. Annals of Internal Medicine 1978;88:819-820.

Annals of Internal Medicine. Diphtheria, tetanus, and pertussis: guidelines for vaccine prophylaxis and other preventive measures. Annals of Internal Medicine 1981;95:723-728.

Annals of Internal Medicine. Mumps vaccine: recommendation of the Immunization Practices Advisory Committee. Annals of Internal Medicine 1983;98:192-194.

Annals of Internal Medicine. Diphtheria, tetanus, and pertussis: guidelines for vaccine prophylaxis and other preventive measures: recommendation of the Immunization Practices Advisory Committee. Annals of Internal Medicine 1985;103:896-905.

Annunziato D, Kaplan MH, Hall WW, Ichinose H, Lin JH, Balsam D et al. Atypical measles syndrome: pathologic and serologic findings. Pediatrics 1982;70:203-209.

Aprile MA, Kadar D, Wilson S. Sensitization of guinea-pigs to measles vaccines. Clinical Experimental Immunology 1969;5:531-539.

Arakawa Y, Amaki S, Miyamoto M, Matsuo Y, Honda T, Shikata T. Safety and efficacy of hepatitis B vaccine in hospital personnel. Japanese Journal of Medicine 1986;25:25-33.

Araujo OE, Flowers FP et al. Stevens-Johnson syndrome. Journal of Emergency Medicine 1984;2:129-135.

Arbeter AM, Arthur JH, Blakeman GJ et al. Measles immunity: reimmunization of children who previously received live measles vaccine and gamma globulin. Journal of Pediatrics 1972;81:737-741.

Arbeter AM, Baker L, Starr SE, Levine BL, Books E, Plotkin SA. Combination measles, mumps, rubella and varicella vaccine. Pediatrics 1986;78(4 Pt. 2):742-747.

Arlazoroff A, Bleicher Z, Klein C, Vure E, Lahat E, Gross B et al. Vaccine-associated contact paralytic poliomyelitis with atypical neurological presentation. Acta Neurologica Scandinavica 1987;76:210-214.

Armenian HK. Case investigation in epidemiology. American Journal of Epidemiology 1991;134:1067-1072.

Arnason BG. Neuroimmunology (editorial). New England Journal of Medicine 1987;316:406-408.

Arnason BG, Soliven B. Acute inflammatory demyelinating polyradiculoneuropathy. In: Syck PJ et al., eds. Peripheral Neuropathy, 3rd edition. W.B. Saunders; 1992.

Arthus M. Injections repetees de serum de cheval chez le lapin. Comptes Rendus des Seances de la Societe de Biologie et ses Filiales 1903;55:817-820.

Asbury AK. Diagnostic considerations in Guillain-Barre syndrome. Annals of Neurology 1981;9(Suppl.):1-5.

Asbury AK. Guillain-Barre syndrome: historical aspects. Annals of Neurology 1990;27(Suppl.):S2-S6.

Asbury AK, Arnason BG, Karp HR, McFarlin DE. Criteria for diagnosis of Guillain-Barre syndrome. Annals of Neurology 1978;3:565-566.

Asbury AK, Arnason BG, Adams RD. The inflammatory lesion in idiopathic polyneuritis. Medicine 1969;48:173-215.

Asbury AK, Cornblath DR. Assessment of current diagnostic criteria for Guillain-Barre syndrome. Annals of Neurology 1992;27(Suppl.):S21-S24.

Asbury AK, Gibbs CJ Jr, eds. Autoimmune neuropathies: Guillain-Barre syndrome. Annals of Neurology 1990;27(Suppl.):S1-S79.

Ashworth N. Health comment. Health Quarterly Magazine (New Zealand Department of Health) 1988;40:2.

Asindi AA, Bell EJ, Browning MJ, Stephenson JB. Vaccine-induced polioencephalomyelitis in Scotland. Scottish Medical Journal 1988;33:306-307.

Askerov VF, Piriev GG. [Clinico-immunological reactions to a live measles vaccine of strain L-16 in children suffering from exudative diathesis and bronchial asthma]. Pediatriya 1977;56:32-33.

Askerov VF, Sadykhova AN. [Effect of measles infection and measles vaccination on the immunological reactivity in the child] Vliianie korevoi infektsii i protivokorevoi vaktsinatsii na immunologicheskuiu reaktivnost' detskogo organizma. Pediatriia 1968;7:34-39.

Assaad FA, Cockburn WC, Perkins FT. The relation between acute persisting spinal paralysis and poliomyelitis vaccine (oral): results of a WHO enquiry. Bulletin of the World Health Organization 1976;53:319-331.

Assis JL. Neurological complication of antirabies vaccination in Sao Paulo, Brazil: clinical and therapeutical aspects. Journal of Neurological Sciences 1975;26:593-598.

Association for the Study of Infectious Disease. A retrospective survey of the complications of mumps. Journal of the Royal College of General Practitioners 1974;24:552-556.

Astabatsian MA, Bolotovskii VM, Gelikman BG, Mikheeva IV. [Reactogenic properties and immunogenicity of measles and mumps vaccines when used by different procedures] Reaktogennye svoistva i immunogennost korevoi i parotitnoi vaktsin pri razlichnoi taktike ikh primenenii. Zhurnal Mikrobiologii, Epidemiologii, i Immunobiologii 1986;6:9-15.

Aukrust L, Almeland TL, Refsum D, Aas K. Severe hypersensitivity or intolerance reactions to measles vaccine in six children: clinical and immunological studies. Allergy 1980;35:581-587.

Australian Family Physician. Tetanus immunoprophylaxis. Australian Family Physician 1978;7:431-435.

Avery OT, Goebel WF. Chemo-immunological studies on conjugated carbohydrate-proteins. II. Immunological specificity of synthetic sugar-protein antigens. Journal of Experimental Medicine 1929;50:533-550.

Ayoola EA, Johnson AO. Hepatitis B vaccine in pregnancy: immunogenicity, safety and transfer of antibodies to infants. International Journal of Gynaecology and Obstetrics 1987;25:297-301.

Azeemuddin S. Thrombocytopenia purpura after combined vaccine against measles, mumps, and rubella (letter). Clinical Pediatrics 1987;26:318.

Azimi PH, Cramblett HG, Haynes RE. Mumps meningoencephalitis in children. Journal of the American Medical Association 1969;207:509-512.

Azzopardi P. Mumps meningitis, possibly vaccine-related—Ontario. Canada Diseases Weekly Report 1988;14:209-211.

Babbott FL Jr., Gordon JE. Modern measles. American Journal of Medical Science 1954;228:334-361.

Bach C, Allard M. [Acute thrombocytopenic purpura after measles vaccination. Report of a case]. Purpura thrombopenique aigu apres vaccination antirougeoleuse. A propos d'une observation. Semaine des Hopitaux de Paris 1974;50:589-593.

Bachand AJ, Rubenstein J, Morrison AN. Thrombocytopenic purpura following live measles vaccine. American Journal of Diseases of Children 1967;113:283-285.

Backes CR. Immunization practices and controversies 1981: Part 1. The "big seven" vaccines. Journal of the American Osteopathic Association 1981;80:595-603.

Bader M. Perspectives on the relative resurgence of mumps in the United States. American Journal of Diseases of Children 1988;142:1021-1022.

Bader M. Polio vaccination during pregnancy (letter). Journal of the American Medical Association 1983;249:2018-2019.

Bader M. Risks from polio vaccination (letter). Journal of the American Medical Association 1984;251:728-729.

Baer CL, Bratt DE, Edwards R, McFarlane H, Utermohlen V. Response of mildly to moderately malnourished children to measles vaccination. West Indian Medical Journal 1986;35:106-111.

Baguley DM, Glasgow GL. Subacute sclerosing panencephalitis and Salk vaccine. Lancet 1973;2:763-765.

Bajoghli M, Naficy AR, Vafai A, Shafa G. Paralytic poliomyelitis in Isfahan. Journal of Tropical Pediatrics and Environmental Child Health 1977;23:236-238.

Bak P. Guillain-Barre syndrome in a Danish county. Neurology 1985;35:207-211.

Bakanov MI. [Development of bronchial asthma attacks in children under the effect of prophylactic immunization] Vozniknovenie pristupov bronkhial'noi astmy u detei pod vliianiem profilakticheskoi immunizatsii. Voprosy Okhrany Materinstva i Detstva 1968;13:78-79.

Balduzzi P, Glasgow LA. Paralytic poliomyelitis in a contact of a vaccinated child. New England Journal of Medicine 1967;276:796-797.

Balfour HH Jr., Amren DP. Rubella, measles and mumps antibodies following vaccination of children: a potential rubella problem. American Journal of Diseases of Children 1978;132:573-577.

Banatvala JE. Insulin-dependent (juvenile-onset, type I) diabetes mellitus: Coxsackie B viruses revisited. Progress in Medical Virology 1987;34:33-54.

Banker DD. Problems in preparation, testing and use of diphtheria, pertussis and tetanus vaccines. Progress in Drug Research 1975;19:229-240.

Banton HJ, Miller PA. An observation of antitoxin titers after booster doses of tetanus toxoid. New England Journal of Medicine 1949;240:13-14.

Bar-Joseph G, Etzioni A, Hemli J, Gershoni-Baruch R et al. Guillain-Barre syndrome in three siblings less than 2 years old. Archives of Disease in Childhood 1991;66:1078-1079.

Baraff LJ, Cherry JD. Nature and rates of adverse reactions associated with pertussis immunization. In: Third International Symposium on Pertussis, National Institutes of Health, 1978. Publication No. (NIH) 79-1830. Bethesda, Md.: Department of Health, Education, and Welfare; 1979:291-296.

Baraff LJ, Cherry JD. Reactogenicity of DTP and DT vaccine. Clinical Research 1979;27:112.

Baraff LJ, Cherry JD. Reactogenicity of DTP and DT vaccines. Pediatric Research 1979;13:794.

Baraff LJ, Cherry JD, Cody CL, March SM, Manclark CR. DTP vaccine reactions: effect of prior reactions on rate of subsequent reactions. Developments in Biological Standardization 1985;61:423-428.

Baraff LJ, Manclark CR, Cherry JD, Christenson P, Marcy SM. Analyses of adverse reactions to diphtheria and tetanus toxoids and pertussis vaccine by vaccine lot, endotoxin content, pertussis vaccine potency and percentage of mouse weight gain. Pediatric Infectious Disease Journal 1989;8:502-507.

Barbanti-Brodano G, Oyanagi S, Katz M, Koprowski H. Presence of two different viral agents in brain cells of patients with subacute sclerosing panencephalitis (SSPE). Proceedings of the Society for Experimental Biology and Medicine 1970;134:230-236.

Barbor PR, Grant DB. Encephalitis after measles vaccination. Lancet 1969;2:55-56.

Barbour ML. *Haemophilus influenzae* type b: carriage and immunity four years after conjugate vaccination. Program Abstracts of the 32nd Interscience Conference on Antimicrobial Agents and Chemotherapy. Abstract 978, p. 273. Washington, DC: American Society for Microbiology; 1992.

Barkin RM, Pichichero ME. Diphtheria-pertussis-tetanus vaccine: reactogenicity of commercial products. Pediatrics 1979;63:256-260.

Barkin RM, Hendley JO, Zahradnik J et al. Capsular polysaccharide *Haemophilus influenzae* type b vaccine: clinical and immunologic responses to two vaccines. Pediatric Infectious Disease Journal 1987;6:20-23.

Barkin RM, Pichichero ME, Samuelson JS, Barkin SZ. Pediatric diphtheria and tetanus toxoids vaccine: clinical and immunologic response when administered as the primary series. Journal of Pediatrics 1985;106:779-781.

Barkin RM, Samuelson JS, Gotlin LP. DTP reactions and serologic response with a reduced dose schedule. Journal of Pediatrics 1984;105:189-194.

Barkin RM, Samuelson JS, Gotlin LP. Diphtheria and tetanus toxoids and pertussis vaccine adsorbed (DTP): response to varying immunizing dosage and schedule. Developments in Biological Standardization 1985;61:297-307.

Barkin RM, Samuelson JS, Gotlin LP, Barkin SZ. Primary immunization with diphtheria-tetanus toxoids vaccine and diphtheria-tetanus toxoids-pertussis vaccine adsorbed: comparison of schedules. Pediatric Infectious Disease 1985;4:168-171.

Barnett LA, Fujinami RS. Molecular mimicry: a mechanism for autoimmune injury. The FASEB Journal 1992;6:840-844.

Barra A, Cordonnier C, Preziosi MP, Intrator L, Hessel L, Fritzell B et al. Immunogenicity of *Haemophilus influenzae* type b conjugate vaccine in allogeneic bone marrow recipients. Journal of Infectious Diseases 1992;166:1021-1028.

Barrucand D, Schmitt J, Schmidt CL. [Neuropsychiatric complications of rabies immunization] Accidents neuro-psychiatriques de la vaccination antirabique. Annales Medicales de Nancy 1977;16:705-714.

Barsky P. Measles: Winnipeg, 1973. Canadian Medical Association Journal 1974;110:931-934.

Bart KJ, Orenstein WA, Hinman AR. The current status of immunization principles: recommendations for use and adverse reactions. Journal of Allergy and Clinical Immunology 1987;79:296-315.

Bartelheimer HK, Mai K. [Tetanus vaccination in relation to the importance of protection by vaccination] Aktuelles zur Tetanusimpfung im Hinblick auf die Erkennung des Impfshcutzes. Monatsschrift fur Kinderheilkunde 1970;118:558-560.

Basillico FC, Bernat JL. Vaccine-associated poliomyelitis in a contact. Journal of the American Medical Association 1978;239:2275.

Basu RN. Measles vaccine: feasibility, efficacy and complication rates in a multicentric study. Indian Journal of Pediatrics 1984;51:139-143.

Basu SN. Paralytic poliomyelitis following inoculation with combined diphtheria-tetanus-pertussis prophylactic: a review of sixteen cases with special reference to immunisation schedules in infancy. Journal of the Indian Medical Association 1973;60:97-99.

Basu SN. A review of paralytic poliomyelitis cases occurring after polio vaccination. Journal of the Indian Medical Association 1986;84:203-206.

Bateman DE, Elrington G, Kennedy P, Saunders M. Vaccine related poliomyelitis in non-immunised relatives and household contacts. British Medical Journal 1987;294:170-171.

Bather R, Furesz J, Fanok AG et al. Long term infection of diploid African green monkey brain cells by Schwarz measles vaccine virus. Journal of General Virology 1973;20:401-405.

Baublis JV, Payne FE. Measles antigen and syncytium formation in brain cell cultures from subacute sclerosing panencephalitis (SSPE). Proceedings of the Society for Experimental Biology and Medicine 1968;129:593-597.

Baust W, Meyer D, Wachsmuth W. Peripheral neuropathy after administration of tetanus toxoid. Journal of Neurology 1979;222:131-133.

Baxley LM. Tetanus is still deadly. Occupational Health and Nursing 1981;29:40-42.

Beale AJ. Hazards of vaccine production. FEMS Microbiology Letters 1992;79:469-473.

Beale AJ. Measles vaccines. Proceedings of the Royal Society of Medicine 1974;67:1116-1119.

Beard CM, Benson RC, Kelalis PP, Elveback LR, Kurland LT. The incidence and outcome of mumps orchitis in Rochester, Minnesota, 1935-1974. Mayo Clinic Proceedings 1977;52:3-7.

Beasley RP, Hwang LY, Lee GC. Prevention of perinatally transmitted hepatitis B virus infections with hepatitis B immune globulin and hepatitis B vaccine. Lancet 1983;2:1099-1102.

Beaussart M, Lacombe A, Fourrier A, Camier P. [Electroencephalographic study during measles vaccination using the Schwarz vaccine] Etude electroencephalographique au cours de la vaccination contre la rougeole par le vaccin Schwarz. Revue Neurologique 1969;121:324-325.

Beck M, Welsz-Malecek R, Mesko-Prejac M, Radman V, Juzbasic M, Rajninger-Miholic M et al. Mumps vaccine L-Zagreb, prepared in chick fibroblasts. I. Production and field trials. Journal of Biological Standardization 1989;17:85-90.

Beck SA, Williams LW, Shirrell MA, Burks AW. Egg hypersensitivity and measles-mumps-rubella vaccine administration. Pediatrics 1991;88:913-917.

Beckmann R, Manz F, Moser R. [Increased occurrence of "sporadic" spinal progressive muscular atrophy in infancy] Gehauftes "sporadisches" Vorkommen spinaler progressiver Muskelatrophien im Kindesalter. Monatsschrift fur Kinderheilkunde 1970;118:41-44.

Becus-Laurentiu M, Szabo-Adorjan E, Pozsgi N, Szabo S. Etude histochimique de l'ovaire de ratte: l'effet du choc anaphylactique et du vaccin pertussis. Archives Roumaines de Pathologie Experimentale et de Microbiologie 1974;33:97-106.

Beede WE, Newcomb RW. Lower motor neuron paralysis in association with asthma. Johns Hopkins Medical Journal 1980;147:186-187.

Beersma MF, Kapsenberg JG, Renier WO, Galama JM, van Druten JA, Lucas CJ. [Subacute sclerosing panencephalitis in The Netherlands (1976-1986)] Subacute scleroserende panencefalitis in Nederland (1976-1986). Nederlands Tijdschrift voor Geneeskunde 1988;132:1194-1199.

Begaud B, ed. Analyse d'Incidence en Pharmacovigilance: Application a la Notification Spontanee. Bordeaux: ARME-Pharmacovigilance Editions; 1991.

Begg NT, Noah ND, Crowley S, Al-Jawad ST, Kovar IZ. Mumps, measles, and rubella vaccination and encephalitis (letter). British Medical Journal 1989;299:978.

Beghi E, Cornelio F, Marconi M, Rizzuto N, Tonali P. The epidemiology of inflammatory polyradiculoneuropathy: a critical review of the distribution, characteristics and outcome of the disease. Plasmapheresis Study Group. Italian Journal of Neurologic Science 1991;12:63-73.

Beghi E, Kurland LT, Mulder DW. Incidence of acute transverse myelitis in Rochester, Minnesota, 1970-1980, and implications with respect to influenza vaccine. Neuroepidemiology 1982;1:176-188.

Beghi E, Kurland LT, Mulder DW, Nicolosi A. Brachial plexus neuropathy in the population of Rochester, Minnesota, 1970-1981. Annals of Neurology 1985;18:320-323.

Beghi E, Kurland LT, Mulder DW, Wiederholt WC. Guillain-Barre syndrome: clinicoepidemiologic features and effect of influenza vaccine. Archives of Neurology 1985;42:1053-1057.

Beghi E, Nicolosi A, Kurland LT, Mulder DW, Hauser WA, Shuster L. Encephalitis and aseptic meningitis, Olmsted County, Minnesota, 1950-1981. I. Epidemiology. Annals of Neurology 1984;16:283-294.

Behan PO. Diffuse myelitis associated with rubella vaccination. British Medical Journal 1977;1:166.

Bell EJ, Riding MH, Grist NR. Paralytic poliomyelitis: a forgotten diagnosis? British Medical Journal 1986;293:193-194.

Bell JF. Canine distemper, measles, and SSPE. American Journal of Epidemiology 1978;107:354-355.

Bellanti JA, Sanga RL, Klutinis B et al. Antibody responses in serum and nasal secretions of children immunized with inactivated and attenuated measles-virus vaccines. New England Journal of Medicine 1969;260:628-633.

Bellini WJ, Rota JS, Greer FW, Zaki SR et al. Measles vaccination death in a child with severe combined immunodeficiency: report of a case. Laboratory Investigation 1992;66:19A.

Bellman MH, Rawson NS, Wadsworth J, Ross EM, Cameron S, Miller DL. A developmental test based on the STYCAR sequences used in the National Childhood Encephalopathy Study. Child: Care, Health and Development 1985;11:309-323.

Bellman MH, Ross EM, Miller DL. Infantile spasms and pertussis immunisation. Lancet 1983;1:1031-1034.

Benacerraf B, Kabat EA. A quantitative study of the Arthus phenomenon induced passively in the guinea pig. Journal of Immunology 1950;64:1-19.

Bendersky-Malbec N. [Mumps in 1982: current situation concerning anti-mumps vaccine] Les oreillons en 1982: mise au point sur le vaccin anti-ourlien. Concours Medecin 1982;104:167-177.

Bengtsson B. [The side effects of the vaccination of 650 children against measles] Biverkningar vid masslingsvaccination av 650 barn. Lakartidningen 1971;68:2235-2244.

Benison S. International medical cooperation: Dr. Albert Sabin, live poliovirus vaccine and the Soviets. Bulletin of the History of Medicine 1982;56:460-483.

Benjamin CM, Chew GC, Silman AJ. Joint and limb symptoms in children after immunisation with measles, mumps, and rubella vaccine. British Medical Journal 1992;204:1075-1078.

Benjamin CM, Silman AJ. Adverse reactions and mumps, measles and rubella vaccine. Journal of Public Health Medicine 1991;13:32-34.

Bennett AD, Modlin J, Orenstein WA, Brandling. Current status of mumps in the United States. Journal of Infectious Diseases 1975;132:106-109.

Bensasson M, Lanoe R, Assan R. [A case of algodystrophy of the upper limb occurring after tetanus vaccination] Un cas de syndrome algodystrophique du membre superieur survenu apres vaccination antitetanique. Semaine des Hopitaux de Paris 1977;53:2965-2966.

Bergeisen GH, Bauman RJ, Gilmore RL. Neonatal paralytic poliomyelitis: a case report. Archives of Neurology 1986;43:192-194.

Berger JR, Ayyar DR, Sheremata WA. Guillain-Barre syndrome complicating acute hepatitis B: A case with detailed electrophysiological and immunological studies. Archives of Neurology 1981;38:366-368.

Bergeson PS. Immunizations to the deltoid region (letter). Pediatrics 1990;85:134-135.

Bergey GK, Bigalke H, Nelson PG. Differential effects of tetanus toxin on inhibitory and excitatory synaptic transmission in mammalian spinal cord neurons in culture: a presynaptic locus of action for tetanus toxin. Journal of Neurophysiology 1987;57:121-131.

Bergmannova V, Stehlikova J, Domorazkova E. [Immunization of children with reactions to the mixed vaccine against diphtheria, tetanus and whooping cough]. Ceskoslovenska Pediatrie 1988;43:522-526.

Bergouignan FX, Saintarailles J, Roux D, Guillon J, Bonnici JF, Fleury H et al. [Prevention of poliomyelitis: live or killed vaccine? Remarks apropos of 2 cases of poliomyelitis] Prevention de la poliomyelite: vaccin vivant ou tue? Reflexions a propos de 2 cas de poliomyelite. Presse Medicale 1984;13:2241-2243.

Berkovich S, Fikrig S, Brunell PA, Steiner M. Effect of live attenuated mumps vaccine virus on the expression of tuberculin sensitivity. Journal of Pediatrics 1972;80:84-87.

Berkowitz CD, Ward JI, Chiu CE, Marcy SM, Gordon L, Hendley JO et al. Persistence of antibody and booster responses to reimmunization with *Haemophilus influenzae* type b polysaccharide and polysaccharide diphtheria toxoid conjugate vaccines in children initially immunized at 15 to 24 months of age. Pediatrics 1990;85:288-293.

Berkowitz CD, Ward JI, Meier K et al. Safety and immunogenicity of *Haemophilus influenzae* type b polysaccharide and polysaccharide diphtheria toxoid conjugate vaccines in children 15 to 24 months of age. Journal of Pediatrics 1987;110:509-514.

Berlin BS. Convulsions after measles immunisation (letter). Lancet 1983;1:1380.

Bernal A, Garcia-Saiz A, Liacer A, De Ory F, Tello O, Najera R. Poliomyelitis in Spain, 1982-1984: virologic and epidemiologic studies. American Journal of Epidemiology 1987;126:69-76.

Bernard KW, Smith PW, Kader FJ, Moran MJ. Neuroparalytic illness and human diploid cell rabies vaccine. Journal of the American Medical Association 1982;248:3136-3138.

Bernier RH. Improved inactivated poliovirus vaccine: an update. Pediatric Infectious Disease 1986;5:289-292.

Bernstein DI, Smith VE, Schiff GM, Rathfon HM, Boscia JA. Comparison of acellular pertussis vaccine with whole cell vaccine as a booster in children 15 to 18 months and 4 to 6 years of age. Pediatric Infectious Disease Journal 1993;12:131-135.

Bernstein L, Ross RK. Prior medication use and health history as risk factors for non-Hodgkin's lymphoma: preliminary results from a case-control study in Los Angeles County. Cancer Research 1992;52(Suppl.):5510s-5515s.

Bernuau J. [Hepatitis B virus vaccination: a neglected, understated risk] Vaccination contre le virus B de l'hepatite: "un risque ignore, sous-evalue, neglige". Concours Medical 1990;112:1062.

Berry S, Hernandez H, Kanashiro R, Campos M, Azabache V, Gomez G et al. Comparison of high titer Edmonston-Zagreb, Biken-CAM and Schwarz measles vaccines in Peruvian infants. Pediatric Infectious Disease Journal 1992;11:822-827.

Bhagwat SM, Samuel MR. Oral polio vaccine (Sabin): vaccine-associated poliolike illnesses. Indian Journal of Medical Science 1966;29:903-906.

Bhaskaram P, Madhusudan J, Radhrakrishna KV, Raj S. Immunological response to measles vaccination in poor communities. Human Nutrition and Clinical Nutrition 1986;40:295-299.

Bhatnagar SK, Mohan M, Kumar P, Balaya S, Prabhakar AK, Bhargava SK. Optimum age for measles immunisation: study of pre- and post-immunization level of HI antibody titres. Indian Pediatrics 1981;18:625-629.

Bianchi R, Dappen U, Hoigne R. [Anaphylactic shock of humans towards foreign species serum: symptomatology, prevention and therapy] Der anaphylaktische Schock des Menschen auf artfremdes Serum: Symptomatologie, Prophylaxe und Therapie. Helvetica Chirurgica Acta 1967;34:257-273.

Biarez O, Sarrut B, Doreau CG, Etienne J. Comparison and evaluation of nine bibliographic databases concerning adverse drug reactions. DICP, The Annals of Pharmacotherapy 1991;25:1062-1065.

Biberi-Moroeanu S, Muntiu A. Commentary on the oral poliomyelitis vaccine (Sabin): associated cases of acute persisting spinal paralysis. Archives Roumaines de Pathologie Experimentale Microbiologie 1978;37:355-368.

Bichel J. Postvaccinial lymphadenitis developing into Hodgkin's disease. Acta Medica Scandinavica 1976;199:523-525.

Bienfang DC, Kantrowitz FG, Noble JL, Raynor A. Ocular abnormalities after influenza immunization. Archives of Ophthalmology 1977;95:1649.

Bilyk MA, Dubchik GK. [Anaphylactic reaction following subcutaneous administration of tetanus anatoxin] Anafilakticheskaia reaktsiia posle podkozhnogo vvedeniia stolbmiachnogo anatoksina. Klinicheskaia Meditsina 1978;56:137-138.

Biron P, Montpetit P, Infante-Rivard C, Lery L. Myasthenia gravis after general anesthesia and hepatitis B vaccine. Archives of Internal Medicine 1988;148:2685.

Bjorkholm B, Bottiger M, Christenson B et al. Antitoxin antibody levels and the outcome of illness during an outbreak of diphtheria among alcoholics. Scandinavian Journal of Infectious Diseases 1986;18:235-239.

Bjorkholm B, Granstrom M, Wahl M, Hedstrom C-E, Hagberg L. Adverse reactions and immunogenicity in adults to regular and increased dosage of diphtheria vaccine. European Journal of Clinical Microbiology 1987;6:637-640.

Black FL, Hierholzer W, Woodall JP, Pinhiero F. Intensified reactions to measles vaccine in unexposed populations of American Indians. Journal of Infectious Diseases 1971;124:306-317.

Black FL, Pinheiro F, Hierholzer WJ, Lee RV. Epidemiology of infectious disease: the example of measles. Ciba Foundation Symposium 1977;49:115-130.

Black FL, Woodall JP, Pinheiro FD. Measles vaccine reactions in a virgin population. American Journal of Epidemiology 1969;89:168-175.

Black SB. Dramatic reduction in invasive Hib disease in a large California population following HbOC conjugate vaccine in infancy. Program Abstracts of the 32nd Interscience Conference on Antimicrobial Agents and Chemotherapy. Abstract 309, p. 162. Washington, DC: American Society for Microbiology; 1992.

Black SB, Cherry JD, Shinefield HR, Fireman B, Christenson P, Lampert D. Apparent decreased risk of invasive bacterial disease after heterologous childhood immunization. American Journal of Diseases of Children 1991;145:746-749.

Black SB, Shinefield HR, Fireman B, Hiatt R, Polen MV, E., Northern California Kaiser Permanente Vaccine Study Center Pediatrics Group. Efficacy in infancy of oligosaccharide conjugate *Haemophilus influenzae* type b (HbOC) vaccine in a United States population of 61,080 children. Pediatric Infectious Disease Journal 1991;10:97-104.

Black SB, Shinefield HR, Fireman B, Hiatt R. Safety, immunogenicity, and efficacy in infancy of oligosaccharide conjugate *Haemophilus influenzae* type b vaccine in a United States population: possible implications for optimal use. Journal of Infectious Diseases 1992;165(Suppl. 1):S139-S143.

Black SB, Shinefield HR, Hiatt RA, Fireman BH, Beekly M, Callas ER et al. Efficacy of *Haemophilus influenzae* type b capsular polysaccharide vaccine. Pediatric Infectious Disease Journal 1988;7:149-156.

Black SB, Shinefield HR, Kaiser Permanente Pediatric Vaccine Study Group. Immunization with oligosaccharide conjugate *Haemophilus influenzae* type b (HbOC) vaccine in a large health maintenance organization population: extended follow-up and impact on *Haemophilus influenzae* disease epidemiology. Pediatric Infectious Disease Journal 1992;11:610-613.

Black SB, Shinefield HR, Lampert D, Fireman B, Hiatt RA, Polen M et al. Safety and immunogenicity of oligosaccharide conjugate *Haemophilus influenzae* type b (HbOC) vaccine in infancy. Pediatric Infectious Disease Journal 1991;10:92-96.

Black SB, Shinefield HR, Northern California Permanente Medical Care Program Departments of Pediatrics Vaccine Study Group. b-CAPSA I *Haemophilus influenzae*, type b, capsular polysaccharide vaccine safety. Pediatrics 1987;79:321-325.

Blake L. Immunizations may pose risks (letter). Nursing BC 1992;24:7-8.

Blanco JD, Gibbs RS. Immunizations in pregnancy. Clinical Obstetrics and Gynecology 1982;25:611-617.

Blattner RJ. Paralytic poliomyelitis: contacts of vaccinated children. Journal of Pediatrics 1967;71:759-762.

Blom L, Nystrom L, Dahlquist G. The Swedish childhood diabetes study: vaccinations and infections as risk determinants for diabetes in childhood. Diabetologia 1991;34:176-181.

Bloom JL, Schiff GM, Graubarth H, Lipp RW Jr, Jackson JE, Osborn RL et al. Evaluation of a trivalent measles, mumps, rubella vaccine in children. Journal of Pediatrics 1975;87:85-87.

Blumberg BS, Sutnick AI, London, WT. Australia antigen and hepatitis. Journal of the American Medical Association 1969;207:1895-1896.

Blumberg S, Bienfang D, Kantrowitz FG. A possible association between influenza vaccination and small-vessel vasculitis. Archives of Internal Medicine 1980;140:847-848.

Blumstein GI, Kreithen H. Peripheral neuropathy following tetanus toxoid administration. Journal of the American Medical Association 1966;198:1030-1031.

Bock LL. Mumps virus vaccine. Pediatrics 1969;43:907.

Bodansky HJ, Dean BM, Grant PJ, McNally J, Schweiger MS, Hambling MH et al. Does exposure to rubella virus generate endocrine autoimmunity? Diabetic Medicine 1990;7:611-614.

Bodansky HJ, Dean BM, Bottazzo GF, Grant PJ, McNally J, Hambling MH et al. Islet-cell antibodies and insulin autoantibodies in association with common viral infections. Lancet 1986;2:1351-1353.

Bodansky HJ, Littlewood JM, Bottazzo GF, Dean BM, Hambling MH. Which virus causes the initial islet lesion in type I diabetes. Lancet 1984;1:401-402.

Bodechtel G. [Juvenile spinal muscular atrophy following polio vaccination?] Juvenile spinale Muskelatrophie nach Polio-Impfung? (letter). Munchener Medizinische Wochenschrift 1975;117:269.

Bodechtel G, Haas R, Joppich G, Lennartz H, Siegert R. [Vaccination complications after oral poliomyelitis vaccination] Zur Frage der Impfschaden nach der Poliomyelitis-Schluckimpfung. Munchener Medizinische Wochenschrift 1977;119:521-528.

Bodian D. A reconsideration of the pathogenesis of poliomyelitis. American Journal of Hygiene 1952;55:414-438.

Bodian D, Morgan I. M., Howe HA. Differentiation of types of poliomyelitis viruses. III. The grouping of fourteen strains into three basic immunological types. American Journal of Hygiene 1949;49:234-245.

Boe E, Nyland H. Guillain-Barre syndrome after vaccination with human diploid cell rabies vaccine. Scandinavian Journal of Infectious Diseases 1980;12:231-232.

Boese T, Lipinski C. [Vaccine-related paralytic poliomyelitis with severe pareses: report of one case] Impfpoliomyelitis mit schwerer Restlahmung: Kasuistischer Beitrag zur Frage der Impfschadigung nach oraler Polioimpfung nach Sabin. Klinische Paediatrie 1978;190:607-609.

Bogli F. [Immunization campaigns in Switzerland] Impfkampagne in der Schweiz. Schweiz Apotheker-Zeitung / Journal suisse de pharmacie 1988;126:160-161.

Bojinov PS, Kirov I, Georgiev I, Miltov G, Kohen M, Ninov N et al. Encephale-myelo-polyradiculonevrites a la suite de l'utilization de vaccin antipoliomyelituque de Sabin a germe vivant. Presse Medicale 1964;72:75-79.

Boletin de la Oficina Sanitaria Panamericana. [Indications and contraindications for immunization] Indicaciones y contraindicaciones de la inmunizacion. Boletin de la Oficina Sanitaria Panamericana 1984;97:72-79.

Boles JM. [Major local reaction after self-injection of diphtheria-tetanus vaccine] Reaction locale majeure apres rappel de vaccination antitetanique et antidiphterique. Medecine et Maladies Infectieuses 1985;15:558-560.

Boling HL. An adult's reaction to measles vaccine. American Journal of Nursing 1980;80:1442-1443.

Bolotovskij VM, Zetilova LP. Comparative study of the reaction-causing properties and the immunological and epidemiological effectiveness of Leningrad-16 and Schwarz live measles vaccines. Bulletin of the World Health Organization 1968;39:293-298.

Bondarev VN, Dadiomova MA. [The changes of the nervous system in children after vaccination] K voprosu o postvaktsinal'nykh izmeneniiakh nervnoi sistemy u detei. Pediatriia 1969;48:20-24.

Bondarev VN, Dadiomova MA, Torosov TM. [On the pathogenesis of several postvaccinal pathologic reactions in children] O patogeneze nekotorykh postvaktsinal'nykh patologicheskikh reaktsii u detei. Voprosy Okhrany Materinstva i Detstva 1968;13:46-48.

Bondarev VN, Dadiomova MA, Pratusevich RM. [Several complications after immunization with associated whooping cough-diphtheria-tetanus, antimeasles and antipoliomyelitis vaccines] Nekotorye oslozhneniia posle immunizatsii assotsiirovannoi kokliushno-difteriino-stolbniachnoi, protivokorevoi i protivopoliomielitnoi vaktsinami. Pediatriia 1968;47:26-29.

Booy R, Moxon ER. Immunisation of infants against *Haemophilus influenzae* type b in the UK. Archives of Disease in Childhood 1991;66:1251-1254.

Booy R, Moxon ER, MacFarlane JA, Mayon-White RT, Slack MP E. Efficacy of *Haemophilus influenzae* type b conjugate vaccine in the Oxford region. Lancet 1992;340:47.

Booy R, Taylor SA, Dobson SR, Isaacs D, Sleight G, Aitken S et al. Immunogenicity and safety of PRP-T conjugate vaccine given according to the British accelerated immunisation schedule. Archives of Disease in Childhood 1992;67:475-478.

Borgono JM, Greiber R, Solari G, Concha F, Carrillo B, Hilleman MR. A field trial of combined measles-mumps-rubella vaccine: satisfactory immunization with 188 children in Chile. Clinical Pediatrics 1973;12:170-172.

Borsche A. [What are the hazards of vaccinations in childhood?] Wie gefahrlich sind Impfungen im Kindesalter. Zeitschrift fur Allemeinmedizin 1976;52:666-674.

Bothig B, Gerike E, Starke G, Giesecke H. [On the simultaneous use of live-virus vaccines, for example measles-polio vaccine] Beitrag zur Frage der simultanen Applikation von Lebendvirus-Impfstoffen am Beispiel Masern—Polio. Revue Roumaine de Virologie 1974;25:15-21.

Bottazzo GF, Gorsuch AN, Dean BM, Cudworth AG, Doniach D. Complement-fixing islet-cell antibodies in type-I diabetes: possible monitors of active beta-cell damage. Lancet 1980;1:668-672.

Bottiger M, Christenson B, Romanus V, Taranger J, Strandell A. Swedish experience of two dose vaccination programme aiming at eliminating measles, mumps, and rubella. British Medical Journal 1987;295:1264-1267.

Bottiger M, Heller L, Kamensky P, Svanberg B. [Measles vaccination of preschool children: reactions and side effects after immunization with vaccine of three different strengths]. Lakartidningen 1974;71:3270-3274.

Bottiger M, Mellin P, Romanus V, Soderstrom H, Wesslen T, von Zeipel G. [Epidemiology of a case of poliomyelitis] Epidemiologin kring ett poliofall i Sverige. Lakartidningen 1979;76:30-34.

Boulton-Jones JM, Sissons JG, Naish PF, Evans DJ, Peters DK. Self-induced glomerulonephritis. British Medical Journal 1974;3:387-390.

Bourke J, Roy CW. Paralytic poliomyelitis. New Zealand Medical Journal 1992;105:36-37.

Bouteille M, Fontaine C, Vedredd CL, Delarue J. Sur un cas d'encephalite subaigue a inclusions: etude anatomo-clinique et ultrastructurate. Revue Neurologique 1965;113:454-458.

Bouter KP, Diepersloot RJ, Wismans PJ, Gmelig Meyling FH, Hoekstra JB, Heijtink RA et al. Humoral immune response to a yeast-derived hepatitis B vaccine in patients with type 1 diabetes mellitus. Diabetic Medicine 1992;9:66-69.

Bouvier-Colle MH, Flahaut A, Messiah A, Jougla E, Hatton F. Sudden infant death and immunization: an extensive epidemiological approach to the problem in France—winter 1986. International Journal of Epidemiology 1989;18:121-126.

Boxall EH, Plester GL, Webber S. Vaccine hypersensitivity or coincidental virus infection (letter). Vaccine 1989;7:77.

Boyd JS. Tetanus in the African and European theatres of war, 1939-1945. Lancet 1946;1:113-119.

Braginskaia VP, Shabad AT, Manvelova MA, Aleksina SG, Podshivalova VA. [Use of reduced doses of diphtheria-tetanus toxoid for revaccination of children with changed reactivity] Primenenie umen'shennykh doz difteriino-stol'bniachnogo anatoksina dlia revaktsinatsii detei s izmenennoi reaktvinost'iu. Voprosy Okhrany Materinstva i Detstva 1974;19:65-69.

Braginskaya VP, Sokolova AF. [Postvaccinal complications and their prevention]. Pediatriya 1974;53:26-31.

Brandt AM. Polio, politics, publicity, and duplicity: ethical aspects in the development of the Salk vaccine. International Journal of Health Services 1978;8:257-270.

Breman JG, Hayner NS. Guillain-Barre syndrome and its relationship to swine influenza vaccination in Michigan, 1976-1977. American Journal of Epidemiology 1984;119:880-889.

Brieger P, Ehrlich P. Beitrage zur Kenntniss der Milch immunisirter Thiere. Zeltschrift fur Hygiene und Infektionskrankheiten 1893;13:336-346.

Brigaud M, Aymard M, Thouvenot D, Chomel JJ, Mahmood RA, Mathew PP et al. Poliomyelitis survey in Middle-East countries. Developments in Biological Standardization 1978;41:149-158.

Brightman CA, Scadding GK, Dumbreck LA, Latchman Y, Brostoff J. Yeast-derived hepatitis B vaccine and yeast sensitivity (letter). Lancet 1989;1:903.

Brindle MJ, Twyman DG. Allergic reactions to tetanus toxoid. British Medical Journal 1962;1:1116-1117.

Brink EW, Wassilak SG. Diseases controlled primarily by vaccination: diphtheria. In: Last JM, Wallace RB, eds. Maxcy-Rosenau-Last Public Health and Preventive Medicine, 13th ed. Norwalk, CT: Appleton & Lange; 1992.

British Medical Journal. Vaccination against measles: a clinical trial of live measles vaccine given alone and live vaccine preceded by killed vaccine. A report to the Medical Research Council by the Measles Vaccines Committee. British Medical Journal 1966;1:441-446.

British Medical Journal. Vaccination against measles. British Medical Journal 1968;1:395-396.

British Medical Journal. Medical news: measles vaccine. British Medical Journal 1969;1:791.

British Medical Journal. A measles vaccine withdrawn. British Medical Journal 1969;1:794-795.

British Medical Journal. Reactions to tetanus toxoid (editorial). British Medical Journal 1974;1:48.

British Medical Journal. Guillain-Barre syndrome and influenza vaccine (editorial). British Medical Journal 1977;1:1373-1374.

British Medical Journal. Subacute sclerosing panencephalitis (editorial). British Medical Journal 1979;2:6198.

British Medical Journal. Prevention of mumps (editorial). British Medical Journal 1980;281:1231-1232.

British Medical Journal. Report from the PHLS Communicable Disease Surveillance Centre. British Medical Journal 1986;293:195-196.

British Medical Journal. Measles, mumps, and rubella vaccine. British Medical Journal 1988;297:780-781.

Broadhurst LE, Erickson RL, Kelley PW. Decreases in invasive *Haemophilus influenzae* diseases in US Army children, 1984 through 1991. Journal of the American Medical Association 1993;269:227-231.

Brodsky L, Stanievich J. Sensorineural hearing loss following live measles virus vaccination. International Journal of Pediatric Otorhinolaryngology 1985;10:159-163.

Brody JA, McAlister R. Depression of tuberculin sensitivity following measles vaccination. American Review of Respiratory Diseases 1964;90:611-617.

Brody JA, Overfield T, Hammes LM. Depression of the tuberculin reaction by viral vaccines. New England Journal of Medicine 1964;271:1294-1296.

Brooks R, Reznik A. Guillain-Barre syndrome following trivalent influenza vaccine in an elderly patient. Mount Sinai Journal of Medicine 1980;47:190-191.

Brouwer R. Vaccination of infants in their first year of life with split inactivated measles vaccine incorporated in a diphtheria-pertussis-tetanus-polio (inactivated) vaccine (DPTP-M), compared with live measles vaccination. Journal of Biological Standardization 1976;4: 13-23.

Brown EG, Furesz J, Dimock K, Yarosh W, Contreras G. Nucleotide sequence analysis of Urabe mumps vaccine strain that caused meningitis in vaccine recipients. Vaccine 1991;9:840-842.

Brown FR, Wolfe HI. Chick embryo grown measles vaccine in an egg-sensitive child. Journal of Pediatrics 1967;71:868-869.

Brown GC, Kendrick PL. Serologic response of infants to combined inactivated measles-poliomyelitis vaccine. American Journal of Public Health/Nations Health 1965;55:1813-1819.

Brummer E, Bhardwaj N, Lawrence HS. A method for eliciting indurated DTH reactions to soluble protein antigens in the flank skin of mice: correlation of visual measurements with 125I-UdR uptake indices. International Archives of Allergy and Applied Immunology 1981;64:266-276.

Brunell PA. The prevention of infectious diseases by immunization. Journal of Allergy and Clinical Immunology 1987;79:848-852.

Brunell PA, Bass JW, Daum RS et al. *Hemophilus* type b polysaccharide vaccine. Pediatrics 1985;76:322-324.

Brunell PA, Novelli VM, Lipton SV, Pollock B. Combined vaccine against measles, mumps, rubella, and varicella. Pediatrics 1988;81:779-784.

Brunell PA, Weigle K, Murphy MD et al. Antibody response following measles-mumps-rubella vaccine under conditions of customary use. Journal of the American Medical Association 1983;250:1409-1412.

Bruno G, Giampietro PG, Grandolfo ME, Milita O, Businco L. Safety of measles immunisation in children with IgE-mediated egg allergy (letter). Lancet 1990;335:739.

Bryett KA, Mathews AH, Bakhshi SS, Schweiger MS. Diphtheria and tetanus vaccine: a comparative study of reactogenicity. British Journal of Clinical Practice 1989;43:52-54.

Buchner H, Ferbert A, Hundgen R. [Polyneuritis cranialis, brain-stem encephalitis and myelitis following influenza] Polyneuritis cranialis, hirnstammenzephalitis und myelitis nach influenzaschutzimpfung. Nervenarzt 1988;59:679-682.

Buck BE, Yang LC, Caleb MH, Green JM, South MA. Measles virus panniculitis subsequent to vaccine administration. Journal of Pediatrics 1982;101:366-373.

Bulletin of the World Health Organization. Evidence on the safety and efficacy of live poliomyelitis vaccines currently in use, with special reference to type 3 poliovirus. Bulletin of the World Health Organization 1969;40:925-945.

Bunch C, Schwartz FC, Bird GW. Paroxysmal cold haemoglobinuria following measles immunization. Archives of Disease in Childhood 1972;47:299-300.

Bunnell CE, Monif GR. Interstitial pancreatitis in the congenital rubella syndrome. Journal of Pediatrics 1972;80:465-466.

Buntain WL, Missall SR. Local subcutaneous atrophy following measles, mumps, and rubella vaccination (letter). American Journal of Diseases of Children 1976;130:335.

Burgess MA. Immunisation: risks vs benefits in the community. Current Therapeutics 1987;28:19-31.

Burkholder JN. Severe vaccine reaction (letter). Canadian Medical Association Journal 1978;118:1027.

Burmester GR, Altstidl U, Kalden JR. Stimulatory response towards the 65 kDa heat shock protein and other mycobacterial antigens in patients with rheumatoid arthritis. Journal of Rheumatology 1991;18:171-176.

Buser F. Side reaction to measles vaccination suggesting the Arthus phenomenon. New England Journal of Medicine 1967;277:250-251.

Bussens P, Pilette J. [Unrecognized complications of oral antipoliomyelitis vaccination] Complications meconnues de la vaccination antipoliomyelitique par voie orale. Revue Medicale de Liege 1976;31:608-611.

Butler H. Hepatitis B in New Zealand. Submitted to Institute of Medicine Vaccine Safety Committee, April 4, 1992. Unpublished.

Buynak EB, Hilleman MR. Live attenuated mumps virus vaccine. I. Vaccine development. Proceedings of the Society for Experimental Biology and Medicine 1966;123:768-775.

Buynak EB, Weibel RE, Whitman JE Jr., Stokes JJ, Hilleman MR. Combined live measles, mumps, and rubella virus vaccines. Journal of the American Medical Association 1969;207:2259-2262.

Bychenko BD, Stroganova MK, Matveev KI, Runova VF, Petrov AN. [Use of tetanus allergen to determine human sensitivity to tetanus toxoid] Primenenie stolbniachnogo allergena dlia opredeleniia chuvstvitelnost liudei k stolbniachnomu anatoksinu. Zhurnal Mikrobiologii, Epidemiologii, i Immunobiologii 1971;48:83-87.

Cabrera J, Griffin DE, Johnson RT. Unusual features of the Guillain-Barre syndrome after rabies vaccine prepared in suckling mouse brain. Journal of Neurological Science 1987;81:239-245.

Cailleba A, Beytout J, Lauras H et al. Shock associated with disseminated intravascular coagulation syndrome after injection of DT-tab vaccine [Choc associe a un syndrome de coagulation intravasculaire disseminee apres une injection de vaccin DT.tab]. Presse Medicale 1984;13:1900.

Campbell AG. Brother-to-sister transmission of measles after MMR immunisation (letter). Lancet 1989;1:442.

Campbell AG. Mumps, measles, and rubella vaccination and encephalitis (letter). British Medical Journal 1989;299:916.

Campbell H, Byass P, Ahonkhai VI, Vella PP, Greenwood BM. Serologic responses to an *Haemophilus influenzae* type b polysaccharide-*Neisseria meningitidis* outer membrane protein conjugate vaccine in very young Gambian infants. Pediatrics 1990;86:102-107.

Campion JJ, Casto DT. *Haemophilus influenzae* type b conjugate vaccine. Journal of Pediatric Health Care 1988;2:215-218.

Canadian Medical Association Journal. Tetanus toxoid. Canadian Medical Association Journal 1968;98:123.

Canadian Medical Association Journal. Anaphylaxis due to vaccination in the office (letters). Canadian Medical Association Journal 1986;134:1109.

Canadian Medical Association Journal. In support of a compensation plan for vaccine-associated injuries. Canadian Medical Association Journal 1986;135:747-749.

Canadian Medical Association Journal. Vaccine-associated poliomyelitis in Quebec. Canadian Medical Association Journal 1987;137:418-419.

Canadian Medical Association Journal. A case of mumps meningitis: a complication of vaccination? Canadian Medical Association Journal 1988;138:135.

Canadian Medical Association Journal. Universal vaccination against hepatitis B. Canadian Medical Association Journal 1992;146:36.

Canadian Medical Association Journal. Alleged link between hepatitis B vaccine and chronic fatigue syndrome. Canadian Medical Association Journal 1992;146:37-38.

Canadian Medical Association Journal. Statement on *Haemophilus influenzae* type b conjugate vaccines for use in infants and children. Canadian Medical Association Journal 1992;146:1363-1366, 1369-1372.

Canadian Medical Association Journal. Adverse events after hepatitis B vaccination. Canadian Medical Association Journal 1992;147:1023-1026.

Canadian Medical Association Journal. Statement on *Haemophilus influenzae* type b conjugate vaccines for use in infants and children. Canadian Medical Association Journal 1993;148:199-214.

Capeding MR, Lazaro JA, Kaneko YY. Pre-discharge immunization among hospitalized Filipino children. Pediatric Infectious Disease Journal 1990;9:570-573.

Carey AB, Meltzer EO. Diagnosis and "desensitization" in tetanus vaccine hypersensitivity. Annals of Allergy 1992;69:336-338.

Cario WR, Schneeweiss B. [Acute thrombocytopenic purpura following virus vaccinations] Akute thrombozytopenische Purpura nach Virusimpfungen. Kinderarztliche Praxis 1972;40:448-453.

Carmeli Y, Oren R. Hepatitis B vaccine side-effect. Lancet 1993;341:250-251.

Carrada-Bravo T. [Epidemiology and control of poliomyelitis. II. Poliovirus vaccines] Epidemiologia y control de la poliomielitis. II. Vacunas antipoliomieliticas. Boletin Medico del Hospital Infantil de Mexico 1983;40:604-612.

Carroll JE, Jedziniak M, Guggenheim MA. Guillain-Barre syndrome: another cause of the "floppy infant." American Journal of Diseases of Children 1977;131:699-700.

Casas Vila MC. [Adverse drug reactions in children: in vivo diagnosis] Reacciones adversas a medicamentos en el nino: diagnostico in vivo. Revista Espanola Alergologia e Immunologia Clinica 1992;7(Suppl. 1):5-7.

Cassata F, Raimondo L. [On the side-effects of poliomyelitis vaccination with the Sabin method] Considerazioni sugli effetti collaterali della vaccinazione antipolio col metodo Sabin. Pediatria (Napoli) 1970;78:26-43.

Castan P, Dehing J. [Coma revealing an acute leukosis in a child, 15 days after an oral antipoliomyelitis vaccination: anatomoclinical study and reflections on cerebral lesions in acute leukoses] Coma revelateur d'une leucose aigue chez un enfant, quinze jours apres une vaccination perorale antipoliomyelitique: etude anatomoclinique et reflexions sur les lesions cerebrales des leucoses aigues. Acta Neurologica et Psychiatrica Belgica 1965;65:349-367.

Castillo Salinas F, Sole Mir E, Ferrer Comalat A, Morales Sanchez M. [Benign intracranial hypertension caused by DTP and polio immunization] Hipertension endocraneal benigna tras inmunizacion con DTP y polio. Anales Espanoles de Pediatria 1990;32:466-467.

Castillo J, Medina G, Carnevale A. Frequency of sister-chromatid exchanges in children vaccinated against measles. Mutation Research 1983;119:65-69.

Cates KL. Serum opsonic activity for *Haemophilus influenzae* type b in infants immunized with polysaccharide-protein vaccines. Journal of Infectious Diseases 1985;152:1076-1077.

Cates KL, Marsh KH, Granoff DM. Serum opsonic activity after immunization of adults with *Haemophilus influenzae* type b-diphtheria toxoid conjugate vaccine. Infection and Immunity 1985;48:183-189.

Cavanagh NP, Brett EM, Marshall WC, Wilson J. The possible adjuvant role of *Bordetella pertussis* and pertussis vaccine in causing severe encephalopathic illness: a presentation of three case histories. Neuropediatrics 1981;12:374-381.

Cencora V, Challoner F, Gooch S, Livingstone A, Widgery D. Immunisation of neonates at risk of hepatitis B. British Medical Journal 1988;297:481.

Centers for Disease Control. Recommendations of the Public Health Service Advisory Committee on Immunization Practices: Measles vaccines. Morbidity and Mortality Weekly Report 1967;16:169-271.

Centers for Disease Control. Poliomyelitis prevention. Morbidity and Mortality Weekly Report 1982;31:22-26, 31-34.

Centers for Disease Control. Vaccine-associated poliomyelitis: United States, 1981. Morbidity and Mortality Weekly Report 1982;31:97-98.

Centers for Disease Control. The safety of hepatitis B virus vaccine. Morbidity and Mortality Weekly Report 1983;32:134-136.

Centers for Disease Control. Adverse Events Following Immunization: Surveillance Report No. 1, 1979-1982. Atlanta, Georgia: U.S. Department of Health and Human Services, Public Health Service; August 1984.

Centers for Disease Control. Paralytic poliomyelitis—United States, 1982 and 1983. Morbidity and Mortality Weekly Report 1984;33:635-638.

Centers for Disease Control. Hepatitis B vaccine: evidence confirming lack of AIDS transmission. Morbidity and Mortality Weekly Report 1984;33:685-687.

Centers for Disease Control, Immunization Practices Advisory Committee. Polysaccharide vaccine for prevention of *Haemophilus influenzae* type b disease. Morbidity and Mortality Weekly Report 1985;34:201-205.

Centers for Disease Control. Recommendations for protection against viral hepatitis. Morbidity and Mortality Weekly Report 1985;34:313-335.

Centers for Disease Control. Adverse Events Following Immunization: Surveillance Report No. 2, 1982-1984. Atlanta, Georgia: U.S. Department of Health and Human Services, Public Health Service; December 1986.

Centers for Disease Control. Update: poliomyelitis outbreak—Finland, 1984-1985. Morbidity and Mortality Weekly Report 1986;35:82-86.

Centers for Disease Control. Poliomyelitis—United States, 1975-1984. Morbidity and Mortality Weekly Report 1986;35:180-182.

Centers for Disease Control. Epidemiologic classification of reported cases of paralytic poliomyelitis, U.S.A., 1975-1986. Unpublished. Received from CDC, 1987.

Centers for Disease Control. Poliomyelitis prevention: enhanced-potency inactivated poliomyelitis vaccine—supplementary statement. Morbidity and Mortality Weekly Report 1987;36:795-798.

Centers for Disease Control. Update: prevention of *Haemophilus influenzae* type b disease. Morbidity and Mortality Weekly Report 1988;37:13-16.

Centers for Disease Control. Adverse Events Following Immunization: Surveillance Report No. 3, 1985-1986. Atlanta, Georgia: U.S. Department of Health and Human Services, Public Health Service; February 1989.

Centers for Disease Control. Update: *Haemophilus influenzae* type b vaccine. Morbidity and Mortality Weekly Report 1989;38:14.

Centers for Disease Control. Mumps prevention. Morbidity and Mortality Weekly Report 1989;38:388-392, 397-400.

Centers for Disease Control. Measles prevention. Morbidity and Mortality Weekly Report 1989;38(Suppl 9):1-18.

Centers for Disease Control. Recommendations of the Immunization Practices Advisory Committee, Supplementary Statement: change in administration schedule for *Haemophilus* b conjugate vaccines. Morbidity and Mortality Weekly Report 1990;39:232-233.

Centers for Disease Control. Food and Drug Administration approval of a *Haemophilus* b conjugate vaccine for infants. Morbidity and Mortality Weekly Report 1990;39:698-699.

Centers for Disease Control. Vaccine Adverse Event Reporting System—United States. Morbidity and Mortality Weekly Report 1990;39:730-733.

Centers for Disease Control. Decline in *Haemophilus influenzae* type b meningitis—Seattle-King County, Washington, 1984-1989. Morbidity and Mortality Weekly Report 1990;39:924-925.

Centers for Disease Control. Food and Drug Administration approval of use of *Haemophilus* b conjugate vaccine for infants. Morbidity and Mortality Weekly Report 1990;39:925-926.

Centers for Disease Control. Protection against viral hepatitis. Recommendations of the Immunization Practices Advisory Committee (ACIP). Morbidity and Mortality Weekly Report 1990;39(RR-2):1-26.

Centers for Disease Control. *Haemophilus* b conjugate vaccines for prevention of *Haemophilus influenzae* type b disease among infants and children two months of age and older. Recommendations of the Immunization Practices Advisory Committee (ACIP). Morbidity and Mortality Weekly Report 1991;40(RR-1):1-7.

Centers for Disease Control. Surveillance of *Escherichia coli* O157 isolation and confirmation, United States, 1988. Morbidity and Mortality Weekly Report 1991;40(SS-1):1-6.

Centers for Disease Control. Misclassification of infant deaths—Alaska, 1990-1991. Morbidity and Mortality Weekly Report 1992;41:584-591.

Centers for Disease Control. Food and Drug Administration approval of use of a new *Haemophilus* b conjugate vaccine and a combined diphtheria-tetanus-pertussis and *Haemophilus* b conjugate vaccine for infants and children. Morbidity and Mortality Weekly Report 1993;42:296-298.

Centers for Disease Control and Prevention. Recommendations of the Advisory Committee on Immunization Practices (ACIP): Use of vaccines and immune globulins in persons with altered immunocompetence. Morbidity and Mortality Weekly Report 1993;42(RR-4):1-18.

Centers for Disease Control and Prevention. Standards for Pediatric Immunization Practices. Morbidity and Mortality Weekly Report 1993;42(RR-5):1-13.

Centers for Disease Control and Prevention, Division of Immunization. Summaries of five cases, from review of records to identify all deaths among confirmed cases of vaccine-associated paralytic poliomyelitis reported to CDC during the period 1980-1991. Unpublished data.

Cernescu C, Cajal N, Popescu-Tismana G. SSPE: epidemiological and serological features in a series of cases recorded between 1975 and 1984. Virologie 1985;36:247-254.

Cernescu C, Milea S, Berbescu C, Pastia M, Popescu L. S.S.P.E.: some clues to pathogenesis from epidemiological data. Virologie 1988;39:247-256.

Cernescu C, Popescu-Tismana G, Alaicescu M, Popescu L, Cajal N. The continuous decrease in the number of SSPE annual cases ten years after compulsory anti-measles immunization. Revue Roumaine de Virologie 1990;41:13-18.

Cesario TC, Nakano JH, Caldwell GG, Youmans RA. Paralytic poliomyelitis in an unimmunized child: apparent result of a vaccine-derived poliovirus. American Journal of Diseases of Children 1969;118:895-898.

Chaiken BP, Williams NW, Preblud SR, Parkin W, Altman R. The effect of a school entry law on mumps activity in a school district. Journal of the American Medical Association 1987;257:2455-2458.

Chaleomchan W, Hemachudha T, Sakulramrung R, Deesomchok U. Anticardiolipin antibodies in patients with rabies vaccination induced neurological complications and other neurological diseases. Journal of Neurological Science 1990;96:143-151.

Champagne S, Thomas E. A case of mumps meningitis: a post-immunization complication? / Cas de meningite ourlienne: complication vaccinale? Canada Diseases Weekly Report / Rapport hebdomadaire des maladies au Canada 1987;13:155-157.

Champsaur HF, Bottazzo GF, Bertrams J, Assan R, Bach C. Virologic, immunologic, and genetic factors in insulin-dependent diabetes mellitus. Journal of Pediatrics 1982;100:15-20.

Chan CY, Lee SD, Tsai YT, Yue MI, Lo KJ. Long-term follow-up of hepatitis B vaccination in infants born to noncarrier mothers in Taiwan. Chinese Medical Journal 1992;50:83-88.

Chan CC, Sogg RL, Steinman L. Isolated oculomotor palsy after measles immunization. American Journal of Ophthalmology 1980;89:446-448.

Chan H-L, Stern RS, Arndt KA, Langlois J, Jick SS, Jick H et al. The incidence of erythema multiforme, Stevens-Johnson syndrome, and toxic epidermal necrolysis. Archives of Dermatology 1990;126:43-47.

Chandra P. Trends in immunisation. Antiseptic 1979;76:729-739.

Chandra RK. Polio-virus vaccines: an iota of risk? Indian Journal of Pediatrics 1965;32:335-336.

Chandra RK. Reactions following measles vaccination. Indian Journal of Pediatrics 1967;34:423-424.

Chandra RK. Reduced secretory antibody response to live attenuated measles and poliovirus vaccines in malnourished children. British Medical Journal 1975;2:583-585.

Chang HH. Immunization problems in measles, rubella and mumps. Journal of the Korean Medical Assocication 1982;25:801-806.

Chang TW, Weinstein L, MacMahon HE. Paralytic poliomyelitis in a child with hypogammaglobulinemia: probable implication of type I vaccine strain. Pediatrics 1966;37:630-636.

Chanukoglu A, Fried D, Gotlieb A. [Anaphylactic shock due to tetanus toxoid]. Harefuah 1975;89:456-457.

Chauplannaz G, Trepo C, Brunon AM, Bady B. [Polyneuropathy following vidarabine therapy of chronic active hepatitis] Neuropathie apres traitement d'une hepatite chronique active par vidarabine. Revue Neurologique 1984;140:743-745.

Chen DS, Hsu HM, Sung JL et al. A mass vaccination program in Taiwan against hepatitis B virus infection in infants of hepatitis B surface antigen-carrier mothers. Journal of the American Medical Association 1987;257:2597-2603.

Chen R. Safety of simultaneous administration of DTP and Hib: Preliminary analysis of VAERS data. Presentation given at meeting of Advisory Commission on Childhood Vaccines, March 10, 1993, Washington, DC.

Chen RT, Moses JM, Markowitz LE, Orenstein WA. Adverse events following measles-mumps-rubella and measles vaccinations in college students. Vaccine 1991;9:297-299.

Chen RT, Rastogi SC, Mullen JR, Hayes SW, Cochi SL, Donlon JA, Wassilak SG. The Vaccine Adverse Event Reporting System (VAERS). Atlanta, Georgia: Centers for Disease Control; submitted for publication.

Chen TQ, Li CZ, Ni SF, Shi M, Luo GX, Dong DX. [Studies on new attenuated strains of type I live poliovirus vaccine. II. Investigation on a series of field trials with "Zhong I9" strain]. Chung Kuo I Hsueh Ko Hsueh Yuan Hsueh Pao 1983;5:373-377.

Cherkeziya SE, Mikhailova GR, Gorshunova LP. [Chromosomal aberrations in mice caused by immunization with a set of antiviral vaccines] Narusheniia v khromosomnom apparate myshei, vyzvannye immunizatsiei kompleksom protivovirusnykh vaktsin. Voprosy Virusologii 1979;:547-550.

Cherry JD, Brunell PA, Golden GS, Karzon DT. Report of the task force on pertussis and pertussis immunization—1988. Pediatrics 1988;81(6, Part 2):939-984.

Cheshik SG, Nefedova LA, Bolotovskii VM. [A clinical study of the reactivity of live antimeasles vaccines] Klinicheskoe izuchenie reaktogennosti zhivykh protivokorevykh vaktsin. Sovetskaia Meditsina 1966;29:126-132.

Chinese Medical Journal. Effects of immunization with live mumps vaccine administered by nasal spraying and atomization. Chinese Medical Journal 1976;2:372-375.

Chinese Medical Journal. Studies on new attenuated strains of type III live poliomyelitis vaccine. I. Development of a new type III attenuated poliovirus. Chinese Medical Journal 1980;93:583-590.

Cho CT, Lansky LJ, D'Souza BJ. Panencephalitis following measles vaccination. Journal of the American Medical Association 1973;224:1299.

Chonmaitree T, Lucia H. Presence of vaccine-strain poliovirus in cerebrospinal fluid of patient with near-miss sudden infant death syndrome (letter). American Journal of Diseases of Children 1986;140:1212-1213.

Christau B, Helin P. [Reactive arthritis following vaccination against hepatitis B] Reaktiv artrit efter vaccination mod hepatitis B. Ugeskrift for Laeger 1987;149:1882.

Christensen PE. Side reactions to tetanus toxoid. Scientific Publication, Pan American Health Organization 1972;253:36-43.

Christenson B, Bottiger M. Changes of the immunological patterns against measles, mumps and rubella: a vaccination programme studied 3 to 7 years after the introduction of a two-dose schedule. Vaccine 1991;9:326-329.

Christenson B, Bottiger M, Heller L. Mass vaccination programme aimed at eradicating measles, mumps, and rubella in Sweden: first experience. British Medical Journal 1983;287:389-391.

Christenson B, Bottiger M. Serological immunity to diphtheria in Sweden in 1978 and 1984. Scandinavian Journal of Infectious Diseases 1986;18:227-233.

Christenson B, Heller L, Bottiger M. The immunizing effect and reactogenicity of two live attenuated mumps virus vaccines in Swedish schoolchildren. Journal of Biological Standardization 1983;11:323-331.

Christian MA. Influenza and hepatitis B vaccine acceptance: a survey of health care workers. American Journal of Infection Control 1991;19:177-184.

Christopher PJ. Measles vaccine failures. Medical Journal of Australia 1988;148:103.

Chumakov MP, Voroshilova MK, Grachev VP, Dzagurov SG, Sinyak KM. The development and the study of live measles vaccine from highly attenuated strain Enders-Schwarz-Chumakov (ESC). Progress in Immunobiological Standardization 1969;3:194-195.

Chumakov MP, Voroshilova MK, Grachev VP, Sinyak KM, Boiko VM, Seibil VB et al. Investigation and application of the USSR AMS live measles vaccine from the ESC strain for mass vaccination against measles. Journal of Hygiene, Epidemiology, Microbiology and Immunology 1970;14:1-18.

Chun H, T'eh-chang H, Kuo-hua T, Shou-teh C, Wen-huan W, Chi-ming C et al. Clinical and immunologic observations on two lines of attenuated measles vaccine virus upon passage in chick embryo cell culture. Chinese Medical Journal 1975;1:283-286.

Chung WK, Yoo JY, Sun HS, Lee HY, Lee IJ, Kim SM, Prince AM. Prevention of perinatal transmission of hepatitis B virus: a comparison between the efficacy of passive and passive-active immunization in Korea. Journal of Infectious Diseases 1985;151:280-286.

Church JA, Richards W. Recurrent abscess formation following DTP immunizations: association with hypersensitivity to tetanus toxoid. Pediatrics 1985;75:899-900.

Ciaccio M, Rebora A. Lichen planus following HBV vaccination: a coincidence? (letter). British Journal of Dermatology 1990;122:424.

Cizewska S, Huber Z, Sluzewski W. [Prophylactic inoculations and seizure activity in the EEG] Szczepienia ochronne a czynnosc napadowa w EEG: doniesienie wstepne. Neurologia i Neurochirurgia Polska 1981;15:554-557.

Cizman M, Mozetic M, Furman-Jakopic M, Pleterski-Rigler D, Radescek-Rakar R, Susec-Michieli M. [Aseptic meningitis following combined vaccination with the Leningrad-3 strain of mumps virus and the Edmonston-Zagreb strain of measles virus] Serozni meningitis po kombiniranem cepljenju s sevom virusa mumpsa Leningrad-3 in sevom virusa ospic Edmonston-Zagreb. Zdravstreni Vestnik 1986;55:587-591.

Cizman M, Mozetic M, Radescek-Rakar R, Pleterski-Rigler D, Susec-Michieli M. Aseptic meningitis after vaccination against measles and mumps. Pediatric Infectious Disease Journal 1989;8:302-308.

Claesson BA, Schneerson R, Lagergard T, Trollfors B, Taranger J, Johansson J et al. Persistence of serum antibodies elicited by *Haemophilus influenzae* type b-tetanus toxoid conjugate vaccine in infants vaccinated at 3, 5 and 12 months of age. Pediatric Infectious Disease Journal 1991;10:560-564.

Claesson BA, Schneerson R, Robbins JB, Johansson J, Lagergard T, Taranger J et al. Protective levels of serum antibodies stimulated in infants by two injections of *Haemophilus influenzae* type b capsular polysaccharide-tetanus toxoid conjugate. Journal of Pediatrics 1989;114:97-100.

Claesson BA, Trollfors B, Lagergard T, Taranger J, Bryla D, Otterman G et al. Clinical and immunologic responses to the capsular polysaccharide of *Haemophilus influenzae* type b alone or conjugated to tetanus toxoid in 18-to 23-month-old children. Journal of Pediatrics 1988;112:695-702.

Clark C, Hashim G, Rosenberg R. Transverse myelitis following rubeola vaccination. Neurology 1977;27:360.

Clements CJ, Von RC F., Mann JM. HIV infection and routine childhood immunization: a review. Bulletin of the World Health Organization 1987;65:905-911.

Clements DA, Rouse JB, London WL, Yancy WS, Moggio MV, Wilfert CM. Antibody response of 18 month old children 1 month and 18 months following *Haemophilus influenzae* type b vaccine administered singly or with DTP vaccine. Journal of Paediatrics and Child Health 1990;26:46-49.

Clinical Pharmacy. Clearinghouse formed for reports of hepatitis B vaccine adverse effects. Clinical Pharmacy 1983;2:297.

Clinical Pediatrics. Influenza vaccination (1977-1978). Clinical Pediatrics 1977;16:867-868.

Cocchi P, Corti R. [Measles vaccination] La vaccinazione anti-morbillo. Pediatria Medica e Chirurgica 1984;6:5-11.

Cochi SL, Broome CV, Hightower AW. Immunization of U.S. children with *H. influenzae* vaccine: a cost-effectiveness model of strategy assessment. Journal of the American Medical Association 1985;253:521-529.

Cochi SL, Preblud SR, Orenstein WA. Perspectives on the relative resurgence of mumps in the United States. American Journal of Diseases of Children 1988;142:499-507.

Cockrell JL. Vaccine reactions: the challenge to pediatricians. Virginia Medicine 1982;109:380-381.

Cockwell P, Allen MB, Page R. Vasculitis related to hepatitis B vaccine (letter). British Medical Journal 1990;301:1281.

Cody CL, Baraff LJ, Cherry JD, Marcy SM, Manclark CR. Nature and rates of adverse reactions associated with DTP and DT immunizations in infants and children. Pediatrics 1981;68:650-660.

Coe CJ. Guillain-Barre syndrome in Korean children. Yonsei Medical Journal 1989;30:81-87.

Coffin CM, Roberts RL, Monafo WJ, Haslam DB, Bellini WJ, Zaki S. Disseminated measles infection following vaccination in severe combined immune deficiency syndrome. Pediatric Pathology 1993;13:102.

Cogne M, Ballet JJ, Schmitt C, Bizzine B. Total and IgE antibody levels following booster immunization with aluminum absorbed and nonabsorbed tetanus toxoid in humans. Annals of Allergy 1985;54:148-151.

Cohen H, Brouwer R, Bijkerk H, Phaff JM. National antimeasles vaccination programme. Nederlands Tijdschrift voor Geneeskunde 1978;122:46-51.

Cohen HI. Safety of measles vaccine in egg-sensitive individuals (letter). Journal of Pediatrics 1978;92:859.

Cohen J. Debate on AIDS origin: Rolling Stone weighs in. Science 1992;255:1505.

Cohen P, Scadron SJ. Effects of active immunization of mother upon offspring. Journal of Pediatrics 1946;29:609-619.

Cohn J. Thrombocytopenia in childhood: an evaluation of 433 patients. Scandinavian Journal of Hematology 1976;16:226-240.

Coleman PJ, Shaw FE Jr., Serovich J, Hadler SC, Margolis HS. Intradermal hepatitis B vaccination in a large hospital employee population. Vaccine 1991;9:723-727.

Coll JR. The incidence and complications of mumps. General Practitioner 1974;24:545-551.

Collier LH. Reactions after plain and adsorbed tetanus vaccines (letter). Lancet 1980;1:148.

Collier LH, Polakoff S, Mortimer J. Reactions and antibody responses to reinforcing doses of adsorbed and plain tetanus vaccines. Lancet 1979;1:1364-1368.

Collingham KE, Pollock TM, Roebuck MO. Paralytic poliomyelitis in England and Wales, 1976-7. Lancet 1978;1:976-977.

Colville A, Pugh S. Mumps meningitis and measles, mumps, and rubella vaccine. Lancet 1992;340:786.

Combes MA, Clark WK. Sciatic nerve injury following intragluteal injection: pathogenesis and prevention. American Journal of Diseases in Children 1960;100:579.

Committee on Infectious Diseases. Prevention of hepatitis B virus infections. Pediatrics 1985;75:362-364.

Concours Medical. [The efficacy and use of *Haemophilus influenzae* type b vaccine combined with PRP-T vaccine] Vaccin PRP-T anti-hemophilus: efficacite et modalites d'emploi. Concours Medical 1992;114:184.

Connolly JH. Subacute sclerosing panencephalitis. Journal of Clinical Pathology 1972;6(Suppl.): 73-77.

Connolly JH. Subacute sclerosing panencephalitis. Postgraduate Medical Journal 1972;48):342-345.

Connolly JH, Allen IV, Hurwitz LJ, Miller JH. Measles-virus antibody and antigen in subacute sclerosing panencephalitis. Lancet 1967;1:542-544.

Connolly JH, Allen IV, Hurwitz LJ, Millar JH. Subacute sclerosing panencephalitis: clinical, pathological, epidemiological, and virological findings in three patients. Quebec Journal of Medicine 1968;37:625-644.

Connolly JH, Robinson FL J., Canavan DA. Mumps or Coxsackie A9 virus antibody in the cerebrospinal fluid of patients with meningitis or encephalitis. Irish Journal of Medical Science 1975;144:60-66.

Connolly KH, Hammer SM. The acute aseptic meningitis syndrome. Infectious Disease Clinics of North America 1990;4:599-622.

Contardi I, Lusardi C, Cattaneo GG. [A comparative study of 3 different types of trivalent measles-mumps-rubella vaccine] Studio comparativo su tre differenti tipi di vaccini trivalenti anti morbillo-parotite-rosolia. Pediatria Medica e Chirurgica 1992;14:421-424.

Contreras G, Furesz J. Possible influence of measles virus infection of cynomolgus monkeys on the outcome of the neurovirulence test for oral poliovirus vaccine. Biologicals 1992;20: 27-33.

Cook JV, Holowach J, Atkins JE Jr., Powers JR. Antibody formation in early infancy against diphtheria and tetanus toxoid. Journal of Pediatrics 1948;33:141-146.

Cooke DR. A study of the side effects of Lirugen measles vaccine in Aboriginal children. Medical Journal of Australia 1972;1:387-388.

Coombs RR, Gell PG. Classification of allergic reactions responsible for clinical hypersensitivity and disease. In: Gell PG, Coombs RR, eds. Clinical Aspects of Immunology, 2nd edition. Oxford and Edinburgh: Blackwell Scientific Publications; 1968.

Cornblath DR, Mellits ED, Griffin JW, and the GBS Study Group. Motor conduction studies in the Guillain-Barre syndrome: description and prognostic value. Annals of Neurology 1988;23:354-359.

Corrigan JJ Jr. Thrombocytopenia: a laboratory sign of septicemia in infants and children. Journal of Pediatrics 1974;83:219-221.

Cosnes A, Flechet ML, Revuz J. Inflammatory nodular reactions after hepatitis B vaccination due to aluminium sensitization. Contact Dermatitis 1990;23:65-67.

Costa M, Giannini V. [Case report of encephalitis occurring during and after measles] Encefalite intra e metamorbillosa: contributo casistico. Giornale di Malattie Infettive e Parassitarie 1975;27:453-455.

Coulehan JL, Hallowell C, Michaels RH et al. Immunogenicity of a *Haemophilus influenzae* type b vaccine in combination with diphtheria-pertussis-tetanus vaccine in infants. Journal of Infectious Diseases 1983;148:530-534.

Coulter HL. Vaccination, Social Violence, and Criminality: The Medical Assault on the American Brain. Berkeley, CA: North Atlantic Books; 1990.

Coulter HL, Fisher BL. DPT: A Shot in the Dark. San Diego: Harcourt Brace Jovanovich; 1985.

Courrier A, Stenbach G, Simonnet P, Rumilly P, Lopez D, Coquillat G et al. Peripheral neuropathy following fetal bovine cell rabies vaccine (letter). Lancet 1986;1:1273.

Coursaget P, Bringer L, Sarr G, Bourdil C, Fritzell B, Blondeau C et al. Comparative immunogenicity in children of mammalian cell-derived recombinant hepatitis B vaccine and plasma-derived hepatitis B vaccine. Vaccine 1992;10:370-382.

Coursaget P, Relyveld E, Brizard A, Frenkiel MP, Fritzell B, Teulieres L et al. Simultaneous injection of hepatitis B vaccine with BCG and killed poliovirus vaccine. Vaccine 1992;10:319-321.

Coursaget P, Yvonnet, B, Chothard J, Sarr M, Vincelot TP, N'doye R, Diop-Mar I, Chiron JP. Seven year study of hepatitis B vaccine efficacy in infants from an endemic area (Senegal). Lancet 1986;2:1143-1145.

Coursaget P, Yvonnet B, Relyveld EH, Barres JL, Diop-Mar I, Chiron JP. Simultaneous administration of diphtheria-tetanus-pertussis-polio and hepatitis B vaccines in a simplified immunization program: immune response to diphtheria toxoid, tetanus toxoid, pertussis, and hepatitis B surface antigen. Infection and Immunity 1986;51:784-787.

Coursaget P, Yvonnet B, Sarr M et al. Clinical trial of hepatitis B vaccine in a simplified immunization programme. Bulletin of the World Health Organization 1986;64:867-871.

Coutinho RA, Lelie N, Albrecht Van Lent P. Efficacy of a heat inactivated hepatitis B vaccine in male homosexuals: outcome of a placebo controlled double blind trial. British Medical Journal 1983;286:1305-1308.

Cox NH, Forsyth A. Thiomersal allergy and vaccination reactions. Contact Dermatitis 1988;18:229-233.

Cox NH, Moss C, Forsyth A. Cutaneous reactions to aluminium in vaccines: an avoidable problem. Lancet 1988;2:43.

Craighead JE. The role of viruses in the pathogenesis of pancreatic disease and diabetes mellitus. Progress in Medical Virology 1975;19:161-214.

Crawford GE, Gremillion DH. Epidemic measles and rubella in Air Force recruits: impact of immunization. Journal of Infectious Diseases 1981;144:403-410.

Cristi G, Dalbuono S. [Probable neurological complications caused by the Sabin type of oral antipoliomyelitis vaccine] Probabili complicazioni neurologiche da vaccino antipoliomielitico orale tipo Sabin. Rivista di Neurologia 1967;37:251-257.

Croft PB. Para-infectious and post-vaccinal encephalomyelitis. Postgraduate Medical Journal 1969;45:392-400.

Crosnier J, Jungers P, Courouce AM. Randomised controlled trial of hepatitis B surface antigen vaccine in French haemophilus units. II. Haemodialysis patients. Lancet 1981;2:797-800.

Crossley KB, Gerding DN, Petzel RA. Acceptance of hepatitis B vaccine by hospital personnel. Infection Control 1985;6:147-149.

Crovari P, Gasparini R, D'Aste E, Culotta C, Romano L. [Case-control study on the association of neurological syndromes and compulsory vaccinations in Liguria during the period January 1980-February 1983] Studio caso-controllo sulla associazione tra sindromi neurologiche e vaccinazioni obbligatorie in Liguria nel periodo Gennaio 1980-Febbraio 1983. Bollettino dell'Istituto Sieroterapico Milanese 1984;63:118-124.

Crowley S, Al-Jawad ST, Kovar IZ. Mumps, measles, and rubella vaccination and encephalitis. British Medical Journal 1989;299:660.

Cruickshank JG, Orme RL, Haas L, Gill NO, Roebuck MO, Magrath DI et al. Two cases of vaccine-associated paralytic poliomyelitis linked in time and place (letter). Lancet 1984;2:804-805.

Curtis T. Did a polio vaccine experiment unleash AIDS in Africa? Washington Post. April 5, 1992:C3.

Cutts FT, Zell ER, Mason D, Bernier RH, Dini EF, Orenstein WA. Monitoring progress toward U.S. Preschool Immunization Goals. Journal of the American Medical Association 1992;267:1952-1955.

D'Alessandro G, Dardanoni L, Albanese M, Brancato P, Cascio G, Romano N et al. [Research on the cases of paralytic poliomyelitis and neurological syndromes observed in Sicily during the 1st phase of the campaign of anti-poliomyelitis vaccination with attenuated viruses] Indagini su casi di poliomielite paralitica e sindromi neurologiche osservati in Sicilia durante la prima fase di attuazione della vaccinazione antipoliomielitica con virus attenuati. Igiene Moderna 1967;60:37-71.

D'Costa DF, Cooper A, Pye IF. Transverse myelitis following cholera, typhoid and polio vaccination. Journal of the Royal Society of Medicine 1990;83:653.

D'Cruz OF, Shapiro ED, Spiegelman KN, Leicher CR, Breningstall GN, Khatri BO et al. Acute inflammatory demyelinating polyradiculoneuropathy (Guillain-Barre syndrome) after immunization with *Haemophilus influenzae* type b conjugate vaccine. Journal of Pediatrics 1989;115:743-746.

Da Villa G, Piazza M, Iorio R, Picciotto L, Peluso P, De Luca G et al. A pilot model of vaccination against hepatitis B virus suitable for mass vaccination campaigns in hyperendemic areas. Journal of Medical Virology 1992;36:274-278.

Dacou-Voutetakis C, Constantinidis M, Moschos S, Vlachou C, Matsaniotis MD. Diabetes mellitus following mumps: insulin reserve. American Journal of Diseases of Children 1974;127:890-891.

Daggett P. Influenza and asthma (letter). Lancet 1992;339:367.

Dahlquist G, Blom L, Lonnberg G. The Swedish childhood diabetes study: a multivariate analysis of risk determinants for diabetes in different age groups. Diabetologia 1991;34:757-762.

Dal Bo S. [Allergic reactions against anti-tetanus toxoid] Reazioni allergiche da tossoide antitetanico. Folia Allergologica 1969;16:63-73.

Dal Canto MC, Rabinowitz SG. Experimental models of virus-induced demyelination of the central nervous system. Annals of Neurology 1982;11:109-127.

Daneault N, Albert G, Girouard Y, Remillard G, Furesz J. Postvaccinal poliomyelitis: a case report. Canadian Journal of Neurological Science 1986;12:202.

Daschbach RJ. Serum sickness and tetanus immunization. Journal of the American Medical Association 1972;220:1619.

Dashefsky B, Wald E, Guerra N, Byers C. Safety, tolerability, and immunogenicity of concurrent administration of *Haemophilus influenzae* type b conjugate vaccine (meningococcal protein conjugate) with either measles-mumps-rubella vaccine or diphtheria-tetanus-pertussis and oral poliovirus vaccines in 14- to 23-month-old infants. Pediatrics 1990;85(4 Pt 2):682-689.

Daum RS, Sood SK, Osterholm MT, Pramberg JC, Granoff PD, White KE et al. Decline in serum antibody to the capsule of *Haemophilus influenzae* type b in the immediate postimmunization period. Journal of Pediatrics 1989;114:742-747.

David D, Zehntner B. [Tetanus vaccination: adverse effects in diverse vaccination sites and mode of administration] Tetanusimpfung: Nebenwirkungen bei verschiedenen Impflokalisationen und Modus. Schweizerische Medizinische Wochenschrift 1971;101:1055-1056.

David MF. Induction of anaphylaxis by commercially prepared pertussis and DPT vaccines in rats. Annals of the Royal College of Physicians and Surgeons of Canada 1975;8:41-42.

Davidson M, Letson W, Ward JI, Ball A, Bulkow L, Christenson P et al. DTP immunization and susceptibility to infectious diseases. American Journal of Diseases of Children 1991;145:750-754.

Davidson NM. S.S.P.E. in New Zealand (letter). Lancet 1973;2:1332-1333.

Davidson WL, Buynak EB, Leagus B, Whitman JE, Hilleman MR. Vaccination of adults with live attenuated mumps virus vaccine. Journal of the American Medical Association 1967;201:995-998.

Davies II. Immunological adjuvants of natural origin and their adverse effects. Adverse Drug Reaction and Acute Poisoning Review 1986;5:1-21.

Davignon L, Lussier G, Quevillon M, Lavergne B, Fauvel M, Aubert D. [Results of clinical trials of the superattenuated measles vaccine of the Institute Armand-Frappier] Resultats d'essais cliniques realises avec le vaccin rougeoleux surattenue I.A.F. Journal of Biological Standardization 1982;10:347-355.

Davis LE, Bodian D, Price D, Butler IJ, Vickers JH. Chronic progressive poliomyelitis secondary to vaccination of an immunodeficient child. New England Journal of Medicine 1977;297:241-245.

Dawson JR. Cellular inclusions in cerebral lesions of lethargic encephalitis. American Journal of Pathology 1933;9:7-15.

Dawson JR. Cellular inclusions in cerebral lesions of epidemic encephalitis (second report). Archives of Neurology and Psychiatry 1934;31:685-700.

De Carli E, Gandolfo G. [Contribution to the statistics of reactions occurring in the subjects vaccinated with the Sabin method in the town of Pordenone from 1 March 1964 to 30 June 1965] Contributo ad una statistica delle reazioni avutesi fra i vaccinati col metodo Sabin nel comune di Pordenone dal 1 marzo 1964 al 30 giugno 1965. Annali della Sanita Pubblica 1966;27:1039-1049.

De la Plaza N, Isola MB. [Infrequent complication of oral anti-poliomyelitis vaccination] Complicacion poco frecuente de la vacunacion antipoliomielitica oral. Prensa Medica Argentina 1966;53:1680-1683.

De Prins F, Van Assche FA, Desmyter J, De Groote G, Gepts W. Congenital rubella and diabetes mellitus. Lancet 1978;1:439-440.

de Quadros CA, Andrus JK, Olive JM, Da Silveira CM, Eikhof RM, Carrasco P et al. Eradication of poliomyelitis: progress in the Americas. Pediatric Infectious Disease Journal 1991;10:222-229.

De Ritis L, Pecorari R. [Thrombocytopenic purpura following measles vaccination] Porpora trombocitopenica in seguito a vaccinazione antimorbillosa. Pediatria Medica e Chirurgica 1990;12:161-163.

De Silva L, Rogers M. Hepatitis B vaccine: urticarial reaction (letter). Medical Journal of Australia 1985;143:323-324.

Deacon SP, Langford DT, Shepherd WM, Knight PA. A comparative clinical study of adsorbed tetanus vaccine and adult-type tetanus-diphtheria vaccine. Journal of Hygiene 1982;89:513-519.

Decker MD, Edwards KM, Bradley R, Palmer P. Comparative trial in infants of four conjugate *Haemophilus influenzae* type b vaccines. Journal of Pediatrics 1992;120(2 Pt. 1):184-189.

Deforest A, Long SS, Lischner HW, Girone JA, Clark JL, Srinivasan R et al. Simultaneous administration of measles-mumps-rubella vaccine with booster doses of diphtheria-tetanus-pertussis and poliovirus vaccines. Pediatrics 1988;81:237-246.

Deibel R. Antigenic variations among type III poliomyelitis viruses. New York State Journal of Medicine 1964;64:2058-2065.

Deibel R, Barron A, Millian S, Smith V. Central nervous system infections in New York State. New York State Journal of Medicine 1974;74:1929-1935.

Deivanayagam N, Nedunchelian K. Epidemiological and clinical features of acute poliomyelitis children admitted in an urban hospital. Indian Pediatrics 1992;29:25-28.

Dekker PA. Paralytic poliomyelitis in children in Ethiopia: a review of 2604 cases. Ethiopian Medical Journal 1986;24:55-62.

Deliyannakis E. Peripheral nerve and root disturbances following active immunization against smallpox and tetanus. Military Medicine 1971;136:458-462.

Dentico P, Buongiorno R, Volpe A, Zavoianni A, Pastore G, Schiraldi O. Long-term immunogenicity, safety and efficacy of a recombinant hepatitis B vaccine in healthy adults. European Journal of Epidemiology 1992;8:650-655.

Department of Health and Social Security. Whooping Cough: Reports from the Committee on the Safety of Medicines and the Joint Committee on Vaccination and Immunisation. London: Her Majesty's Stationery Office; 1981.

Derenne F, Vanderheyden JE, Bain H, Jocquet P, Jacquy J, Yane F et al. [Acute maternal anterior poliomyelitis in a non-endemic zone] Poliomyelite anterieure aigue maternelle en zone non endemique. Acta Neurologica et Psychiatrica Belgica 1989;89:358-365.

Desai BV, Dixit S, Pope RM. Limited proliferative response to type II collagen in rheumatoid arthritis. Journal of Rheumatology 1989;16:1310-1314.

Desmyter J. [Bogaert's disease and vaccination against measles] De ziekte van van Bogaert en de mazelenvaccinatie. Tijdschrift voor Geneeskunde 1978;34:339-341.

Deutsche Medizinische Wochenschrift. [Safety of hepatitis B vaccine] Sicherheit von Impfstoffen gegen Hepatitis B. Deutsche Medizinische Wochenschrift 1983;108:754-755.

Devey ME, Bleasdale K, Isenberg DA. Antibody affinity and IgG subclass of responses to tetanus toxoid in patients with rheumatoid arthritis and systemic lupus erythematosus. Clinical and Experimental Immunology 1987;68:562-569.

Di Cristofano A. [Measles vaccination in children allergic to eggs] La vaccinazione contro il morbillo in bambini allergici all'uovo. Professioni Infermieristiche 1989;42:24-30.

Di Giusto CA, Bernhard JD. Erythema nodosum provoked by hepatitis B vaccine (letter). Lancet 1986;2:1042.

Di Stasio L, Esposito G, Di Stasio M. [Contribution to the study of neonatal, fulminating laryngo-tracheo-bronchitis after antidiphtheria antitetanus prophylaxis] Contributo allo studio delle laringo-tracheo-bronchiti fulminanti neonati dopo profilassi antidifterico-antitetanica. Osp Ital Pediatr Spec Chir 1979;14(Suppl. 2):143-148.

Diamond S. Childhood routine immunizations. On Contin Pract 1990;17:9-16.

Dickersin K. The existence of publication bias and risk factors for its occurrence. Journal of the American Medical Association 1990;263:1385-1389.

Dickersin K, Berlin JA. Meta-analysis: state-of-the-science. Epidemiological Reviews 1992;14:154-176.

Dickersin K, Hewitt P, Mutch L, Chalmers I, Chalmers TC. Perusing the literature: comparison of MEDLINE searching with a Perinatal Trials Database. Controlled Clinic Trials 1985;6:306-317.

Dickersin K, Min YI, Meinert CL. Factors influencing publication of research results: follow-up of applications submitted to two institutional review boards. Journal of the American Medical Association 1992;267:374-378.

Dieckhoefer K, Scholl R, Wolf R. [Neurological disorders after protective tetanus vaccination]. Neurologische Storungen nach Tetanusschutzi. Medizinische Welt 1978;29:1710-1712.

Dietzsch HJ, Kiehl W. [Central nervous complications after measles vaccination] Zentralnervose Komplikationen nach Masern-Schutzimpfung. Deutsche Gesundheitswesen 1976;31:2489-2491.

Dietzsch HJ, Leupold W, Rogner G. [Occurrence and importance of complications in measles] Haufigkeit und Bedeutung der Masernkomplikationen. Zeitschrift fur Aerztliche Fortbildung 1971;65:138-140.

Diop Mar I, Conde K, Sow A, Badiane S. [Neuropathies in the course of diphtheria] Les neuropathies au cours de la diphterie. Bulletin de la Societe Medicale d'Afrique Noire de Langue Francaise 1976;21:455-464.

Dittmann S. [Smallpox vaccination: atypical course] Die Pockenschutzimpfung und ihre atypischen Verlaufsformen. Beitrage zur Hygiene und Epidemiologie 1981;25:26-76.

Dittmann S. [Measles immunization: atypical course] Die Masernschutzimpfung und ihre atypischen Verlaufsformen. Beitrage zur Hygiene und Epidemiologie 1981;25:76-94.

Dittmann S. [Diphtheria immunization: atypical course] Die Diphtherieschutzimpfung und Ihre atypischen Verlaufsformen. Beitrage zur Hygiene und Epidemiologie 1981;25:143-154.

Dittmann S. [Measles immunization] Masernschutzimpfung. Beitrage zur Hygiene und Epidemiologie 1981;25:213-217.

Dittmann S. [Diphtheria immunization] Diphterieschutzimpfung. Beitrage zur Hygiene und Epidemiologie 1981;25:237-239.

Dittmann S. [Tetanus immunization] Tetanusschutzimpfung. Beitrage zur Hygiene und Epidemiologie 1981;25:239-240.

Dodson WE. Metabolic encephalopathies in neurological pathophysiology. In: Eliasson SG, Prensky AL, Hardin WB Jr., eds. Neurological Pathophysiology. New York: Oxford; 1978.

Dodson WE, Pasternak J, Trotter JL. Rapid deterioration in subacute sclerosing panencephalitis after measles immunisation (letter). Lancet 1978;1:767-768.

Dolinova L. [Bilateral uveoretinoneuritis following DTP vaccination] Bilateralni uveoretinoneuritida po ockovani DITEPE. Ceskoslovenska Oftalmologie 1974;30:114-116.

Dolovich J, Hargreave FE, Chalmeis R, Shier KJ, Cauldie J, Bienenstock J. Late cutaneous allergic responses in isolated-IgE-dependent reactions. Journal of Allergy and Clinical Immunology 1973;52:38-46.

Domok I. Experiences associated with the use of live poliovirus vaccine in Hungary, 1959-1982. Reviews of Infectious Diseases 1984;6(Suppl. 2):S413-S418.

Domorazkova E, Drevo M, Bergmannova V, Stehlikova J, Vodickova M, Slonim D. [Comparison of clinical and serological results after the intravenous and subcutaneous administration of measles vaccine]. Ceskoslovenska Pediatrie 1982;37:19-22.

Domorazkova E, Janotova J, Vodickova M, Drevo M. [Relationship between the age of the child and the degree of body temperature and antibody titre after vaccination against measles] Vztah veku ditete k vysce teploty a titru protilatek po ockovani proti spalnickam. Ceskoslovenska Pediatrie 1975;30:468-470.

Donaghy M, Gray JA, Squier W, Kurtz JB, Higgins RM, Richardson AJ et al. Recurrent Guillain-Barre syndrome after multiple exposures to cytomegalovirus. American Journal of Medicine 1989;87:339-341.

Donchev D, Arabadzhieva T, Zhukovets V, Iancheva B. [A comparative study of live measles vaccines in controlled epidemiologic trials] Sravnietl'noe izuchenie zhivykh korevykh vaktsin v kontroliruemom epidemiologicheskom opyte. Voprosy Virusologii 1969;14:104-107.

Donner M, Halonen H, Haltia M. [Subacute sclerosing panencephalitis] Subakuutti sklerosoiva panenkefaliitti. Duodecim 1969;85:541-553.

Dontschev D, Gatscheva N, Kossev B. [On the epidemiological effectiveness of mass vaccination against mumps in the People's Republic of Bulgaria] Uber die Epidemiologische wirksamkeit der Massenimpfung gegen Mumps in der VR Bulgarien. Padiatrie und Grenzgebiete 1980;19:151-156.

Dorfman RF, Herweg JC. Live, attenuated measles virus vaccine. Inguinal lymphadenopathy complicating administration. Journal of the American Medical Association 1966;198:320-321.

Dorndorf W, van Rey W, Arndt T. Zur Frage neurologischer komplikationen nach der oralen poliomyelitisimpfung (Sabin). Nervenarzt 1963;34:473-480.

Dosik H, Tricarico F. Haemolytic-uraemic syndrome following mumps vaccination. Lancet 1970;1:247.

Douglas SD, Anolik R. Postvaccination paralysis in a 20-month-old child. Hospital Practice 1981;16:40A.

Drucker J, Soula G, Diallo O, Fabre P. Evaluation of a new combined inactivated DPT-polio vaccine. Developments in Biological Standardization 1986;65:145-151.

Drug and Therapeutics Bulletin. Contraindications to childhood immunisation. Drug and Therapeutics Bulletin 1988;26:81-84.

Drug and Therapeutics Bulletin. *Haemophilus influenzae* b immunisation. Drug and Therapeutics Bulletin 1993;31:1-2.

Drug and Therapeutics Bulletin. Update on MMR vaccination. Drug and Therapeutics Bulletin 1991;29:61-62.

Deutsche Apotheker Zeitung. [*Haemophilus influenzae* type b vaccination] *Haemophilus influenzae* typ b Impfprophylaxe mit hib-vakzine. Deutsche Apotheker Zeitung 1991;131:2179-2180.

Duclos P, Koch J, Hardy M. Immunizing Agent-Associated Adverse Events, Canada, 1987-1990. Ottawa, Ontario: Laboratory Centre for Disease Control; 1992.

Ducos J, Colombies P, Ohayon E. [Oral administration of polio vaccine: subsequent hypersensitivity reaction—blast transformation test for etiologic diagnosis] Administration orale de vaccin antipoliomyelitique: reaction d'hypersensibilite consequente—interet du test de transformation blastique pour le diagnostic etiologique. Presse Medicale 1968;76:2347-2348.

Dudgeon JA. Antibody response and clinical reactions in children given measles vaccine with immunoglobulin. British Medical Journal 1986;293:206.

Dufour FD, Arce MA, St. Geme JW Jr. Correlation between the potency of mumps virus skin test antigen and cutaneous delayed hypersensitivity. Journal of Pediatrics 1972;81:742-746.

Dunlop JM, RaiChoudhury K, Roberts JS, Bryett KA. An evaluation of measles, mumps and rubella vaccine in a population of Yorkshire infants. Public Health 1989;103:331-335.

Dunmire C, Ruckdeschel JC, Mardiney MR Jr. Suppression of in vitro lymphocyte responsiveness to purified protein derivative by measles virus: a reexploration of the phenomenon. Cellular Immunology 1975;20:205-217.

Duplay H, Monnier B, Bracco J, Dellamonica P. [Acute glomerulonephritis associated with Fisher's syndrome after tetanus prophylaxis (letter)] Glomerulonephrite aigue associee a un syndrome de M. Fisher apres prevention anti-tetanique. Nouvelle Presse Medicale 1980;9:315.

Durrer A. [Vaccination of children against bacterial meningitis] La vaccination des enfants contre la meningite bacterienne. Schweizerische Apotheker-Zeitung / Journal Suisse de Pharmacie 1992;130:89-90.

Duverne J, Volle H, Gogue Y. [Hyperergic accidents of the Sanarelli-Shwartzman type caused by DT-polio vaccination in children] Accidents hyperergiques du type Sanarelli-Shwartzman par vaccination DT-polio chez l'enfant. Bulletin de la Societe Francaise de Dermatologie et de Syphiligraphie 1966;73:221-223.

Duvina PL, Bini E. [Complications due to oral poliomyelitis vaccination] Complicazioni in corso di vaccinazione antipoliomielitica orale. Giornale di Malattie Infettive e Parassitarie 1970;22:307.

Duvina PL, Bini R. [Reactions caused by the Sabin poliovirus vaccine in infants. (Considerations on 134 cases hospitalized in 1965)] Le reazioni da poliovaccino Sabin nel lattante. (Considerazioni su 134 casi ricoverati nel 1965). Rivista di Clinica Pediatrica 1966;78:400-411.

Dyken PR, Cunningham SC, Ward LC. Changing character of subacute sclerosing panencephalitis in the United States. Pediatric Neurology 1989;5:339-341.

Dyrberg T, Schwimmbeck PL, Oldstone MB A. et al. Inhibition of diabetes in BB rats by virus infection. Journal of Clinical Investigation 1988;81:928-931.

Dyro FM. Vaccination mononeuropathy. Annals of Neurology 1978;3:468.

Easton JG. Egg-derived vaccines (letter). Annals of Allergy 1991;66:519.

Edees S, Pullan CR, Hull D. A randomised single blind trial of a combined mumps measles rubella vaccine to evaluate serological response and reactions in the UK population. Public Health 1991;105:91-97.

Eden AN. Guillain-Barre syndrome in a six-month-old infant. American Journal of Diseases of Children 1961;102:224-227.

Edsall G. The current status of tetanus immunization. Hospital Practice 1971;6:57-66.

Edsall G et al. Diphtheria, tetanus, and pertussis immunization. Archives of Environmental Health 1967;15:473-477.

Edsall G et al. Specific Prophylaxis of tetanus. Journal of the American Medical Association 1959;171:417-428.

Edsall G, Altman JS, Gaspar AJ. Combined tetanus-diphtheria immunization of adults: use of small doses of diphtheria toxoid. American Journal of Public Health 1954;44:1537-1545.

Edsall G, Elliott MW, Peebles TC, Levine L, Eldred MC. Excessive use of tetanus toxoid boosters. Journal of the American Medical Association 1967;202:17-19.

Edsall G, Elliott MW, Peebles TC, Eldred MC. Excessive use of tetanus toxoid boosters. Journal of the American Medical Association 1967;202:111-113.

Edwards KM, Decker MD, Halsey NA, Koblin BA, Townsend T, Auerbach B et al. Differences in antibody response to whole-cell pertussis vaccines. Pediatrics 1991;88:1019-1023.

Edwards KM, Decker MD, Porch CR, Palmer P, Bradley R. Immunization after invasive *Haemophilus influenzae* type b disease: serologic response to a conjugate vaccine. American Journal of Diseases of Children 1989;143:31-33.

Edwards R. A report on the incidence of adverse events following low dose hepatitis B vaccination. 1989. Unpublished.

Egashira Y. On some problems of complications in the central nervous system due to vaccination. Japanese Journal of Medical Sciences and Biology 1968;21:297-298.

Eggers HJ, Mertens T. Polio vaccination (letter). Journal of the American Medical Association 1987;258:322-323.

Eggers HJ, Weyer J. Provocation paralysis (letter). Lancet 1993;341:62.

Ehrengut W. [Present problems of tetanus vaccination] Gegenwartige Fragen der Tetanusschutzimpfung. Monatsschrift fur Kinderheilkunde 1969;117:117-118.

Ehrengut W. Diabetes mellitus durch impfenzephalitis? [Diabetes mellitus from post-vaccinal encephalitis?]. Deutsche Medizinische Wochenschrift 1970;95:1135.

Ehrengut W. Susceptibility to infection after vaccination. British Medical Journal 1972;1:683.

Ehrengut W. [Immunization in allergic patients: 1] Schutzimpfungen bei Allergikern: 1. Medizinische Klinik 1973;68:939-942.

Ehrengut W. [Immunization in allergic patients: 2] Schutzimpfungen bei Allergikern: 2. Medizinische Klinik 1973;68:972-974.

Ehrengut W. [Convulsive reactions after pertussis immunization] Uber konvulsive Reaktionen nach Pertussis-Schutzimpfung. Deutsche Medizinische Wochenschrift 1974;99:2273-2279.

Ehrengut W. [Complications of immunizations] Impfkomplikationen. Deutsche Medizinische Wochenschrift 1975;100:499.

Ehrengut W. [Multiple immunizations and their complications] Mehrfachschutzimpfungen und ihre Komplikationen. Deutsches Arzteblatt 1976;15:1009-1012.

Ehrengut W. Dermatomyositis and vaccination (letter). Lancet 1978;1:1040-1041.

Ehrengut W. Whooping-cough vaccination: comment on report from Joint Committee on Vaccination and Immunisation. Lancet 1978;2:370-371.

Ehrengut W. Die parenteral Pertussis-Schutzimfung: Schaden-Nutzen Relation. Monatsschrift fur Kinderheilkunde 1981;129:67-69.

Ehrengut W. Central nervous sequelae of vaccinations (letter). Lancet 1986;1:1275-1276.

Ehrengut W. [Neural complications following immunization against diphtheria] Neurale komplikastionen nach diphtherie-schutzumpfung und impfungen mit diphtherietoxoid-mischimpfstoffen. Deutsche Medizinische Wochenschrift 1986;111:939-942.

Ehrengut W. Mumps vaccine and meningitis (letter). Lancet 1989;2:751.

Ehrengut W. Attenuation and antigenicity of mumps vaccine: significance for vaccination praxis. Padiat Prax 1990;40:379-381.

Ehrengut W. Central nervous system sequelae of immunization against measles, mumps, rubella and poliomyelitis. Acta Paediatrica Japonica 1990;32:8-11.

Ehrengut W, Allerdist H. [Neurological complications after influenza vaccination] Uber neurologische Komplikationen nach der Influenza-schutzimpfung. Munchener Medizinische Wochenschrift 1977;119:705-710.

Ehrengut W, Ehrengut J. Convulsions following oral polio immunisation. Developments in Biological Standardization 1979;43:165-171.

Ehrengut W, Ehrengut-Lange J. [Intercurrent fatal diseases after oral polio vaccination and smallpox vaccination] Interkurrente todliche Erkrankungen nach Polioschluckimpfung und Pockenschutzimpfung. Munchener Medizinische Wochenschrift 1969;111:1092-1099.

Ehrengut W, Ehrengut-Lange J. [On convulsive reactions following oral vaccination against polio] Uber konvulsive Reaktionen nach Polioschluckimpfung. Klinische Paediatrie 1979;191:261-270.

Ehrengut W, Staak M. [Anaphylactic reaction following injection of tetanus toxoid] Anaphylaktische Reaktion nach Tetanustoxoid-Injektion. Deutsche Medizinische Wochenschrift 1973;98:517.

Ehrengut W, Zastrow K. [Complications "following" mumps vaccinations in the Federal Republic of Germany (including combined vaccine immunizations)] Komplikationen "nach" Mumpsschutzimpfungen in der Bundesrepublik Deutschland (einschliesslich Mehrfachschutzimpfungen). Monatsschrift fur Kinderheilkunde 1989;137:398-402.

Ehrengut W, Georges AM, Andre FE. The reactogenicity and immunogenicity of the Urabe Am 9 live mumps vaccine and persistence of vaccine induced antibodies in healthy young children. Journal of Biological Standardization 1983;11:105-113.

Eicher W, Neundorfer B. [Paralysis of the recurrent laryngeal nerve following a booster injection of tetanus toxoid (associated with local allergic reaction)] Rekurrenslahmung nach Tetanustoxoid-Auffrischimpfung (mit allergischer Lokalreaktion). Munchener Medizinische Wochenschrift 1969;111:1692-1695.

Einarson TR, Leeder JS, Koren G. A method for meta-analysis of epidemiological studies. Drug Intelligence and Clinical Pharmacy 1988;22:813-824.

Einhorn MS, Weinberg GA, Anderson EL et al. Immunogenicity in infants of Haemophilus influenzae type b polysaccharide in a conjugate vaccine with Neisseria meningitidis outer-membrane protein. Lancet 1986;2:299-302.

Eisen AH, Cohen JJ, Rose B. Reaction to tetanus toxoid. New England Journal of Medicine 1963;269:1408-1411.

Ekunwe EO. Immunization by inhalation of aerosolized measles vaccine. Annals of Tropical Paediatrics 1990;10:145-149.

Eller JJ. Inactivated myxovirus vaccines, atypical illness, and delayed hypersensitivity. Journal of Pediatrics 1969;74:664-666.

Elliman D. Adverse reactions and immunization schedules. Current Opinion in Infectious Disease 1989;2:773-778.

Elliman D, Dhanraj B. Safe MMR vaccination despite neomycin allergy (letter). Lancet 1991;337:365.

Elliman D, Miller CL. Antibody response and clinical reactions in children given measles vaccine with immunoglobulin (letter). British Medical Journal 1986;292:1597-1598.

Elliott RB, Martin M. Dietary protein: a trigger of insulin-dependent diabetes in the BB rat. Diabetologia 1984;26:297-299.

Emanuel I, Ansell JS. Congenital abnormalities after mumps vaccination in pregnancy. Lancet 1971;2:156-157.

Emini EA, Ellis RW, Miller WJ. Production and immunological analysis of recombinant hepatitis B vaccine. Journal of Infection 1986;13(Suppl. A.):3-9.

Enders JF. Techniques of laboratory diagnosis, tests for susceptibility, and experiments on specific prophylaxis. Journal of Pediatrics 1946;29:129-142.

Enders JF, Peebles TC. Propagation in tissue culture of cytopathic agents from patients with measles. Proceedings of the Society for Experimental Biology and Medicine 1954;86:277-286.

Enders JF, Weller TH, Robbins FC. Cultivation of the Lansing strain of poliomyelitis virus in cultures of various human embryonic tissues. Science 1949;109:85-87.

Enders-Ruckle G. Frequency, serodiagnosis and epidemiological features of subacute sclerosing panencephalitis (SSPE) and epidemiology and vaccination policy for measles in the Federal Republic of Germany (FRG). Developments in Biological Standardization 1978;41:195-207.

Enders-Ruckle G, Spiess H, Wolf H. [First results with a quintuple vaccine against measles, diphtheria, whooping cough, tetanus and poliomyelitis] Erste Ergebnisse mit einem Funffachimpistoff gegen Masern, Diphtherie, Pertussis, Tetanus, Poliomyelitis. Deutsche Medizinische Wochenschrift 1966;91:575-580.

Enell H, Simonsson H. [Vaccination against measles—adverse effects, cause of reduced protective effect in investigated material] Masslingsvaccinering—biverkningar, orsak till minskad skyddseffekt i ett studerat material. Lakartidningen 1973;70:3357-3358.

Englund JA, Suarez CS, Kelly J, Tate DY, Balfour HH Jr. Placebo-controlled trial of varicella vaccine given with or after measles-mumps-rubella vaccine. Journal of Pediatrics 1989;114:37-44.

Erdmann G. [Vaccination allergy] Impfallergie. Allergologie 1987;10:48-55.

Eskola J, Kayhty H, Takala AK, Peltola H, Ronnberg PR, Kela E et al. A randomized, prospective field trial of a conjugate vaccine in the protection of infants and young children against invasive *Haemophilus influenzae* type b disease. New England Journal of Medicine 1990;323:1381-1387.

Eskola J, Kayhty H, Takala A, Ronnberg PR, Kela E, Peltola H. Reactogenicity and immunogenicity of combined vaccines for bacteraemic diseases caused by *Haemophilus influenzae* type b, meningococci and pneumococci in 24-month-old children. Vaccine 1990;8:107-110.

Eskola J, Peltola H, Takala AK, Kayhty H, Hakulinen M. Efficacy of *Haemophilus influenzae* type b polysaccharide-diphtheria toxoid conjugate vaccine in infancy. New England Journal of Medicine 1987;317:717-722.

Eskola J, Takala AK, Kayhty H, Peltola H, Makela PH. Protection achieved by *Haemophilus influenzae* type b (Hib) conjugate vaccines is better than expected on the basis of efficacy trials. Program Abstracts of the 32nd Interscience Conference on Antimicrobial Agents and Chemotherapy. Abstract 979, p. 273. Washington, DC: American Society for Microbiology; 1992.

Evans OB. Guillain-Barre syndrome in children. Pediatrics in Review 1986;8:69-74.

Evans OB et al. Pediatrics for the clinician. Pediatrics 1979;64:96-105.

Eyquem E, de Saint Martin J. [Anti-tetanus immunization: complexity and polymorphism of humoral and cellular manifestations] Immunisation anti-tetanique: complexite et polymorphisme des manifestations humorales et cellulaires. Revue Francaise de Transfusion et Immunohematologie 1987;30:193-221.

Fabiani F, Cioffi P. [On some neurologic complications during vaccination with the Sabin vaccine] Su alcune complicanze neurologiche in corso di vaccinazione alla Sabin. Rivista di Neurobiologia 1967;13:127-130.

Facktor MA, Bernstein RA, Fireman P. Hypersensitivity to tetanus toxoid. Journal of Allergy and Clinical Immunology 1973;52:1-12.

Faden H, Duffy L. Effect of concurrent viral infection on systemic and local antibody responses to live attenuated and enhanced-potency inactivated poliovirus vaccines. American Journal of Diseases of Children 1992;146:1320-1323.

Fagan EA, Williams R. Hepatitis B vaccination. British Journal of Clinical Practice 1987;41:569-576.

Faich GA. Adverse drug reaction monitoring. New England Journal of Medicine 1986;314:1589-1592.

Fajans SS. Diabetes Mellitus. In: DeGroot LJ et al., ed. Endocrinology. Philadelphia: W.B. Saunders; 1989.

Family Practice News. HHS urged to tighten definitions of vaccine injuries. Family Practice News 1992;22:37.

Family Practice News. Not yet clear if new Hib vaccines can be mixed. Family Practice News 1991;21:20.

Fankhauser R, Freudiger U, Vandevelde M, Fatzer R. [Atrophy of Purkinje cells following measles virus vaccination in the dog] Purkinjezellatrophie nach Masernvirus-Vakzinierung beim Hund. Schweizer Archiv fur Neurologie, Neurochirurgie und Psychiatrie 1973;112:353-363.

Fardon DF. Unusual reactions to tetanus toxoid. Journal of the American Medical Association 1967;199:125-126.

Farizo KM, Cochi SL, Patriarca PA. Poliomyelitis in the United States: a historical perspective and current vaccination policy. Journal of American College Health 1990;39:137-143.

Farkkila M, Kinnunen E, Weckstrom P. Survey of Guillain-Barre syndrome in southern Finland. Neuroepidemiology 1991;10:236-241.

Farwell JR, Dohrmann GJ, Marrett LD, Meigs JW. Effect of SV40 virus-contaminated polio vaccine on the incidence and type of CNS neoplasms in children: a population-based study. Transactions of the American Neurological Association 1979;104:261-264.

Fasano MB, Wood RA, Cooke SK, Sampson HA. Egg hypersensitivity and adverse reactions to measles, mumps, and rubella vaccine. Journal of Pediatrics 1992;120:878-881.

FDA Drug Bulletin. Hib vaccine recommendations. FDA Drug Bulletin 1985;15:18-19.

Feasby TE, Gilbert JJ, Brown WF, Bolton CF, Hahn AF, Koopman WF et al. An acute axonal form of Guillain-Barre polyneuropathy. Brain 1986;109:1115-1126.

Feasby TE, Hahan AF, Brown WF, Bolton CF, Gilbert J. J., Koopman WJ. Severe axonal degeneration in acute Guillain-Barre syndrome: evidence of two different mechanisms? Journal of the Neurological Sciences 1993;116:185-192.

Feery BJ. Incidence and type of reactions to triple antigen (DTP) and DT (CDT) vaccines. Medical Journal of Australia 1982;2:511-515.

Feigin RD, Guggenheim MA, Johnsen SD. Vaccine-related paralytic poliomyelitis in an immunodeficient child. Journal of Pediatrics 1971;79:642-647.

Feldman R, Kamath D, Christopher S. Oral poliovaccine and paralysis. Indian Pediatrics 1968;5:475-478.

Feldman S, Gigliotti F, Shenep JL, Roberson PK, Lott L. Risk of *Haemophilus influenzae* type b disease in children with cancer and response of immunocompromised leukemic children to a conjugate vaccine. Journal of Infectious Diseases 1990;161:926-931.

Feldshon SD, Sampliner RE. Reaction to hepatitis B virus vaccine (letter). Annals of Internal Medicine 1984;100:156-157.

Fenichel GM. Neurological complications of immunization. Annals of Neurology 1982;12:119-128.

Fenichel GM. Neurologic complications of tetanus toxoid (letter). Archives of Neurology 1983;40:390.

Fenichel GM, Lane DA, Livengood JR, Horwitz SJ, Menkes JH, Schwartz JF. Adverse events following immunization: assessing probability of causation. Pediatric Neurology 1989;5:287-290.

Fenner F. Vaccination: its birth, death and resurrection; eighth Burnet lecture of the Australian Academy of Science, 1985. Australian Journal of Experimental Biology and Medical Science 1985;63((Pt. 6):607-622.

Fernandez de Castro J, Kumate J. [Vaccination against measles. The situation in Mexico and America. Advances in the method of aerosol immunization] La vacunacion contra el sarampion. Situacion en Mexico y America. Avances en el metodo de inmunizacion por aerosol. Boletin Medico del Hospital Infantil de Mexico 1990;47:449-461.

Fernandez Bracho JG, Roldan Fernandez SG. [Early reactions in pupils vaccinated with an aerosol measles vaccine] Reacciones tempranas en escolares vacunados con antisarampionosa en aerosol. Salud Publica de Mexico 1990;32:653-657.

Ferreccio C, Clemens J, Avendano A, Horwitz I, Flores C, Avila L et al. The clinical and immunologic response of Chilean infants to *Haemophilus influenzae* type b polysaccharide-tetanus protein conjugate vaccine coadministered in the same syringe with diphtheria-tetanus toxoids-pertussis vaccine at two, four and six months of age. Pediatric Infectious Disease Journal 1991;10:764-771.

Fescharek R, Quast U, Maass G, Merkle W, Schwarz S. Measles-mumps vaccination in the FRG: an empirical analysis after 14 years of use. I. Efficacy and analysis of vaccine failures. Vaccine 1990;8:333-336.

Fescharek R, Quast U, Maass G, Merkle W, Schwarz S. Measles-mumps vaccination in the FRG: an empirical analysis after 14 years of use. II. Tolerability and analysis of spontaneously reported side effects. Vaccine 1990;8:446-456.

Field EJ, Caspary EA, Shenton BK, Madgwick H. Lymphocyte sensitization after exposure to measles, and influenza: possible relevance to pathogenesis of multiple sclerosis. Journal of the Neurological Sciences 1973;19:179-187.

Fillastre C, Bregere P, Guerin N. [Tetravalent diphtheria, tetanus, pertussis and inactivated poliomyelitis vaccine] Vaccination tetravalente diphterique, tetanique, coquelucheuse et poliomyelitique inactivee. Archives Francaises de Pediatrie 1989;46:693-700.

Fine PM, Chen RT. Confounding in studies of adverse reactions to vaccines. American Journal of Epidemiology 1992;136:121-135.

Fischmeister M. [Acute reaction following injection with tetanus toxoid (letter).]. Akute Reaktion nach Tetanustoxoi-Injektion. Deutsche Medizinishe Wochenschrift 1974;99:850.

Fisher M. Anaphylaxis. Diseases of Man 1987;33:433-479.

Fishman PS, Carigan DR. Motoneuron uptake from the circulation of the binding fragment of tetanus toxin. Archives of Neurology 1988;45:558-561.

Flahault A, Messiah A, Jougla E, Bouvet E, Perin J, Hatton F. Sudden infant death syndrome and diphtheria/tetanus toxoid/pertussis/poliomyelitis immunisation (letter). Lancet 1988;1:582-583.

Floyd CB, Freeling P. Survey to establish the incidence of minor side effects in infants following protective immunization. Journal of the Royal College of General Practitioners 1989;39:359-363.

Foege WH, Eddins DL. Mass vaccination programs in developing countries. Progress in Medical Virology 1973;15:205-243.

Foege WH, Foster SO. Multiple antigen vaccine strategies in developing countries. American Journal of Tropical Medicine and Hygiene 1974;23:685-689.

Folie Pharmacother. Hypersensibilite aux vaccins contre l'hepatite B. Folie Pharmacother 1992;19:31-32.

Food and Drug Administration. No AIDS risk from polio vaccines. FDA Talk Paper, No. T92-19, April 6, 1992.

Food and Drug Administration. Unapproved DTP vaccine vials. FDA Talk Paper, No. T92-17, March 27, 1992.

Forsey T, Bentley ML, Minor PD, Begg N. Mumps vaccines and meningitis. Lancet 1992;340:980.

Forsey T, Mawn JA, Yates PJ, Bentley ML, Minor PD. Differentiation of vaccine and wild mumps viruses using the polymerase chain reaction and dideoxynucleotide sequencing. Journal of General Virology 1990;71(Pt. 4):987-990.

Forsey T, Minor PD. Mumps viruses and mumps, measles, and rubella vaccine (letter). British Medical Journal 1989;299:1340.

Forster J, Urbanek R. [Encephalitis following measles-mumps vaccination simultaneous to an EBV-infection] Encephalitis nach masern-mumps-impfung und gleichzeitiger EBV-infektion. Klinische Paediatrie 1982;194:29-30.

Forstrom L, Hannuksela M, Kousa M, Lehmuskallio E. Merthiolate hypersensitivity and vaccination. Contact Dermatitis 1980;6:241-245.

Fort P, Sekaran C, Stone P, Teichberg S, Wapnir RA, Lifshitz F. Mumps vaccine effects on glucose tolerance in genetically susceptible diabetes mellitus mice (DBA) (abstract no. 173). Diabetes 1977;26(Sup. 1):396.

Fothergill LD, Wright J. Influenzal meningitis: the relation of age incidence to the bactericidal power of blood against the causal organism. Journal of Immunology 1933;24:273-284.

Foulis AK. In type 1 diabetes, does a non-cytopathic viral infection of insulin-secreting B-cells initiate the disease process leading to their autoimmune destruction. Diabetic Medicine 1989;6:666-674.

Fourrier A, Valet PM, Mouton Y. [Encephalitis due to viral vaccines] Les encephalites des vaccins a virus. Journal de Medicine de Montpellier 1974;9:39-46.

Francis DP, Feorino PM, Mcdougal S. The safety of the hepatitis B vaccine: inactivation of the AIDS virus during routine vaccine manufacture. Journal of the American Medical Association 1986;256:869-872.

Francis DP, Hadler SC, Thompson SE et al. The prevention of hepatitis B with vaccine: report of the Centers for Disease Control multi-center efficacy trial among homosexual men. Annals of Internal Medicine 1982;97:362-366.

Frank AL, Labotka RJ, Rao S, Frisone LR, McVerry PH, Samuelson JS et al. Haemophilus influenzae type b immunization of children with sickle cell diseases. Pediatrics 1988;82:571-575.

Frank J, Loh K. SSPE: but we thought measles was gone! Journal of Pediatric Nursing 1991;6:87-92.

Frantzidou-Adamopoulou F. Poliomyelitis cases in northern Greece during 1976-1990. European Journal of Epidemiology 1992;8:112-113.

Fra Sundhedsstyrelsen. [Complications in poliovaccination with Sabin vaccine in Spring, 1966] Komplikationer ved poliovaccinationen med Sabin-vaccine forangaret 1966. Fra Sundhedsstyrelsen 1967;4:201-208.

Frayha HH, Dent P, Shannon HS, Johnson SE, Gordon L. Safety and immunogenicity of subcutaneous H. influenzae vaccines in 15-17 month-old children. Clinical and Investigative Medicine [Medicine Clinique et Experimentale] 1991;14:379-387.

Freeman T. Erythema multiforme in children taking amoxicillin after vaccination. Canadian Medical Association Journal 1982;127:818-820.

Fried M, Conen D, Conzelmann M, Steinemann E. Uveitis after hepatitis B vaccination (letter). Lancet 1987;2:631-632.

Friedland IR, Snipelisky M. Contraindications to immunisation. South African Medical Journal 1990;78:169-170.

Fritz RB, McFarlin DE. Encephalitogenic epitopes of myelin basic protein. Chemical Immunology 1989;46:101-125.

Fritzell B, Plotkin S. Efficacy and safety of a Haemophilus influenzae type b capsular polysaccharide-tetanus protein conjugate vaccine. Journal of Pediatrics 1992;121:355-362.

Froeschle JE, Connaught Laboratories. Presentation to the Institute of Medicine Vaccine Safety Committee. Public Meeting. Washington, DC, May 11, 1992.

Frontera Izquierdo P. [Should we modify antipoliomyelitis vaccination?] Debemos modificar la vacunacion antipoliomielitica? Anales Espanoles de Pediatria 1986;24:209-211.

Frosner GG. [Hepatitis B immunization: results of clinical trial and one year's use] Impfung gegen Hepatitis B: Ergebnisse der klinischen Prufung und der einjahrigen Anwendung. Monatsschrift fur Kinderheilkunde 1984;132:495-498.

Fujii H, Moriyama K, Sakamoto N, Kondo T, Yasuda K, Hiraizumi Y et al. Gly145 to Arg substitution in HBs antigen of immune escape mutant of hepatitis B virus. Biochemical and Biophysical Research Communications 1992;184:1152-1157.

Fujinaga T, Motegi Y, Tamura H, Kuroume T. A prefecture-wide survey of mumps meningitis associated with measles, mumps and rubella vaccine. Pediatric Infectious Disease Journal 1991;10:204-209.

Fujinami RS. Molecular mimicry. In: The Autoimmune Diseases. Academic Press, Inc.; 1992.

Fujinami RS, Oldstone MB. Molecular mimicry as a mechanism for virus-induced autoimmunity. Immunologic Research 1989;8:3-15.

Fujiyama S, Yoshida K, Sato T, Shimada H, Deguchi T. Immunogenicity and safety of recombinant yeast-derived hepatitis B vaccine in haemodialysis patients. Hepatogastroenterology 1990;37(Suppl. 2):140-144.

Fukumi H. [Viral vaccine: immunity and vaccine]. [Japanese Journal of Clinical Medicine] Nippon Rinsho 1971;29:1218-1224.

Fukuyama Y, Shirki K. [Current problems of measles encephalitis]. Naika 1970;25:416-420.

Fukuyama Y, Tomori N, Sugitate M. Critical evaluation of the role of immunization as an etiological factor of infantile spasms. Neuropadiatrie 1977;8:224-237.

Fulginiti VA. The problems of poliovirus immunization. Hospital Practice 1980;15:61-67.

Fulginiti VA. How safe are pertussis and rubella vaccines? A commentary on the Institute of Medicine report. Pediatrics 1992;89:334-336.

Fulginiti VA, Kempe CH. Killed-measles-virus vaccine. Lancet 1967;2:468.

Fulginiti VA, Arthur JH, Pearlman DS, Kempe CH. Altered reactivity to measles virus: local reactions following attenuated measles virus immunization in children who previously received a combination of inactivated and attenuated vaccines. American Journal of Diseases of Children 1968;115:671-676.

Fulginiti VA, Nelson JD, McCracken GH Jr. Panel on immunizations. Pediatric Infectious Disease Journal 1983;2(3 Suppl.):S64-S69.

Furesz J. Serologic diagnosis of measles in subacute sclerosing panencephalitis (letter). New England Journal of Medicine 1971;284:729-730.

Furesz J, Contreras G. Vaccine-related mumps meningitis—Canada / Meningite ourlienne vaccinale—Canada. Canada Diseases Weekly Report / Rapport hebdomadaire des maladies au Canada 1990;16:253-254.

Furlow TW Jr. Neuropathy after influenza vaccination (letter). Lancet 1977;1:253-254.

Gaebler JW, Kleiman MB, French ML, Chastain G, Barrett C, Griffin C. Neurologic complications in oral polio vaccine recipients. Journal of Pediatrics 1986;108:878-881.

Galazka AM, Lauer BA, Henderson RH, Keja J. Indications and contraindications for vaccines used in the Expanded Programme on Immunization. Bulletin of the World Health Organization 1984;62:357-366.

Galazka AM, Lauer BA, Henderson RH, Keja J. [Indications and contraindications of vaccines used in the Extended Programme on Immunization] Indications et contre-indications des vaccins utilises dans le Programme elargi de vaccination. [Bulletin of the World Health Organization] Bulletin de l'Organisation mondiale de la Sante 1984;62:517-526.

Galazka AM, Lauer BA, Henderson RH, Keja J. [Indications and contraindications of vaccines used in the Expanded Programme on Immunization] Indications et contre-indications des vaccins utilises dans le Programme elargi de vaccination. Medecine et Hygiene 1985;43:1718-1725.

Galbraith NS, Crosby G, Barnes JM, Fernandes R. Simultaneous immunization with B.C.G., diphtheria-tetanus, and oral poliomyelitis vaccines in children aged 13-14. British Medical Journal 1971;2:193-197.

Galbraith NS, Young SE, Pusey JJ, Crombie DL, Sparks JP. Mumps surveillance in England and Wales 1962-81. Lancet 1984;1:91-94.

Gale JL, Thapa PB, Bobo JK, Wassilak SG, Mendelman PM, Foy HM. Acute neurological illness and DTP: report of a case-control study in Washington and Oregon. Sixth International Symposium on Pertussis Abstracts. DHHS Publication No. (FDA) 90-1162. Bethesda, MD: U.S. Public Health Service, U.S. Department of Health and Human Services; 1990.

Galili S. A mild form of Stevens-Johnson syndrome following measles vaccination. Israel Journal of Medical Sciences 1967;3:903-905.

Gambia Hepatitis Study Group. Hepatitis B vaccine in the Expanded Program on Immunization: the Gambian experience. Lancet 1989;1:1057-1060.

Gamble DR. Relation of antecedent illness to development of diabetes in children. British Medical Journal 1980;281:99-101.

Gamboa ET, Cowen D, Eggers A, Cogan P, Ganti R, Brust JC. Delayed onset of post-rabies vaccination encephalitis. Annals of Neurology 1983;13:676-678.

Ganguly R, Cusumano CL, Waldman RH. Suppression of cell-mediated immunity after infection with attenuated rubella virus. Infection and Immunity 1976;13:464-469.

Ganiats TG, Bowersox MT, Ralph LP. Universal neonatal hepatitis B immunization—are we jumping on the bandwagon too early? (editorial). Journal of Family Practice 1993;36:147-149.

Ganry O, Lerailler F, Vercelletto M, Chiffoleau A, Larousse C. [Peripheral facial paralysis following immunization for hepatitis b vaccine: a case report] Paralysie faciale peripherique faisant suite a une vaccination contre l'hepatite b: a propos d'un cas. Therapie 1992;47:437-438.

Garber HJ, Witte JJ, Tayback M, Latta R, Kelley E. Clinical reactions following vaccination with two types of live virus measles vaccines. Journal of the American Medical Association 1968;205:309-311.

Garenne M, Leroy O, Beau JP, Sene I. Child mortality after high-titre measles vaccines: prospective study in Senegal. Lancet 1991;338:903-907.

Gateff C, Relyveld EH, Le Gonidec G, Vincent J, McBean AM, Durand B et al. [A simplified tetanus immunization associated with live viral vaccines] Vaccination antitetanique simplifiee associee a des vaccins viraux vivants. Medecine Tropicale 1974;34:171-181.

Gathier JC, Bruyn GW. Peripheral neuropathies following the administration of heterologous immune sera: a critical evaluation. Psychiatria, Neurologia, Neurochirurgia 1968;71:351-371.

Gear MW. Immunization against tetanus. Postgraduate Medical Journal 1965;41:10-14.

Geffen T. Poliovaccination in the Gambia (letter). Lancet 1987;2:511-512.

Geier MR, Stanbro H, Merril CR. Endotoxins in commercial vaccines. Applied and Environmental Microbiology 1978;36:445-449.

Geissler E, Staneczek W. SV40 and human brain tumors. Archiv fur Geschwulstforschung 1988;58:129-134.

Gerber P. Patterns of antibodies to SV40 in children following the last booster with inactivated poliomyelitis vaccines. Proceedings of the Society for Experimental Biology and Medicine 1967;125:1284-1287.

Gerbrandy JL, Bienenstock J. Kinetics and localization of IgE tetanus antibody response in mice immunized by the intratracheal, intraperitoneal and subcutaneous routes. Immunology 1976;31:913-919.

Gerety RJ, Tabor E. Newly licensed hepatitis B vaccine: known safety and unknown risks. Journal of the American Medical Association 1983;249:745-746.

Gerichter C, Lasch E, Sever I, el-Massri M, Skalska P. Paralytic poliomyelitis in the Gaza Strip and West Bank during recent years. Developments in Biological Standardization 1978;41:173-177.

Gersbach P, Waridel D. [Paralysis after tetanus prevention] Paralysie apres preevention antitetanique. Schweizerische Medizinische Wochenschrift 1976;106:150-153.

Gershon AA. Immunization practices in children. Hospital Practice 1990;25:91-94, 97-103, 107.

Gerson K, Haslam RH A. Subtle immunologic abnormalities in four boys with subacute sclerosing panencephalitis. New England Journal of Medicine 1971;285:78-82.

Gervaix A, Caflisch M, Suter S, Haenggeli CA. Guillain-Barre syndrome following immunization with *Haemophilus influenzae* type b conjugate vaccine. European Journal of Pediatrics 1993;152:613-614.

Gezondheidsraad. Report on Hepatitis B. The Hague, The Netherlands: Gezondheidsraad [Health Council of the Netherlands]; 1983.

Gezondheidsraad. Adverse Reactions to Vaccines in the National Vaccination Programme in 1986. The Hague, The Netherlands: Gezondheidsraad [Health Council of the Netherlands]; 1987.

Gezondheidsraad. Adverse Reactions to Vaccines in the National Vaccination Programme in 1987. The Hague, The Netherlands: Gezondheidsraad [Health Council of the Netherlands]; 1988.

Gezondheidsraad. Adverse Reactions to Vaccines in the National Immunization Programme in 1988. The Hague, The Netherlands: Gezondheidsraad [Health Council of the Netherlands]; 1989.

Gezondheidsraad. Adverse Reactions to Vaccines in the National Vaccination Programme in 1989. The Hague, The Netherlands: Gezondheidsraad [Health Council of the Netherlands]; 1990.

Gezondheidsraad. Adverse Reactions to Vaccines in the National Vaccination Programme in 1990. The Hague, The Netherlands: Gezondheidsraad [Health Council of the Netherlands]; 1991.

Gezondheidsraad. Adverse Reactions to Vaccinations in the National Immunization Programme in 1991. The Hague, The Netherlands: Gezondheidsraad [Health Council of the Netherlands]; 1993.

Ghosh S, Kumari S, Bhargava SK. Antibody titres after measles vaccine. Indian Journal of Medical Research 1977;66:165-171.

Giammanco G, Li Volti S, Mauro L, Ciccia M, De Maria C, Patania S et al. Antibody responses of children to a measles mumps and rubella vaccine administered alone or simultaneously with booster doses of diphtheria-tetanus and oral poliovirus vaccines. Igiene Moderna 1989;92:1212-1218.

Giammanco G, Li Volti S, Mauro L, Giammanco Bilancia G, Salemi I, Barone P et al. Immune response to simultaneous administration of a recombinant DNA hepatitis B vaccine and multiple compulsory vaccines in infancy. Vaccine 1991;9:747-750.

Gigliotti F, Feldman S, Wang WC, Day SW, Brunson G. Immunization of young infants with sickle cell disease with a *Haemophilus influenzae* type b saccharide-diphtheria CRM 197 protein conjugate vaccine. Journal of Pediatrics 1989;114:1006-1010.

Gigliotti F, Feldman S, Wang WC, Day SW, Brunson G. Serologic follow-up of children with sickle cell disease immunized with a *Haemophilus influenzae* type b conjugate vaccine during early infancy. Journal of Pediatrics 1991;118:917-919.

Gilbert GL. *Haemophilus influenzae* type b vaccines in Australia. Australian Paediatric Journal 1989;25:185-186.

Gill D. Measles: going, going, gone? (editorial). Irish Medical Journal 1986;79:174-175.

Gillie C, Hodgkin K. An effective measles immunisation programme in a general practice. Journal of the Royal College of General Practitioners 1968;15:258-260.

Gillum JE, Garrison MW, Crossley KB, Rotschafer JC. Current immunization practices. 1. Polio, diphtheria, tetanus, pertussis, measles, mumps, rubella, and influenza. Postgraduate Medicine 1989;85:183-186, 188-190, 195, 198.

Gilmartin RC, Ch'ien LT. Guillain-Barre syndrome with hydrocephalus in early infancy. Archives of Neurology 1977;34:567-569.

Gilsdorf JR. *Haemophilus influenzae* type b vaccine. Indian Journal of Pediatrics 1988;55:218-224.

Gimeno de Sande A, Najera R, Najera E, Ortiz Berrocal A, Perez Gallardo F. [Results of the 1968 measles vaccination campaign] Resultados de la Campana de Vacunacion antisarampion 1968. Revista de Sanidad e Higiene Publica 1972;46:805-821.

Ginting R, Schilling G, Eis-Hubinger AM, Gerritzen A. [Hepatitis B vaccines: protective action and side effects] Hepatitis-B-Impfstoffe: Schutzwirkung und Nebenwirkungen. Arbeitsmedizin, Sozialmedizin, Praventivmedizin 1990;25:517-519.

Giroud M, Page G, Genelle B, Lacroix X. Les thrombopenies post vaccinales avec purpura [Post-vaccinal thrombopenia with purpura]. Journal de Medecine de Lyon 1983;64:97-100.

Girsh LS. Current neurological trends with allergic implications. Immunology and Allergy Practice 1981;3:19-28.

Gladisch R., Hofmann W, Waldherr R. Myokarditis und insulitis nach Coxsackie virus infekt. Zeitschrift fur Kardiologie 1976;65:837-849.

Gladwell M. It's possible, but not likely: this theory leaves even more mysterious questions. Washington Post. April 5, 1992:C3.

Glenn MP, McKendrick DW. Varicella bullosa associated with measles vaccine. British Journal of Dermatology 1970;83:595-596.

Gluck R, Hoskins JM, Wegmann A, Just M, Germanier R. Rubini, a new live attenuated mumps vaccine virus strain for human diploid cells. Developments in Biological Standardization 1986;65:29-35.

Gocke DJ. Extrahepatic manifestations of viral hepatitis. American Journal of Medical Science 1975;270:49-52.

Gocke JD. Immune complex phenomena associated with hepatitis. In: Vyas GN, Cohen SN, Schmid R, eds. Viral Hepatitis: A Contemporary Assessment of Etiology, Epidemiology, Pathogenesis and Prevention. Philadelphia: Franklin Institute Press; 1977.

Goepp JG, Hohenboken M, Almeidohill J, Santosham M. Persistent urinary antigen excretion in infants vaccinated with *Haemophilus influenzae* type b capsular polysaccharide conjugated with outer membrane protein from *Neisseria meningitidis*. Pediatric Infectious Disease Journal 1992;11:2-5.

Goetz O. [Preventive vaccination against measles and rubella] Masernschutzimpfung und Rotelnschutzimpfung. Medizinische Klinik 1972;67:217-221.

Gogolin J. [A study to determine the neuropathogenicity of mumps vaccine on dwarf pigs] Untersuchungen zur Neuropathogenitatsbestimmung von Mumps-Impfstoff an Zwergschweinen. Zeitschrift fur die Gesamte Hygiene Ihre Grenzgebiete 1981;27:239-241.

Gold H. Sensitization induced by tetanus toxoid, alum precipitated. Journal of Laboratory and Clinical Medicine 1941;27:26-36.

Gold R, Scheifele D, Fast M, Contreras G, Gagnon A, Sidorowicz E et al. Evaluation of poliovirus-related cases occurring in Canada in 1989 / Etude des cas lies a des poliovirus survenus au Canada en 1989. Canada Diseases Weekly Report / Rapport hebdomadaire des maladies au Canada 1991;17:75-78.

Goldblatt D, Turner MW, Levinsky RJ. Branhamella catarrhalis: antigenic determinants and the development of the IgG subclass response in childhood. Journal of Infectious Diseases 1990;162:1128-1135.

Golden JA. No increased incidence of AIDS in recipients of hepatitis B vaccine (letter). New England Journal of Medicine 1983;308:1163-1164.

Goldsmith MF. Vaccine information pamphlets here, but some physicians react strongly. Journal of the American Medical Association 1992;267:2005-2007.

Goldwater PN. The cost of hepatitis B vaccine: money or morbidity? (letter). New Zealand Medical Journal 1983;96:588.

Goldwater PN. Hypersensitivity to intradermal hepatitis B vaccine (letter). Lancet 1984;2:1156.

Golub N, Bogdanov I, Vashchenko M. [Possibility of diseases affecting the central nervous system caused by vaccine strains of poliovirus, type 3] O vozmozhnosti zabolevanii s porazheniem tsentral'noi nervnoi sistemy, vyzvannykh vaktsinopodobnymi shtammami poliovirusa tipa 3. Zhurnal Mikrobiologii, Epidemiologii, i Immunobiologii 1972;49:134-136.

Gonzalez E, Cordero J. [Poliomyelitis associated with a vaccine: two clinical cases] Poliomielitis asociada a vacuna: dos casos clinicos. Revista Medica de Chile 1988;116:461-464.

Goolsby PL. Erythema nodosum after Recombivax HB hepatitis B vaccine (letter). New England Journal of Medicine 1989;321:1198-1199.

Gordon EH, Krouse HA, Kinney JL, Stiehm JR, Klaustermeyer WB. Delayed cutaneous hypersensitivity in normals: choice of antigens and comparison to in vitro assays of cell-mediated immunity. Journal of Allergy and Clinical Immunology 1983;72:487-494.

Gordon LK. Characterization of a hapten-carrier conjugate vaccine: *H. influenzae*-diphtheria conjugate vaccine. In: Chanock RM, Lerner RA, eds. Modern Approaches to Vaccines. Cold Spring Harbor, NY: Cold Spring Harbor Laboratory; 1984.

Gorshunova LP, Mikhailova GR. [Effect of viral vaccines on animal bone marrow cell chromosomes] Issledovanie vliianiia protivovirusnykh vaktsin na khromosomy kletok kostnogo mozga zhivotnykh. Voprosy Virusologii 1976;5:521-526.

Gorshunova LP, Bektemirov TA, Koshtoyan SE. [On production of interferon and nonspecific protective reactions in the central nervous systems of animals vaccinated with live measles vaccine] O produktsii interferona i nespetsificheskikh zashchitnykh reaktsiiakh v tsentralnoi nervnoi sisteme zhivotnykh pri vaktsiantsii zhivoi protivokorevoi vaktsinoi. Voprosy Virusologii 1971;16:735-739.

Gorshunova LP, Mikhailova GR, Cherkezia SE. [Effect of mice immunization with live antiviral vaccines on bone marrow cell chromosomes in the first generation progeny] Vliianie immunizatsii myshei zhivymi protivovirusnymi vaktsinami na khromosomy kletok kostnogo mozga potomstva pervogo pokoleniia. Tsitologiia i Genetika 1975;9:542-545.

Goubau P. Immunogenicity and safety of measles vaccine in ill African children (letter). International Journal of Epidemiology 1989;18:467.

Grabenstein JD. Delayed-hypersensitivity testing: guide to product selection. Hospital Pharmacy 1990;25:1102-1107.

Graham DY, Brown CH, Benrey J, Butel JS. Thrombocytopenia. Journal of the American Medical Association 1974;227:1161-1164.

Granoff DM, Cates KL. *Haemophilus influenzae* type b polysaccharide vaccines. Journal of Pediatrics 1985;107:330-336.

Granoff DM, Munson RS Jr. Prospects for prevention of *Haemophilus influenzae* type b disease by immunization. Journal of Infectious Diseases 1986;153:448-461.

Granoff DM, Osterholm MT. Safety and efficacy of *Haemophilus influenzae* type b polysaccharide vaccine. Pediatrics 1987;80:590-592.

Granoff DM, Anderson EL, Osterholm MT et al. Differences in the immunogenicity of three *Haemophilus influenzae* type b conjugate vaccines in infants. Journal of Pediatrics 1992;121:187-194.

Granoff DM, Boies EG, Munson RS. Immunogenicity of *Haemophilus influenzae* type b polysaccharide-diphtheria toxoid conjugate vaccine in adults. Journal of Pediatrics 1984;105:22-27.

Granoff DM, Chacko A, Lottenbach KR, Sheetz KE. Immunogenicity of *Haemophilus influenzae* type b polysaccharide-outer membrane protein conjugate vaccine in patients who acquired Haemophilus disease despite previous vaccination with type b polysaccharide vaccine. Journal of Pediatrics 1989;114:925-933.

Granoff DM, Holmes SJ, Osterholm MT. Induction of immunologic memory in infants primed with *Haemophilus influenzae* type b conjugate vaccines. Journal of Infectious Diseases; in press.

Granoff DM, Pandey JP, Boies E et al. Response to immunization with *Haemophilus influenzae* type b polysaccharide-pertussis vaccine and risk of *haemophilis* meningitis in children with the km(1) immunoglobulin allotype. Journal of Clinical Investigation 1984;74:1708-1714.

Granoff DM, Shackelford PG, Suarez BK et al. *Haemophilus influenzae* type b disease in children vaccinated with type b polysaccharide vaccine. New England Journal of Medicine 1986;315:1584-1590.

Granoff DM, Weinberg GA, Shackelford PE. IgG subclass response to immunization with *Haemophilus influenzae* type b polysaccharide-outer membrane protein conjugate vaccine. Pediatric Research 1988;24:180-185.

Grant KL. Recombinant hepatitis B vaccine-induced central nervous system demyelination. P & T 1992;17:297.

Grattan-Smith PJ, Procopis PG, Wise GA, Grigor WG. Serious neurological complications of measles: a continuing preventable problem. Medical Journal of Australia 1985;143:385-387.

Gray BM. Opsonophagocidal activity in sera from infants and children immunized with *Haemophilus influenzae* type b conjugate vaccine (meningococcal protein conjugate). Pediatrics 1990;85(4 Pt 2):694-697.

Gray JA, Burns SM. Mumps meningitis after mumps, measles, and rubella vaccination (letter). British Medical Journal 1989;299:1464-1465.

Gray JA, Burns SM. Mumps meningitis following measles, mumps, and rubella immunisation (letter). Lancet 1989;2:98.

Gray JA, Burns SM. Mumps vaccine meningitis (letter). Lancet 1989;2:927.

Grazhdanov NP, Popov VF, Sokhin AA, Salmin LV, Frolov AK, Ektova LK et al. [Safety, antigenic activity and epidemiologic effectiveness of live parotitis vaccine from strain Leningrad-3. I. Study of the reactogenic, allergenic and mutagenic properties of the vaccine and its effect on systemic resistance against intercurrent diseases] Bezvrednost, antigennaia aktivnost i epidemiologicheskaia effektivnost zhivoi parotitnoi vaktsiny iz shtamma Leningrad-3. Soobshchenie I. Reaktogennye, allergennye i mutagennye svoistva vaktsiny i ee vliianie na rezistentnost organizma k interkurrentnym zabolevaniiam. Zhurnal Mikrobiologii, Epidemiologii, i Immunobiologii 1981;1:69-74.

Greco D. Case-control study on encephalopathy associated with diphtheria-tetanus immunization in Campania, Italy. Bulletin of the World Health Organization 1985;63:919-925.

Green A, Gale EA, Patterson CC. Incidence of childhood-onset insulin-dependent diabetes mellitus: the EURODIAB ACE study. Lancet 1992;339:905-909.

Green C, Lakshmipathi T. A case of hepatitis related to etretinate therapy and hepatitis B vaccine. Dermatologica 1991;182:119-120.

Green MS, Handsher R, Cohen D, Melnick JL, Slepon R, Mendelsohn E et al. Age differences in immunity against wild and vaccine strains of poliovirus prior to the 1988 outbreak in Israel and response to booster immunization. Vaccine 1993;11:75-81.

Green MS, Melnick JL, Cohen D, Slepon R, Danon YL. Response to trivalent oral poliovirus vaccine with and without immune serum globulin in young adults in Israel in 1988. Journal of Infectious Diseases 1990;162:971-974.

Greenberg DP, Vadheim CM, March SM, Ward JI, Kaiser-UCLA Hib Vaccine Study Group. Evaluation of the safety, immunogenicity, and efficacy of *Haemophilus* b (Hib) PRP-T conjugate vaccine in a prospective, randomized, and placebo-controlled trial in young infants. Program Abstracts of the 32nd Interscience Conference on Antimicrobial Agents and Chemotherapy. Abstract 65, p. 109. Washington, DC: American Society for Microbiology; 1991.

Greenberg DP, Ward JI, Burkart K et al. Factors influencing immunogenicity and safety of two *Haemophilus influenzae* type b polysaccharide vaccines in children 18 and 24 months of age. Pediatric Infectious Disease Journal 1987;6:660-665.

Greenberg MA, Birx DL. Safe administration of mumps-measles-rubella vaccine in egg-allergic children. Journal of Pediatrics 1988;113:504-506.

Greenstreet R. Adjustment of rates of Guillain-Barre syndrome among recipients of swine flu vaccine, 1976-1977 (letter). Journal of the Royal Society of Medicine 1983;76:620-621.

Greenwood BM, Greenwood AM, Bradley AK et al. Studies with combined meningococcal vaccines. I. A combined meningococcal, measles and tetanus vaccine. Annals of Tropical Medicine and Parasitology 1981;75:217-226.

Grenier B, Viarme F, Roumiantzeff M, Xueref C, Demont F. [Antipoliomyelitis vaccination of young children with a new inactivated vaccine: serological results] Vaccination antipoliomyelitique de jeunes enfants par un nouveau vaccin inactive: resultats serologiques. Archives Francaises de Pediatrie 1985;42:321-323.

Griffin DE. Monophasic autoimmune inflammatory diseases of the CNS and PNS. Research Publications—Association for Research in Nervous and Mental Disease 1990;68:91-104.

Griffin MR, Ray WA, Livengood JR, Schaffner W. Risk of sudden infant death syndrome after immunization with the diphtheria-tetanus-pertussis vaccine. New England Journal of Medicine 1988;319:618-623.

Griffin MR, Ray WA, Mortimer EA, Fenichel GM, Schaffner W. Risk of seizures and encephalopathy after immunization with the diphtheria-tetanus-pertussis vaccine. Journal of the American Medical Association 1990;263):1641-1645.

Griffin MR, Ray WA, Mortimer EA, Fenichel GM, Schaffner W. Risk of seizures after measles-mumps-rubella immunization. Pediatrics 1991;88:881-885.

Griffin MR, Taylor JA, Daugherty JR, Ray WA. No increased risk for invasive bacterial infection found following diphtheria-tetanus-pertussis immunization. Pediatrics 1992;89(4 Pt. 1):640-642.

Griffith RD, Miller OF III. Erythema multiforme following diphtheria and tetanus toxoid vaccination. Journal of the American Academy of Dermatology 1988;19:758-759.

Grilli G, Cimini D, Vacca F. [Antimeasles vaccine: incidence of side-effects using two different vaccine strains] Vaccinazione antimorbillo: incidenza di effetti collaterali utilizzando due diversi ceppi di vaccino. Giornale di Malattie Infettive e Parassitarie 1991;43:147-149.

Grilli G, Cimini D, Vacca F et al. [Vaccination against measles, mumps and rubella: incidence of side effects using different vaccine strains] Vaccinazione contro morbillo, parotite e rosolia: incidenza di effetti collaterali utilizzando vaccini di diversa composizione. Giornale di Malattie Infettive e Parassitarie 1992;44:38-42.

Gronski P, Seiler FR, Schwick HG. Discovery of antitoxins and development of antibody preparations for clinical uses from 1890 to 1990. Molecular Immunology 1991;28:1321-1332.

Grose C. Guillain-Barre syndrome (letter). American Journal of Diseases of Children 1974;127(3):444.

Grose C, Henle W, Henle G, Feorino PM. Primary Epstein-Barr-virus infections in acute neurologic diseases. New England Journal of Medicine 1975;292:392-395.

Grose C, Spigland I. Guillain-Barre syndrome following administration of live measles vaccine. American Journal of Medicine 1976;60:441-443.

Gross TP, Hayes SW. *Haemophilus* conjugate vaccine and Guillain-Barre syndrome (letter). Journal of Pediatrics 1991;118:161.

Gross TP, Khurana RK, Higgins T, Nkowane BS, Hirsch RL. Vaccine-associated poliomyelitis in a household contact with Netherton's syndrome receiving long-term steroid therapy. American Journal of Medicine 1987;83:797-800.

Gross TP, Milstien JB, Kuritsky JN. Bulging fontanelle after immunization with diphtheria-tetanus-pertussis vaccine and diphtheria-tetanus vaccine. Journal of Pediatrics 1989;114:423-425.

Guerin A, Buisson Y, Nutini MT, Saliou P, London G, Marchais S. Response to vaccination against tetanus in chronic haemodialysed patients. Nephrology, Dialysis, Transplantation 1992;7:323-326.

Guillain G, Barre JA, Strohl A. Sur un syndrome de radiculonevrite avec hyperalbuminose due liquide cephalo-rachidien sans reaction cellulaire: remarques sure les caracteres cliniques et graphiques des reflexes tendineux. Bulletins et Memoires Societe Medicale des Hopitaux de Paris 1916;40:1462-1470.

Gunby P. 'Atypical' mumps may occur after immunization. Journal of the American Medical Association 1980;243:2374-2375.

Gunby P. SSPE incidence, therapy receive renewed attention. Journal of the American Medical Association 1981;246:927, 931-932.

Gunderman JR. Guillain-Barre syndrome: occurrence following combined mumps-rubella vaccine. American Journal of Diseases of Children 1973;125:834-835.

Gunderson E. Is diabetes of infectious origin? Journal of Infectious Diseases 1927;41:197-202.

Gunn TR, Bosley A, Woodfield DG. The safety and immunogenicity of a recombinant hepatitis B vaccine in neonates. New Zealand Medical Journal 1989;102:1-3.

Gupta RK, Relyveld EH. Adverse reactions after injection of adsorbed diphtheria-pertussis-tetanus (DPT) vaccine are not due only to pertussis organisms or pertussis components in the vaccine. Vaccine 1991;9:699-702.

Gupte SC, Bhatia HM. Anti-A and anti-B titre response after tetanus toxoid injections in normal adults and pregnant women. Indian Journal of Medical Research 1979;70:221-228.

Gupte SC, Bhatia HM. Increased incidence of haemolytic disease of the new-born caused by ABO-incompatibility when tetanus toxoid is given during pregnancy. Vox Sanguinis 1980;38:22-28.

Gutierrez K, Abzug MJ. Vaccine-associated poliovirus meningitis in children with ventriculoperitoneal shunts. Journal of Pediatrics 1990;117:424-427.

Gutierrez-Lopez MD, Bertera S, Chantres MT, Vavassori C, Dorman JS, Trucco M et al. Susceptibility to Type 1 (insulin-dependent) diabetes mellitus in Spanish patients correlates quantitatively with expression of HLA-DQ(alpha) ARG 52 and HLA-DQ(beta) non-Asp 57 alleles. Diabetologia 1992;35:583-588.

Haas D, Krause-Wichmann D. [Important notice concerning information on damage caused by oral polio vaccination] Wichtige Hinweise zur Impfschaden-Aufklarung nach Polio-Schluckimpfung. Offentliche Gesundheitswesen 1968;30:291-293.

Hachulla E, Houvenagel E, Mingui A, Vincent G, Laine A. Reactive arthritis after hepatitis B vaccination. Journal of Rheumatology 1990;17:1250-1251.

Hadler SC, Margolis HS. Hepatitis B immunization: vaccine types, efficacy, and indications for immunization. Current Clinical Topics in Infectious Diseases 1992;12:282-308.

Hagen-Coenen J, Drinka PJ, Siewert M. Tetanus-diphtheria vaccinations in a veterans nursing home. Journal of the American Geriatric Society 1992;40:513-514.

Hagge W, Enders-Ruckle G, von Brenndorff AI. [Atypical measles following immunization with inactivated measles vaccine (split vaccine)] Atypische Masern nach Immunisierung mit inaktiviertem Masernimpfstoff (Spaltvakzine). Monatsschrift fur Kinderheilkunde 1974;122:504-506.

Hajeri H. [Vaccinations and pregnancy] Vaccins et grossesse. Revue de Medecine 1978;19:947-950.

Hallam LA. Role of aluminium sensitivity in delayed persistent immunisation reactions (letter). Journal of Clinical Pathology 1991;44:877.

Halliday ML, Kang LY, Rankin JG, Coates RA, Corey PN, Hu ZH et al. An efficacy trial of a mammalian cell-derived recombinant DNA hepatitis B vaccine in infants born to mothers positive for HBsAg, in Shanghai, China. International Journal of Epidemiology 1992;21:564-573.

Halsey NA. Risk of subacute sclerosing panencephalitis from measles vaccination. Pediatric Infectious Disease Journal 1990;9:857-858.

Halsey NA. Case material on subacute sclerosing panencephalitis. Submitted to the Institute of Medicine Vaccine Safety Committee, November 1992.

Halsey NA, Holt E. Confounders are always a problem. Pediatrics 1990;86:490-491.

Halsey NA, Boulos R, Mode F, Andre J, Bowman L, Yaeger RG et al. Response to measles vaccine in Haitian infants 6 to 12 months old: influence of maternal antibodies, malnutrition, and concurrent illnesses. New England Journal of Medicine 1985;313:544-549.

Halsey NA, Modlin JF, Dyken PR. Subacute sclerosing panencephalitis (letter). Pediatric Neurology 1991;7:151.

Halsey NA, Modlin JF, Jabbour JT, Dubey L, Eddins DL, Ludwig DD. Risk factors in subacute sclerosing panencephalitis: a case-control study. American Journal of Epidemiology 1980;111:415-424.

Halsey NA, Modlin JF, Jabbour JT. Subacute sclerosing panencephalitis (SSPE): an epidemiologic review. In: Stevens JG et al., eds. Persistent Viruses. New York: Academic Press; 1978:101-114.

Halsey NA, Schubert W, Jabbour JT, Preblud SR. Measles vaccine and the course of subacute sclerosing panencephalitis (letter). Lancet 1978;2:783.

Halsey NA, Weiner LB, Meyers MG, Herrmann KL, Hinman A. Clinical evaluation of a new live measles vaccine derived in chick chorioallantoic membranes. Journal of Biological Standardization 1981;9:507-511.

Hamilos DL, Young RM, Peter JB, Agopian MS, Ikle DN, Barka N. Hypogammaglobulinemia in asthmatic patients. Annals of Allergy 1992;68:472-481.

Hammon WM, Coriell LL, Stokes J. Evaluation of Red Cross gamma globulin as a prophylactic agent for poliomyelitis. Journal of the American Medical Association 1952;150:739-760.

Hammon WM, Coriell LL, Wehrle PF, Stokes J. Evaluation of Red Cross gamma globulin as a prophylactic agent for poliomyelitis. 4. Final report of results based on clinical diagnoses. Journal of the American Medical Association 1953;151:1272-1285.

Haneberg B, Matre R, Winsnes R, Dalen A, Vogt H, Finne PH. Acute hemolytic anemia related to diphtheria-pertussis-tetanus vaccination. Acta Paediatrica Scandinavica 1978;67:345-350.

Haneberg B, Orstavik I. Poliomyelitis associated with oral poliovaccine: report on two cases. Acta Paediatrica Scandinavica 1972;61:105-108.

Hankey GJ. Guillain-Barre syndrome in Western Australia, 1980-1985. Medical Journal of Australia 1987;146:130-133.

Hankins RW, Black FL. Western blot analyses of measles virus antibody in normal persons and in patients with multiple sclerosis, subacute sclerosing panencephalitis, or atypical measles. Journal of Clinical Microbiology 1986;24:324-329.

Hansen J, Lennarzt H. Die virusdiagnostik zur atiologischen klarung. Deutsche Zeitscrift fur Nervenheilkunde 1961;182:185-200.

Hansson H, Moller H. Cutaneous reactions to merthiolate and their relationship to vaccination with tetanus toxoid. Acta Allergologica 1971;26:150-156.

Hara M, Saito Y, Komatsu T, Kodama H, Abo W, Chiba S et al. Antigenic analysis of polioviruses isolated from a child with agammaglobulinemia and paralytic poliomyelitis after Sabin vaccine administration. Microbiology and Immunology 1981;25:905-913.

Harcus AW, Ward AE, Roberts JS, Bryett KA. An evaluation of diphtheria-tetanus (adult) vaccine in unselected human volunteers. Journal of International Medical Research 1989;17:262-267.

Harjulehto T, Aro T, Hovi T, Saxen L. Congenital malformations and oral poliovirus vaccination during pregnancy. Lancet 1989;1:771-772.

Harrer G, Melnizky U, Wendt H. [Accommodation paresis and swallowing paralysis following tetanus toxoid booster inoculation] Akkommodationsparese und Schlucklahmung nach Tetanus-Toxoid-Auffrischungsimpfung. Wiener Medizinische Wochenschrift 1971;121:296-297.

Harris G. Can injection technique reduce vaccine reactions? Practitioner 1983;227:299-300.

Harris HF. A case of diabetes mellitus quickly following mumps. Boston Medical and Surgical Journal 1899;140:465-469.

Harris MF. The safety of measles vaccine in severe illness (letter). South African Medical Journal 1979;55:38.

Harris RW, Isacson P, Karzon DT. Vaccine-induced hypersensitivity: reactions to live measles and mumps vaccine in prior recipients of inactivated measles vaccine. Journal of Pediatrics 1969;74:552-563.

Harrison HR, Fulginiti VA. Bacterial immunizations. American Journal of Diseases of Children 1980;134:184-193.

Harrison LH, Broome CV, Hightower AW, Hoppe CC, Makintubee S, Sitze SL et al. A day care-based study of the efficacy of *Haemophilus* b polysaccharide vaccine. Journal of the American Medical Association 1988;260:1413-1418.

Hartman S. Convulsion associated with fever following hepatitis B vaccination (letter). Journal of Paediatrics and Child Health 1990;26:65.

Hartsock R. Postvaccinal lymphadenitis. Hyperplasia of lymphoid tissue that simulates malignant lymphomas. Cancer 1968;21:632-649.

Hartung HP, Toyka KV. T-cell and macrophage activation in experimental autoimmune neuritis and Guillain-Barre syndrome. Annals of Neurology 1990;27(Suppl.):S57-S63.

Hasselbacher P et al. Neuropathy after influenza vaccination. Lancet 1977;1:551-552.

Hassin H. Ophthalmoplegic migraine wrongly attributed to measles immunization. American Journal of Ophthalmology 1987;104:192-193.

Hatem J. Fallout from Washington: the IOM report continues to be misinterpreted. NVIC News (National Vaccine Information Center) 1992;2(1):4.

Hatem J. IOM given new contract to review remaining vaccines. NVIC News 1992;2(1):4.

Haun U, Ehrhardt G. [Postvaccinal complications following protective vaccination against measles]. Zur problematik postvakzinaler komplikationen nach Masernschutzimpfung. Deutsche Gesundheitswesen 1973;28:1306-1308.

Hauser P, Voet P, Simoen E. Immunological properties of recombinant HBsAg produced in yeast. Postgraduate Medical Journal 1987;63(Suppl. 2):83-91.

Hayward JC, Gillespie SM, Kaplan KM, Packer R, Pallansch M, Plotkin S et al. Outbreak of poliomyelitis-like paralysis associated with enterovirus 71. Pediatric Infectious Disease Journal 1989;8:611-616.

Healy CE. Mumps vaccine and nerve deafness. American Journal of Diseases of Children 1972;123:612.

Heaton KW. Measles inoculation. British Medical Journal 1968;2:435.

Hecht FM. *H. influenzae* vaccines in HIV (letter). New England Journal of Medicine 1992;326:1569-1571.

Hedges LV, Cooper H, Bushman BJ. Testing the null hypothesis in meta-analysis: a comparison of combined probability and confidence interval procedures. Psychological Bulletin 1992;111:188-194.

Heidel G, Demmler M. [Neurological syndromes as atypical courses of vaccination after protective influenza a vaccination] Neurologische syndrome als atypische impfverlaufe nach influenza-a-schutzimpfung. Zeitschrift fur die Gesamte Hygiene und Ihre Grenzgebiete 1985;31:218-220.

Heidel G, Olbricht H, Ely K, Henkler J. [Influence of measles vaccination using the live measles virus vaccine SSW-L 16 on the complication rate in measles] Der Einfluss der Masernimpfung mit Masern-Lebendvirus-Impfstoff SSW-L 16 auf die Komplikationsrate bei Masernerkrankungen. Zeitschrift fur Arztliche Fortbildung 1972;66:171-174.

Heinonen OP, Shapiro S, Monson RR, Hartz SC, Rosenberg L, Slone D. Immunization during pregnancy against poliomyelitis and influenza in relation to childhood malignancy. International Journal of Epidemiology 1973;2:229-235.

Held JR, Adaros HL. Neurological disease in man following administration of suckling mouse brain antirabies vaccine. Bulletin of the World Health Organization 1972;46:321-327.

Helle EP, Koskenvuo K, Heikkila J, Pikkarainen J, Weckstrom P. Myocardial complications of immunisations. Annals of Clinical Research 1978;10:280-287.

Helmke K, Otten A, Willems WR, Brockhaus R, Mueller-Eckhardt G, Stief T et al. Islet cell antibodies and the development of diabetes mellitus in relation to mumps infection and mumps vaccination. Diabetologia 1986;29:30-33.

Hemachudha T, Griffin DE, Chen WW, Johnson RT. Immunologic studies of rabies vaccination-induced Guillain-Barre syndrome. Neurology 1988;38:375-378.

Hemachudha T, Griffin DE, Giffels JJ, Johnson RT, Moser AB, Phanuphak P. Myelin basic protein as an encephalitogen in encephalomyelitis and polyneuritis following rabies vaccination. New England Journal of Medicine 1987;316:369-374.

Hemachudha T, Phanuphak P, Johnson RT, Griffin DE, Ratanavongsiri J, Siriprasomsup W. Neurologic complications of Semple-type rabies vaccine: clinical and immunologic studies. Neurology 1987;37:550-556.

Hempel HC, Grimm J. [Measles vaccination in children with brain damage] Masernschutzimpfung bei hirngeschadigten Kindern. Deutsche Gesundheitswesen 1968;23:2106-2107.

Henderson DA, Witte JJ, Morris L, Langmuir AD. Paralytic disease associated with oral polio vaccines. Journal of the American Medical Association 1964;190:41-48.

Hendley JO, Wenzel JG, Ashe KM, Samuelson JS. Immunogenicity of *Haemophilus influenzae* type b capsular polysaccharide vaccines in 18-month-old infants. Pediatrics 1987;80:351-354.

Henry P, Vital C, Du Pasquier P, Loiseau P, Barat M. [Subacute anterior poliomyelitis after oral polio vaccination: anatomo-clinical study] Poliomyelite anterieure subaigue apres vaccination antipoliomyelitique par voie orale: etude anatomo-clinique. Revue Neurologique 1972;127:364-370.

Henson PM. Antibody and immune-complex-mediated allergic and inflammatory reactions. In: Lachmann PJ, Peters DK, eds. Clinical Aspects of Immunology, 4th edition. Oxford: Blackwell; 1982.

Hepsen LS, Thomsen AC. Profylaktisk hepatitis B vaccinaton af et hospitalspersonale. Ugeskrift for Laeger 1992;154:2421-2423.

Herman JH, Bradley J, Ziff M, Smiley JD. Response of the rheumatoid synovial membrane to exogenous immunization. Journal of Clinical Investigation 1971;50:266-273.

Herman JJ, Radin R, Schneiderman R. Allergic reactions to measles (rubeola) vaccine in patients hypersensitive to egg protein. Journal of Pediatrics 1983;102:196-199.

Herroelen L, De Keyser J, Ebinger G. Central-nervous-system demyelination after immunisation with recombinant hepatitis B vaccine. Lancet 1991;338:1174-1175.

Hersch BS, Fine PE, Kent WK, Cochi SL, Kahn LH, Zell ER et al. Mumps outbreak in a highly vaccinated population. Journal of Pediatrics 1991;119:187-193.

Hess G, Hingst V, Cseke J, Bock HL, Clemens R. Influence of vaccination schedules and host factors on antibody response following hepatitis B vaccination. European Journal of Clinical Microbiology and Infectious Diseases 1992;11:334-340.

Hetherington SB, Lepow ML. Correlation between antibody affinity and serum bactericidal activity in infants. Journal of Infectious Diseases 1992;165:753-756.

Heyne K. [Paralytic poliomyelitis following vaccination contact in the 1st trimester of an infant] Paralytische Impfkontakt-Poliomyelitis im 1. Trimenon eines Sauglings. Medizinische Welt 1977;28:1439-1441.

Heywood JL. Clinical observations following the introduction of a mass immunization programme for hepatitis B. Submitted to the National Institutes of Health, April 4, 1992. Unpublished.

Hickling S. Tetanus immunisation. New Zealand Medical Journal 1977;86:529-530.

Hill A. Measles, mumps, and rubella vaccination (letter). British Medical Journal 1992;304:779.

Hill AB. Inoculation and Poliomyelitis. In: Statistical Methods in Clinical and Preventive Medicine. Edinburgh: E. & S. Livingstone Ltd.; 1962.

Hill AB. The environment and disease: association or causation. Proceedings of the Royal Society of Medicine 1965;58:295-300.

Hill JC. Summary of a workshop on *Haemophilus influenzae* type b vaccines. Journal of Infectious Diseases 1983;148:167-175.

Hilleman MR. Past, present, and future of measles, mumps, and rubella virus vaccines. Pediatrics 1992;90(1 Pt 2):149-153.

Hilleman MR, Buynak EB, Weibel RE, Stokes JJ, Whitman JE Jr, Leagus MB. Development and evaluation of the Moraten measles virus vaccine. Journal of the American Medical Association 1968;206:587-590.

Hilleman MR, Buynak EB, Weibel RE et al. Live attenuated mumps-virus vaccine. New England Journal of Medicine 1968;278:227-232.

Hinden E. Mumps followed by diabetes. Lancet 1962;1:1381.

Hiner EE, Frasch CE. Spectrum of disease due to *Haemophilus influenzae* type b occurring in vaccinated children. Journal of Infectious Diseases 1988;158:343-348.

Hinman AR. Landmark perspective: mass vaccination against polio. Journal of the American Medical Association 1984;251:2994-2996.

Hinman AR, Koplan JP, Orenstein WA, Brink EW, Nkowane BM. Live or inactivated poliomyelitis vaccine: an analysis of benefits and risks. American Journal of Public Health 1988;78:291-295.

Hinman AR, Koplan JP, Orenstein WA, Brink EW. Decision analysis and polio immunization policy. American Journal of Public Health 1988;78:301-303.

Hinton GG, Duncan IB, Rathbun JC. Paralysis after oral poliomyelitis vaccine. Canadian Medical Association Journal 1962;87:915-916.

Hirayama M. Measles vaccines used in Japan. Reviews of Infectious Diseases 1983;5:495-503.

Hirsch RL, Mokhtarian F, Griffin DE, Brooks BR, Hess J, Johnson RT. Measles virus vaccination of measles seropositive individuals suppresses lymphocyte proliferation and chemotactic factor production. Clinical Immunology and Immunopathology 1981;21:341-350.

Hirtz DG, Nelson KB, Ellenberg JH. Seizures following childhood immunizations. Journal of Pediatrics 1983;102:14-18.

Hisano S, Miyazaki C, Hatae K, Kaku Y, Yamane I, Ueda K et al. Immune status of children on continuous ambulatory peritoneal dialysis. Pediatric Nephrology 1992;6:179-181.

Hitsch RL, Griffin DE, Johnson RT, Cooper SJ, Lindo de Soriano I, Roedenbeck S et al.

Cellular immune responses during complicated and uncomplicated measles virus infections of man. Clinical Immunology and Immunopathology 1984;31:1-12.

Ho MS, Floyd RL, Glass RI, Pallansch MA, Jones B, Hamby B et al. Simultaneous administration of rhesus rotavirus vaccine and oral poliovirus vaccine: immunogenicity and reactogenicity. Pediatric Infectious Disease Journal 1989;8:692-696.

Hoffman HJ, Hunter JC, Damus K, Pakter J, Peterson DR, van Belle G et al. Diphtheria-tetanus-pertussis immunization and sudden infant death: results of the National Institute of Child Health and Human Development Cooperative Epidemiological Study of Sudden Infant Death Syndrome Risk Factors. Pediatrics 1987;79:598-611.

Hofmann F, Sydow B. [Considering the question of mumps-immunity of hospital personnel] Zur Frage der Mumps-Immunitat bei Krankenhausbeschaftigen. Arbeitsmed Sozialmed Praventivmed 1989;24:115-117.

Holden JM, Strang DU. Reactions to tetanus toxoid: comparison of fluid and adsorbed toxoids. New Zealand Medical Journal 1965;64:574-577.

Holland P, Hutchinson CE. Uptake of hepatitis B vaccination amongst West Midlands radiologists. Clinical Radiology 1992;45:335-337.

Holliday PL, Bauer RB. Polyradiculoneuritis secondary to immunization with tetanus and diphtheria toxoids. Archives of Neurology 1983;40:56-57.

Holmes SJ, Lucas AH, Osterholm MT, Froeschle JE, Granoff DM, Collaborative Study Group. Immunoglobulin deficiency and idiotype expression in children developing *Haemophilus influenzae* type b disease after vaccination with conjugate vaccine. Journal of the American Medical Association 1991;266:1960-1965.

Holmes SJ, Murphy TV, Anderson RS, Kaplan SL, Rothstein EP, Gan VN et al. Immunogenicity of four *Haemophilus influenzae* type b conjugate vaccines in 17- to 19-month old children. Journal of Pediatrics 1991;118:364-371.

Holmes WH. Diphtheria: History. Bacillary and Rickettsial Infections. New York: Macmillan; 1940.

Holt S, Hudgins D, Krisnan KR, Critchley EM. Diffuse myelitis associated with rubella vaccination. British Medical Journal 1976;2:1037-1038.

Hong R, Gilbert EF, Opitz JM. Omenn disease: termination in lymphoma. Pediatric Pathology 1985;3:143-154.

Honovar M, Tharakan JK, Hughes RA, Leibowitz S, Winer JB. A clinicopathological study of the Guillain-Barre syndrome: nine cases and literature review. Brain 1991;114:1245-1269.

Hopf HC. [Guillain-Barre syndrome following tetanus toxoid administration: survey and report of a case.]. Guillain-Barre-Syndrom nach Tetanus-Schutzimpfung: Ubersicht und Fallmitteilung. Aktuelle Neurologie 1980;7:195-200.

Hopkins CC, Dismukes WE, Glick TH, Warren RJ. Surveillance of paralytic poliomyelitis in the United States: 1966 and 1967 cases, and 1965-1967 cases associated with oral poliovirus vaccine. Journal of the American Medical Association 1969;210:694-700.

Horowitz SD, Nagatani MS, Bowen GS, Holloway AW, St. Geme JW Jr. The acquisition of delayed hypersensitivity following attenuated mumps virus infection. Pediatrics 1970;45:77-82.

Horstmann DM. The Sabin live poliovirus vaccination trials in the USSR, 1959. Yale Journal of Biology and Medicine 1991;64:499-512.

Horta-Barbosa L, Fucillo DA, Sever JL. Subacute sclerosing panencephalitis: isolation of measles virus from a brain biopsy. Nature 1969;221:974.

Horta-Barbosa L, Hamilton R, Wittig B, Fuccillo DA, Sever JL. Subacute sclerosing panencephalitis: isolation of suppressed measles virus from lymph node biopsies. Science 1971;173:840-841.

Hospital Employee Health. Hepatitis B: anaphylactic shock after Recombivax underscores need to question staff. Hospital Employee Health, December 1987.

House A. Alleged link between hepatitis B vaccine and chronic fatigue syndrome. Canadian Medical Association Journal 1992;146:1145.

Hovi T, Cantell K, Huovilainen A, Kinnunen E, Kuronen T, Lapinleimu K et al. Outbreak of paralytic poliomyelitis in Finland: widespread circulation of antigenically altered poliovirus type 3 in a vaccinated population. Lancet 1986;1:1427-1432.

Howson CP, Fineberg HV. Adverse events following pertussis and rubella vaccines: summary of a report of the Institute of Medicine. Journal of the American Medical Association 1992;267:392-396.

Howson CP, Fineberg HV. The ricochet of magic bullets: summary of the Institute of Medicine report, Adverse Effects of Pertussis and Rubella Vaccines. Pediatrics 1992;89:318-324.

Hoyeraal HM, Mellbye OJ. Humoral immunity in juvenile rheumatoid arthritis. Annals of the Rheumatic Diseases 1974;33:248-253.

Hu XM. [Recent advance in research on the incidence of paralysis following immunization with live oral polio vaccine]. Chung Hua Liu Hsing Ping Hsueh Tsa Chih 1985;6:125-127.

Huber EG, Rannon L, Galffy G. [Long-term-follow-up-study after measles-vaccination] Langzeitstudie nach Masernimpfung. Padiatrie und Padologie 1976;11:72-76.

Hudson JB, Weinstein L, Chang T. Thrombocytopenic purpura in measles. Journal of Pediatrics 1956;48:48-56.

Hudson TJ, Newkirk M, Gervais F, Shuster J. Adverse reaction to the recombinant hepatitis B vaccine. Journal of Allergy and Clinical Immunology 1991;88:821-822.

Hughes RA. Guillain-Barre Syndrome. London: Springer-Verlag; 1990.

Hughes WT, Smith JS, Kim MH. Suppression of the histoplasmin reaction with measles and smallpox vaccines. American Journal of Diseases of Children 1968;116:402-406.

Huisman J. [Adverse effects of the state vaccination program in 1986] Bijwerkingen van het rijksvaccinatieprogramma in 1986. Nederlands Tijdschrift voor Geneeskunde 1988;132:5-6.

Hulbert TV, Larsen RA, Davis CL, Holtom PD. Bilateral hearing loss after measles and rubella vaccination in an adult (letter). New England Journal of Medicine 1991;325:134.

Hunt A. Tuberous sclerosis: a survey of 97 cases. I. Seizures, pertussis immunisation and handicap. Developmental Medicine and Child Neurology 1983;25:346-349.

Huovila R. Adverse reactions in children vaccinated with DPT and pertussis vaccine. Acta Paediatrica Scandinavica 1982;71(Suppl. 298):26-29.

Hurt RD, Hogan MJ, Hagmeier CH, Wright PF, Kim-Farley RJ, Robertson S et al. The eradication of poliomyelitis. New England Journal of Medicine 1992;326:1295.

Hurwitz ES, Holman RC, Nelson DB, Schonberger LB. National surveillance for Guillain-Barre syndrome: January 1978-March 1979. Neurology 1983;33:150-157.

Hurwitz ES, Schonberger LB, Nelson DB, Holman RC. Guillain-Barre syndrome and the 1978-1979 influenza vaccine. New England Journal of Medicine 1981;304:1557-1561.

Hutcheson R. DTP immunization and sudden infant death—Tennessee. Morbidity and Mortality Weekly Report 1979;28:131-132.

Hutcheson R. Follow-up on DTP immunization and sudden infant death—Tennessee. Morbidity and Mortality Weekly Report 1979;28:134-135.

Hutchinson TA, Lane DA. Assessing methods for causality assessment of suspected adverse drug reactions. Journal of Clinical Epidemiology 1989;42:5-16.

Hutteroth TH, Quast U. [Aluminum hydroxide-induced granulomas after hepatitis B vaccination] Aluminiumhydroxid-Granulome nach Hepatitis-B-Impfung. Deutsche Medizinische Wochenschrift 1990;115:476.

Ifekwunigwe AE, Grasset N, Glass R, Foster S. Immune response to measles and smallpox vaccinations in malnourished children. American Journal of Clinical Nutrition 1980;33:621-624.

Iglehart JK. Compensating children with vaccine-related injuries. New England Journal of Medicine 1987;316:1282-1288.

Ikic D, Jancikic B, Branica M, Manhalter T. The safety of human diploid cell strains for man: a controlled study of symptoms occurring after the administration of WM-3 living attenuated poliovirus vaccine prepared in the WI-38 human diploid cell strain. American Journal of Epidemiology 1968;87:411-418.

Ilinskikh NN. [Chromosome breaks and changes in the mitotic regime of human and animal cells under the influence of a measles virus vaccinal strain (L-16)] Khromosomnye narusheniia i izmenenie mitoticheskogo rezhima v kletkakh cheloveka i zhivotynykh pod vliianiem vaktsinogo shtamma virusa kori (L-16). Tsitologiia 1975;17:131-136.

Ilinskikh NN. [Chromosome disorders in the leukocytes of healthy children and children with Down's syndrome vaccinated and unvaccinated against measles] Khromosomnye narusheniia v leikotsitakh krovi zdorovykh detei i detei, bol'nykh sindromom Dauna, v norme i posle vaktsinatsii protiv kori. Tsitologiia 1981;23:67-73.

Ilinskikh NN. [Chronobiological studies of the antimutagenic action of methyluracil in cytogenetic lesions induced in mice by the vaccinal strain of the poliomyelitis virus] Khronobiologicheskie issledovaniia antimutagennoi aktivnosti metiluratsila pri tsitogeneticheskikh porazheniiakh, indutsirovannykh u myshei vaktsinnym shtammom virusa poliomielita. Biulletin Eksperimentalnoi Biologii i Meditsiny 1982;94:102-104.

Ilinskikh NN. [Human intraspecific genetic polymorphism and the sensitivity of the chromosome apparatus to the mutagenic action of vaccinal viral strains] Vnutrividovoi geneticheskii polimorfizm u cheloveka i chuvstvitel'nost' khromosomnogo apparata k mutagennomu deistviiu vaktsinnykh shtammov virusov. Izvestiia Akademii Nauk SSSR (Biol) 1984;1:31-39.

Illis LS, Taylor FM. Neurological and electroencephalographic sequelae of tetanus. Lancet 1971;1:826-830.

Immunization Practices Advisory Committee, Centers for Disease Control. Poliomyelitis prevention. Annals of Internal Medicine 1982;96:630-634.

Inami S. Appearance of enterovirus in the Takatsuki district. Nippon Shonika Gakkai Sasshi [Journal of the Japan Pediatric Society] 1966;70:539-553.

Ing DJ, Glass RI, Woods PA, Simonetti M, Pallansch MA, Wilcox WD et al. Immunogenicity of tetravalent rhesus rotavirus vaccine administered with buffer and oral polio vaccine. American Journal of Diseases of Children 1991;145:892-897.

Innis MD. Oncogenesis and poliomyelitis vaccine. Nature 1968;219:972-973.

Inoue A, Tsukada N, Koh C-S, Yanagisawa N. Chronic relapsing demyelinating polyneuropathy associated with hepatitis B infection. Neurology 1987;37:1663-1666.

Insel RA, Anderson PW. Response to oligosaccharide-protein conjugate vaccine against Haemophilus influenzae b in two patients with IgG2 deficiency unresponsive to capsular polysaccharide vaccine. New England Journal of Medicine 1986;315:499-503.

Institute of Medicine. Adverse Effects of Pertussis and Rubella Vaccines. Washington, DC: National Academy Press. 1991.

Institute of Medicine. Evaluation of Poliomyelitis Vaccines. Washington, DC: National Academy of Sciences; 1977.

Institute of Medicine. An Evaluation of Poliomyelitis Vaccine Policy Options. Washington, DC: National Academy of Sciences; 1988.

Institute of Medicine. New Vaccine Development: Establishing Priorities. Volume I. Diseases of Importance in the United States. Washington, DC: National Academy Press; 1985.

Institute of Medicine. Vaccine Supply and Innovation. Washington, DC: National Academy Press; 1985.

Interagency Committee to Improve Access to Immunization Services. The Public Health Service action plan to improve access to immunization services. Public Health Reports 1992;107:243-251.

Ipp MM, Gold R, Greenberg S, Goldbach M, Kupfert BB, Lloyd DD et al. Acetaminophen prophylaxis of adverse reactions following vaccination of infants with diphtheria-pertussis-tetanus toxoids-polio vaccine. Pediatric Infectious Disease Journal 1987;6:721-725.

Ipp MM, Gold R, Goldbach M, Maresky DC, Saunders N, Greenberg S et al. Adverse reactions to diphtheria, tetanus, pertussis-polio vaccination at 18 months of age: effect of injection site and needle length. Pediatrics 1989;83:679-682.

Ipp M, Goldbach M, Greenberg S, Gold R. Effect of needle change and air bubble in syringe on minor adverse reactions associated with diphtheria-tetanus toxoids-pertussis-polio vaccination in infants. Pediatric Infectious Disease Journal 1990;9:291-293.

Irtel Von Brenndorff A, Enders Ruckle G, Hagge W. [Atypical measles after immunization with inactivated measles vaccine (split vaccine)] Atypische masern nach immunisierung mit inaktiviertem masernimpfstoff (spaltvakzine). Medizinische Monatsschrift 1973;27:265-268.

Isaacs D, Menser M. Measles, mumps, rubella, and varicella. Lancet 1990;335:1384-1387.

Isacson P, Stone A. Allergic reactions associated with viral vaccines. Progress in Medical Virology 1971;13:239-270.

Ishitobi A. Studies on diphtheria-tetanus combined vaccine. Acta Paediatrica Japonica 1980;22:66-67.

Ishizaki A, Noda Y. [Neurological complications of immunization]. No To Hattatsu 1986;18:105-113.

Isomura S. Measles and measles vaccine in Japan. Acta Paediatrica Japonica 1988;30:154-162.

Isomura S, Asano Y, Hon AS et al. Studies on live attenuated mumps vaccine. I. Comparative field trials with two different live vaccines. Biken Journal 1973;16:39-42.

Isozaki M, Kuno-Sakai H, Hoshi N, Takesue R, Takakura I, Kimura M et al. Effects and side effects of a new trivalent combined measles-mumps-rubella (MMR) vaccine. Tokai Journal of Experimental and Clinical Medicine 1982;7:547-550.

Iwai T, Matumoto M, Kawana R. Unusual clinical reactions to live measles vaccine in a child previously immunized with killed measles vaccine. Japanese Journal of Experimental Medicine and Biology 1968;38:139-142.

Iwarson S. The main five types of viral hepatitis: an alphabetical update. Scandinavian Journal of Infectious Diseases 1992;24:129-135.

Izuora GI. Acute paralytic poliomyelitis among Nigerian children in Enugu. East Africa Medical Journal 1981;58:405-411.

Jabbour JT, Duenas DA, Sever JL, Krebs HM, Horta-Barbosa L. Epidemiology of subacute sclerosing panencephalitis (SSPE). Journal of the American Medical Association 1972;220:959-962.

Jabbour JT, Garcia JH, Lemmi H, Ragland J, Duenas DA, Sever JL. Subacute sclerosing panencephalitis. Journal of the American Medical Association 1969;207:2248-2254.

Jabbour JT, Roane JA, Sever JL. Studies of delayed dermal hypersensitivity in patients with subacute sclerosing panencephalitis. Neurology 1969;19:929-931.

Jaber L, Shohat M, Mimouni. Infectious episodes following diphtheria-pertussis-tetanus vaccination: a preliminary observation in infants. Clinical Pediatrics 1988;27:491-494.

Jackson H. A fatal case of purpura with a few notes on the recent literature of this disease. Archives of Pediatrics 1890;7:951.

Jacobs RL, Lowe RS, Lanier BQ. Adverse reactions to tetanus toxoid. Journal of the American Medical Association 1982;247:40-42.

Jacquest D, Stout I. Reactions to Haemophilus influenzae type b vaccine. Canadian Journal of Public Health 1989;80:304-305.

Jagdis F, Langston C, Gurwith M. Encephalitis after administration of live measles vaccine. Canadian Medical Association Journal 1975;112:972-975.

Jahnke U, Fischer EH, Alvord EC Jr. Sequence homology between certain viral proteins and proteins related to encephalomyelitis and neuritis. Science 1985;229:282-284.

Jakacki R, Luery N, McVerry P, Lange B. *Haemophilus influenzae* diphtheria protein conjugate immunization after therapy in splenectomized patients with Hodgkin disease. Annals of Internal Medicine 1990;112:143-144.

James G, Longshore WA, Hendry JL. Diphtheria immunization studies of students in an urban high school. American Journal of Hygiene 1951;53:178-201.

Janzen R, Balzereit F, Jannakis C. [Is there a panoramic variation in inflammatory nerve diseases since the introduction of poliomyelitis vaccination? Observations on rare courses of virus induced encephalitis, myelitis and polyneuritis] Gibt es einen Panoramawandel bei entzundlichen Nervenkrank-heiten seit Einfuhrung der Poliomyelitis-Schutzimpfung? Beobachtungen uber ungewohnliche Verlaufsformen von virusbedingten Enzephalitiden, Myelitiden, Polyneuritiden. Deutsche Medizinische Wochenschrift 1968;93:860-867.

Japan Measles Vaccine Research Commission. A field trial of further attenuated live measles virus vaccines in Japan, 1968. Japanese Journal of Medical Science and Biology 1969;22:191-200.

Jawad AS, Scott DG. Immunisation triggering rheumatoid arthritis? (letter). Annals of the Rheumatic Diseases 1989;48:174.

Jean-Joseph P, Sow S, Casey HL, Imperato PJ, Henderson RH, Noble JJ. A comparison of Edmonston-B and Schwarz measles vaccine in Malian children. Lancet 1969;1:665-667.

Jenson AB, Rosenberg HS, Notkins AL. Pancreatic islet cell damage in children with fatal viral infections. Lancet 1980;2:354-358.

Jilg W et al. [Vaccination for hepatitis B virus: unresolved questions] Hepatitis-B impfung: ungelöste probleme. Schweizerische Rundschau fur Medizin Praxis 1992;81:795-797.

Jimenez Puente A, Cejas Hermoso P, Luna del Castillo JD, Valles Casado LM, Benitez Bocanegra S, Cortes Martinez C et al. [Postvaccinal reactions to simultaneous administration of the triple viral, oral polio and diphtheria-tetanus vaccines compared with their administration in sequence] Reacciones posvacunales tras la administracion simultanea de vacunas triple virica y antipolio oral-difteria-tetanos, frente a su administracion secuencial. Atencion Primaria 1992;10:825-830.

Job JS, Halsey NA, Boulos R, Holt E, Farrell D, Albrecht P et al. Successful immunization of infants at 6 months of age with high dose Edmonston-Zagreb measles vaccine. Pediatric Infectious Disease Journal 1991;10:303-311.

Joffe LS, Glode MP, Gutierrez MK, Wiesenthal A, Luckey DW, Harken L. Diphtheria-tetanus toxoids-pertussis vaccination does not increase the risk of hospitalization with an infectious illness. Pediatric Infectious Disease Journal 1992;11:730-735.

John TJ, Moore R, Gibson JJ et al. Choice between inactivated and oral poliovirus vaccines in India. Lancet 1992;339:504.

John TJ, Nambiar A, Samuel BU, Rajasingh J. Ulnar nerve inoculation of poliovirus in bonnet monkey: a new primate model to investigate neurovirulence. Vaccine 1992;10:529-532.

Johnson DE. Guillain-Barre syndrome in the US Army. Archives of Neurology 1982;39:21-24.

Johnson DW, Fleming SJ. The use of vaccines in renal failure. Clinical Pharmacokinetics 1992;22:434-446.

Johnson RT. Neurologic diseases associated with viral infections. Postgraduate Medicine 1971;50:158-163.

Johnson RT. Viral aspects of multiple sclerosis. 3. Vinken PJ, Bruyn GW, Klawans HL, eds. Handbook of Clinical Neurology. New York: Elsevier Science Publishing Co., Inc.; 1985:319-336.

Johnson RT, Griffin DE, Gendelman HE. Postinfectious encephalomyelitis. Seminars in Neurology 1985;5:180-190.

Johnson RT, Griffin DE, Hirsch RL, Wolinsky JS, Roedenbeck S, Lindo de Soriano I, Vaisberg

A. Measles encephalomyelitis: clinical and immunologic studies. New England Journal of Medicine 1984;310:137-141.

Jones AE, Melville-Smith M, Watkins J. Adverse reactions in adolescents to reinforcing doses of plain and adsorbed tetanus vaccines. Community Medicine 1985;7:99-106.

Jones RG, Bass JW, Weisse ME, Vincent JM. Antigenuria after immunization with *Haemophilus influenzae* oligosaccharide CRM197 conjugate (HBOC) vaccine. Pediatric Infectious Disease Journal 1991;10:557-559.

Jorch G, Kleine M, Erwig H. [Coincidence of virus encephalitis and measles-mumps vaccination] Koinzidenz von Virusenzephalitis und Masern-Mumps-Impfung. Monatsschrift fur Kinderheilkunde 1984;132:299-300.

Joseph VJ, Yeshwanth M. Poliomyelitis and immunization status (letter). Indian Pediatrics 1992;29:241-244.

Journal of the American Medical Association. Evaluation of a new mumps vaccine: mumps virus vaccine, live, attenuated (Mumpsvax). Journal of the American Medical Association 1969;209:2042.

Journal of the American Medical Association. Update: prevention of *Haemophilus influenzae* type b disease. Journal of the American Medical Association 1988;259:798-804.

Journal of the American Medical Association. Paralytic poliomyelitis—Senegal, 1986-1987: update on the N-IPV efficacy study. Journal of the American Medical Association 1988;259:2974.

Journal of the American Medical Association. Update: *Haemophilus influenzae* type b vaccine. Journal of the American Medical Association 1989;261:1118.

Journal of the American Medical Association. *Haemophilus influenzae* declining among young? Journal of the American Medical Association 1991;266:3398-3399.

Journal of the Indian Medical Association. Paralytic poliomyelitis. Journal of the Indian Medical Association 1973;60:309-310.

Journal of Pediatrics. Neurologic complications of oral poliomyelitis vaccine (letter). Journal of Pediatrics 1987;110:996-998.

Jung S, Schluesener HJ, Toyka K, Hartung HP. T cell vaccination does not induce resistance to experimental autoimmune neuritis. Journal of Neuroimmunology 1991;35:1-11.

Jungkunz G, Kohler P, Holbach M, Schweisfurth H. [Case representation: two cases of strong local reaction after active hepatitis B-vaccination with sensitisation to thiomersal] Kasuistik: zwei falle mit heftiger lokaler reaktion nach aktiver hepatitis B-impfung bei sensibilisierung auf thiomersal. Hygiene + Medizin 1990;15:418-420.

Juntunen-Backman K, Peltola H, Backman A, Salo OP. Safe immunization of allergic children against measles, mumps, and rubella. American Journal of Diseases of Children 1987;141:1103-1105.

Just M, Berger R. [Immunogenicity of vaccines: a comparative study of a mumps-measles-rubella vaccine given with or without oral polio vaccine] Immunantwort auf impfstoffe: Vergleichende studie mit mumps-, masern- und roteln-impfstoff allein oder zusammen mit polio-impfstoff appliziert. Munchener Medizinische Wochenschrift 1987;129:78-82.

Just M, Berger R, Gluck R, Wegmann A. Evaluation of a combined vaccine against measles-mumps-rubella produced on human diploid cells. Developments in Biological Standardization 1986;65:25-27.

Just M, Berger R, Just V. Evaluation of a combined measles-mumps-rubella-chickenpox vaccine. Developments in Biological Standardization 1986;65:85-88.

Just M, Berger R, Just V. Reactogenicity and immunogenicity of a recombinant hepatitis B vaccine compared with a plasma-derived vaccine in young adults. Postgraduate Medical Journal 1987;63(Suppl. 2):121-123.

Kaaber K, Nielsen AO, Veien NK. Vaccination granulomas and aluminium allergy: course and prognostic factors. Contact Dermatitis 1992;26:304-306.

Kaaber K, Samuelsson IS, Larsen SO. [Reactions after MMR vaccination] Reaktioner efter MFR-vaccination. Ugeskrift for Laeger 1990;152:1672-1676.

Kabat EA, Wolf A, Bezer AE. The rapid production of acute disseminated encephalomyelitis in rhesus monkeys by injection of heterologous and homologous brain tissue with adjuvants. Journal of Experimental Medicine 1947;85:117-130.

Kafidi KT, Rotschafer JC. Bacterial vaccines for splenectomized patients. Drug Intelligence and Clinical Pharmacy 1988;22:192-197.

Kaiser GC, King RD, Lempke RE, Ruster MH. Delayed recall of active tetanus immunization. Journal of the American Medical Association 1961;178:914-916.

Kakakios AM, Burgess MA, Bransby RD, Quinn AA, Allars HM. Optimal age for measles and mumps vaccination in Australia. Medical Journal of Australia 1990;152:472-474.

Kalet A, Berger DK, Bateman WB, Dubitsky J, Covitz K. Allergic reactions to MMR vaccine (letter). Pediatrics 1992;89:168-169.

Kamin PB, Fein BT, Britton HA. Live, attenuated measles vaccine. Journal of the American Medical Association 1963;185:99-102.

Kamin PB, Fein BT, Britton HA. Use of live, attenuated measles virus vaccine in children allergic to egg protein. Journal of the American Medical Association 1965;193:143-144.

Kamin PB, Fein BT, Britton HA. Use of live, attenuated measles virus vaccine in children allergic to egg protein. Journal of the American Medical Association 1965;193:1125-1126.

Kanesaki T, Baba K, Tsuda N, Yabuuchi H, Yamanishi K, Takahashi M. Protection of mumps in children with various underlying diseases: application of a live attenuated mumps and trivalent measles-rubella-mumps (MRM) vaccines in these children. Biken Journal 1986;29:63-71.

Kantoch M, Naruszewicz LD, Polna I, Litynska J. Immunologic response and reactions to vaccination in children during the campaign of vaccinations against measles. II. Antibody levels and seroconversion after vaccination. Przeglad Epidemiologiczny 1974;28:325-331.

Kantoch M, Naruszewicz LD, Polna I, Litynska J. Immunologic response and reactions to vaccination in children vaccinated against measles. III. Persistence of measles antibodies in children vaccinated in 1972. Przeglad Epidemiologiczny 1976;30:235-241.

Kaplan BS, Proesmans W. The hemolytic uremic syndrome of childhood. Seminars in Hematology 1987;24:148-160.

Kaplan C, Morinet F, Cartron J. Virus-induced autoimmune thrombocytopenia and neutropenia. Seminars in Hematology 1992;29:34-44.

Kaplan JE, Katona P, Hurwitz ES, Schonberger LB. Guillain-Barre syndrome in the United States, 1979-1980 and 1980-1981: lack of an association with influenza vaccination. Journal of the American Medical Association 1982;248:698-700.

Kaplan JE, Schonberger LB, Hurwitz ES, Katona P. Guillain-Barre syndrome in the United States, 1978-1981: additional observations from the national surveillance system. Neurology 1983;33:633-637.

Kaplan KM, Marder DC, Cochi SL, Preblud SR. Mumps in the workplace: further evidence of the changing epidemiology of a childhood vaccine-preventable disease. Journal of the American Medical Association 1988;260:1434-1438.

Kaplan SA. Clinical Pediatric Endocrinology. Philadelphia: W. B. Saunders; 1990.

Kaplan SL, Duckett T, Mahoney DH Jr., Kennedy LL, Dukes CM, Schaffer DM et al. Immunogenicity of *Haemophilus influenzae* type b polysaccharide-tetanus protein conjugate vaccine in children with sickle hemoglobinopathy or malignancies, and after systemic *Haemophilus influenzae* type b infection. Journal of Pediatrics 1992;120:367-370.

Kaplan SL, Zahradnik JM, Mason EO Jr., Dukes CM. Immunogenicity of the *Haemophilus influenzae* type b capsular polysaccharide conjugate vaccine in children after systemic *Haemophilus influenzae* type b infections. Journal of Pediatrics 1988;113:272-277.

Karchmer AW, Friedman JP, Casey HL, Shope TC, Riker JB, Kappelman MM et al. Simultaneous administration of live virus vaccines: measles, mumps, poliomyelitis, and smallpox. American Journal of Diseases of Children 1971;121:382-388.

Karjalainen J, Martin JM, Knip M, Ilonen J, Robinson B, Savilahti E et al. A bovine albumin peptide as a possible trigger of insulin-dependent diabetes mellitus. New England Journal of Medicine 1992;327:302-307.

Karzon D, Edwards K. Diphtheria outbreaks in immunized populations. New England Journal of Medicine 1988;318:41-43.

Kaslow RA, Sullivan-Bolyai JZ, Hafkin B, Schonberger LB, Kraus L, Moore MJ et al. HLA antigens in Guillain-Barre syndrome. Neurology 1984;34:240-242.

Kaslow RA, Sullivan-Bolyai JZ, Holman RC, Hafkin B, Dicker RC, Schonberger LB. Risk factors for Guillain-Barre syndrome. Neurology 1987;37:685-688.

Kasper JM, Waesser ST. [Value of EEG studies in connection with vaccinations] Uber den Wert von EEG-Untersuchungen im zusammenhang mit Schutzimpfungen. Zeitschrift fur Aerztliche Fortbildung 1978;72:457-461.

Kass B, Nyberg-Hansen R. Acute brachial neuropathy. Tidsskrift for den Norske Laegeforening 1983;103:7-9, 26.

Katz M, Oyanagi S, Koprowski H et al. Structures resembling myxovirus nucleocapsids in cells cultures from brains. Nature 1969;222:888-890.

Katz SL. Immunization with live attenuated measles virus vaccine: five years' experience. Archiv Fur Die Gesamte Virusforschung 1965;16:222-230.

Katz SL. How does measles virus cause subacute sclerosing panencephalitis? New England Journal of Medicine 1969;281:615-616.

Katz SL. International Symposium on Measles Immunization: summary and recommendations. Pediatrics 1983;71:653-654.

Kaufman DL, Erlander MG, Slare-Salzler M, Atkinson MA, Maclaren NK, Tobin AJ. Autoimmunity to two forms of flutamate decarboxylase in insulin-dependent diabetes mellitus. Journal of Clinical Investigation 1992;89:283-292.

Kawamura S. [An analytical study on the clinical reactions to measles vaccine]. Nippon Eiseigaku Zasshi 1968;23:406-411.

Kawanishi K. [Clinical and serological studies of live attenuated mumps virus vaccine—inoculation of mumps vaccine singly and in combination with measles vaccine]. Kansenshogaku Zasshi 1971;45:54-66.

Kayhty H, Eskola J, Peltola H, Ronnberg PR, Kela E, Karanko V et al. Antibody responses to four *Haemophilus influenzae* type b conjugate vaccines. American Journal of Diseases of Children 1991;145:223-227.

Kayhty H, Peltola H, Eskola J. Immunogenicity and reactogenicity for four *Haemophilus influenzae* type b capsular polysaccharide vaccines in Finnish 24-month-old children. Pediatric Infectious Disease Journal 1988;7:574-577.

Kayhty H, Peltola H, Eskola J, Ronnberg PR, Kela E, Karanko V et al. Immunogenicity of *Haemophilus influenzae* oligosaccharide-protein and polysaccharide-protein conjugate vaccination of children at 4, 6, and 14 months of age. Pediatrics 1989;84:995-999.

Kazarian EL, Gager WE. Optic neuritis complicating measles, mumps, and rubella vaccination. American Journal of Ophthalmology 1978;86:544-547.

Kekomaki R, Nieminen U, Peltola H. Acute idiopathic thrombocytopenic purpura following measles, mumps and rubella vaccination (abstract). 13th Congress of the International Society on Thrombosis and Haemostatis, Amsterdam, The Netherlands, Abstract No. 600, p. 866.

Kellaway P, Krachoby RA, Frost JD, Zion T. Precise characterization and quantification of infantile spasms. Annals of Neurology 1979;6:214-218.

Kelton JG. Vaccination-associated relapse of immune thrombocytopenia. Journal of the American Medical Association 1981;245:369-371.

Kelton JG, Neame PB, Gauldie J, Hirsch J. Elevated platelet-associated IgG in the thrombocytopenia of septicemia. New England Journal of Medicine 1979;300:760-764.

Kemp A, Van Asperen P, Mukhi A. Measles immunization in children with clinical reactions to egg protein. American Journal of Diseases of Children 1990;144:33-35.

Kernbaum S. [Acute myelitis and vaccination] Myelite aigue et vaccination. Concours Medical 1991;113:1760.

Kernbaum S. [Meningoencephalitis after DTP vaccination] Meningo-encephalite apres DT-polio. Concours Medical 1992;114:156.

Keuth U. [Cerebral damage caused by enteritis (so-called toxicosis) following oral poliomyelitis vaccination, recognized as vaccination damage (letter)] Zerebralschaden durch Enteritis (sogenannte Toxikose) nach oraler Poliomyelitis-Impfung als Impfschaden anerkannt. Deutsche Medizinische Wochenschrift 1974;99:110.

Kibel MA et al. Guillain-Barre syndrome in childhood. South African Medical Journal 1983;63:715.

Kibel MA, Hay I, Donald P. Contraindications to immunisation. South African Medical Journal 1990;77:537-538.

Kiefaber RW. Thrombocytopenic purpura after measles vaccination (letter). New England Journal of Medicine 1981;305:225.

Kim KS, Wong VK, Adler R, Steinberg EA. Comparative immune responses to *Haemophilus influenzae* type b polysaccharide and a polysaccharide-protein conjugate vaccine. Pediatrics 1990;85(4 Pt 2):648-650.

Kim-Farley R. Global immunization. Annuual Reviews of Public Health 1992;13:223-237.

Kim-Farley R, Bart S, Stetler H, Orenstein W, Bart K, Sullivan K et al. Clinical mumps vaccine efficacy. American Journal of Epidemiology 1985;121:593-597.

Kinder J, Teare L, Rao M, Bridgman G, Kurian A. False contraindications to childhood immunization. British Journal of General Practice 1992;42:160-161.

King SD, Ramlal A, Wynter H, Moodie K, Castle D, Kuo JS et al. Safety and immunogenicity of a new *Haemophilus influenzae* type b vaccine in infants under one year of age. Lancet 1981;2:705-709.

Kinnunen E, Farkkila M, Hovi T, Juntunen J, Weckstrom P. Incidence of Guillain-Barre syndrome during a nationwide oral poliovirus vaccine campaign. Neurology 1989;39:1034-1036.

Kinnunen E, Farkkila M, Hovi T, Juntunen J, Weckstrom P. Polio vaccine and GBS. Neurology 1990;40:729.

Kirkland LR. Ocular sensitivity to thimerosal: a problem with hepatitis B vaccine? Southern Medical Journal 1990;83:497-499.

Kitamura I, Hirai S, Kurashige T. Poliomyelitis from a vaccine. Lancet 1969;1:465.

Kitsiou S, Saxoni-Papageorgiou P, Haidemenaki T, Gala A, Koukoutsakis P, Stavrinadis C et al. Sister chromatid exchanges in peripheral lymphocytes of children vaccinated against rubella and measles-mumps-rubella. Acta Paediatrica Scandinavica 1988;77:879-884.

Kittler FJ, Smith PJ, Hefley BF, Cazort AG. Reactions to tetanus toxoid. Southern Medical Journal 1966;59:149-153.

Kiwit JC. Neuralgic amyotrophy after administration of tetanus toxoid. Journal of Neurology, Neurosurgery and Psychiatry 1984;47:320.

Klajman A, Sternbach M, Ranon L, Drucker M, Geminder D, Sadan N. Impaired delayed hypersensitivity in subacute sclerosing panencephalitis. Acta Paediatrica Scandinavica 1973;62:523-526.

Kletz MR, Holland CL, Mendelson JS, Bielory L. Administration of egg-derived vaccines in patients with history of egg sensitivity. Annals of Allergy 1990;64:527-529.

Kniker WT. Anaphylaxis in children and adults. In: Bierman CW, Pearlman DW, eds. Allergic Diseases from Infancy to Adulthood. Philadelphia: W. B. Saunders Co.; 1988.

Koch J, Leet C, McCarthy R, Carter A, Cuff W. Adverse events temporally associated with immunizing agents—1987 report/Manifestations facheuses associees dans le temps a des agents immunisants—rapport de 1987. Canada Diseases Weekly Report/Rapport hebdomadaire des maladies au Canada 1989;15:151-158.

Kok PW, Leeuwenburg J, Tukei P, van Wezel AL, Kapsenberg JG, van Steenis G et al. Serological and virological assessment of oral and inactivated poliovirus vaccines in a rural population in Kenya. Bulletin of the World Health Organization 1992;70:93-103.

Kolmer JA. Vaccination against acute anterior poliomyelitis. American Journal of Public Health and the Nations Health 1936;26:126-135.

Koplan JP, Preblud SR. A benefit-cost analysis of mumps vaccine. American Journal of Diseases of Children 1982;136:362-364.

Koprowski H, Jervis GA, Norton TW. Immune responses in human volunteers upon oral administration of a rodent-adapted strain of poliomyelitis virus. American Journal of Hygiene 1952;55:108-126.

Korger G, Quast U, Dechert G. [Tetanus vaccination: tolerance and avoidance of adverse reactions] Tetanusimpfung: Vertraglichkeit und Vermeidung von Nebenreaktionen. Klinische Wochenschrift 1986;64:767-775.

Korman SH. Thrombocytopenic purpura during the incubation of hepatitis B. Acta Pediatrica Scandinavica 1991;80:975-976.

Kostrzewski JM. [Case of poliomyelitis in unvaccinated children in contact with persons vaccinated with attenuated virus] Zachorowania na poliomyelitis w otoczeniu szczepionych wirusem atenuowanym. Przeglad Epidemiologiczny 1973;27:259-265.

Kostrzewski J, Kantoch M. [Reactions to vaccination and measles antibody levels in children inoculated with vaccine prepared from the L-16 strain from Japanese quail embryonic fibroblast cultures] Odczyny i poziom przeciwcial odrowych u dzieci po podaniu szczepionki ze szczepu L-16 przygotowanej w hodowli fibroblastow zarodka przepiorki Japonskiej. Przeglad Epidemiologiczny 1975;29:291-300.

Kovalskaya SI. [The anaphylactogenic properties of absorbed and non-absorbed pertussis-diphtheria-tetanus vaccines] Anafilaktogennye svoistva adsorbipovannoi i neadsorbirovannoi kokliusnodifterino-stolbniachnoi vaktsin. Zhurnal Mikrobiologii, Epidemiologii, i Immunobiologii 1967;44:105-109.

Kovalskaya SI. [Anaphylactogenic properties of ADT-, PDT- and APDT vaccines under experimental conditions] Anafilaktogennye svoistva ADS, KDS- i AKDS-baktsin v eksperimente. Zhurnal Mikrobiologii, Epidemiologii, i Immunobiologii 1969;46:65-71.

Kovel A, Wald ER, Guerra N, Serdy C, Meschievitz CK. Safety and immunogenicity of acellular diphtheria-tetanus-pertussis and haemophilus conjugate vaccines given in combination or at separate injection sites. Journal of Pediatrics 1992;120:84-87.

Kramer MS. Assessing causality of adverse drug reactions: global introspection and its limitations. Drug Information Journal 1986;20:433-437.

Kramer MS. A Bayesian approach to assessment of adverse drug reactions: evaluation of a case of fatal anaphylaxis. Drug Information Journal 1986;20:505-517.

Kramer MS. Difficulties in assessing the adverse effects of drugs. British Journal of Clinical Pharmacology 1981;11:105S-110S.

Kramer MS, Lane DA. Causal propositions in clinical research and practice. Journal of Clinical Epidemiology 1992;45:639-649.

Kramer MS, Leventhal JM, Hutchinson TA, Feinstein AR. An algorithm for the operational assessment of adverse drug reactions. I. Background, description, and instructions for use. Journal of the American Medical Association 1979;242:623-632.

Krasinski K, Borkowsky W. Measles and measles immunity in children infected with human immunodeficiency virus. Journal of the American Medical Association 1989;261:2512-2516.

Krause DS, Cook L. Prevalence of hepatitis B in pregnant women (letter). Journal of the American Medical Association 1992;267:1919-1920.

Krause PJ, Cherry JD, Deseda-Tous J, Champion JG, Strassburg M, Sullivan C et al. Epidemic measles in young adults: clinical, epidemiologic, and serologic studies. Annals of Internal Medicine 1979;90:873-876.

Kremer HU. Juvenile diabetes as a sequel to mumps. American Journal of Medicine 1947;3:257-258.

Kringelbach J, Senstius J. [Hypsarrhythmia after triple vaccination] Hypsarrhytmia efter tripelvakcination. Nordisk Medicin 1966;76:1433-1436.

Krober MS, Stracener CE, Bass JW. Decreased measles antibody response after measles-mumps-rubella vaccine in infants with colds. Journal of the American Medical Association 1991;265:2095-2096.

Krugman S. Hepatitis B vaccine. In: Plotkin SA, Mortimer EA, eds. Vaccines. Philadelphia: W.B. Saunders Co.; 1988.

Krugman S, Giles JP. Viral hepatitis type B(MS-2 strain): further observations on natural history and prevention. New England Journal of Medicine 1973;288:755-760.

Krugman S, Giles JP, Friedman H, Stone S. Studies on immunity to measles. Journal of Pediatrics 1965;66:471-488.

Krugman S, Giles JP, Hammond J. Hepatitis virus: effect of heat on the infectivity and antigenicity of the MS-1 and MS-2 strains. Journal of Infectious Diseases 1970;122:432-436.

Krugman S, Giles JP, Hammond J. Viral hepatitis, type B(MS-2 strain): studies on active immunization. Journal of the American Medical Association 1971;217:41-45.

Krugman S, Giles JP, Jacobs AM, Friedman H. Studies with live attenuated measles-virus vaccine. American Journal of Diseases of Children 1962;103:353-363.

Kruppenbacher JP, Mertens T, Adrian M, Smolenski S, Leidel J, Eggers HJ. [Vaccine poliomyelitis as a complication of oral vaccination] Die Impfpoliomyelitis als Komplikation der Oralvakzination. Offentliche Gesundheitswesen 1983;45:528-531.

Kucharska Z, Sramova H, Zdrazilek J. Excretion of attenuated polioviruses in children vaccinated with live oral poliovirus vaccine. Journal of Hygiene, Epidemiology, Microbiology and Immunology 1982;26:74-82.

Kuhns WJ, Pappenheimer AM Jr. Immunochemical studies of antitoxin produced in normal and allergic individuals hyperimmunized with Diphtheria toxoid. Journal of Experimental Medicine 1952;95:363-374, 375-392.

Kulhanjian J. The decline in invasive Haemophilus Influenzae type b (Hib) disease in a large pediatric referral hospital following introduction to Hib conjugate vaccines. Program Abstracts of the 32nd Interscience Conference on Antimicrobial Agents and Chemotherapy. Abstract 1727, p. 398. Washington, DC: American Society for Microbiology; 1992.

Kumar A. New vaccines for prevention of *Hemophilus influenzae* type b diseases. Drugs Today 1986;22(9):469-472.

Kumar R, Chandra R, Bhushan V, Srivastava BC. Adverse reaction after measles immunization in a rural population. Indian Pediatrics 1982;19:605-610.

Kupers TA, Petrich JM, Holloway AW, St. Geme JW Jr. Depression of tuberculin delayed hypersensitivity by live attenuated mumps virus. Journal of Pediatrics 1970;76:716-721.

Kurokawa T, Mizuno Y, Tomita S, Ueda K, Mitsudome A, Yokota K et al. [Neurological complications related to immunization]. No To Hattatsu 1986;18:98-104.

Kurz VM. Zwei falle von kurzfristiger diplopie nach poliomyelitis-schluckimpfung bei kindern. Wiener Medizinische Wochenschrift 1966;116:135.

Kuwert E, Thraenhart O, Hoher PG, Dorndorf W, Voit D, Blumenthal W. [Spinal poliomyelitis due to contact with polio vaccine virus] Spinale Kinderlahmung nach Kontakt mit Polioimpfvirus. Deutsche Medizinische Wochenschrift 1971;96:1562-1568.

Kwiatkowska E, Pajor Z. [Remarks on the preventive vaccination in children with damaged central nervous system] Uwagi o stosowaniu szczepien ochronnych u dzieci z uszkodzeniem osrodkowego ukladu nerwowego. Neurologia, Neurochirurgia i Psychiatria Polska 1965;15:635-637.

Kwittken PL, Rosen S, Sweinberg SK. MMR vaccine and neomycin allergy (letter). American Journal of Diseases of Children 1993;147:128-129.

Kyle WS. Simian retrovirus, poliovaccine, and origin of AIDS. Lancet 1992;339:600-601.

Labauge R, Marty-Double C, Pages M, Boukobza M, Monstrey J. [Postvaccinal encephalitis in an adult: a case with anatomo-clinical report] Encephalite post-vaccinale de l'adulte: etude anatomo-clinique d'une observation. Revue Neurologique 1979;135:803-813.

Label LS, Batts DH. Transverse myelitis caused by duck embryo rabies vaccine. Archives of Neurology 1982;39:426-430.

LaForce FM. Poliomyelitis vaccines: success and controversy. Infectious Disease Clinics of North America 1990;4:75-83.

Lahelle O. [Vaccination against poliomyelitis] Vaksinasjon mot poliomyelitt. Tidsskrift for den Norske Laegeforening 1973;93:598-600.

Lahrech MT, Caudrelier P. Immunological response of Moroccan children and newborns to oral poliovirus vaccine prepared on Vero cells. Vaccine 1990;8:306-307.

Lancet. N.Z. and S.S.P.E (editorial). Lancet 1973;2:772-773.

Lancet. Identification of the origin of poliovirus isolates: report of World Health Organisation informal meetings 1979—80. Lancet 1981;2:968-970.

Lancet. Correction: mumps meningitis following measles, mumps, and rubella immunisation. Lancet 1989;2:696.

Lancet. Mumps meningitis and MMR vaccination. Lancet 1989;2:1015-1016.

Landay AL, Jessop C, Lennette ET, Levy JA. Chronic fatigue syndrome: clinical condition associated with immune activation. Lancet 1991;338:707-712.

Lancet. Safety of high-titre measles vaccine (editorial). Lancet 1991;338:920.

Landrigan PJ, Witte JJ. Neurologic disorders following live measles-virus vaccination. Journal of the American Medical Association 1973;223:1459-1462.

Lane DA. A probabilist's view of causality assessment. Drug Information Journal 1984;18:323-330.

Lane DA, Kramer MS, Hutchinson TA, Jones JK, Naranjo C. The causality assessment of adverse drug reactions using a Bayesian approach. Pharmaceutical Medicine 1987;2:265-283.

Langholz E, Nielsen OH. Induction of endogenous Arachidonic acid metabolism in human neutrophils with snake venom phospholipase A2, immune complexes, and A23187. Prostaglandins, Leukotrienes and Essential Fatty Acids 1990;39:227-229.

Langmuir AD, Bregman DJ, Kurland LT, Nathanson N, Victor M. An epidemiologic and clinical evaluation of Guillain-Barre syndrome reported in association with the administration of swine influenza vaccines. American Journal of Epidemiology 1984;119:841-879.

Langsjoen PH, Stinson JC. Acute fatal allergic myocarditis: report of a case. Diseases of the Chest 1965;48:440-441.

Langue J, Preziosi MP, Boutitie F, Langue S, Schulz D, Hessel L et al. Vaccination of 3-month-old children with the capsular polysaccharide *Haemophilus influenzae* type b (Hib) combined with tetanus proteins (PRP-T). Medecine et Hygiene 1991;49:422-429.

Lasch EE, Livni E, Englander T, el-Massri M, Marcus O, Joshua H. The cell mediated immune response in acute poliomyelitis and its use in early diagnosis. Developments in Biological Standardization 1978;41:179-182.

Last JM, ed. A Dictionary of Epidemiology, 2nd edition. New York: Oxford University Press; 1988.

Last JM, Wallace RB, eds. Maxcy-Rosenau-Last Public Health and Preventive Medicine, 13th ed. Norwalk, CT: Appleton & Lange; 1992.

Lau YL, Tam AY, Ng KW, Tsoi NS, Lam B, Yeung CY. Response to preterm infants to hepatitis B vaccine. Journal of Pediatrics 1992;121:962-965.

Lavi S, Zimmerman B, Koren G, Gold R. Administration of measles, mumps, and rubella virus vaccine (live) to egg-allergic children. Journal of the American Medical Association 1990;263:269-271.

Lazzari G. [Post-vaccinal encephalopathy] Sullencefalopatia postvaccinale. Minerva Pediatrica 1970;22:581-584.

Leake JP. Poliomyelitis following vaccination against this disease. Journal of the American Medicial Association 1935;105:2152.

Lederle-Praxis Biologicals. Oral poliovirus vaccine. Report to the Institute of Medicine Vaccine Safety Committee. May 4, 1992.

Lee CT. Parental knowledge of their own immunization to poliomyelitis. Journal of the American Medical Association 1985;254:608-609.

Lee DA, Eby WC, Molinaro GA. HIV false positivity after hepatitis B vaccination (letter). Lancet 1992;339:1060.

Lee GR, Foerster J, Athens JW, Lukens JN, eds. Wintrobe's Clinical Hematology, 9th edition. London: Lea & Febiger; 1993.

Leen CL, Barclay GR, McClelland DB et al. Double-blind comparative trial of standard (commercial) and antibody-affinity-purified tetanus toxoid vaccines. Journal of Infection 1987;14:119-124.

Le Goff P, Fauquert P, Youinou P, Hoang S. [Periarteritis nodosa following vaccination against hepatitis B (letter)] Periarterite noueuse apres vaccination contre l'hepatite B. Presse Medicale 1988;17:1763.

Le Goff P, Fauquert P, Youinou P, Hoang S. [Periarteritis nodosa (PAN) following vaccine against B hepatitis]. Rhumatologie 1991;43:79.

Lemaire V. No risk of seizures or encephalopathy after DTP vaccination. Concours Medical 1991;113:177.

LeMay M. Infection after *Haemophilus* vaccine (letter). Pediatric Infectious Disease Journal 1986;5:387.

Leneman F. The Guillain-Barre syndrome. Archives of Internal Medicine 1966;118:139-144.

Lennartz H. [Enterovirus infections] Die Infektion mit Enteroviren. Ergebnisse der Inneren Medizin und Kinderheilkunde 1963;20:89-126.

Lenoir AA, Granoff PD, Granoff DM. Immunogenicity of *Haemophilus influenzae* type b polysaccharide-*Neisseria meningitidis* outer membrane protein conjugate vaccine in 2- to 6-month-old infants. Pediatrics 1987;80:283-287.

Lenz TR. Foreign body granuloma caused by jet injection of tetanus toxoid. Rocky Mountain Medical Journal 1966;63:48.

Lepage P, Dabis F, Msellati P, Hitimana DG, Stevens AM, Mukamabano B et al. Safety and immunogenicity of high-dose Edmonston-Zagreb measles vaccine in children with HIV-1 infection: a cohort study in Kigali, Rwanda. American Journal of Diseases of Children 1992;146:550-555.

Lepow M. Clinical trials of the *Haemophilus influenzae* type b capsular polysaccharide-diphtheria toxoid conjugate vaccine. Pediatric Infectious Disease Journal 1987;6:804-807.

Lepow ML. Pediatric immunizations and adverse events. Current Opinion in Infectious Disease 1991;4:463-468.

Lepow ML, Barkin RM, Berkowitz CD, Brunell PA, James D, Meier K et al. Safety and immunogenicity of *Haemophilus influenzae* type b polysaccharide-diphtheria toxoid conjugate vaccine (PRP-D) in infants. Journal of Infectious Diseases 1987;156:591-596.

Lepow ML, Peter G, Glode MP et al. Response of infants to *Haemophilus influenzae* type b polysaccharide and diphtheria-tetanus-pertussis vaccines in combination. Journal of Infectious Diseases 1984;149:950-955.

Lepow M, Randolph M, Cimma R et al. Persistence of antibody and response to booster dose of *Haemophilus influenzae* type b polysaccharide diphtheria toxoid conjugate vaccine in infants immunized at 9 to 15 months of age. Journal of Pediatrics 1986;108:882-886.

Lepow ML, Samuelson JS, Gordon LK. Safety and immunogenicity of *Haemophilus influenzae* type b polysaccharide-diphtheria toxoid conjugate vaccine in adults. Journal of Infectious Diseases 1984;150:402-406.

Lepow ML, Samuelson JS, Gordon LK. Safety and immunogenicity of *Haemophilus influenzae* type b-polysaccharide diphtheria toxoid conjugate vaccine in infants 9 to 15 months of age. Journal of Pediatrics 1985;106:185-189.

Lerman SJ, Bollinger M, Brunken JM. Clinical and serologic evaluation of measles, mumps, and rubella (HPV-77;DE-5 and RA 27/3) virus vaccines, singly and in combination. Pediatrics 1981;68:18-22.

Lerner S. Overdose of tetanus toxoid (letter). Journal of the American Medical Association 1974;228:159.

Lernmark A, Freedman ZR, Hofmann C, Rubinstein AH, Steiner DF, Jackson RL et al. Islet-cell-surface antibodies in juvenile diabetes mellitus. New England Journal of Medicine 1978;299:375-380.

Lesser RP, Hauser WA, Kurland LT, Mulder DW et al. Epidemiologic features of the Guillain-Barre syndrome: Experience in Olmsted County, Minnesota, 1935 through 1968. Neurology 1973;23:1269-1272.

Leung A. Anaphylaxis to tetanus toxoid. Irish Medical Journal 1984;77:306.

Leung AK. Congenital heart disease and DPT vaccination (letter). Canadian Medical Association Journal 1984;131:541.

Leung AK. Erythema multiforme following DPT vaccination. Journal of the Royal Society of Medicine 1984;77:1066-1067.

Leung AK. Anaphylaxis to DPT vaccine (letter). Journal of the Royal Society of Medicine 1985;78:175.

Leung AK, Jadavji T. Polysaccharide vaccine for prevention of *Haemophilus influenzae* type b disease. Journal of the Royal Society of Health 1988;108:180-181.

Leung AK, Szabo TF. Erythema multiforme following diphtheria-pertussis-tetanus vaccination. Kobe Journal of Medical Science 1987;33:121-124.

Levin M, Walter MD S., Barratt TM. Hemolytic uremic syndrome. Advances in Pediatric Infectious Disease 1989;4:51-81.

Levine BE, Lavi S. Perils of childhood immunization against measles, mumps, and rubella. Pediatric Nursing 1991;17:159-161, 215.

Levine L, Edsall G. Tetanus toxoid: what determines reaction proneness? Journal of Infectious Diseases 1981;144:376.

Levine L, Ibsen J, McComb JA. Adult immunization: preparation and evaluation of combined fluid tetanus and diphtheria toxoids for adult use. American Journal of Hygiene 1961;73:20-35.

Levy M, Koren G. Hepatitis B vaccine in pregnancy: maternal and fetal safety. American Journal of Perinatology 1991;8:227-232.

Levy NL, Notkins AL. Viral infections and diseases of the endocrine system. Journal of Infectious Diseases 1971;124:94-103.

Lewis JE, Chernesky MA, Rawls ML, Rawls WE. Epidemic of mumps in a partially immune population. Canadian Medical Association Journal 1979;121:751-754.

Lewis K, Jordan SC, Cherry JD et al. Petechiae and urticaria after DTP vaccination: detection of circulating immune complexes containing vaccine-specific antigens. Journal of Pediatrics 1986;109:1009-1012.

Lhuillier M, Mazzariol MJ, Zadi S, Le Cam N, Bentejac MC, Adamowicz L et al. Study of combined vaccination against yellow fever and measles in infants from six to nine months. Journal of Biological Standardization 1989;17:9-15.

Libbey MA. New vaccination: measles, mumps, rubella (letter). British Dental Journal 1988;165:160.

Lidin-Janson G, Strannegard O. Two cases of Guillain-Barre syndrome and encephalitis after measles. British Medical Journal 1972;2:572.

Liebenau JM. Public health and the production and use of diphtheria antitoxin in Philadelphia. Bulletin of the History of Medicine 1987;61:216-236.

Light RJ, Pillemer DB. Summing up: the science of reviewing research. Cambridge, Mass.: Harvard University Press; 1984.

Lightsey AL. Thrombocytopenia in children. Pediatric Clinics of North America 1980;27:293-308.

Limongi JC, Machado LR, Spina-Franca A. [Demyelinating diseases and the cerebrospinal fluid cytoproteinogram] Afeccoes desmielinizantes e citoproteinograma do liquido cefalorraqueano. Arquivos de Neuropsiquiatria 1981;39:296-300.

Lin JJ, Chang MK, Hsu CT, Tang HS. A rare association between hepatitis B virus vaccination and Guillain-Barre syndrome: a case report. Chinese Journal of Gastroenterology 1989;6:229-232.

Ling CM, Loong SC. Injection injury of the radial nerve. Injury 1976;8:60-62.

Lingam S, Miller CL, Clarke M, Pateman J. Antibody response and clinical reactions in children given measles vaccine with immunoglobulin. British Medical Journal 1986;292:1044-1045.

Linnemann CC Jr, May DB, Schubert WK, Caraway CT, Schiff GM. Fatal viral encephalitis in children with X-linked hypogammaglobulinemia. American Journal of Diseases of Children 1973;126:100-103.

Lione A. More on aluminum in infants. New England Journal of Medicine 1986;314:923.

Lipton et al. Autoimmunity and genetics contribute to the risk of insulin-dependent diabetes mellitus in families: islet cell antibodies and HLA DQ heterodimers. American Journal of Epidemiology 1992;136:503-512.

Little RE, Peterson DR. Sudden infant death syndrome epidemiology: a review and update. Epidemiologic Reviews 1990;12:241-246.

Livengood JR, Mullen JR, White JW, Brink EW, Orenstein WA. Family history of convulsions and use of pertussis vaccine. Journal of Pediatrics 1989;115:527-531.

Lleonart-Bellfill R, Cistero-Bahima A, Cerda-Trias MT, Olive-Perez A. Tetanus toxoid anaphylaxis. DICP Annals of Pharmacotherapy 1991;25:870.

Loffel M, Meienberg O, Diem P, Mombelli G. [Vaccine poliomyelitis in an adult undergoing chemotherapy for non-Hodgkin lymphoma] Impfpoliomyelitis bei einem Erwachsenen unter Chemotherapie wegen Non-Hodgkin-Lymphoms. Schweizerische Medizinische Wochenschrift 1982;112:419-421.

Lohiya G. Asthma and urticaria after hepatitis B vaccination (letter). Western Journal of Medicine 1987;147:341.

Lohr JM, Oldstone MB A. Detection of cytomegalovirus nucleic acid sequences in pancreas in type 2 diabetes. Lancet 1990;336:644-648.

Lokietz H, Fulginiti VA. Diphtheria and tetanus toxoids and pertussis vaccine litigation. American Journal of Diseases of Children 1991;145:425.

Long AP, Sartwell PE. Tetanus in the U.S. Army in World War II. Bulletin of the U.S. Army Medical Department 1947;7:371-385.

Lopez C, Biggar WD, Park BH, Good RA. Nonparalytic poliovirus infections in patients with severe combined immunodeficiency disease. Journal of Pediatrics 1974;84:497-502.

Lopez Adaros H, Held JR. Guillain-Barre syndrome associated with immunization against rabies: epidemiological aspects. Research Publications—Association for Research in Nervous and Mental Disease 1971;49:178-186.

Lorentz IT, McLeod JG. Post-vaccinial sensory polyneuropathy with myoclonus. Proceedings of the Australian Association of Neurologists 1969;6:81-86.

Louchet E, Tamalet J, Dufour Y, Chippaux. [Fleeting paralysis after oral anti-poliomyelitic agent: role of Echo 11 virus isolated in the patient] Paralysie fugace apres anti-poliomyelitique par voie buccale: role d'un virus Echo 11 isole chez le malade. Marseille Medical 1969;106:701-703.

Loughlin AM, Marchant CD, Lett S, Shapiro ED. Efficacy of *Haemophilus influenzae* type b vaccines in Massachusetts children 18 to 59 months of age. Pediatric Infectious Disease Journal 1992;11:374-379.

Lu WL, Zhao BX. Postvaccinal neurological complication: report of 12 cases. Chinese Medical Journal 1984;97:447-50.

Luby JP, Jones SR, Wohl AJ, Toben HR. Adverse reaction to duck embryo rabies vaccine (letter). Annals of Internal Medicine 1974;81:400-401.

Lumbiganon P, Kowsuwan P, Lumbiganon P, Taksaphan S, Panamonta M, Assateerawatts A. Comparison of immunogenicity of hepatitis B vaccine between low and normal birth weight infants. Asian Pacific Journal of Allergy and Immunology 1992;10:61-63.

Lynch TP, Cherry JD, Fulginiti VA. Vaccine myth and physician handouts. American Journal of Diseases of Children 1991;145:426-427.

Lyons R, Howell F. Pain and measles, mumps, and rubella vaccination. Archives of Disease in Childhood 1991;66:346-347.

Maass G, Quast U. Acute spinal paralysis after the administration of oral poliomyelitis vaccine in the Federal Republic of Germany (1963-1984). Journal of Biological Standardization 1987;15:185-191.

Macchia P, Terrosi F. [On an unusual case of encephalitis in a Sabin vaccinated infant] Su di un particolare caso di encefalite in bambino vaccinato secondo Sabin. Rivista di Clinica Pediatrica 1967;80:22-26.

Macko MB, Powell CE. Comparison of the morbidity of tetanus toxoid boosters with tetanus-diphtheria toxoid boosters. Annals of Emergency Medicine 1985;14:33-35.

Maclaren N, Atkinson M. Is insulin-dependent diabetes mellitus environmentally induced? New England Journal of Medicine 1992;327:348-349.

MacLennan R, Schoefield FD, Pittman M, Hardegree MC, Barile MF. Immunization against neonatal tetanus in New Guinea. Bulletin of the World Health Organization 1965;32:683-697.

Madden DL, Fuccillo DA, Traub RG, Ley AC, Sever JL, Beadle EL. Juvenile onset diabetes mellitus in pregnant women: failure to associate with Coxsackie B1-6, mumps, or respiratory syncytial virus infections. Journal of Pediatrics 1978;92:959-960.

Madore DV, Johnson CL, Phipps DC, Pennridge Pediatric Associates, Popejoy LA, Eby R et al. Safety and immunologic response to *Haemophilus influenzae* type b oligosaccharide-CRM197 conjugate vaccine in 1- to 6-month-old infants. Pediatrics 1990;85:331-337.

Madore DV, Johnson CL, Phipps DC, Pennridge Pediatric Associates, Myers MG, Eby R et al. Safety and immunogenicity of *Haemophilus influenzae* type b oligosaccharide-CRM197 conjugate vaccine in infants aged 15 to 23 months. Pediatrics 1990;86:527-534.

Madsen T, Jensen C, Ipsen J et al. Problems in active and passive immunity. Bulletin of the Johns Hopkins Hospital 1937;61:221-245.

Magdzik W. [Surveillance of adverse effects following immunization (AEFI)] Surveillance niepoangzadanych odczynow poszczepiennych (AEFI). Przeglad Epidemiologiczny 1992;46:27-33.

Mahmoud Abdel Azeem M, Imam ZE, Sohair SA. A study of a case of acute paralytic poliomyelitis. Journal of the Egyptian Public Health Association 1973;47:198-209.

Mahnke PF. [On the pathogenesis of vaccination damage in childhood] Zur Pathogenese des Impfschadens im Kindesalter. Zeitschrift fur die Gesamte Innere Medizin und Ihre Grenzgebiete 1967;22:806-811.

Mair IW, Elverland HH. Sudden deafness and vaccination. Journal of Laryngology and Otolaryngology 1977;91:323-329.

Majeron MA, Salvatores U. [Neuritic complications of antitetanus seroprophylaxis] Complicanze neuritiche della sieroprofilassi antitetanica. Rivista Sperimentale di Freniatria e Medicina Legale delle Alienazioni Mentali 1968;92:1904-1915.

Makela H, Eskola J, Peltola H, Takala AK, Kayhty H. Clinical experience with *Haemophilus influenzae* type b conjugate vaccines. Pediatrics 1990;85(4 Pt 2):651-653.

Makela PH, Peltola H, Kayhty H, Jousimies H, Perray O, Ruoslahti E et al. Polysaccharide vaccines of group A *Neisseria meningitidis* and *Haemophilus influenzae* type b: a field trial in Finland. Journal of Infectious Diseases 1977;136(Supplement):S43-S50.

Makino S, Sasaki K, Nakayama T, Oka S, Urano T, Kimura M et al. A new combined trivalent live measles (AIK-C strain), mumps (Hoshino strain), and rubella (Takahashi strain) vaccine. Findings in clinical and laboratory studies. American Journal of Diseases of Children 1990;144:905-910.

Mandal GS, Mukhopadhyay M, Bhattacharya AR. Adverse reactions following tetanus toxoid injection. Journal of the Indian Medical Association 1980;74:35-37.

Manfredi M. [A fatal case following antitetanic serum prophylaxis] Su un caso mortale da sieroprofilassi antitetanica. Bollettino Societa Medico Chirurgica Cremona 1968;22:19-35.

Mansfield LE, Ting S, Rawls DO, Frederick R. Systemic reactions during cutaneous testing for tetanus toxoid hypersensitivity. Annals of Allergy 57;:135-137.

Mantel N. Re: An epidemiologic and clinical evaluation of Guillain-Barre syndrome reported in association with the administration of swine influenza vaccines. American Journal of Epidemiology 1985;121:620-623.

Mantel N, Haenszel W. Statistical aspects of the analysis of data from retrospective studies of disease. Journal of the National Cancer Institute 1959;22:719-748.

Marchant CD, Band E, Froeschle JE, McVerry PH. Depression of anticapsular antibody after immunization with *Haemophilus influenzae* type b polysaccharide-diphtheria conjugate vaccine. Pediatric Infectious Disease Journal 1989;8:508-511.

Marchand JC. [The anti-measles vaccination] La vaccination antirougeoleuse. Cahiers du Medecine 1970;11:1105-1108.

Marcinak JF, Frank AL, Labotka RL, Fao S, Frisone LR, Yogev R et al. *Haemophilus influenzae* after vaccination at age one and one-half to six years. Pediatric Infectious Disease Journal 1991;10:157-159.

Marcuse EK, Wentz KR. The NCES reconsidered: summary of a 1989 workshop. Vaccine 1990;8:531-535.

Margileth AM, Mella GW, Di Moia F. Live measles vaccine: effect of age and preservative upon seroconversion. Medical Annals of the District of Columbia 1966;35:297-301.

Margileth AM, Mella GW, Di Moia F. Live mumps virus vaccine: clinical reactions and serological response in 615 children. Medical Annals of the District of Columbia 1968;37:197-201.

Mariner WK. The National Vaccine Injury Compensation Program: update. Health Affairs 1992;(Spring):255-265.

Mark A, Christenson B, Granstrom M, Strandell A, Wickbom B, Bottiger M. Immunity and immunization of children against diphtheria in Sweden. European Journal of Clinical Microbiology and Infectious Disease 1989;8:214-219.

Markland LD, Riley HD. The Guillain-Barre syndrome in childhood: a comprehensive review, including observations on 19 additional cases. Clinical Pediatrics 1967;6:162-170.

Markowitz LE, Sepulveda J, Diaz-Ortega JL, Valdespino JL, Albrecht P, Zell ER et al. Immunization of six-month-old infants with different doses of Edmonston-Zagreb and Schwarz measles vaccines. New England Journal of Medicine 1990;322:580-587.

Marks JS, Halpin TJ. Guillain-Barre syndrome in recipients of A/New Jersey influenza vaccine. Journal of the American Medical Association 1980;243:2490-2494.

Marshall GS, Wright PF, Fenichel GM, Karzon DT. Diffuse retinopathy following measles, mumps, and rubella vaccination. Pediatrics 1985;76:989-991.

Marti-Masso JF, Obeso JA, Cosme A. Guillain-Barre syndrome associated with a type B acute hepatitis. Medicina Clinica (Barcelona) 1979;73:447.

Martin GI, Weintraub MI. Brachial neuritis and seventh nerve palsy: a rare hazard of DPT vaccination. Clinical Pediatrics 1973;12:506-507.

Martin R, McFarland H, McFarlin D. Immunological aspects of demyelinating diseases. Annual Review of Immunology 1992;10:153-183.

Martinez E, Domingo P. Evans's syndrome triggered by recombinant hepatitis B vaccine. Clinical Infectious Diseases 1992;15:1051.

Marwick C. Expert panel convened by FDA recommends *Haemophilus influenzae* type b vaccine should continue in use for children older than 2 years. Journal of the American Medical Association 1987;257:3182-3183.

Marwick C. *H. influenzae* vaccines gain favor. Journal of the American Medical Association 1990;264:1375.

Marwick C. *Haemophilus influenzae* declining among young? Journal of the American Medical Association 1991;266:3398-3399.

Marzetti G, Bertolini L, Midulla M. [Virological and clinical study of morbid manifestations connected with anti-poliomyelitis vaccination with the oral Sabin vaccine] Studio virologico-clinico delle manifestazioni morbose in rapporto con la vaccinazione antipoliomielitica orale di Sabin. Minerva Pediatrica 1967;19:2236-2245.

Mason JO. From the Assistant Secretary for Health, US Public Health Service: protecting physicians from vaccine liability. Journal of the American Medical Association 1991;266:2951.

Mason JO. Addressing the measles epidemic (editorial). Public Health Reports 1992;107:241-242.

Maspero A, Cancellieri V, Della Rosa C. [Adverse reactions to measles vaccine] Reazioni secondarie alla vaccinazione contro il morbillo. Giornale di Malattie Infettive e Parassitarie 1991;43:499-503.

Maspero A, Sesana B, Ferrante P. Adverse reactions to measles vaccine. Bollettino dell'Istituto Sieroterapico Milanese 1984;63:125-129.

Mastaglia FL, Ojeda VJ. Inflammatory myopathies: part 1. Annals of Neurology 1985;17:215-227.

Mastaglia FL, Ojeda VJ. Inflammatory myopathies: part 2. Annals of Neurology 1985;17:317-323.

Mastaglia FL, Walton JN. Inflammatory myopathies. In: Mastaglia FL, Walton JN, eds. Skeletal Muscle Pathology. Edinburgh: Churchill; 1982.

Mathias RG, Routley JV. Paralysis in an immunocompromised adult following oral polio vaccination (letter). Canadian Medical Association Journal 1985;132:738-739.

Matuhasi T, Ikegami H. Elevation of levels of IgE antibody to tetanus toxin in individuals vaccinated with diphtheria-pertussis-tetanus vaccine. Journal of Infectious Diseases 1982;146:290.

Mawhinney H, Allen IV, Beare JM, Bridges JM, Connolly HH, Haire M et al. Dysgammaglobulinaemia complicated by disseminated measles. British Medical Journal 1971;2:380-381.

Maynard JE. Viral hepatitis as an occupational hazard in the health care profession. In: Vyas GN, Cohen SN, Schmid R, eds. Viral Hepatitis. Philadelphia: Franklin Institute Press; 1978.

McBean AM, Thoms ML, Albrecht P, Cuthie JC, Bernier R. Serologic response to oral polio vaccine and enhanced-potency inactivated polio vaccines. American Journal of Epidemiology 1988;128:615-628.

McBean AM, Thoms ML, Johnson RH, Gadless BR, MacDonald B, Nerhood L et al. A comparison of the serologic responses to oral and injectable trivalent poliovirus vaccines. Reviews of Infectious Diseases 1984;6(Suppl. 2):S552-S555.

McChesney MB, Oldstone MBA. Viruses perturb lymphocyte functions: selected principles characterizing virus-induced immunosuppression. Annual Review of Immunology 1987;5:279-304.

McChesney MB, Oldstone MBA. Virus-induced immunosuppression: infections with measles virus and human immunodeficiency virus. Advances in Immunology 1989;45:335-380.

McComb J, Levine L. Adult immunization. II. Dosage reduction as a solution to increasing reactions to tetanus toxoid. New England Journal of Medicine 1961;265:1152.

McCrae WM. Diabetes mellitus following mumps. Lancet 1963;1:1300-1301.

McDonald JC, Moore DL, Quennec P. Clinical and epidemiologic features of mumps meningoencephalitis and possible vaccine-related disease. Pediatric Infectious Disease Journal 1989;8:751-755.

McDonald R. SSPE (subacute sclerosing panencephalitis): is measles vaccination promotive or preventive? Clinical Pediatrics 1977;16:124-127.

McEwen J. Early-onset reaction after measles vaccination: further Australian reports. Medical Journal of Australia 1983;2:503-505.

McFarlin DE. Immunological parameters in Guillain-Barre syndrome. Annals of Neurology 1990;27(Suppl.):S25-S29.

McIntosh K. Feasible improvements in vaccines in the Expanded Programme on Immunization. Reviews of Infectious Diseases 1989;11(Suppl. 3):S530-S537.

McKendrick GD W., Nishtar T. Mumps orchitis and sterility. Public Health 1966;80:277-278.

McKhann GM, Cornblath DR, Griffin JW, Ho TW, Li CY, Jiang Z et al. Acute motor axonal neuropathy: a frequent cause of acute flaccid paralysis in China. Annals of Neurology 1993;33:in press.

McKhann GM, Cornblath DR, Ho TL, Li CY, Bai AY, Wu HS, Yei QF et al. Clinical and electrophysiological aspects of acute paralytic disease of children and young adults in northern China. Lancet 1991;38:593-597.

McKhann GM, Griffin JW, Cornblath DR, Mellits ED, Fisher RS, Quaskey SA. Plasmapheresis and Guillain-Barre syndrome: analysis of prognostic factors and the effect of plasmapheresis. Annals of Neurology 1988;23:347-353.

McLaughlin M, Thomas P, Onorato I, Rubinstein A, Oleske J, Nicholas S et al. Live virus vaccines in human immunodeficiency virus-infected children: a retrospective survey. Pediatrics 1988;82:229-233.

McLean AA, Hilleman MR, McAleer WJ, Buynak EB. Summary of world wide experience with HB-Vax. Journal of Infectious Diseases 1983;7(Suppl.):95-104.

McMahon B et al. Hepatitis B associated polyarteritis in Alaskan eskimos: clinical and epidemiologic features and long-term follow-up. Hepatology 1989;9:97-101.

McMahon BJ, Helminiak C, Wainwright RB, Bulkow L, Trimble BA, Wainwright K. Frequency of adverse reactions to hepatitis B vaccine in 43,618 persons. American Journal of Medicine 1992;92:254-256.

Medecine et Hygiene. [Compulsory immunizations: side effects and responsibility] Vaccinations obligatoires, effets secondaires et responsabilite. Medecine et Hygiene 1981;39:3501-3502.

Medical Journal of Australia. Vaccine-associated poliomyelitis (editorial). Medical Journal of Australia 1973;2:795-796.

Medical Journal of Australia. Measles vaccination: thrombocytopenia. Medical Journal of Australia 1980;1:561.

Medical Letter on Drugs and Therapeutics. *Haemophilus influenzae* type b vaccine. Medical Letter on Drugs and Therapeutics 1985;27:61-62.

Medical Letter on Drugs and Therapeutics. Conjugated *Haemophilus influenzae* type b vaccine. Medical Letter on Drugs and Therapeutics 1988;30:47-48.

Medical Letter on Drugs and Therapeutics. Routine immunization for adults. Medical Letter on Drugs and Therapeutics 1990;32:54-56.

Medical Letter on Drugs and Therapeutics. *H. influenzae* vaccine for infants. Medical Letter on Drugs and Therapeutics 1991;33:5-7.

Medical Research Council. Vaccination against measles: Clinical trial of live measles vaccine given alone and live vaccine preceded by killed vaccine. Practitioner 1971;206:458-466.

Medical Research Council, Measles Vaccines Committee. Vaccination against measles: a study of clinical reactions and serological responses of young children—a report to the Medical Research Council by the Measles Vaccines Committee. British Medical Journal 1965;1:817-863.

Medical Research Council, Measles Vaccines Committee. Vaccination against measles: a clinical trial of live measles vaccine given alone and live vaccine preceded by killed vaccine—a report to the Medical Research Council by the Measles Vaccines Committee. British Medical Journal 1966;1:441-446.

Medical Research Council, Measles Vaccines Committee. Vaccination against measles: a clinical trial of live measles vaccine given alone and live vaccine preceded by killed vaccine—second report to the Medical Research Council by the Measles Vaccines Committee. British Medical Journal 1968;2:449-452.

Mekler-Lupolover Y. [Uveitis and hepatitis B vaccination] Uveitis bei Hepatitis-B-Impfung. Klinische Monatsblatter fur Augenheilkunde 1987;190:297-298.

Melamed I, Romem Y, Shimoni T et al. Overdose of booster tetanus toxoid given in error: a clinical study. Scandinavian Journal of Infectious Diseases 1983;15:303-306.

Mellin H, Neff JM, Garber H, Lane JM. Complications of smallpox vaccination, Maryland 1968. Johns Hopkins Medical Journal 1970;126:160-168.

Melnick JL. Advantages and disadvantages of killed and live poliomyelitis vaccines. Bulletin of the World Health Organization 1978;56:21-38.

Melnick JL. Toward eradication of poliomyelitis by combined use of killed and live vaccines. Cardiovascular Research Center Bulletin 1982;20:49-60.

Melnick JL. Live attenuated poliovaccines. In: Plotkin SA, Mortimer EA, eds. Vaccines. Philadelphia: W.B. Saunders Co.; 1988.

Melnick JL. Vaccination against poliomyelitis: present possibilities and future prospects. American Journal of Public Health 1988;78:304-305.

Menser MA, Forrest JM, Bransby RD. Rubella infection and diabetes mellitus. Lancet 1978;1:57-60.

Meric AL. The safety of the hepatitis B vaccine (letter). Journal of the American Medical Association 1987;257:315-316.

Mertens T, Eggers HJ, Urteaga-Ballon O et al. Vaccine-associated poliomyelitis (letter). Lancet 1984;2:1390-1391.

Mertens T, Schurmann W, Kruppenbacher J, Rheingans K, Kellermann K, Maass G et al. Problems of live virus vaccine-associated poliomyelitis a paralytic case with isolation of all three poliovirus types. Medical Microbiology and Immunology 1983;172:13-21.

Mertens T, Schurmann W, Kruppenbacher JP, Eggers HJ, Rheingans K, Kellermann K et al. Two cases of vaccine-induced poliomyelitis. Acta Paediatrica Scandinavica 1984;73:133-134.

Messaritakis J. Toxic epidermal necrolysis in children. Annales Paediatrici 1966;207:236-246.

Messaritakis J. Diabetes following mumps in sibs. Archives of Disease in Childhood 1971;46:561.

Meyer JC, Trachsel H. Precipitating antibodies in sera of normal blood donors against some antigens related to type III allergy, detected by counterimmunoelectrophoresis. Allergologia et Immunopathologia 1979;7:205-210.

Meyer MB. An epidemiologic study of mumps: its spread in school and families. American Journal of Hygiene 1962;75:259.

Miadonna A. [Biological characteristics of specific IgE for tetanus toxoid] Caratteristiche biologiche delle IgE specifiche per il tossoide tetanico. Bollettino dell Istituto Sieroterapico Milanese 1980;59:554-559.

Miadonna A, Falagiani P. Determinazione delle IgE specifiche in 15 soggetti con sospetta allergia al tossoide tetanico. Folia Allergologica et Immunologica Clinica 1978;25:609-611.

Michielsen W. [Reactions to tetanus vaccination] Reacties bij tetanusvaccinatie. Tijdschrift voor Geneeskunde 1992;48:475-476.

Middaugh JP. Side effects of diphtheria-tetanus toxoid in adults. American Journal of Public Health 1979;69:246-249.

Mieli-Vergani G, Sutherland S, Mowat AP. Measles and autoimmune chronic active hepatitis (letter). Lancet 1989;2:688.

Miles RN, Hosking GP. Pertussis: should we immunise neurologically disabled and developmentally delayed children. British Medical Journal 1983;287:318-320.

Miller CL. Ten years of measles vaccinations: a review of the advantages and hazards of vaccination. Nursing Times 1978;74:2059-2060.

Miller CL. Surveillance after measles vaccination in children. Practitioner 1982;226:535-537.

Miller CL. Convulsions after measles vaccination. Lancet 1983;2:215.

Miller C, Farrington CP, Harbert K. The epidemiology of subacute sclerosing panencephalitis in England and Wales 1970-1989. International Journal of Epidemiology 1992;21:998-1006.

Miller C, Miller E, Rowe K, Bowie C, Judd M, Walker D. Surveillance of symptoms following MMR vaccine in children. Practitioner 1989;233:69-73.

Miller DL, Ross EM. ABC of 1 to 7: whooping cough. British Medical Journal 1982;284:1874.

Miller DL et al. Frequency of complications of measles, 1963. British Medical Journal 1964;2:75-78.

Miller DL, Alderslade R, Ross EM. Whooping cough and whooping cough vaccine: the risks and benefits debate. Epidemiologic Reviews 1982;4:1-24.

Miller DL, Reid D, Diamond JR. Poliomyelitis surveillance in England and Wales, 1965-8. Public Health 1970;84:265-285.

Miller DL, Ross EM, Alderslade R, Bellman MH, Rawson NS B. Pertussis immunisation and serious acute neurological illness in children. British Medical Journal 1981;282:1595-1599.

Miller DL, Wadsworth J, Diamond J, Ross E. Pertussis vaccine and whooping cough as risk factors in acute neurological illness and death in young children. Developments in Biological Standardization 1985;61:389-394.

Miller DL, Wadsworth MJH, Ross EM. Pertussis vaccine and severe acute neurological illnesses: response to a recent review by members of the NCES team. Vaccine 1989;7:487-489.

Miller DL, Wadsworth J, Ross E. Severe neurological illness: further analyses of the British National Childhood Encephalopathy Study. Tokai Journal of Experimental and Clinical Medicine 1988;13(Suppl.):145-155.

Miller E, Nokes DJ, Anderson RM. Measles, mumps, and rubella vaccination (letter). British Medical Journal 1992;304:1440-1441.

Miller G, Gale J, Villarejos V, James W, Arteaga CG, Casey H et al. Edmonston B and a further attenuated measles vaccine: a placebo controlled double blind comparison. American Journal of Public Health / Nations Health 1967;57:1333-1340.

Miller HG, Stanton JB. Neurological sequelae of prophylactic inoculation. Quarterly Journal of Medicine 1954;23:1-27.

Miller JE, Harding-Cox B. Measles vaccination in general practice. Practitioner 1969;203:352-354.

Miller JR, Orgel HA, Meltzer EO. The safety of egg-containing vaccines for egg-allergic patients. Journal of Allergy and Clinical Immunology 1983;71:568-573.

Miller NZ. Vaccines: Are They Really Safe and Effective? A Parents' Guide to Childhood Shots. Santa Fe, NM: New Atlantean Press; 1992.

Miller RG. Guillain-Barre syndrome: current methods of diagnosis and treatment. Postgraduate Medicine 1985;77:57-64.

Millson DS. Brother-to-sister transmission of measles after measles, mumps, and rubella immunisation. Lancet 1989;1:271.

Milstien JB, Kuritsky JN. Erythema multiforme and hepatitis B immunization (letter). Archives of Dermatology 1986;122:511-512.

Milstien JB, Gross TP, Kuritsky JN. Adverse reactions reported following receipt of Haemophilus influenzae type b vaccine: an analysis after 1 year of marketing. Pediatrics 1987;80:270-274.

Mirchamsy H. Measles immunization in Iran. Reviews of Infectious Diseases 1983;5:491-494.

Mirchamsy H, Nilforoushan MA, Shafyi A, Razavi J, Ashtiani MP, Youssofi I et al. Comparative evaluation of two combined measles-mumps-rubella vaccines based on AIK and Edmonston-Zagreb strains of measles virus. Kitasato Archives of Experimental Medicine 1991;64:141-147.

Mittelmeier VH. Generalisierte anaphylaktisch-toxische Gefabwandschadigung mit sinusthrombose nach aktiver Diphtherie-Schutzimpfung. Monatsschrift fur Kinderheilkunde 1959;107:288-293.

Mitus A. Vaccination of college students with attenuated live measles vaccine (letter). New England Journal of Medicine 1985;312:1326.

Mitus A, Holloway A, Evans AE, Enders JF. Attenuated measles vaccine in children with acute leukemia. American Journal of Diseases of Children 1962;103:243-248.

Mizutani H, Gerson KL, Haslam RH. Skin-test reactions in patients with SSPE. New England Journal of Medicine 1972;286:48.

Mobius G, Wiedersberg H, Wunscher W, Backer F. [Pathological-anatomical findings in cases of death following poliomyelitis and diphtheria-pertussis-tetanus vaccination] Pathologisch-anatomische Befunde bei Todesfallen nach Poliomyelitis- und Dreifach-Schutzimpfung. Deutsche Gesundheitswesen 1972;27:1382-1386.

Modlin JF, Jabbour JT, Witte JJ, Halsey NA. Epidemiologic studies of measles, measles vaccine, and subacute sclerosing panencephalitis. Pediatrics 1977;59:505-512.

Modlin JF, Onorato IM, McBean AM, Albrecht P, Thoms ML, Nerhood L et al. The humoral immune response to type 1 oral poliovirus vaccine in children previously immunized with enhanced potency inactivated poliovirus vaccine or live oral poliovirus vaccine. American Journal of Diseases of Children 1990;144:480-484.

Mohle-Boetani J. Oropharyngeal carriage of Haemophilus influenzae type b (Hib) in a heavily vaccinated population of 2-5 year olds. Program Abstracts of the 32nd Interscience Conference on Antimicrobial Agents and Chemotherapy. Abstract 1729, p. 399. Washington, DC: American Society for Microbiology; 1992.

Mok JQ, De Rossi A, Ades AE, Giaqunito C, Grosch-Wörner I, Peckham CS et al. Infants born to mothers seropositive for human immunodeficiency virus. Lancet 1987;1:1164-1168.

Monif GR. Can diabetes mellitus result from an infectious disease. Hospital Practice 1973;18:124-130.

Monif GR. Rubella virus and the pancreas. Medecine et Chirurgie Digestives 1974;3:195-197.

Monnet P. [Vaccinating children] Les vaccinations chez l'enfant. Rev Pediatr 1981;17:429-438.

Montanaro D, De Ruggiero N, Triassi M, D'Ambrosio R. [Reactions to required vaccinations:

a year of surveillance in Naples] Reazioni a vaccinazioni obbligatorie: un anno di sorveglianza in Napoli. Nuovi Annali Igiene e Microbiologia 1982;33:725-740.

Morens DM, Halsey NA, Schonberger LB, Baublis JV. Reye syndrome associated with vaccination with live virus vaccines: an exploration of possible etiologic relationships. Clinical Pediatrics 1979;18:42-44.

Morgan M, Nathwani D. Facial palsy and infection: the unfolding story. Clinical Infectious Diseases 1992;14:263-271.

Mori I, Torii S, Hamamoto Y, Kanda A, Tabata Y, Nagafuji H. [Virological evaluation of mumps meningitis following vaccination against mumps]. Kansenshogaku Zasshi [Journal of the Japanese Association for Infectious Diseases] 1991;65:226-283.

Mori I, Torii S, Mochida Y, Hatano Y, Nagafuji H. Poliovirus in cerebrospinal fluid from an infant with adenovirus infection. Clinical Infectious Diseases 1993;16:342-343.

Morley DC. Measles in the developing world. Proceedings of the Royal Society of Medicine 1974;67:1112-1115.

Morley D. Severe measles in the tropics. II. British Medical Journal 1969;1:363-365.

Morris JA, Butler H. Nature and frequency of adverse reactions following hepatitis B vaccine injection in children in New Zealand, 1985-1988. Submitted to Institute of Medicine Vaccine Safety Committee, May 4, 1992.

Morrison H, Mao Y, Semenciw R, Carter A, Davies J. Vaccine adverse reactions in young children in Ontario. Canadian Journal of Public Health 1988;79:459-460.

Morrow JI, Dowey KE, Swallow MW. Subacute sclerosing panencephalitis in Northern Ireland: twenty years' experience. Ulster Medical Journal 1986;55:124-130.

Morse LJ. Poliomyelitis from a vaccine. Lancet 1968;1:1312-1313.

Morse LJ, Rubin HE, Blount RE Jr. Vaccine-acquired paralytic poliomyelitis in an unvaccinated mother. Journal of the American Medical Association 1966;197:1034-1035.

Mortimer EA. Diphtheria toxoid. In: Plotkin SA, Mortimer EA, eds. Vaccines. Philadelphia: W.B. Saunders Co.; 1988.

Mortimer J, Melville-Smith M, Sheffield F. Diphtheria vaccine for adults. Lancet 1986;2:1182-1183.

Moss PD, Robertson L, Durbe NG, Cowburn GR. The Blackburn poliomyelitis epidemic: an analysis of the 109 cases admitted to hospital. Lancet 1968;2:555-558.

Mougrabi MM, Zarate AM, Alvarado GA, Reyes CA, Valdez DA. [Epidemiological field study of a poliomyelitis outbreak occurring in the state of Coahuila in 1977] Estudio epidemiologico de campo de un brote de poliomielitis ocurrido en el esdado de Coahuila duirante 1977. Salud Publica de Mexico 1980;22:39-44.

Moulignier A, Richer A, Fritzell C, Foulon D, Khoubesserian P, De Recondo J. [Meningoradiculitis after second injection of an anti-rabies vaccine 13 obtained from human diploid cell culture] Meningo-radiculite secondaire a une vaccination antirabique a partir d'un vaccin prepare sur culture de cellules diploides humaines. Presse Medicale 1991;20:1121-1123.

Moutard CML, Lejeune C. [Techniques, indications, contraindications and supervision of vaccination] Techniques, indications, contre-indications et surveillance des vaccinations. Revue du Praticien 1983;33:355-359.

Mouton Y, Chidiac C, Fourrier A. [Tetanus and diphtheria vaccinations in children] Vaccinations antitetanique et antidiphterique chez l'enfant. Semaine des Hopitaux de Paris 1985;61:1535-1538.

Moyner K. Specific IgE antibodies in sera from individuals with adverse reactions following diphtheria-tetanus-pertussis (DTP) or diphtheria-tetanus (DT) immunization. Allergy 1982;37(Suppl. 1):12.

Moynihan NH. Serum-sickness and local reactions in tetanus prophylaxis. Lancet 1955;2:264-266.

Mueller-Eckhardt G, Stief T, Otten A, Helmke K, Willems WR, Mueller-Eckhardt C. Complications of mumps infection, islet-cell antibodies, and HLA. Immunobiology 1984;167:338-344.

Mullen J, Centers for Disease Control. Questions and answers about vaccine safety and large-linked databases (LLDB). Submission to the Institute of Medicine Vaccine Safety Committee. Public Meeting, Washington, DC, May 11, 1992.

Mullen J, Centers for Disease Control. The Vaccine Adverse Events Reporting System (VAERS). Presentation to the Institute of Medicine Vaccine Safety Committee. Public Meeting, Washington, DC, May 11, 1992.

Mullen JR, Chen RT, Swint E, Hayes SW, Rastogi S, Knapp G. The Vaccine Adverse Event Reporting System (VAERS): A single post-marketing surveillance system for vaccines in the United States. Presented at the 7th International Conference on Pharmacoepidemiology, Basel, Switzerland, August 26-29, 1991.

Muller HE. [Local reactions after tetanus vaccination] Lokalreaktion nach tetanus-schutzimpfung. Deutsche Medizinische Wochenschrift 1990;115:235.

Muller HE. [Tetanus vaccination] Tetanus-schutzimpfung. Deutsche Medizinische Wochenschrift 1990;115:998.

Muller K. [Endangering of children with brain damage by measles vaccination] Zur Frage der Gefahrdung von hirngeschadigten Kindern durch Masernschutzimpfung. Deutsche Gesundheitswesen 1968;23:2104-2105.

Muller K, Eckoldt G. [Measles vaccination and EEG: evaluation of measles vaccination from the electroencephalographic point] Masern-Schutzimpfung und EEG: die Beurteilung der Masernimpfungen aus elektrencephalographischer Sicht. Zeitschrift fur Kinderheilkunde 1966;96:172-180.

Munoz O, Benitez-Diaz L, Martinez MC, Guiscafre H. Hearing loss after *Hemophilus influenzae* meningitis: follow-up study with auditory brainstem potentials. Annals of Otolaryngology Rhinology and Laryngology 1983;92:272-275.

Munoz JJ, Peacock MG, Hadlow WJ. Anaphylaxis or so-called encephalopathy in mice sensitized to an antigen with the aid of pertussigen (pertussis toxin). Infection and Immunity 1987;55:1004-1008.

Munyer TP, Mange RJ, Dolan T, Kantor FS. Depressed lymphocyte function after measles-mumps-rubella vaccination. Journal of Infectious Diseases 1975;134:75-78.

Murph JR, Grose C, McAndrew P, Mickiewicz C, Mento S, Cano F et al. Sabin inactivated trivalent poliovirus vaccine: first clinical trial and seroimmunity survey. Pediatric Infectious Disease Journal 1988;7:760-765.

Murphy TV. *Haemophilus* b polysaccharide vaccine: need for continuing assessment. Pediatric Infectious Disease Journal 1987;6:701-703.

Murphy TV. Is *Haemophilus influenzae* type b colonization of children in day care reduced by Hib conjugate (Conj) and plain polysaccharide (PPRP) vaccine (Vac)? Program Abstracts of the 31st Interscience Conference on Antimicrobial Agents and Chemotherapy. Abstract 66, p. 121. Washington, DC: American Society for Microbiology; 1991.

Murphy TV, Pastor P, Medley F, Osterholm MT, Granoff DM. Decreased *Haemophilus* colonization in children vaccinated with *Haemophilus influenzae* type b conjugate vaccine. Journal of Pediatrics 1993;122:517-523.

Murphy TV, White KE, Pastor P et al. Declining incidence of *Haemophilus influenzae* type b disease since introduction of vaccination. Journal of the American Medical Association 1993;269:246-248.

Murray MW, Lewis MJ. Mumps meningitis after measles, mumps, and rubella vaccination (letter). Lancet 1989;2:677.

Musgrove J. Measles vaccine. New Zealand Medical Journal 1971;73:309.

Musher DM, Watson DA, Lepow ML, McVerry P, Hamill R, Baughn RE. Vaccination of 18-month-old children with conjugated polyribosyl ribitol phosphate stimulates production of functional antibody to *Haemophilus influenzae* type b. Pediatric Infectious Disease Journal 1988;7:156-159.

Myers MG, Beckman CW, Vosdingh RA, Hankins WA. Primary immunization with tetanus and diphtheria toxoids: reaction rates and immunogenicity in older children and adults. Journal of the American Medical Association 1982;248:2478-2480.

Nabe-Nielsen J, Walter B. Unilateral total deafness as a complication of the measles-mumps-rubella vaccination. Scandinavian Audiology, Supplementum 1988;30:69-70.

Nabe-Nielsen J, Walter B. Unilateral deafness as a complication of the mumps, measles, and rubella vaccination. British Medical Journal 1988;297:489.

Nader PR, Warren RJ. Reported neurologic disorders following live measles vaccine. Pediatrics 1968;41:997-1001.

Nagel J, Svec D, Waters T, Fireman P. IgE synthesis in man. I. Development of specific IgE antibodies after immunization with tetanus diphtheria (TD) toxoids. Journal of Immunology 1977;118:334-341.

Nakayama T, Oka S, Komase K, Mori T, Nakagawa M, Sasaki K et al. The relationship between the mumps vaccine strain and parotitis after vaccination. Journal of Infectious Diseases 1992;165:186-187.

Nalin DR. Evaluating mumps vaccine (letter). Lancet 1992;339:305.

Nalin DR. Mumps vaccine complications: which strain? (letter). Lancet 1989;2:1396.

Nalin DR. Mumps, measles, and rubella vaccination and encephalitis. British Medical Journal 1989;299:1219.

Naruszewicz-Lesiuk D, Kantoch M, Polna I. [Immunological responses and postvaccination reactions in children vaccinated against measles. I. Assessment of postvaccination reactions] Odpowiedz immunologiczna i odczyny poszczepienne u dzieci objetych akcja szczepien przeciw odrze. I. Ocena odczynow poszczepiennych. Przeglad Epidemiologiczny 1974;28:315-324.

Naruszewicz-Lesiuk D, Wieczorkiewicz M, Iwinska B, Kulczycki J, Gut W. [Subacute sclerosing panencephalitis (SSPE) in Poland 1984-1986. Stage III of epidemiologic studies] Podostre stwardniajace zapalenie mozgu (SSPE) w Polsce w latach 1984-1986. III. Etap badan epidemiologicznych. Przeglad Epidemiologiczny 1988;42:205-210.

Nassif X, Haroche G, Lafaix C. [Problems of measles vaccination] Problemes poses par la vaccination morbilleuse. Medecine et Hygiene 1985;43:1144-1150.

Nategh R, Naficy K, Shahriary M. Mass trivalent oral polio vaccination in primary school age children in Teheran. Tropical and Geographical Medicine 1970;22:303-306.

Nathanson N, Horn SD. Neurovirulence tests of type 3 oral poliovirus vaccine manufactured by Lederle Laboratories, 1964-1988. Vaccine 1992;10:469-474.

Nathanson N, Langmuir AD. The Cutter incident: poliomyelitis following formaldehyde-inactivated poliovirus vaccination in the United States during the spring of 1955. I. Background. American Journal of Hygiene 1963;78:16-28.

National Center for Health Statistics. Current Estimates from the National Health Interview Survey, United States, 1988. Vital and Health Statistics, Series 10, No. 173. Washington, DC: U.S. Government Printing Office; 1989.

National Library of Medicine. Vaccine-Preventable Diseases of Childhood: Current Bibliographies in Medicine, No. 88-12. Washington, DC: U.S. Department of Health and Human Services; 1988.

National Vaccine Information Center, Dissatisfied Parents Together. NVIC News 1992;2(1):1-12.

Navarrete-Navarro S, Alvarez-Munoz MT, Bustamante-Calvillo ME, Vallejo-Aguilar OJ, Munoz O, Santos-Preciado JI et al. [Protection of health personnel against hepatitis B by DNA recombinant vaccine] Proteccion contra hepatitis B en trabajadores de salud con vacuna de DNA recombinante. Boletin Medico del Hospital Infantil de Mexico 1992;49:739-742.

Nederlands Tijdschrift voor Geneeskunde. [Vaccination and the Guillain-Barre syndrome] Vaccinatie en het syndroom van Guillain-Barre. Nederlands Tijdschrift voor Geneeskunde 1978;122:1780.

Neiderud J. Thrombocytopenic purpura after a combined vaccine against morbilli, parotitis and rubella. Acta Paediatrica Scandinavica 1983;72:613-614.

Nelson PG, Pyke DA, Gamble DR. Viruses and the aetiology of diabetes: a study in identical twins. British Medical Journal 1975;4:249-251.

Neuman E. Vaccines and victims. Washington Times. April 5, 1992:(Insight)6-11, 26, 28.

Neumann-Haefelin D, Newmann-Haefelin C, Baumeister HG, Knocke KW, Petersen EE, Haas R. [Poliomyelitis in the Federal Republic of Germany: a retrospective study of 1973] Poliomyelitis in der Bundesrepublik Deutschland: Ruckblick auf das Jahr 1973. Deutsche Medizinische Wochenschrift 1974;99:2597-2602.

New Zealand Department of Health. Hepatitis B: why we have to immunize. Health Quarterly Magazine (New Zealand Department of Health) 1988;40(3):3-5.

Newell KW, Duenas Lehmann A, LeBlanc DR, Garces Osorio N. The use of toxoid for the prevention of tetanus neonatorum: final report of a double-blind controlled field trial. Bulletin of the World Health Organization 1966;35:863-871.

Newell KW, Leblanc DR, Edsall G, Levine L, Christensen H, Montouri MH et al. The serological assessment of a tetanus toxoid field trial. Bulletin of the World Health Organization 1971;45:773-785.

Newman SL, Waldo B, Johnston RB Jr. Separation of serum bactericidal and opsonizing activities for Haemophilus influenzae type b. Infection and Immunity 1973;8:488-490.

Newton NJ, Janati A. Guillain-Barre syndrome after vaccination with purified tetanus toxoid. Southern Medical Journal 1987;80:1053-1054.

Ng PL, Powell LW, Campbell CP. Guillain-Barre syndrome during the Pre-icteric phase of acute type B viral hepatitis. Australia and New Zealand Journal of Medicine 1975;5:367-369.

Nicholson JK A., Holman RC, Jones BM, McDougal SM A., Markowitz LE. The effect of measles-rubella vaccination on lymphocyte populations and subpopulations in HIV-infected and healthy individuals. Journal of Acquired Immune Deficiency Syndromes 1992;5:528-529.

Nicoll A. Vaccine related poliomyelitis in non-immunised relatives and household contacts (letter). British Medical Journal 1987;294:374.

Nicoll A, Begg N. Immunizations in children. Current Opinion in Pediatrics 1993;5:60-67.

Nicolosi A, Hauser WA, Beghi E, Kurland LT. Epidemiology of central nervous system infections in Olmsted County, Minnesota, 1950-1981. Journal of Infectious Diseases 1986;154:399-408.

Nieminen U, Peltola H, Syrjala MT, Makipernaa A, Kekomaki R. Acute thrombocytopenic purpura following measles, mumps and rubella vaccination: a report on 23 patients. Acta Paediatrica 1993;82:267-270.

Niermeijer P, Gips CH. Guillain-Barre syndrome in acute HBs Ag-positive hepatitis. British Medical Journal 1975;4:732-733.

Nightingale SL. From the Food and Drug Administration. Journal of the American Medical Association 1990;264:2863.

Nishio O, Ishihara Y, Sakae K, Nonomura Y, Kuno A, Yasukawa W et al. The trend of acquired immunity with live poliovirus vaccine and the effect of revaccination: follow-up of vaccinees for ten years. Journal of Biological Standardization 1984;12:1-10.

Niv M. Mumps vaccine: possible reaction. Pediatrics 1969;44:146.

Nkowane BM, Wassilak SG, Orenstein WA, Bart KJ, Schonberger LB, Hinman AR et al. Vaccine-associated paralytic poliomyelitis, United States: 1973 through 1984. Journal of the American Medical Association 1987;257:1335-1340.

Noah ND. Vaccination today. British Journal of Hospital Medicine 1980;24:533-536.

Noel I, Galloway A, Ive FA. Hypersensitivity to thiomersal in hepatitis B vaccine (letter). Lancet 1991;338:705.

Nokes DJ, Anderson RM. Measles, mumps, and rubella vaccine: what coverage to block transmission? (letter). Lancet 1988;2:1374.

Nokes DJ, Anderson RM. Vaccine safety versus vaccine efficacy in mass immunisation programmes. Lancet 1991;338:1309-1312.

Nokes DJ, Anderson RM. Evaluation of mumps vaccine (letter). Lancet 1992;339:1052-1053.

Norden CW, Michaels RH, Melish M. Serologic responses of children with meningitis due to *Haemophilus influenzae* type b. Journal of Infectious Diseases 1976;134:495-499.

Norrby R. Polyradiculitis in connection with vaccination against morbilli, parotitis and rubella. Lakartidningen 1984;81:1636-1637.

Novak M, Kvicalova E, Friedlanderova B. Reactions to merthiolate in infants. Contact Dermatitis 1986;15:309-310.

Novello F, Lombardi F, Amato C, Santoro R, Fiore L, Grandolfo ME et al. Paralytic poliomyelitis in Italy (1981-85). European Journal of Epidemiology 1987;3:54-60.

Nutini MT, Marie FN, Loucq C, Tron F. Hepatitis B vaccine: clinical experience and safety (letter). Lancet 1983;2:1301.

Nyerges G, Zimonyi I, Nyerges G et al. Efficiency of tetanus toxoid booster in leukaemic children. Acta Paediatrica Academiae Scientiarum Hungaricae 1981;22:237-241.

Obodowska-Zysk W. [Reaction after vaccination against poliomyelitis and discussion of 3 cases] Odczynypo szczepieniu przeciw poliomyelitis z omowieniem 3 przypadkow. Przeglad Epidemiologiczny 1970;24:249-254.

Ochsenfahrt H. [Adverse reactions of drugs: collection and evaluation of reported data by the committee on safety of medicines] Unerwunschte Arzneimittelwirkungen: Sammlung und Auswertung durch die Arzneimittelkommission. Fortschritte der Medizin 1984;102:355-360.

Office of Technology Assessment. Compensation for Vaccine-Related Injuries: A Technical Memorandum. Washington, DC: U.S. Government Printing Office; 1980.

Offor E, Obi JO. Paralytic poliomyelitis in Benin City in Nigeria. Public Health 1986;100:297-301.

Ogra PL, Faden HS. Poliovirus vaccines: live or dead. Journal of Pediatrics 1986;108:1031-1033.

Okuno Y, Nakao T, Ishida N, Konno T, Mizutani H, Sato T et al. An epidemiological study of subacute sclerosing panencephalitis in Japan, 1976. Biken Journal 1978;21(A):9-14.

Okuno Y, Nakao T, Ishida N, Konno T, Mizutani H, Fukuyama Y et al. Incidence of subacute sclerosing panencephalitis following measles and measles vaccination in Japan. International Journal of Epidemiology 1989;18:684-689.

Oldstone MB. Prevention of type I diabetes in nonobese diabetic mice by virus infection. Science 1988;239:500-502.

Oldstone MB. Viruses can cause disease in the absence of morphological evidence of cell injury: implication for uncovering new diseases in the future. Journal of Infectious Diseases 1989;159:384-389.

Oldstone MB, Ahmed R, Salvato M. Viruses as therapeutic agents II. Viral reassortants map prevention of insulin-dependent diabetes mellitus to the small RNA of lymphocytic choriomeningitis virus. Journal of Experimental Medicine 1990;171:2091-2100.

Oldstone MB, Nerenberg M, Southern P, Price J, Lewicki H. Virus infection triggers insulin-dependent diabetes mellitus in a transgenic model: role of anti-self (virus) immune response. Cell 1991;65:319-331.

Oldstone MB, Tishon A, Schwimmbeck PL, Shyp S, Lewicki H, Dryberg T. Cytotoxic T lymphocytes do not control lymphocytic choriomeningitis virus infection of BB diabetes-prone rats. Journal of General Virology 1990;71(Pt. 4):785-791.

Olivares M, Walter T, Osorio M, Chadud P, Schlesinger L. Anemia of a mild viral infection: the measles vaccine as a model. Pediatrics 1989;84:851-855.

Onisawa S, Sekine I, Ichimura T, Homma N. Guillain-Barre syndrome secondary to immunization with diphtheria toxoid. Dokkyo Journal of Medical Science 1985;12:227-229.

Onorato IM, Markowitz LE, Oxtoby MJ. Childhood immunization, vaccine-preventable diseases and infection with human immunodeficiency virus. Pediatric Infectious Disease Journal 1988;7:588-595.

Onorato IM, Modlin JF, McBean A. M., Thoms ML, Losonsky GA, Bernier RH. Mucosal immunity induced by enhanced-potency inactivated and oral polio vaccines. Journal of Infectious Diseases 1991;163:1-6.

Openshaw H, Lieberman JS. Vaccine-related poliomyelitis (editorial). Archives of Internal Medicine 1982;142:1617.

Openshaw H, Lieberman JS. Vaccine-related poliomyelitis: serum IgM and cerebrospinal fluid antibodies. Western Journal of Medicine 1983;138:420-422.

Oppenheimer DR. A case of so-called demyelinating encephalitis. Neuropatologia Polska 1966;4(Suppl.):717-21.

Orenstein WA. Safety of combined schedules of OPV and IPV. Prepared for Meeting of Immunization Practices Advisory Committee. October 24-25, 1985.

Orenstein WA, Markowitz LE, Hinman AR. Diseases controlled primarily by vaccination: measles. In: Last JM, Wallace RB, eds. Maxcy-Rosenau-Last Public Health and Preventive Medicine, 13th ed. Norwalk, CT: Appleton & Lange; 1992.

Orgel HA, Hamburger RN, Mendelson LM et al. Antibody responses in normal infants and in infants receiving chemotherapy for congenital neuroblastoma. Cancer 1977;40:994-997.

Ornoy A, Arnon J, Feingold M, Ben Ishai P. Spontaneous abortions following oral poliovirus vaccination in first trimester (letter). Lancet 1990;335:800.

Orzechowska-Wolczyk M, Szulc-Kuberska J, Zawadzki Z. [Case of poliomyelitis in the mother of a child vaccinated against poliomyelitis] Przypadek zapalenia rogow przednich rdzenia kregowego u matki dziecka szczepionego przeciw polio. Wiadomosci Lekarskie 1976;29:1007-1010.

Osawa J, Kitamura K, Ikezawa Z, Nakajima H. A probable role for vaccines containing thimerosal in thimerosal hypersensitivity. Contact Dermatitis 1991;24:178-182.

Osawa J, Kitamura K, Ikezawa Z, Nakajima H. A study on hypersensitivity reactions to piroxicam in experimentally induced thimerosal allergy. Skin Research 1991;33(Suppl. 10):154-159.

Osetowska E, Biernacki M, Pietrzyk J. "Spontaneous" changes in the brains of monkeys used for vaccine production. Polish Medical Journal 1966;5:1132-1151.

Oski FA, Naiman JL. Effect of live measles vaccine on the platelet count. New England Journal of Medicine 1966;275:352-356.

Osorio M, Olivares M, Chadud P, Schlesinger L, Arevalo M, Stekel A. [Clinical manifestations and leukocyte response induced by measles vaccination] Manifestaciones clinicas y respuesta leucocitaria producidas por la vacunacion antisarampion. Revista Chilena de Pediatria 1987;58:74-77.

Osterholm MT, Rambeck JH, White KE, Jacobs JL, Pierson LM, Neaton JD et al. Lack of efficacy of *Haemophilus* b polysaccharide vaccine in Minnesota. Journal of the American Medical Association 1988;260:1423-1428.

Osuntokun BO. The neurological complications of vaccination against smallpox and measles. West African Medical Journal and Nigerian Practitioner 1968;17:115-121.

Otsuki A. [Current status and problems of measles vaccine and vaccination]. Hokenfu Zasshi 1970;26:50-51.

Ott K. [Iatrogenic disease in the prevention of tetanus] Iatrogenie v prevenci tetanu. Rozhledy v Chirurgii 1967;46:493-495.

Otten A, Helmke K, Stief T, Mueller-Eckhard G, Willems WR, Federlin K. Mumps, mumps vaccination, islet cell antibodies and the first manifestation of diabetes mellitus type I. Behring Institute Mitteilungen 1984;75:83-88.

Ovens H. Anaphylaxis due to vaccination in the office. Canadian Medical Association Journal 1986;134:369-370.

Ozaki T, Miwata H, Kodama H, Matsui Y, Asano Y. Henoch-Schonlein purpura after measles immunization. Acta Paediatrica Japonica 1989;31:484-486.

Ozeretskovskii NA, Gurvich EB. [The side effects of vaccines used in prophylactic inoculation schedules] Pobochnoe deistvie vaktsin kalendaria profilakticheskikh privivok. Zhurnal Mikrobiologii, Epidemiologii, i Immunobiologii 1991;5:59-63.

Pachman DJ. Mumps occurring in previously vaccinated adolescents. American Journal of Diseases of Children 1988;142:478-479.

Palumbo P, Hoyt L, Demasio K, Oleske J, Connor E. Population-based study of measles and measles immunization in human immunodeficiency virus-infected children. Pediatric Infectious Disease Journal 1992;11:1008-1014.

Pampiglione G, Griffith AH, Bramwell EC. Transient cerebral changes after vaccination against measles. Lancet 1971;2:5-8.

Pappenheimer AM Jr. Diphtheria. In: Germanier R, ed. Bacterial Vaccines. Orlando: Academic Press; 1984.

Pappenheimer AM Jr. A study of reactions following administration of crude and purified diphtheria toxoid in an adult population. American Journal of Hygiene 1950;52:353-370.

Paradiso G, Micheli F, Fernandez Pardal M, Casas Parera I. [Multifocal demyelinating neuropathy after tetanus vaccine] Neuropatia desmielinizante multifocal siguiendo vacunacion antitetanica. Medicina 1990;50:52-54.

Parish HJ, Oakley CL. Anaphylaxis after injection of tetanus toxoid. British Medical Journal 1940;1:294-295.

Parish WE. Eosinophilia. I. Eosinophilia in guinea-pigs mediated by passive anaphylaxis and by antigen-antibody complexes containing homologous IgG1a and IgG1b. Immunology 1972;22:1087-1098.

Parke JC Jr, Schneerson R, Reimer C, Black C, Welfare S, Bryla D et al. Clinical and immunologic responses to *Haemophilus influenzae* type b-tetanus toxoid conjugate vaccine in infants injected at 3, 5, 7, and 18 months of age. Journal of Pediatrics 1991;118:184-190.

Parker JC, Klintworth GK, Graham DG, Griffith JF. Uncommon morphologic features in subacute sclerosing panencephalities (SSPE). American Journal of Pathology 1970;61:275-291.

Parkkonen P, Hyoty H, Koskinen L, Leinikki P. Mumps virus infects beta cells in human fetal islet cell cultures upregulating the expression of HLA class I molecules. Diabetologia 1992;35:63-69.

Pasetto N. Problems of vaccinations in pregnancy. Clinica Terapeutica 1988;125:65-70.

Pataky L. [Late vaccination complications in the prevention of tetanus and rabies] Spate Impfkomplikationen bei der Prophylaxe gegen Tetanus und Tollwut. Zeitschrift fur die Gesamte Hygiene 1977;23:917-918.

Patan B. [Postvaccinal severe diabetes mellitus]. Posvaktsinoznyi tiazhelyi sakharnyi diabet. Terapevticheskii Arkhiv (Moskva) 1968;40:117-118.

Pathak UN, Dilawari JB, Chawla Y, Sokhey CS, Sharma BK, Ganguly NK. Immunogenicity and side effects of low dose intradermally administered hepatitis B vaccine. Indian Journal of Gastroenterology 1988;7:113-114.

Patriarca PA, Sutter RW. Diseases controlled primarily by vaccination: poliomyelitis. In: Last JM, Wallace RB, eds. Maxcy-Rosenau-Last Public Health and Preventive Medicine, 13th ed. Norwalk, CT: Appleton & Lange; 1992.

Patrick A. Acute diabetes following mumps. British Medical Journal 1924;2:802.

Patterson K, Chandra RS, Jenson AB. Congenital rubella, insulitis, and diabetes mellitus in an infant. Lancet 1981;1:1048-1049.

Pauksen K, Duraj V, Ljungman P, Sjolin J, Oberg G, Lonnerholm G et al. Immunity to and immunization again measles, rubella and mumps in patients after autologous bone marrow transplantation. Bone Marrow Transplantation 1992;9:427-432.

Paulson GW. The Landry-Guillain-Barre-Strohl syndrome in childhood. Developmental Medicine and Child Neurology 1970;12:604-607.

Paux G, Chretien P, Hermier C, Moore N, Boismare F. [Minor and major side-effects from vaccination: interest of a precise inquiry done by a pharmacovigilance center] Incidents et accidents vaccinaux: interet de l'enquete precise faite a l'initiative du centre de pharmacovigilance aupres des praticiens. Therapie 1983;38:583-585.

Pawlowski B, Gries FA. [Mumps vaccination and type-I diabetes]. Mumpsimpfung und Typ-I-Diabetes. Deutsche Medizinische Wochenschrift 1991;116:635.

Payne FE, Baublis JV, Itabashi HH. Isolation of measles virus from cell cultures of brain from a patient with subacute sclerosing panencephalitis. New England Journal of Medicine 1969;281:585-589.

Pearlman DS, Bierman CW. Allergic disorders. In: Stiehm ER, ed. Immunologic Disorders in Infants and Children, 3rd edition. Philadelphia: W. B. Saunders Co.; 1989.

Peebles TC, Levine L, Eldred ML. Tetanus-toxoid emergency boosters: a reappraisal. New England Journal of Medicine 1969;280:575-581.

Peel MM, Edsall G, White WG, Barnes GM. Relationship between lymphocyte response to tetanus toxoid and age of lymphocyte donor. Journal of Hygiene 1978;80:259-265.

Peig M, Ercilla G, Millan M, Gomis R. Post-mumps diabetes mellitus (letter). Lancet 1981;1:1007.

Peltola H. Rapid effect on endemic measles, mumps, and rubella of nationwide vaccination programme in Finland. Lancet 1986;1:137-139.

Peltola H. Clinical efficacy of the PRP-D versus HbOC conjugate vaccine Haemophilus influenzae type b (Hib). Program Abstracts of the 32nd Interscience Conference on Antimicrobial Agents and Chemotherapy. Abstract 975, p. 273. Washington, DC: American Society for Microbiology; 1992.

Peltola H, Heinonen OP. Frequency of true adverse reactions to measles-mumps-rubella vaccine: a double-blind placebo-controlled trial in twins. Lancet 1986;1:939-942.

Peltola H, Kayhty H, Sivonen A, Makela PH. Haemophilus influenzae type b capsular polysaccharide vaccine in children: a double-blind field study of 100,000 vaccinees 3 months to 5 years of age in Finland. Pediatrics 1977;60:730-737.

Peltola H, Kayhty H, Virtanen M, Makela PH. Prevention of Hemophilus influenzae type b bacteremic infections with the capsular polysaccharide vaccine. New England Journal of Medicine 1984;310:1561-1566.

Penner E, Maida E, Mamoli B, Gangl A. Serum and cerebrospinal fluid immune complexes containing hepatitis B surface antigen in Guillain-Barre syndrome. Gastroenterology 1982;82:576-580.

Pennie RA, O'Connor AM, Dulberg CS, Bottiglia A, Manga P, Kang CY. Low-cost hepatitis B vaccine improves uptake among self-paying health-care students. Journal of Medical Virology 1992;37:48-53.

Penttinen K. Benefits and risks of killed polio vaccine. Experiences in Finland. Developments in Biological Standardization 1979;43:159-163.

Penttinen K, Cantell K, Somer P, Poikolainen A. Mumps vaccination in the Finnish defense forces. American Journal of Epidemiology 1968;88:234-244.

Pere JC. Estimation du numerateur en notification spontanee. In: Begaud B, ed. Analyse d'Incidence en Pharmacovigilance: Application a la Notification Spontanee. Bordeaux, France: ARME-Pharmacovigilance Editions; 1991.

Perez-Martin R. Reactions to booster doses of tetanus vaccine. Pediatrics 1968;42:711-712.

Perkins LD. Complying with the National Childhood Vaccine Injury Act. American Journal of Hospital Pharmacy 1990;47:1260, 1262, 1266.

Perlman EC. Purpuric and cerebral manifestations following measles. Archives of Pediatrics 1934;51:596-604.

Peter G. Vaccine crisis: an emerging societal problem. Journal of Infectious Diseases 1985;151:981-983.

Peter G. Measles immunization: recommendations, challenges, and more information (editorial). Journal of the American Medical Association 1991;265:2111-2112.

Peterson JC, Christie A. Immunization in the young infant. American Journal of Diseases of Children 1951;81:518-529.

Pharmacy International. Vaccination and drug interactions. Pharmacy International 1985;6:291-292.

Philip RN, Reinhard KR, Lackman DB. Observations on a mumps epidemic in a "virgin" population. American Journal of Hygiene 1959;69:91-111.

Physicians' Desk Reference, 46th edition. Montvale, NJ: Medical Economics Company Inc.; 1992.

Piazza M, Picciotto L, Villari R et al. Hepatitis B immunisation with a reduced number of doses in newborn babies and children. Lancet 1985;1:949-951.

Pichichero ME, Barkin RM, Samuelson JS. Pediatric diphtheria and tetanus toxoids-adsorbed vaccine: immune response to the first booster following the diphtheria and tetanus toxoids vaccine primary series. Pediatric Infectious Disease 1986;5:428-430.

Pierce EJ, Davison MD, Parton RG, Habig WH, Critchley DR. Characterization of tetanus toxin binding to rat brain membranes. Biochemical Journal 1986;236:845-852.

Pierchalla P, Petri H, Ruping KW, Stary A. [Urticaria after H-B-vax injection due to hypersensitivity to thiomersal (merthiolate)] Urtikarielle Reaktion nach Injektion von H-B-Vax bei Sensibilisierung auf Thiomersal (Merthiolat). Allergologie 1987;10:97-99.

Pietroski N. Viral hepatitis: advances in pharmacy therapy. American Druggist 1992;206:71-85.

Pilotti G. [Thrombopenia and acute hemolytic anemia in the course of poliomyelitis vaccination] Piastrinopenia ed anemia emolitica acuta in corso di vaccinazione antipoliomielitica. Minerva Pediatrica 1975;27:637-639.

Pincus DJ, Morrison D, Andrews C, Lawrence E, Sell SH, Wright PF. Age-related response to two *Haemophilus influenzae* type b vaccines. Journal of Pediatrics 1982;100:197-201.

Pineau A, Durand C, Guillard O, Bureau B, Stalder JF. Role of aluminium in skin reactions after diphtheria-tetanus-pertussis-poliomyelitis vaccination: an experimental study in rabbits. Toxicology 1992;73:117-125.

Pinson JB, Weart CW. New considerations for *Haemophilus influenzae* type b vaccination. Clinical Pharmacy 1992;11:332-336.

Piriev GG, Liashchenko VA. [Possibilities of measles vaccination in children with counterindications and duration of preservation of postvaccinal immunity] Izuchenie vozmozhnosti vaktsinatsii protiv kori detei s nekotorymi protivopokazaniiami i prodolzhitel'nost' sokhraneniia postvaktsinal'nogo immuniteta. Pediatriia 1990;12:27-30.

Plotkin SA, Mortimer EA, eds. Vaccines. Philadelphia: W.B. Saunders Co.; 1988.

Plotkin SL, Plotkin SA. A short history of vaccination. In: Plotkin SA, Mortimer EA, eds. Vaccines. Philadelphia: W.B. Saunders Co.; 1988.

Pohl KR, Farley JD, Jan JE, Junker AK. Ataxia-telangiectasia in a child with vaccine-associated paralytic poliomyelitis. Journal of Pediatrics 1992;121:405-407.

Pokrovskii VI, Bolotovskii VM, Titova NS, Pokrovskaia NI. [Subacute sclerosing panencephalitis] Podostryi skleroziruiushchii panentsefalit. Sovetskaia Meditsina 1982;7:53-59.

Pol KM. Measles: the epidemiology and control of an outbreak. Journal of the American College Health Association 1983;31:158-161.

Polakoff S. Immunisation of infants at high risk of hepatitis B. British Medical Journal 1982;285:1294-1295.

Poland GA, Love KR, Hughes CE. Routine immunization of the HIV-positive asymptomatic patient. Journal of General Internal Medicine 1990;5:147-152.

Pollard JD, Selby G. Relapsing allergic neuritis. Proceedings of the Australian Association of Neurologists 1977;14:133-136.

Pollard JD, Selby G. Relapsing neuropathy due to tetanus toxoid: report of a case. Journal of Neurological Science 1978;37:113-125.

Pollard JD, Selby G, McLeod JG. Chronic relapsing polyneuritis (abstract). Electroencephalography and Clinical Neurophysiology 1977;43:617.

Pollock TM. Measles control in the United Kingdom. Reviews of Infectious Diseases 1983;5:574-576.

Pollock TM, Morris J. A 7-year survey of disorders attributed to vaccination in North West Thames region. Lancet 1983;1:753-757.

Pollock TM, Morris J. Vaccine reactions. Lancet 1983;1:1380-1381.

Pollock TM, Miller E, Mortimer JY, Smith G. Symptoms after primary immunisation with DTP and with DT vaccine. Lancet 1984;2:146-149.

Pollock TM, Miller E, Mortimer JY, Smith G. Post-vaccination symptoms following DTP and DT vaccination. Developments in Biological Standardization 1985;61:407-410.

Poole FT. Abnormal result of treatment. Occupational Health 1974;26:55-57.

Pope RM, Pahlavani MA, LaCour E. Antigenic specificity of rheumatoid synovial fluid lymphocytes. Arthritis and Rheumatism 1989;32:1371-1380.

Popejoy LA, Rivera AI, Gonzales-Torres I. Side-effects and immunogenicity of *Haemophilus influenzae* type b polysaccharide vaccine in a multi-ethnic pediatric population. Military Medicine 1989;154:25-29.

Popow-Kraupp T, Kundi M, Ambrosch F, Vanura H, Kunz C. A controlled trial for evaluating two live attenuated mumps-measles vaccines (Urabe Am 9-Schwarz and Jeryl Lynn-Moraten) in young children. Journal of Medical Virology 1986;18:69-79.

Porter D, Porter R. The politics of prevention: anti-vaccinationism and public health in nineteenth-century England. Medical History 1988;32:231-252.

Poser CM. Disseminated vasculomyelinopathy: a review of the clinical and pathologic reactions of the nervous system in hyperergic diseases. Acta Neurologica Scandinavica 1969;37(Suppl.):3-44.

Poser CM. Postvaccinal encephalitis (letter). Annals of Neurology 1983;13:341-342.

Poser CM. Neurological complications of infections and vaccinations. Saudi Medical Journal 1992;13:379-386.

Pounder DJ. Sudden, unexpected death following typhoid-cholera vaccination. Forensic Science International 1984;24:95-98.

Pozzetto B, Genin C, Gaudin OG, Berthoux FC, Alloin B, Laurent B et al. Live poliovirus vaccine in patients with chronic glomerulonephritis: effects on renal function and specific antibody response. Clinical Nephrology 1987;28:194-198.

Preblud SR, Katz SL. Measles vaccine. In: Plotkin SA, Mortimer EA, eds. Vaccines. Philadelphia: W.B. Saunders Co.; 1988.

Press E. Desirability of the routine use of tetanus toxoid. New England Journal of Medicine 1948;239:50-56.

Price DL, Griffin JW. Immunocytochemical localization of tetanus toxin to synapses of spinal cord. Neuroscience Letters 1981;23:149-155.

Prilutskaya AF, Feldman EV, Votyakov VI, Protas II. [Diagnosis of poliomyelitis and polio like paralysis in children under conditions of mass vaccination with live poliovaccine in Byelorussia]. Zdravookhr Beloruss 1974;20:73-76.

Prince GA, Jenson AB, Billups LC, Notkins AL. Infection of human pancreatic beta cell cultures with mumps virus. Nature 1978;271:158-161.

Profeta ML. [Characteristics of the virus and of measles vaccines] Generalita sul virus del morbillo e sui relativi vaccini. Annali Sclavo 1979;21(Suppl. 1):377-383.

Prost J. [Remarks on 10,000 anti-poliomyelitis vaccinations made in the factories of a business] Remarques sur 10,000 vaccinations anti-poliomyelitiques effectuees dans les ateliers d'une entreprise. Archives des Maladies Professionnelles de Medecine du Travail et de Securite Sociale 1967;28:871-875.

Purcell RH, Gerin JL. Hepatitis B subunit vaccine: a preliminary report of safety and efficacy tests in chimpanzees. American Journal of Medical Science 1975;270:395-399.

Puvvada L, Silverman B, Bassett C, Chiaramonte LT. Systemic reactions to measles-mumps-rubella vaccine skin testing. Pediatrics 1993;91:835-836.

Quagliarello V, Scheld WM. Bacterial meningitis: pathogenesis, pathophysiology, and progress. New England Journal of Medicine 1992;327:864-872.

Quast U, Hennessen W, Widmark RM. Mono- and polyneuritis after tetanus vaccination (1970-1977). Developments in Biological Standardization 1979;43:25-32.

Quast U, Hennessen W, Widmark RM. Vaccine induced mumps-like diseases. Developments in Biological Standardization 1979;43:269-272.

Quast U, Herder C, Zwisler O. Vaccination of patients with encephalomyelitis disseminata. Vaccine 1991;9:228-230.

Querfurth H, Swanson PD. Vaccine-associated paralytic poliomyelitis: regional case series and review. Archives of Neurology 1990;47:541-544.

Racaniello VR. Poliovirus vaccines. Biotechnology 1992;20:205-222.

Radl H. [Virus meningitis: newer clinical and epidemiological observations] Virus-Meningitiden: neuere klinische und epidemiologische Beobachtungen. Munchener Medizinische Wochenschrift 1967;109:1900-1904.

Raettig H. Provokation einer infektion durch Schutzimpfung. Zentralblatt fur Bakteriologie, Parasitendunde, Infektionskrankheiten und Hygiene 1959;174:192-217.

Raj B, Dubey YD. A study of sensitivity induced by certain drugs by intradermal skin tests. Indian Journal of Medical Research 1969;57:1769-1775.

Ramon G. Mecedine experimentale: sur le pouvoir floculant et sur les proprietes immunisantes d'une toxine diphtherique rendue anatoxique (anatoxine). Comptes Rendus Hebdomadaires des Seances de l'Academie des Sciences 1923;177:1338-1340.

Ramon G, Zoeller C. Medecine experimentale: de la valeur antigene de l'anatoxine tetanique chez l'homme. Comptes Rendues Hebdomadaires des Seances de l'Academie des Sciences 1926;182:245-247.

Ramon G, Zoeller C. L'anatoxine tetanique et l'immunisation active de l'homme vis-a-vis du tetanos. Annales Institut Pasteur 1927;41:803-833.

Ramsay ME, Rao M. Meningoencephalitis after measles-mumps-rubella vaccine (letter). Archives of Disease in Childhood 1991;66:1365.

Ramsay ME, Rao M, Begg NT. Symptoms after accelerated immunisation. British Medical Journal 1992;304:1543-1536.

Ramsey M, Rao M, Symons J, Virdee S, Gogarty M, Ryan J et al. Vaccine reaction: "guilty until proven innocent". Commun Dis Rep 1990;90:3.

Ranieri R, Passaretti B, Vecchi L, Milella AM. Hepatitis B vaccination in a group of 50 Italian prisoners. Medical Science Research 1992;20:115-116.

Rantala H, Uhari M, Niemela M et al. Occurrence, clinical manifestations, and prognosis of Guillain-Barre syndrome. Archives of Disease in Childhood 1991;66:706-709.

Rantala H, Uhari M, Tuokko H, Stenvik M, Kinnunen L. Poliovaccine virus in the cerebrospinal fluid after oral polio vaccination. Journal of Infection 1989;19:173-176.

Rapicetta M. Hepatitis B vaccination in dialysis centres: advantages and limits. Nephron 1992;61:284-286.

Rappouli R, Perugini M, Falsen E. Molecular epidemiology of the 1984-1986 outbreak of diphtheria in Sweden. New England Journal of Medicine 1988;318:12-14.

Rasmussen JE. Erythema multiforme in children: response to treatment with systemic corticosteroids. British Journal of Dermatology 1976;95:181-186.

Ratliff DA, Burns-Cox CJ. Anaphylaxis to tetanus toxoid. British Medical Journal 1984;288:114.

Ratzmann KP, Strese J, Witt S, Berling H, Keilacker H, Michaelis D. Mumps infection and insulin-dependent diabetes mellitus (IDDM). Diabetes Care 1984;7:170173.

Rau R, Karger T, Herborn G. Zwei falle chronischer polyarthritis nach Hepatitis B impfung. Zeitschrift fur Rheumatologie (Tagung der Deutschen Gesellschaft fur Rheumatologie) 1984;43:213.

Rayfield EJ, Kelly KJ, Yoon JW. Rubella virus-induced diabetes in the hamster. Diabetes 1986;35:1278-1281.

Rayfield EJ, Seto Y. Viruses and the pathogenesis of diabetes mellitus. Diabetes 1978;27:1126-1139.

Read SJ, Schapel GJ, Pender MP. Acute transverse myelitis after tetanus toxoid vaccination (letter). Lancet 1992;339:1111-1112.

Reed D, Brown G, Merrick R, Sever J, Feltz E. A mumps epidemic on St. George Island, Alaska. Journal of the American Medical Association 1967;199:113-117.

Regamey RH. Die Tetanus-Schutzimpfung. In: Herrlick A, ed. Handbuch der Schutzimpfungen. Berlin-Heidelberg-New York: Springer; 1965.

Reinstein L, Pargament JM, Goodman JS. Peripheral neuropathy after multiple tetanus toxoid injections. Archives of Physical Medicine and Rehabilitation 1982;63:332-334.

Reisman RE, Rose NR, Witebsky E, Arbesman CE. Serum sickness: II. Demonstration and characteristics of antibodies. Journal of Allergy 1961;32:531-543.

Relihan M. Reactions to tetanus toxoid. Journal of the Irish Medical Association 1969;62:430-434.

Relyveld EH. Current developments in production and testing of tetanus and diphtheria vaccines. Progress in Clinical and Biological Research 1980;47:51-76.

Relyveld EH. Preparation and use of calcium phosphate adsorbed vaccines. Developments in Biological Standardization 1986;65:131-136.

Relyveld EH, Henocq E, Bizzini B. Studies on untoward reactions to diphtheria and tetanus toxoids. Developments in Biological Standardization 1979;43:33-37.

Reutens DC, Dunne JW, Leather H. Neuralgic amyotrophy following recombinant DNA hepatitis B vaccination (letter). Muscle and Nerve 1990;13:461.

Revista de Igiena. [The national program to eliminate poliomyelitis (NPEP)] Programul national pentru eliminarea poliomielitei (PNEP). Revista de Igiena (Bacteriol) 1988;33:372-380.

Reviews of Infectious Diseases. Seroconversion rates and measles antibody titers induced by measles vaccination in Latin American children six to 12 months of age. Reviews of Infectious Diseases 1983;5:596-605.

Revue du Practicien—Medecine Generale. [Haemophilus vaccine] Vaccination anti-haemophilus. Revue du Practicien—Medecine Generale 1992;6:1231.

Rhoads JL, Birx DL, Wright DC, Brundage JF, Brandt BL, Redfield RR et al. Safety and immunogenicity of multiple conventional immunizations administered during early HIV infection. Journal of Acquired Immune Deficiency Syndrome 1991;4:724-731.

Ribera EF, Dutka AJ. Polyneuropathy associated with administration of hepatitis B vaccine (letter). New England Journal of Medicine 1983;309:614-615.

Ricciardi G, Graziano G. [Safety and immunogenicity of an anti-hepatitis-B vaccine obtained using the recombinant DNA technique: results of a longitudinal study in hospital personnel] Sicurezza ed immunogenicita di un vaccino anti-epatite B ottenuto con la tecnica del DNA-ricombinante: risultati di un'indagine longitudinale su personale ospedaliero. Bollettino dell Istituto Sieroterapico Milanese 1990;69:385-390.

Richens ER, Jones WG. Islet-cell antibodies and mumps. Lancet 1981;1:507-508.

Rietschel RL, Adams RM. Reactions to thimerosal in hepatitis B vaccines. Dermatologic Clinics 1990;8:161-164.

Riikonen R. The role of infection and vaccination in the genesis of optic neuritis and multiple sclerosis in children. Acta Neurologica Scandinavica 1989;80:425-431.

Riikonen R, Donner M. Incidence and aetiology of infantile spasms from 1960 to 1976: a population study in Finland. Developmental Medicine and Child Neurology 1979;21:333-343.

Riker JB, Brandt CD, Chandra R, Arrobio JO, Nakano JH. Vaccine-associated poliomyelitis in a child with thymic abnormality. Pediatrics 1971;48:923-929.

Riley HD Jr. Immunization against measles (rubeola). Journal of the Oklahoma State Medical Association 1969;62:107-110.

Ring J. Exacerbation of eczema by formalin-containing hepatitis B vaccine in formaldehyde-allergic patient (letter). Lancet 1986;2:522-523.

Rivers TM, Schwenker FF. Encephalomyelitis accompanied by myelin destruction experimentally produced in monkeys. Journal of Experimental Medicine 1935;61:689-702.

Rizzuto N, Napoleone-Capra A, Ferrari G. [Atonic diplegia caused by antipoliomyelitic oral vaccination: anatomo-clinical study] Diplegia atonica insorta dopo vaccinazione antipoliomielitica per via orale: studio anatomo-clincio. Acta Neurologica 1969;24:248-258.

Robbins FC. Measles: clinical features, pathogenesis, pathology, and complications. American Journal of Diseases of Children 1962;103:266-273.

Robbins FC, Robbins JB. Current status and prospects for some improved and new bacterial vaccines. Annual Review of Public Health 1986;7:105-125.

Robbins JB, Parke JC Jr., Schneerson R, Whisnant JK. Quantitative measurement of "natural" and immunization-induced *Haemophilus influenzae* type b capsular polysaccharide antibodies. Pediatric Research 1973;7:103-110.

Robbins JB, Schneerson R. Evaluating the *Haemophilus influenzae* type b conjugate vaccine PRP-D (editorial). New England Journal of Medicine 1990;323:1415-1416.

Robbins JB, Schneerson R. Polysaccharide-protein conjugates: a new generation of vaccines. Journal of Infectious Diseases 1990;161:821-832.

Robertson CM, Bennett VJ, Jefferson N, Mayon-White RT. Serological evaluation of a measles, mumps, and rubella vaccine. Archives of Disease in Childhood 1988;63:612-616.

Robinson IG. Unusual reaction to tetanus toxoid (letter). New Zealand Medical Journal 1981;94:359.

Rocchi G, Giannini V, Provvidenza G, Andreoni G. [Poliomyelitis due to poliovirus 3, with fatal outcome in an infant vaccinated with Sabin vaccine] Poliomielite da virus polio 3 ad esito letale in vaccinazto con vaccino Sabin. Giornale di Malattie Infettive e Parassitarie 1967;19:463-465.

Roden A. Convulsive disorders in young children. Proceedings of the Royal Society of Medicine 1974;67:380.

Roedenbeck SD, Diaz C. [Poliomyelitis and oral vaccine] Poliomielitis y vacuna oral. Revista de Neuropsiquiatria 1967;30:38-56.

Rogerson SJ, Nye FJ. Hepatitis B vaccine associated with erythema nodosum and polyarthritis. British Medical Journal 1990;301:345.

Rohde W. [Possibilities of reactions and complications from the part of CNS in vaccinations] Reaktionsmiglichkeiten und Komplikationen von seiten des ZNS bei Schutzimpfungen. Zeitschrift fur Arztliche Fortbildung 1974;68:202-208.

Ronne T. Measles virus infection without rash in childhood is related to disease in adult life. Lancet 1985;1:1-5.

Ropper AH. The Guillain-Barre syndrome. New England Journal of Medicine 1992;326:1130-1136.

Ropper AG, Wijdicks EF, Truax BT. Guillain-Barre syndrome. Philadelphia: F. A. Davis; 1991.

Roscelli JD, Bass JW, Pang L. Guillain-Barre syndrome and influenza vaccination in the US Army, 1980-1988. American Journal of Epidemiology 1991;133:952-955.

Rose I. Adverse reactions to tetanus toxoid. Lancet 1973;1:380.

Rosen HR, Stierer M, Wolf HM, Eibl MM. Impaired primary antibody responses after vaccination against hepatitis B in patients with breast cancer. Breast Cancer Research and Treatment 1992;23:233-240.

Ross JS, Smith NP, White IR. Role of aluminium sensitivity in delayed persistent immunisation reactions (letter). Journal of Clinical Pathology 1991;44:876-877.

Rothstein RJ. Tetanus toxoid boosters (letter). Journal of the American Medical Association 1978;239:1133.

Rousseau SA. Symptomatic reaction to hepatitis B vaccine with abnormal liver function values (letter). British Medical Journal 1985;290:1989.

Rowe JE, Messinger IK, Schwendeman CA, Popejoy LA. Three-dose vaccination of infants under 8 months of age with a conjugate *Haemophilus influenzae* type b vaccine. Military Medicine 1990;155:483-486.

Rowe PC, Orrbine E, Wells GA, McLaine PN. Epidemiology of hemolytic-uremic syndrome in Canadian children from 1986 to 1988. Journal of Pediatrics 1991;119:218-224.

Rowe PC, Orrbine E, Wells GA, McLaine PN, and the members of the Canadian Pediatric Kidney Disease Reference Centre. Epidemiology of hemolytic-uremic syndrome in Canadian children from 1986 to 1988. Journal of Pediatrics 1991;119:218-224.

Rowland A. Vaccination against measles. Community Health 1971;2:235-239.

Rozina EE, Hilgenfeldt M. Comparative study on the neurovirulence of different vaccine strains of parotitis virus in monkeys. Acta Virologica 1985;29:225-230.

Ruben FL, Nagel J, Fireman P. Antitoxin responses in the elderly to tetanus-diphtheria (TD) immunization. American Journal of Epidemiology 1978;108:145-149.

Rubin LG, Voulalas D, Carmody L. Immunization of children with sickle cell disease with *Haemophilus influenzae* type b polysaccharide vaccine. Pediatrics 1989;84:509-513.

Rubin LG, Voulalas D, Carmody L. Immunogenicity of *Haemophilus influenzae* type b conjugate vaccine in children with sickle cell disease. American Journal of Diseases of Children 1992;146:340-342.

Rubinstein P, Walker ME, Fedun B, Witt ME, Cooper LZ, Ginsberg-Fellner F. The HLA system in congenital rubella patients with and without diabetes. Diabetes 1982;31:1088-1091.

Ruddock DG, Dickson A. Intradermal hepatitis B vaccine: pilot study. Canadian Family Physician 1992;38:59-64.

Rumke HC. Contraindications for vaccinations in the state vaccination program. Nederlands Tijdschrift voor Geneeskunde 1989;133:1975-1977.

Rutledge SL, Snead OC. Neurologic complications of immunizations. Journal of Pediatrics 1986;109:917-924.

Ruuskanen O, Salmi TT, Stenvik M, Lapinleimu K. Inactivated poliovaccine: adverse reactions and antibody responses. Acta Paediatrica Scandinavica 1980;69:397-401.

Saballus MK, Lake KD, Wager GP. Immunizing the pregnant woman: risks versus benefits. Postgraduate Medicine 1987;81:103-113.

Sabin AB. Immunization of chimpanzees and human beings with avirulent strains of poliomyelitis virus. Annals of the New York Academy Sciences 1956;61:1050-1056.

Sabin AB. Oral poliovirus vaccine: history of its development and prospects for eradication of poliomyelitis. Journal of the American Medical Association 1965;194:872-876.

Sabin AB. Oral poliomyelitis vaccine: achievements and problems in worldwide use. Bulletin of the International Pediatric Association 1977;2:6-18.

Sabin AB. Poliomyelitis vaccination. Evaluation and direction in continuing application. American Journal of Clinical Pathology 1978;70(1 Suppl.):136-140.

Sabin AB. Oral poliovirus vaccine: history of its development and use and current challenge to eliminate poliomyelitis from the world. Journal of Infectious Diseases 1985;151:420-436.

Saez-Llorens X, Ramilo O, Mustafa MM, Mertsola J. Molecular pathophysiology of bacterial meningitis: current concepts and therapeutic implications. Journal of Pediatrics 1990;116:671-684.

Safranek TJ, Lawrence DN, Kurland LT, Culver DH, Wiederholt WC, Hayner NS et al. Reassessment of the association between Guillain-Barre syndrome and receipt of swine influenza vaccine in 1976-1977: results of a two-state study. Expert Neurology Group. American Journal of Epidemiology 1991;133:940-951.

Saggese G, Federico G, Carzelli C, Toniolo A. Insulin-dependent diabetes: a possible viral disease. Pediatrician 1985;12:179-193.

Sagman D. Guillain-Barre syndrome. Journal of the American Medical Association 1972;221:301.

Saisbren BA. Swine-influenza vaccine (letter). Annals of Internal Medicine 1982;97:149.

Sakano T, Kittaka E, Tanaka Y, Yamaoka H, Kobayashi Y, Usui T. Vaccine-associated poliomyelitis in an infant with agammaglobulinemia. Acta Paediatrica Scandinavica 1980;69:549-551.

Salk D. Eradication of poliomyelitis in the United States. III. Poliovaccines—practical considerations. Reviews of Infectious Diseases 1980;2:258-273.

Salk D. Polio immunization policy in the United States: a new challenge for a new generation. American Journal of Public Health 1988;78:296-300.

Salk D, Salk J. Vaccinology of poliomyelitis. Vaccine 1984;2:59-74.

Salk J. The virus of poliomyelitis: from discovery to extinction. Journal of the American Medical Association 1983;250:808-810.

Salk J, Drucker J. Noninfectious poliovirus vaccine. In: Plotkin SA, Mortimer EA, eds. Vaccines. Philadelphia: W.B. Saunders Co.; 1988.

Salk JE. The logic of the magic of vaccination. Allergy Proceedings 1988;9:689-692.

Salk JE. Recent studies on immunization against poliomyelitis. Pediatrics 1953;12:471-482.

Salk JE, Bennett BL, Lewis LJ, Ward EN, Youngner JS. Studies in human subjects on active immunization against poliomyelitis 1. A preliminary report of experiments in progress. Journal of the American Medical Association 1953;151:1081-1098.

Salomonsen CJ, Madsen TH. Bulletin de l'Academie de Sciences et des Lettres de Danemark. 1896.

Sanchez-Lanier M, Guerin P, McLaren LC, Bankhurst AD. Measles virus-induced suppression of lymphocyte proliferation. Cellular Immunology 1988;116:367-381.

Sandler B. Recovery from sterility after mumps orchitis. British Medical Journal 1954;11:795.

Santosham M, Hill J, Wolff M, Reid R, Lukacs L, Ahonkhai V. Safety and immunogenicity of a *Haemophilus influenzae* type b conjugate vaccine in a high risk American Indian population. Pediatric Infectious Disease Journal 1991;10:113-117.

Santosham M, Reid R, Letson GW, Wolff MC, Siber G. Passive immunization for infection with *Haemophilus influenzae* type b. Pediatrics 1990;85(4 Pt 2):662-666.

Santosham M, Rivin B, Wolff M, Reid R, Newcomer W, Letson GW et al. Prevention of *Haemophilus influenzae* type b infections in Apache and Navajo children. Journal of Infectious Diseases 1992;165(Suppl. 1):S144-S151.

Santosham M, Wolff M, Reid R, Hohenboken M, Bateman M, Goepp J et al. The efficacy in Navajo infants of a conjugate vaccine consisting of *Haemophilus influenzae* type b polysaccharide and Neisseria meningitidis outer-membrane protein complex. New England Journal of Medicine 1991;324:1767-1772.

Sarnaik S, Kaplan J, Schiffman G, Bryla D, Robbins JB, Schneerson R. Studies on pneumococcus vaccine alone or mixed with DTP and on pneumococcus type 6b and *Haemophilis influenzae* type b capsular polysaccharide-tetanus toxoid conjugates in two- to five-year-old children with sickle cell anemia. Pediatric Infectious Disease Journal 1990;9:181-186.

Sassini A, Mirchamsy H, Ahourai SP, Razavi J, Gholami MR, Mohammadi A et al. Development of a new live attenuated mumps virus vaccine in human diploid cells. Biologicals 1991;19:203-211.

Satar M, Savas N, Kozanoglu MN. Prophylaxis of babies born to HBsAg+ mothers. Mikrobiyoloji Bulteni 1992;26:37-40.

Saulsbury FT, Winkelstein JA, Davis LE, Hsu SH, D'Souza BJ, Gutcher GR et al. Combined immunodeficiency and vaccine-related poliomyelitis in a child with cartilage-hair hypoplasia. Journal of Pediatrics 1975;86:868-872.

Saxonhouse WJ. Hepatitis vaccine (letter). Journal of the American Dental Association 1985;110:670.

Saxton NL. Thrombocytopenic purpura following the administration of attenuated live measles vaccine. Journal of the Iowa Medical Society 1967;57:1017-1018.

Schacher SA. An epidemiological approach to subacute sclerosing panencephalitis. Neurology 1968;18(1 Pt. 2):76-77.

Schaltenbrand G, Hopf HC. Neurologische komplikationen nach schluckimpfung. Nervenarzt 1964;35:120-132.

Schattner A, Ben-Chetrit E, Schmilovitz H. Poliovaccines and the course of systemic lupus erythematosus—a retrospective study of 73 patients. Vaccine 1992;10:98-100.

Scheifele DW. Postmarketing surveillance of adverse reactions to ProHIBit vaccine in British Columbia. Canadian Medical Association Journal 1989;141:927-929.

Scheifele D, Bjornson G, Barreto L, Meekison W, Guasparini R. Controlled trial of *Haemophilus influenzae* type b diphtheria toxoid conjugate combined with diphtheria, tetanus and pertussis vaccines, in 18-month-old children, including comparison of arm versus thigh injection. Vaccine 1992;10:455-460.

Scheinberg L, Allensworth M. Sciatic neuropathy in infants related to antibiotic injections. Pediatrics 1957;19:261-265.

Scherer RW, Dickersin K, Kaplan E. The accessible biomedical literature represents a fraction of all studies in a field. Unpublished manuscript.

Schettini F, Manzionna MM, De MD, Amendola F, Di BG. Clinical and immunological evaluation of a bivalent vaccine against measles and rubella. Minerva Pediatrica 1990;42:531-536.

Schick B. Die diphtherietoxin-Hautreaktion des menschen als vorprobe der prophylaktischen diphtherieheilseruimnektion. Munchener Medizinische Wochenschrift 1913;60:2606.

Schlech WF, Ward JI, Bard JD et al. Bacterial meningitis in the United States, 1978-81: the National Bacterial Meningitis Surveillance Study. Journal of the American Medical Association 1985;253:1749-1754.

Schlenska GK. Unusual neurological complications following tetanus toxoid administration. Journal of Neurology 1977;215:299-302.

Schlesinger Y, Granoff DM. Avidity and bactericidal activity of antibody elicited by different *Haemophilus influenzae* type b conjugate vaccines. Journal of the American Medical Association 1992;267:1489-1494.

Schneck SA. Vaccination with measles and central nervous system disease. Neurology 1968;18(Part 2):79-82.

Schneerson R, Barrera O, Sutton A, Robbins JB. Preparation, characterization, and immunogenicity of *H. influenzae* type b polysaccharide-protein conjugates. Journal of Experimental Medicine 1980;152:361-376.

Schneerson R, Rodrigues LP, Parke JC Jr., Robbins JB. Immunity to disease caused by *Hemophilus influenzae* type b. II. Specificity and some biologic characteristics of "natural," infection-acquired, and immunization-induced antibodies to the capsular polysaccharide of *Hemophilus influenzae* type b. Journal of Immunology 1971;107:1081-1089.

Schneider CH. Reactions to tetanus toxoid: a report of five cases. Medical Journal of Australia 1964;1:303-305.

Schonberger LB, Bregman D, Sullivan-Bolyai JZ, Bryan L, Noble GR. Guillain-Barre syndrome after administration of killed vaccines. Developments in Biological Standardization 1977;39:295-296.

Schonberger LB, Bregman DJ, Sullivan-Bolyai JZ, Keenlyside RA, Ziegler DW, Retailliau HF et al. Guillain-Barre syndrome following vaccination in the National Influenza Immunization Program, United States, 1976-1977. American Journal of Epidemiology 1979;110:105-123.

Schonberger LB, McGowan JE Jr., Gregg MB. Vaccine-associated poliomyelitis in the United States, 1961-1972. American Journal of Epidemiology 1976;104:202-211.

Schoub BD, Johnson S. Contraindications to immunisation (letter). South African Medical Journal 1990;78:169.

Schreiber JR, Barrus V, Cates KL, Siber GR. Functional characterization of human IgG, IgM, and IgA antibody directed to the capsule of *Haemophilus influenzae* type b. Journal of Infectious Diseases 1986;153:8-16.

Schreurs AJ, Terpstra GK, Raaijmakers JA, Nijkamp FP. The effects of *Haemophilus influenzae* vaccination on anaphylactic mediator release and isoprenaline-induced inhibition of mediator release. European Journal of Pharmacology 1980;62:261-268.

Schroder JP. [Complications of tetanus vaccinations in juveniles] Tetanus: Keine blindimpfungen bei jugendlichen. Therapiewoche 1992;42:202.

Schroder JP, Gessler M, Kuhlmann WD, Trendelenburg C. [Avoidance of hyperergic reactions after tetanus immunization by using a knowledge base system for questions concerning the necessity for vaccination] Vermeidung hyperergischer reaktionen bei tetanus-impfungen durch einsatz eines wissensbasierten systems bei fragen der impfnotwendigkeit. Klinisches Labor 1992;38:229-233.

Schulman SL, Deforest A, Kaiser BA, Polinsky MS, Baluarte HJ. Response to measles-mumps-rubella vaccine in children on dialysis. Pediatric Nephrology 1992;6:187-189.

Schulz TF, Hoad JG, Whitby D, Tizard EJ, Dillon MJ, Weiss RA. A measles virus isolate from a child with Kawasaki disease: sequence comparison with contemporaneous isolates from 'classical' cases. Journal of General Virology 1992;73(Pt 6):1581-1586.

Schumacher HR, Gall EP. Arthritis in acute hepatitis and chronic active hepatitis: pathology of the synovial membranes with evidence of Australian antigen in synovial membranes. American Journal of Medicine 1974;57:655-664.

Schwarz AJ. Immunization against measles: development and evaluation of a highly attenuated live measles vaccine. Annales de Paediatrie 1964;202:241-252.

Schwarz AJ, Anderson JT. Immunization with a further attenuated live measles virus vaccine. Archiv fur die Gesamte Virusforschung 1965;16:273-278.

Schwarz AJ, Jackson JE, Ehrenkranz NJ, Ventura A, Schiff GM, Walters VW. Clinical evaluation of a new measles-mumps-rubella trivalent vaccine. American Journal of Diseases of Children 1975;129:1408-1412.

Schwarz G, Lanzer G, List WF. Acute midbrain syndrome as an adverse reaction to tetanus immunization. Intensive Care Medicine 1988;15:53-54.

Schwimmbeck PL, Dyrberg T, Oldstone MB A. et al. Abrogation of diabetes in BB rats by acute virus infection. Journal of Immunology 1988;140:3394-3400.

Scott GB. HIV infection in children: clinical features and management. Journal of the Acquired Immune Deficiency Syndrome 1991;4:109-115.

Scottish Medical Journal. Clinico-pathological conference from the University of Aberdeen and the Grampian Health Board. Scottish Medical Journal 1982;27:343-350.

Seeff LB, Beebe GW, Hoofnagle JH, Norman JE, Buskell-Bales Z, Waggoner JG et al. A serologic follow-up of the 1942 epidemic of post-vaccination hepatitis in the United States Army. New England Journal of Medicine 1987;316:965-970.

Seki T, Miyazaki Y, Chiba H, Fukazawa J. [Atypical measles accompanying radiculitis]. Nippon Shonika Gakkai Zasshi 1971;75:251-254.

Sell E, Katzmann GW. Reaktive arthritis und immunvasculitis mit cardiovascularem Schock nach Dreifach-(Diphtherie-Pertussis-Tetanus) Schutzimpfund? Kinderarztliche Praxis 1990;58:547-549.

Senecal J, Roussey M. [Combined vaccination against measles, mumps and rubella] Vaccination associee contre la rougeole, les oreillons et la rubeole (R.O.R.). Bulletin de l'Academie Nationale de Medecine 1987;171:325-332.

Serdaru M, Lacomblez L, Danze F, Agid Y. [Meningo-myelitis with a favorable course after measles vaccination] Meningo-myelite d'evolution favorable apres vaccination antirubeolique. Revue Neurologique 1984;140:226-227.

Settergren B, Broholm KA, Norrby SR, Christenson B. Schick test as a predictor of immunity to diphtheria and of side effects after revaccination with diphtheria vaccine. British Medical Journal 1986;292:524-525.

Seyal M, Ziegler DK, Couch JR. Recurrent Guillain-Barre syndrome following influenza vaccine. Neurology 1978;28:725-726.

Shackelford PG, Granoff DM. IgG subclass composition of the antibody response of healthy adults, and normal or IgG2-deficient children to immunization with H. influenzae type b polysaccharide vaccine or Hib PS-protein conjugate vaccines. Monographs in Allergy 1988;23:269-281.

Shaikh N, Raut SK, Bedekar SS, Phadke MA, Banerjee K. Experience with a measles vaccine manufactured in India. Indian Pediatrics 1992;29:883-887.

Shapiro ED. New vaccines against Haemophilus influenzae type b. Pediatric Clinics of North America 1990;37:567-583.

Shapiro ED, Berg AT. Protective efficacy of Haemophilus influenzae type b polysaccharide vaccine. Pediatrics 1990;85(4 Pt 2):643-647.

Shapiro ED, Dobyns WB. Polio vaccine and GBS (letter). Neurology 1990;40:729.

Shapiro ED, Murphy TV, Wald ER, Brady CA. The protective efficacy of Haemophilus b polysaccharide vaccine. Journal of the American Medical Association 1988;260:1419-1422.

Shaw EB, Cesario TC. Vaccine-derived poliomyelitis. American Journal of Diseases of Children 1970;119:546.

Shaw FE Jr, Graham DJ, Guess HA, Milstien JB, Johnson JM, Schatz GC et al. Postmarketing surveillance for neurologic adverse events reported after hepatitis B vaccination: experience of the first three years. American Journal of Epidemiology 1988;127:337-352.

Shaw FE, Guess HA, Roets JM. The effect of anatomic injection site, age and smoking on the immune response to hepatitis B vaccination. Vaccine 1989;7:425-430.

Sheffield FW, Ironside AG, Abbott JD. Immunisation of adults against diphtheria. British Medical Journal 1978;2:249-250.

Shelley WB. Bacterial endotoxin (lipopolysaccharide) as a cause of erythema multiforme. Journal of the American Medical Association 1980;243:58-60.

Shimizu H, Baba K, Abe J et al. Vaccination to the handicapped children. Brain and Development 1981;13:329-336.

Shimojo H. Poliomyelitis control in Japan. Reviews of Infectious Diseases 1984;6(Suppl. 2):S427-S430.

Shoss RG, Rayhanzadeh S. Toxic epidermal necrolysis following measles vaccination. Archives of Dermatology 1974;110:766-770.

Shyamalan NC, Singh SS, Bisht DB. Transverse myelitis after vaccination. British Medical Journal 1964;1:434-435.

Siber GR, Santosham M, Reid GR, Thompson C, Almeido-Hill J, Morell A et al. Impaired antibody response to *Haemophilus influenzae* type b polysaccharide and low IgG2 and IgG4 concentrations in Apache children. New England Journal of Medicine 1990;323:1387-1392.

Sibley WA, Bamford CA, Clark K. Clinical viral infections and multiple sclerosis. Lancet 1985;1:1313-1315.

Sicot C. Urticaire apres hevac B. Concours Medical 1988;110:4083-4084.

Sigmund J, Guggenbichler JP. [Flaccid paralysis following oral poliomyelitis vaccination] Schlaffe Parese nach oraler Poliomyelitisimpfung. Padiatrie und Padologie 1985;20:77-82.

Silva CA, Sa MJ, Cruz C. Tetanus antibody production in serum and cerebrospinal fluid in the rabbit and correlated histopathological features of the central nervous system. Journal of Neurological Science 1977;33:213-227.

Simoes EA, Balraj V, Selvakumar R, John TJ. Antibody response of children to measles vaccine mixed with diphtheria-pertussis-tetanus or diphtheria-pertussis-tetanus-poliomyelitis vaccine. American Journal of Diseases of Children 1988;142:309-311.

Simoes EA F., Padmini B, Steinhoff MC, Jadhav M, John TJ. Antibody response of infants to two doses of inactivated poliovirus vaccine of enhanced potency. American Journal of Diseases of Children 1985;139:977-980.

Simonsen O, Klaerke M, Klaerke A, Block AB, Hansen BR, Hald N et al. Revaccination of adults against diphtheria. II. Combined diphtheria and tetanus revaccination with different doses of diphtheria toxoid 20 years after primary vaccination. Acta Pathologica, Microbiologica, et Immunologica Scandinavica 1986;94:219-225.

Simpson LL. Molecular pharmacology of botulinum toxin and tetanus toxin. Annual Review of Pharmacology and Toxicology 1986;26:427-453.

Sinaniotis CA, Daskalopoulou E, Lapatsanis P, Doxiadis S. Diabetes mellitus after mumps vaccination (letter). Archives of Disease in Childhood 1975;50:749-750.

Singhi SC, Kaur A, Khajuria R, Datta N, Kumar V. Side effects of measles vaccine—as perceived by mothers. Indian Pediatrics 1987;24:215-219.

Sinha SK, Carlson SD. Immune responses of mentally retarded subjects to measles, mumps and rubella vaccines. Wisconsin Medical Journal 1975;74:S75-S77.

Sinyak KM, Chumakov MP, Voroshilova MK, Livanova LV, Zlatkovskaya NM, Ralko LP et al. [Controlled observation of the incidence of disease and post-vaccinal reactions in children during three weeks after vaccination with live measles vaccine developed by the USSR Academy of Medical Sciences from ESC strain] Kontrolirovanie nabliudeniia za chastotoi zabolevanii i postvaktsinalnykh reaktsii u detei v trekhnedelnyi period posle nachala privivok zhivoi korevoi vaktsinoi AMN SSSR iz shtamma EShCh. Voprosy Virusologii 1967;12:406-415.

Sipila R, Hortling L, Hovi T. Good seroresponse to enhanced-potency inactivated poliovirus vaccine in patients on chronic dialysis. Nephrology, Dialysis, Transplantation 1990;5:352-355.

Sisk CW, Lewis CE. Reactions to tetanus-diphtheria toxoid (adult). Archives of Environmental Health 1965;11:34-36.

Sisk M, Griffith JF. Normal electroencephalograms in subacute sclerosing panencephalitis (letter). Archives of Neurology 1975;32:575-576.

Sitzmann FC. [Vaccination against measles and poliomyelitis with attenuated living virus in children with brain damage: problematic vaccinations] Masern- und Poliolebend-Impfung bei vorgeschadigten Kindern: Problem-Impfungen. Monatsschrift fur Kinderheilkunde 1981;129:69-71.

Skovrankova J, Domorazkova E. [Neurological complications after immunization] Neurologicke komplikace po ockovani. Ceskoslovenska Pediatrie 1991;46:169-172.

Skovrankova J, Komarek V, Domorazkova E. [Neurologic complications after vaccination against diphtheria, tetanus and whooping cough] Neurologicke komplikace po ockovani proti zaskrtu, tetanu a davivemu kasli. Ceskoslovenska Pediatrie 1992;47:122-124.

Smith DH, Madore DV, Eby RJ, Anderson PW, Insel RA, Johnson CL. *Haemophilus* b oligosaccharide-CRM197 and other *Haemophilus* b conjugate vaccines: a status report. Advances in Experimental Medicine and Biology 1989;251:65-82.

Smith JW. Diphtheria and tetanus toxoids. British Medical Bulletin 1969;25:177-182.

Smith JS. Suspended judgment: remembering the role of Thomas Francis, Jr. in the design of the 1954 Salk vaccine test. Controlled Clinical Trials 1992;13:181-184.

Smith JW, Wherry PJ. Poliomyelitis surveillance in England and Wales, 1969-1975. Journal of Hygiene 1978;80:155-167.

Smith MH. Mumps virus vaccine. Pediatrics 1969;43:907-909.

Smith PW. CRS Issue Brief: Vaccine Injury Compensation. Washington, DC: Congressional Research Service, The Library of Congress; 1987.

Smith P. Tetanus prophylaxis. Journal of the Arkansas Medical Society 1966;63:226-230.

Smith RE, Wolnisty C. Allergic reactions to tetanus, diphtheria, influenza and poliomyelitis immunization. Annals of Allergy 1962;20:809-813.

Snider GB, Gogate SA. A possible systemic reaction to hepatitis B vaccine (letter). Journal of the American Medical Association 1985;253:1260-1261.

Snyder RD. Facial palsy following measles vaccination, a possible connection. Pediatrics 1968;42:215-216.

Soderstron K, Halapi E, Nilsson E. Synovial cells responding to a 65-kDa mycobacterial heat shock protein have a high proportion of TcR-gamma-delta subtype uncommon in peripheral blood. Scandinavian Journal of Immunology 1990;32:503-515.

Soffer D, Feldman S, Alter M. Epidemiology of Guillain-Barre syndrome. Neurology 1978;28:686-690.

Sokhey J. Adverse events following immunization: 1990. Indian Pediatrics 1991;28:593-607.

Solberg LK. [DPT vaccination, visit to child health center and sudden infant death syndrome (SIDS)] DPT-Vaksinasjon, helsestasjonsbesok og plutselig spedbarnsdod (SIDS): evaluering av DPT-vaksinasjon. Oslo: Oslo Helserad; 1985.

Solomon GF, Rubbo SD, Batchelder E. Secondary immune response to tetanus toxoid in psychiatric patients. Journal of Psychiatric Research 1970;7:201-207.

Solomonova K, Damiyanova K, Damiyanova M, Betovska M. Active immunization against tetanus of children suffering with diabetes mellitus. Zeitschrift fur Immunitatsforschung—Immunobiology 1976;151:383-390.

Sood SK, Daum RS. Disease caused by *Haemophilus influenzae* type b in the immediate period after homologous immunization: immunologic investigation. Pediatrics 1990;85(4 Pt 2):698-704.

Sood SK, Schreiber JR, Siber GR, Daum RS. Postvaccination susceptibility to invasive *Haemophilus influenzae* type b disease in infant rats. Journal of Pediatrics 1988;113:814-819.

Soothill JF, Dudgeon JA. Immunization reactions and immunodeficiency. Birth Defects: Original Article Series 1983;19:339-341.

Sosin DM, Cochi SL, Gunn RA, Jennings CE, Preblud SR. Changing epidemiology of mumps and its impact on university campuses. Pediatrics 1989;84:779-784.

South African Medical Journal. Poliomyelitis vaccines (editorial). South African Medical Journal 1977;52:868.

Spiess H, Staak M. [Anaphylactic reaction following active tetanus immunization] Anaphylaktische Reaktionen nach aktiver Tetanus-Immunisierung. Deutsche Medizinische Wochenschrift 1973;98:682.

Spinola SM, Sheaffer CI, Philbrick KB, Gilligan PH. Antigenuria after *Haemophilus influenzae* type b polysaccharide immunization: a prospective study. Journal of Pediatrics 1986;109:835-838.

Squires S. Hepatitis B vaccinations: pediatricians begin immunizing infants to curb the spread of the disease. Washington Post, Health. May 5, 1992:9.

Srivastava RN, Bagga A. Hemolytic uremic syndrome: recent developments. Indian Pediatrics 1992;29:11-24.

Staak M, Wirth E. [Anaphylactic reactions following active tetanus immunization] Zur problematik anaphylaktischer Reaktionen nach aktiver Tetanus-Immunisierung. Deutsche Medizinische Wochenschrift 1973;98:110-111.

Starke G, Hlinak P, Nobel B, Winkler C, Kaesler G. [Measles control—a possibility? Results and experiences with measles vaccination from 1967 to 1969 in the German Democratic Republic]. Maserneradikation—eine Moglichkeit? Ergebnisse und Erfahrungen mit der Masernschutzimpfung 1967 bis 1969 in der DDR. Deutsche Gesundheitswesen 1970;25:2384-2390.

Starr S, Berkovich S. Effects of measles, gamma-globulin-modified measles and vaccine measles on the tuberculin test. New England Journal of Medicine 1964;270:386-391.

Steele RW, Suttle DE, LeMaster PC. Screening for cell-mediated immunity in children. American Journal of Diseases of Children 1976;130:1218-1221.

Steffen R, Woodall JP, Nagel J, Desaules M. Evaluation of immunization policies for peacekeeping missions. International Journal of Technology Assessment in Health Care 1991;7:354-360.

Stehlikova J, Bergmannova V, Domorazkova E. [Immunization against diphtheria and tetanus in children with serious neurological disease] Ockovani proti zaskrtu a tetanu u deti se zavaznym neurologickym onemocnenim. Ceskoslovenska Pediatrie 1992;47:417-420.

Stehr-Green PA, Cochi SL. Diseases controlled primarily by vaccination: mumps. In: Last JM, Wallace RB, eds. Maxcy-Rosenau-Last Public Health and Preventive Medicine, 13th ed. Norwalk, CT: Appleton & Lange; 1992.

Steigman A. Allergic reactions to tetanus toxoid. Journal of Pediatrics 1968;73:648-649.

Steigman AJ. Abuse of tetanus toxoid. Journal of Pediatrics 1968;72:753-754.

Steinhoff MC, Auerbach BS, Nelson KE, Vlahov D, Becker RL, Graham NMH et al. Antibody responses to *Haemophilus influenzae* type b vaccines in men with human immunodeficiency virus infection. New England Journal of Medicine 1991;325:1837-1842.

Steinman L. Neurologic complications of routine immunization. Western Journal of Medicine 1982;137:315-316.

Stephenne J. Development and production aspects of a recombinant yeast derived hepatitis vaccine. Vaccine 1990;8(Suppl.):S69-S73.

Stetler HC, Gens RD, Seastrom GR. Severe local reactions to live measles virus vaccine following an immunization program. American Journal of Public Health 1983;73:899-900.

Stevens CE. No increased incidence of AIDS in recipients of hepatitis B vaccine. New England Journal of Medicine 1983;308:1163-1164.

Stickl H. [Iatrogenic immunosuppression through vaccination] Iatrogene Immunosuppression durch Schutzimpfungen. Fortschritte der Medezin 1981;99:289-292.

Stiehm ER. Skin testing prior to measles vaccination for egg-sensitive patients (editorial). American Journal of Diseases of Children 1990;144:32.

Stoeckel P, Schlumberger M, Parent G, Maire B, van Wezel A, van Steenis G et al. Use of killed poliovirus vaccine in a routine immunization program in West Africa. Reviews of Infectious Diseases 1984;6(Suppl. 2):S463-S466.

Stoehr M. [Para infectious cerebral nerve mononeuritis and mononeuritis multiplex: a selectively located type of para infectious, postvaccination, serogenetic neuritis] Parainfektiose hirnnerven mononeuritis und -mononeuritis multiplexa: ein besonderer lokalisationstyp parainfektioser, postvaccinaler und serogenetischer neuritiden. Nervenarzt 1977;48:359-364.

Stokes JJ. Use of mumps vaccine. New England Journal of Medicine 1968;278:682.

Stokes JJ, Maris EP, Gelles SS. Chemical, clinical, and immunologic studies on the products of human plasma fractionation: XI. The use of concentrated normal human serum gamma globulin (human immune serum globulin) in the prevention and attenuation of measles. Journal of Clinical Investigations 1944;23:531-540.

Stokes JJ, Weibel RE, Villarejos VM, Arguedas JA, Buynak EB, Hilleman MR. Trivalent combined measles-mumps-rubella vaccine: findings in clinical-laboratory studies. Journal of the American Medical Association 1971;218:57-61.

Stolley PD. How to interpret studies of adverse drug reactions. Clinical Pharmacology and Therapeutics 1990;48:337-339.

Stolley PD, Joseph JM, Allen JC, Deane G, Janney JH. Poliomyelitis associated with type-2 poliovirus vaccine strain: possible transmission from an immunised child to a non-immunised child. Lancet 1968;1:661-663.

Stopfkuchen H, Juengst BK, Wilutzky H. [Purpura fulminans associated with varicella and polyvalent protective inoculations] Purpura fulminans nach varizellen und polyvalenter impfung. Klinische Paediatrie 1976;188:190-193.

Storsaeter J, Olin P, Renemar B, Lagergard T, Norberg R, Romanus V et al. Mortality and morbidity from invasive bacterial infections during a clinical trial in acellular pertussis vaccines in Sweden. Pediatric Infectious Disease Journal 1988;7:637-645.

Strebel PM, Sutter RW, Cochi SL, Biellik RJ, Brink EW, Kew OM et al. Epidemiology of poliomyelitis in the United States one decade after the last reported case of indigenous wild virus-associated disease. Clinical Infectious Diseases 1992;14:568-579.

Struve J, Aronsson B, Frenning B, Granath F, von Sydow M, Weiland O. Intramuscular versus intradermal administration of a recombinant hepatitis B vaccine: a comparison of response rates and analysis of factors influencing the antibody response. Scandinavian Journal of Infectious Diseases 1992;24:423-429.

Sugg WC, Finger JA, Levine RH, Pagano JS. Field evaluation of live virus mumps vaccine. Journal of Pediatrics 1968;72:461-466.

Sugiura A, Yamada A. Aseptic meningitis as a complication of mumps vaccination. Pediatric Infectious Disease Journal 1991;10:209-213.

Sullivan KM, Halpin TJ, Marks JS, Kim-Farley R. Effectiveness of mumps vaccine in a school outbreak. American Journal of Diseases of Children 1985;139:909-912.

Sultz HA, Hart BA, Zielezny M, Schlesinger ER. Is mumps virus an etiologic factor in juvenile diabetes mellitus? Journal of Pediatrics 1975;86:654-656.

Sultz HA, Schlesinger ER, Mosher WE, Feldman JG. Long-term childhood illness. Pittsburgh: University of Pittsburgh Press; 1972.

Sun T-T, Chu Y-R, Ni Z-Q et al. A pilot study on universal immunization of newborn infants in an area of hepatitis B virus and primary hepatocellular carcinoma prevalence with a low dose of hepatitis B vaccine. Journal of Cellular Physiology 1986;129(Suppl. 4):83-90.

Sundar PS. Allergy to diphtheria and tetanus toxoid (a case report). Antiseptic 1978;75:458-459.

Sunderland S. Nerves and Nerve Injuries. Baltimore: The Williams and Wilkins Company; 1968.

Susser M. Causal Thinking in the Health Sciences. New York: Oxford; 1973.

Sussman GL, Dolovich J. Prevention of anaphylaxis. Seminars in Dermatology 1989;8:158-165.

Sutter RW, Patriarca PA, Suleiman AJ, Brogan S, Malankar PG, Cochi SL et al. Attributable risk of DTP (diphtheria and tetanus toxoids and pertussis vaccine) injection in provoking paralytic poliomyelitis during a large outbreak in Oman. Journal of Infectious Diseases 1992;165:444-449.

Sutton GC. Mumps, measles and rubella vaccination: a pragmatic study. Public Health 1991;105:133-138.

Swaak AJ. [Local reactions following booster injections with DWTP-vaccine (diphtheria-whooping cough-tetanus-poliovirus vaccine) in children born in 1960 and 1961] Lokale klachten bij kinderen van de jaarklassen 1960 en 1961 na een herbalingsinjectie met DKTP-entstof. Nederlands Tijdschrift voor Geneeskunde 1966;110:332-334.

Swaak AJ. [A study of children born in 1962 on the relation between local complaints and the type of vaccine used in the immunization for whooping cough, diphtheria, tetanus and poliomyelitis] Een onderzoek bij kinderen van de jaarklasse 1962 naar het verband tussen de lokale klachten en de aard van de entstof bij de immunisatie tegen kinkhoest, difterie, tetanus en poliomyelitis. Nederlands Tijdschrift voor Geneeskunde 1966;110:1696-1699.

Swanson PD, McAlister R, Peterson DR. Poliomyelitis associated with type 2 virus: paralytic disease in the father of a recently immunized child. Journal of the American Medical Association 1967;201:771-773.

Swartz TA, Klingberg W, Klingberg MA. Combined trivalent and bivalent measles, mumps and rubella virus vaccination: a controlled trial. Infection 1974;2:115-117.

Syrogiannopoulos GA, Hansen EJ, Erwin AL et al. *Haemophilus influenzae* type b lipooligosaccharide induced meningeal inflammation. Journal of Infectious Diseases 1988;157:237-244.

Szillat K, Meyke M, Kopsel G. [Sequelae following triple vaccination (epidemic parotitis, measles, rubella)?] Enzephalitis, Meningitis serosa und Parotitis nach MMR-Schutzimpfung? Kinderarztliche Praxis 1992;60:203.

Szmuness W, Stevens CE, Harley EJ, Zang EA, Oleszko WR, William DC et al. Hepatitis B vaccine: demonstration of efficacy in a controlled clinical trial in a high-risk population in the United States. New England Journal of Medicine 1980;303:833-841.

Szmuness W, Stevens CE, Harley EJ, Zang EA, Alter HJ, Taylor PE et al. Hepatitis B vaccine in medical staff of hemodialysis units: efficacy and subtype cross-protection. New England Journal of Medicine 1982;307:1481-1486.

Tabor E. Guillain-Barre syndrome and other neurologic syndromes in hepatitis A, B, and Non-A, Non-B. Journal of Medical Virology 1987;21:207-216.

Takala AK, Eskola J, Leinonen M, Kayhty H, Nissinen A, Pekkanen E. Reduction of oropharyngeal carriage of *Haemophilus influenzae* type b (Hib) in children immunized with an Hib conjugate vaccine. Journal of Infectious Diseases 1991;164:982-986.

Takasu T, Kondo K, Ahmed A, Yoshikawa Y, Yamanouchi K, Tsuchiya M et al. Elevated ratio of late measles among subacute sclerosing panencephalitis patients in Karachi, Pakistan. Neuroepidemiology 1992;11:282-287.

Takayama N, Kidokoro M, Suzuki K, Morita M. [Immunization of healthy children with measles-mumps-rubella trivalent vaccine simultaneously given with varicella vaccine]. Kansenshogaku Zasshi [Journal of the Japanese Association for Infectious Diseases] 1992;66:776-780.

Takeuchi K, Tanabayashi K, Hishiyama M, Yamada A, Sugiura A. Variations of nucleotide sequences and transcription of the SH gene among mumps virus strains. Virology 1991;181:364-366.

Tan KL, Oon CJ, Goh KT, Wong LY, Chan SH. Immunogenicity and safety of low doses of recombinant yeast-derived hepatitis B vaccine. Acta Paediatrica Scandinavica 1990;79:593-598.

Tanabayashi K, Takeuchi K, Hishiyama M, Yamada A, Tsurudome M, Ito Y et al. Nucleotide sequence of the leader and nucleocapsid protein gene of mumps virus and epitope mapping with the in vitro expressed nucleocapsid protein. Virology 1990;177:124-130.

Taranger J, Wiholm BE. [The low number of reported adverse effects after vaccination against measles, mumps, rubella] Litet antal biverkningar rapporterade efter vaccination mot massling-passjuka-roda hund. Lakartidningen 1987;84:948-950.

Tarlov IM. Paralysis caused by penicillin injection; mechanism complication—a warning. Journal of Neuropathology and Experimental Neurology 1951;10:158-176.

Taylor EM, Emery JL. Immunisation and cot deaths (letter). Lancet 1982;2:721.

Telzak E, Wolff SM, Dinarello CA et al. Clinical evaluation of the immunoadjuvant murabutide, a derivative of MDP, administered with a tetanus toxoid vaccine. Journal of Infectious Diseases 1986;153:628-633.

Terpstra GK, Raaijmakers JA, Kreukniet J. Comparison of vaccination of mice and rats with *Haemophilus influenzae* and *Bordetella pertussis* as models of atopy. Clinical and Experimental Pharmacology and Physiology 1979;6:139-149.

Terpstra GK, Raaijmakers JA, Hamelink M, Kreukniet J. Effects of *Haemophilus influenzae* vaccination on the (para-)sympathic-cyclic nucleotide-histamine axis in rats. Annals of Allergy 1979;42:36-40.

Thacker SB. Meta-analysis: a quantitative approach to research integration. Journal of the American Medical Association 1988;259:1685-1689.

Themann J. Hepatitis B aktuell: erst lust—dann frust. Therapiewoche 1991;41:2154.

Thesen R. [*Haemophilus influenzae* type b vaccines] Hib-vakzine. Pharmazeutische Zeitung 1990;135:30, 32, 34, 36.

Thier SO. Importance of the single case. New England Journal of Medicine 1968;278:1347.

Thomas GA, O'Brien RT. Thrombocytosis in children with *Haemophilus influenzae* meningitis. Clinical Pediatrics 1986;25:610-611.

Thomas P. Immunization of children infected with HIV: a public health perspective. Pediatric Annals 1988;17:347-351.

Thomison JB. The price of safety (editorial). Southern Medical Journal 1990;83:494-496.

Thompson WL. Adverse drug reactions: finding sharp safety signals in a noisy haystack. Food Drug Cosmetic Law Journal 1991;46:487-502.

Thormar H, Mehta PD, Barshatzky MR, Brown HR. Measles virus encephalitis in ferrets as a model for subacute sclerosing panencephalitis. Laboratory Animal Science 1985;35:229-232.

Thraenhart O, Kuwert E. [Intratypic differentiation of poliovirus strains with special regard to complication after oral vaccination in West-Germany]. Intratypische charakterisierung von poliovirussammen unter besonderer Berucksichtigung der impfreaktion nach schluckimpfung. Sentralblatt fur Bakteriologic, Parasitunkunde, Infektionskrankheiten und Hygiene 1972;221:143-156.

Thurston A. Anaphylactic shock reaction to measles vaccine (letter). Journal of the Royal College of General Practice 1987;37:41.

Tidjani PO, Grunitzky B, Guerin N, Levy-Bruhl D, Lecam N, Xuereff C et al. [Comparative serological efficacy of anti-measles vaccine strains Edmonston-Zagreb, Schwarz and AIK-C in Togolese infants of 4-5 months and 8-10 months]. Efficacité sérologique comparative des souches de vaccin antirougeoleux Edmonston-Zagreb, Schwarz et AIK-C chez des enfants togolois de 4-5 moise et 8-10 mois. Bulletin de la Societe de Pathologie Exotique 1991;84(5 Pt 5):873-884.

Tishon A, Oldstone MB. Persistent virus infection associated with chemical manifestations of diabetes. American Journal of Pathology 1987;126:61-72.

Todd JK, Bruhn FW. Severe *Haemophilus influenzae* infections: spectrum of disease. American Journal of Diseases in Children 1975;129:607-611.

Toffler WL, Olenick JS, Wolf NE, Retzlaff ZH, Swanson JR, Kenny TA. The immunogenicity and safety of intradermal hepatitis B vaccine. Journal of Family Practice 1991;33:149-154.

Topaloglu H, Berker M, Kansu T, Saatci U, Renda Y. Optic neuritis and myelitis after booster tetanus toxoid vaccination (letter). Lancet 1992;339:178-179.

Topley WW. The role of active or passive immunization in the control of enteric infection. Lancet 1938;1:181-186.

Toraldo R, Tolone C, Catalanotti P, Ianniello R, D'Avanzo M, Canino G et al. Effect of measles-mumps-rubella vaccination on polymorphonuclear neutrophil functions in children. Acta Paediatrica 1992;81:887-890.

Toreki W. Risk management: National Childhood Vaccine Injury Act of 1986. Trends in Health Care, Law and Ethics 1992;7:41-44.

Torinuki W. Mucha-Habermann disease in a child: possible association with measles vaccination. Journal of Dermatology 1992;19:253-255.

Tosti A, Melino M, Bardazzi F. Systemic reactions due to thiomersal. Contact Dermatitis 1986;15:187-188.

Trinca JC. Active immunization against tetanus: the need for a single all-purpose toxoid. Medical Journal of Australia 1965;2:116-120.

Trinca JC. Combined diphtheria-tetanus immunization of adults. Medical Journal of Australia 1975;2:543-546.

Trinca JC. Over-immunization: an ever present problem. Australian Family Physician 1976;5:734-755.

Trollfors B, Lagergard T, Claesson BA, Thornberg E, Martinell J, Schneerson R. Characterization of the serum antibody response to the capsular polysaccharide *Haemophilus influenzae* type b in children with invasive infections. Journal of Infectious Diseases 1992;166:1335-1339.

Trump RC, White TR. Cerebellar ataxia presumed due to live, attenuated measles virus vaccine. Journal of the American Medical Association 1967;199:129-130.

Tsairis P, Dyck PJ, Mulder DW. Natural history of brachial plexus neuropathy: report on 99 patients. Archives of Neurology 1972;27:109-117.

Tsukada N, Koh C-S, Owa M, Yanagisawa N. Chronic neuropathy associated with immune complexes of hepatitis B virus. Journal of the Neurological Sciences 1983;61:193-211.

Tsukada N, Koh C-S, Inoue A, Yanagisawa N. Demyelinating neuropathy associated with hepatitis B infection: detection of immune complexes composed of hepatitis B virus surface antigen. Journal of the Neurological Sciences 1987;77:203-216.

Tubert P, Begaud B, Pere JC, Haramburu F, Lellouch J. Power and weakness of spontaneous reporting: a probabilistic approach. Journal of Clinical Epidemiology 1992;45:283-286.

Tudela P, Marti S, Bonal J. Systemic lupus erythematosus and vaccination against hepatitis B (letter). Nephron 1992;62:236.

Tudor-Williams G, Frankland J, Isaacs D, Mayon-White RT, MacFarlane JA, Rees DG et al. *Haemophilus influenzae* type b conjugate vaccine trial in Oxford: implications for the United Kingdom. Archives of Disease in Childhood 1989;64:520-524.

Tuft L et al. Allergic reactions following immunization procedures. Archives of Environmental Health 1966;13:91-95.

Tuohy PG. Guillain-Barre syndrome following immunisation with synthetic hepatitis B vaccine (letter). New Zealand Medical Journal 1989;102:114-115.

Turner PC, Forsey T, Minor PD. Comparison of the nucleotide sequence of the SH gene and flanking regions of mumps vaccine virus (Urabe strain) grown on different substrates and isolated from vaccinees. Journal of General Virology 1991;72(Pt 2):435-437.

Tyufanov AV, Stefanov SB. [Seasonal differences in the pathomorphological reactions of monkeys to poliomyelitis vaccine] Sezonnye razlichiia patomorfologicheskikh reaktsii obez'ian na vaktsinu protiv poliomielita. Voprosy Virusologii 1983;2:238-240.

U.S. Department of Health, Education, and Welfare. Smoking and Health: Report of the Advisory Committee to the Surgeon General. PHS Publ. No. 1003. Washington, DC: U.S. Public Health Service, U.S. Department of Health, Education, and Welfare; 1964.

U.S. Department of Health and Human Services, U.S. Public Health Service. National Vaccine Injury Compensation Program; Revision of the Vaccine Injury Table; Proposed Rule. Federal Register, 42 CFR Part 100, August 14, 1992;57(158):36877-36885.

U.S. Public Health Service. Interim document gives advice on use of Salk and Sabin vaccines. Journal of the American Medical Association 1962;180:23-26.

Uchida T. Diphtheria toxin. In: Dorner F, Drews J, eds. Pharmacology of Bacterial Toxins IEPT Section 199. Oxford: Pergamon Press; 1986.

Uhari M, Rantala H, Niemela M. Cluster of childhood Guillain-Barre cases after an oral poliovaccine campaign (letter). Lancet 1989;2:440-441.

Ullberg-Olsson K. [Vaccination reactions after injection of tetanus toxoid with and without diphtheria toxoid] Vaccinationsreaktioner efter injektion av tetanustoxoid med och utan tillsats av difteritoxoid. Lakartidningen 1979;76:2976.

Vaandrager GJ, Molenaar JL, Bruining GJ, Plantinga AD, Ruitenberg EJ. Islet cell antibodies, mumps infection and mumps vaccination (letter). Diabetologia 1986;29:406-407.

Vadheim CM. Reduction of Hib disease in Southern California, 1983-1991. Program Abstracts of the 32nd Interscience Conference on Antimicrobial Agents and Chemotherapy. Abstract 1726, p. 398. Washington, DC: American Society for Microbiology; 1992.

Vadheim CM, Greenberg DP, Marcy SM, Froeschle J, Ward JI. Safety evaluation of PRP-D *Haemophilus influenzae* type b conjugate vaccine in children immunized at 18 months of age and older: follow-up study of 30,000 children. Pediatric Infectious Disease Journal 1990;9:555-561.

Vallancourt RJ. Current poliovirus vaccines. Reviews of Infectious Diseases 1984;6(Suppl. 2):S328-S330.

Valman HB. Convulsions in the older infant. British Medical Journal 1989;299:1331-1333.

Valmari P, Lanning M, Tuokko H, Kouvalainen K. Measles virus in the cerebrospinal fluid in postvaccination immunosuppressive measles encephalopathy. Pediatric Infectious Disease Journal 1987;6:59-63.

van Alphen L, Bijlmer HA. Molecular epidemiology of *Haemophilus influenzae* type b. Pediatrics 1990;85(4 Pt 2):636-642.

Van Asperen PP, McEniery J, Kemp AS. Immediate reactions following live attenuated measles vaccine. Medical Journal of Australia 1981;2:330-331.

van Bogaert L. Une leucoencephalite sclerosante subaigue. Journal de Neurologie et de Psychiatrie 1945;8:101-120.

Van de Voorde A. Eye of the needle. Westword 1992;15:10-12, 15-16.

van der Meché FG, Schmitz PI, Dutch Guillain-Barre Study Group. A randomized trial comparing intravenous immune globulin and plasma exchange in Guillain-Barre syndrome. New England Journal of Medicine 1992;326:1123-1129.

van Heyningen S. Tetanus toxin. In: Dorner F, Drews J, eds. Pharmacology of Bacterial Toxins IEPT Section 199. Oxford: Pergamon Press; 1986.

van Ramshorst JD, Cohen H, Levine L, Edsall G. The relation between animal potency tests and the human response to adsorbed tetanus toxoids. Journal of Biological Standardization 1973;1:215-220.

Varughese PV, Carter AO, Acres SE, Furesz J. Eradication of indigenous poliomyelitis in Canada: impact of immunization strategies. Canadian Journal of Public Health 1989;80:363-368.

Vassilev TL. Aluminium phosphate but not calcium phosphate stimulates the specific IgE response in guinea pigs to tetanus toxoid. Allergy 1978;33:155-159.

Vella PP, Staub JM, Armstrong J, Dolan KT, Rusk CM, Szymanski S et al. Immunogenicity of a new *Haemophilus influenzae* type b conjugate vaccine (meningococcal protein conjugate) (PedvaxHIB). Pediatrics 1990;85(4 Pt 2):668-675.

Vellayappan K, Lee CY. Tetanus toxoid hypersensitivity. Journal of the Singapore Paediatric Society 1976;18:17-19.

Venulet J. Assessing Causes of Adverse Drug Reactions with Special Reference to Standardized Methods. London: Academic Press; 1982.

Verduzco Guerrero E, Calderon C, Velazquez Franco E. [Repercussions of vaccination against measles] Repercusiones de la vacunacion contra el sarampion. Salud Publica de Mexico 1974;16:707-720.

Vesikari T, Ala-Laurila EL, Heikkinen A, Kuusinen H, Terho A. [Efficacy and side effects of live attenuated single mumps and measles vaccines, and bivalent mumps-measles vaccine in young infants] Elava sikotautirokote yksin ja tuhkarokko-rokotteeseen yhdistettyna pienilla lapsilla. Duodecim 1982;98:839-847.

Vesikari T, Ala-Laurila EL, Heikkinen A, Terho A, D'Hondt E, Andre FE. Clinical trial of a new trivalent measles-mumps-rubella vaccine in young children. American Journal of Diseases of Children 1984;138:843-847.

Vesikari T, Andre FE, Simoen E, Florent G, Ala-Laurila EL, Heikkinen A et al. Evaluation in young children of the Urabe Am 9 strain of live attenuated mumps vaccine in comparison with the Jeryl Lynn strain. Acta Paediatrica Scandinavica 1983;72:37-40.

Vesikari T, Andre FE, Simoen E, Florent G, Ala-Laurila EL, Heikkinen A et al. Comparison of the Urabe Am 9-Schwarz and Jeryl Lynn-Moraten combinations of mumps-measles vaccines in young children. Acta Paediatrica Scandinavica 1983;72:41-46.

Vessal S, Kravis LP. Immunologic mechanisms responsible for adverse reactions to routine immunizations in children. Clinical Pediatrics 1976;15:688-696.

Vijay HM, Huang H, Young NM, Bernstein IL et al. Studies on alternaria allergens. I. Isolation of allergens from alternaria tenuis and alternaria solani. International Archives of Allergy and Applied Immunology 1979;60:229-239.

Vijay HM, Lavergne G, Huang H, Bernstein IL et al. Preferential synthesis of IgE reaginic antibodies in rats immunized with alum-adsorbed antigens. International Archives of Allergy and Applied Immunology 1979;59:227-232.

Villaca LM, de Macedo DD. [Subacute sclerosing panencephalitis with partial remission] Panencefalite esclerosante subaguda com remissao parcial. Arquivos de Neuropsiquiatria 1979;37:435-442.

Vivell O. [Oral vaccination against poliomyelitis] Poliomyelitis-Schluckimpfung. Deutsche Medizinische Wochenschrift 1973;98:1049.

Vogel C. [Complication by contact after vaccination against poliomyelitis]. Zum Thema Impfkomplikation (am beispiel einer impf-kontakt-poliomyelitis). Kinderarztliche Praxis 1980;48:296-299.

Volk VK. Safety and effectiveness of multiple antigen preparations in a group of free-living children. American Journal of Public Health 1949;39:1299-1313.

Volk VK, Gottshall RY, Anderson HD et al. Antibody response to booster dose of diphtheria and tetanus toxoids: reactions in institutionalized adults and noninstitutionalized children and young adults. Public Health Reports 1963;78:161-164.

Volk VK, Gottshall RY, Anderson HD, Top FH, Bunney WE, Serfling RE. Antigenic response to booster dose of diphtheria and tetanus toxoids: seven to thirteen years after primary inoculation of noninstitutionalized children. Public Health Reports 1962;77:185-194.

von Muhlendahl KE. [Side effects and complications of measles-mumps vaccination] Nebenwirkungen und Komplikationen der Masern-Mumps-Impfung. Monatsschrift fur Kinderheilkunde 1989;137:440-446.

von Muhlendahl KE. Side-effects of measles-mumps vaccination (letter). Lancet 1990;335:540-541.

von Muhlendahl KE, Eguiluz GC, Trallero EP, Thalayasingam B. Mumps meningitis following measles, mumps, and rubella immunization. Lancet 1989;2:394-395.

von Reyn CF, Clements CJ, Mann JM. Human immunodeficiency virus infection and routine childhood immunisation. Lancet 1987;2:669-672.

Von Seefried A, Chun JH, Grant JA, Letvenuk L, Pearson EW. Inactivated poliovirus vaccine and test development at Connaught Laboratories LTD. Reviews of Infectious Diseases 1984;6(Suppl. 2):S345-S349.

von Wirth G. Reversible kochlearisschadigung nach Tetanol-Injektion? Munchener Medizinische Wochenschrift 1965;107:379-381.

Voss L, Lennon D, Gillies M. *Haemophilus influenzae* type b disease in Auckland children 1981-87. New Zealand Medical Journal 1989;102:149-151.

Wahl M, Hermodsson S. Intradermal, subcutaneous or intramuscular administration of hepatitis B vaccine: side effects and antibody response. Scandinavian Journal of Infectious Diseases 1987;19:617-621.

Waight PA, Pollock TM, Miller E, Coleman EM. Pyrexia after diphtheria/tetanus/pertussis and diphtheria/tetanus vaccines. Archives of Disease in Childhood 1983;58:921-923.

Waisbren BA. A commentary regarding personal observations of demyelinizing disease caused by viral vaccines, borrelia infections, and proteolytic enzymes. Submitted to the Institute of Medicine Committee on Vaccine Safety, August 11, 1992.

Wakeel RA, White MI. Erythema multiforme associated with hepatitis B vaccine (letter). British Journal of Dermatology 1992;126:94-95.

Waksman BH, Adams RD. Allergic neuritis: an experimental disease of rabbits induced by the injection of peripheral nervous tissue and adjuvants. Journal of Experimental Medicine 1955;102:213-235.

Walker AM, Jick H, Perera DR, Thompson RJ, Knauss TA. Diphtheria-tetanus-pertussis immunization and sudden infant death syndrome. American Journal of Public Health 1987;77: 945-951.

Walker AM, Martin-Moreno JM, Artalejo FR. Odd man out: a graphical approach to meta-analysis. American Journal of Public Health 1988;78:961-966.

Walter EB, Moggio MV, Drucker RP, Wilfert CM. Immunogenicity of *Haemophilus* b conjugate vaccine (meningococcal protein conjugate) in children with prior invasive *Haemophilus influenzae* type b disease. Pediatric Infectious Disease Journal 1990;9:632-635.

Walter Z, Walter T. [Six cases of poliomyelitis associated with oral immunization] Szesc przypadkow zachorowan na polio w powiazaniu ze szczepieniami doustnymi przeciw polio. Wiadomosci Lekarskie 1973;26:901-905.

Wands JR, Mann E, Alpert E. The pathogenesis of arthritis associated with acute hepatitis B surface antigen-positive hepatitis: complement activation and characterization of circulating immune complexes. Journal of Clinical Investigation 1975;55:930-939.

Ward BJ, Johnson RT, Vaisberg A, Jauregui E, Griffin DE. Cytokine production in vitro and the lymphoproliferative defect of natural measles infection. Clinical Immunology and Immunopathology 1991;61:236-248.

Ward JI. Commentary: results of efficacy trials in Alaska and Finland of *Haemophilus influenzae* type b conjugate vaccine. Pediatrics 1990;85(4 Pt 2):667.

Ward JI, Broome CV, Harrison LH, Shinefield H, Black S. *Haemophilus influenzae* type b vaccines: lessons for the future. Pediatrics 1988;81:886-893.

Ward JI, Cochi S. *Haemophilus influenzae* vaccines. In: Plotkin SA, Mortimer EA, eds. Vaccines. Philadelphia: W.B. Saunders; 1988.

Wassilak SG. Adverse events following IPV. Prepared for Meeting of Immunization Practices Advisory Committee. October 24-25, 1985.

Wassilak SG, Brink EW. Diseases controlled primarily by vaccination: tetanus. In: Last JM, Wallace RB, eds. Maxcy-Rosenau-Last Public Health and Preventive Medicine, 13th ed. Norwalk, CT: Appleton & Lange; 1992.

Wassilak SG, Orenstein WA. Tetanus. In: Plotkin SA, Mortimer EA, eds. Vaccines. Philadelphia: W.B. Saunders Co.; 1988.

Wassilak SG, Brink EW, Orenstein WA et al. Neurologic complications of oral poliomyelitis vaccine. Journal of Pediatrics 1987;110:996-998.

Watemberg N, Dagan R, Arbelli Y, Belmaker I, Morag A, Hessel L et al. Safety and immunogenicity of *Haemophilus* type b-tetanus protein conjugate vaccine, mixed in the same syringe with diphtheria-tetanus-pertussis vaccine in young infants. Pediatric Infectious Disease Journal 1991;10:758-763.

Watson GI. The roseolar reaction (letter). British Medical Journal 1974;4:719-720.

Watson JG. A child of 3 years who developed an encephalitic reaction to MMR (mumps, measles, rubella) immunisation at age 15 months (letter). International Journal of Pediatric Otorhinolaryngology 1990;19:189-190.

Weber G, Falk U. Vaccinations in the presence of skin diseases. International Journal of Dermatology 1975;14:136-140.

Weckx LY, Schmidt BJ, Herrmann AA, Miyasaki CH, Novo NF. Early immunization of neonates with trivalent oral poliovirus vaccine. Bulletin of the World Health Organization 1992;70:85-91.

Weekly Epidemiological Record. Expanded Programme on Immunization: reactions to tetanus toxoids. Weekly Epidemiological Record 1982;57:193-194.

Weekly Epidemiological Record. Poliomyelitis: evaluation of poliovirus-related cases. Weekly Epidemiological Record 1990;65:159-162.

Weekly Epidemiological Record. Expanded Programme on Immunization: serological and virological assessment of oral and inactivated poliovirus vaccines in a rural population. Weekly Epidemiological Record 1992;6:179-182.

Weekly Epidemiological Record. Expanded Programme on Immunization (EPI): safety of high titre measles vaccines. Weekly Epidemiological Record 1992;67:357-361.

Wehrle PF. Injury associated with the use of vaccines. Clinical Therapeutics 1985;7:282-284.

Weibel RE. Mumps vaccine. In: Plotkin SA, Mortimer EA, eds. Vaccines. Philadelphia: W.B. Saunders Co.; 1988.

Weibel RE, Stokes J, Buynak EB, Whitman JE, Hilleman MR. Live, attenuated mumps-virus vaccine. 3. Clinical and serologic aspects in a field evaluation. New England Journal of Medicine 1967;276:245-251.

Weibel RE, Villarejos VM, Hernandez G, Stokes JJ, Buynak EB, Hilleman MR. Combined live measles-mumps virus vaccine. Archives of Disease in Childhood 1973;48:532-536.

Weidmeier SE, Chung HT, Cho BH, Kim UH, Daynes RA. Murine responses to immunization with pertussis toxin and bovine albumin. I. Mortality observed after bovine albumin challenge is due to an anaphylactic reaction. Pediatric Research 1987;22:262-267.

Weinberg GA, Granoff DM. Polysaccharide-protein conjugate vaccines for the prevention of *Haemophilus influenzae* type b disease. Journal of Pediatrics 1988;113:621-631.

Weinberg GA, Granoff DM. Immunogenicity of *Haemophilus influenzae* type polysaccharide-protein conjugate vaccines in children with conditions associated with impaired antibody responses to type b polysaccharide vaccine. Pediatrics 1990;85(4 Pt 2):654-661.

Weinberg GA, Einhorn MS, Lenoir AA, Granoff PD, Granoff DM et al. Immunologic priming to capsular polysaccharide in infants immunized with *Haemophilus influenzae* type b polysaccharide-*Neisseria meningitidis* outer membrane protein conjugate vaccine. Journal of Pediatrics 1987;111:22-27.

Weisman SJ, Cates KL, Allegretta GJ, Quinn JJ, Altman AJ. Antibody response to immunization with *Haemophilus influenzae* type b polysaccharide vaccine in children with cancer. Journal of Pediatrics 1987;111:727-729.

Weiss R. Change the U.S. polio vaccine or leave it alone? ASM News (American Society for Microbiology) 1988;54:560-562.

Weisse AB. Polio: the not-so-twentieth-century disease. Hospital Practice 1992;27:97-100, 104, 113-115, 119-120.

Wells EC. Neurological note on vaccination against influenza. British Medical Journal 1971;3:755-756.

Wenger JD, Fraser DW, Broome CV. Diseases controlled primarily by vaccination: *Haemophilus influenzae* infections. In: Last JM, Wallace RB, eds. Maxcy-Rosenau-Last Public Health and Preventive Medicine, 13th ed. Norwalk, CT: Appleton & Lange; 1992.

Wentz KR, Marcuse EK. Diphtheria-tetanus-pertussis vaccine and serious neurologic illness: an updated review of the epidemiologic evidence. Pediatrics 1991;87:287-297.

Werne J, Garrow I. Fatal anaphylactic shock occurrence in identical twins following second injection of diphtheria toxoid and pertussis antigen. Journal of the American Medical Association 1946;131:730-735.

Werner CA. Mumps orchitis and testicular atrophy: I. Occurrence. Annals of Internal Medicine 1950;32:1066-1074.

Werner CA. Mumps orchitis and testicular atrophy. II. A factor in male sterility. Annals of Internal Medicine 1950;32:1075-1086.

West DH, Calandra GB, Ellis RW. Vaccination of infants and children against hepatitis B. Pediatric Clinics of North America 1990;37:585-601.

Westall FC, Root-Bernstein R. Cause and prevention of postinfectious and postvaccinal neuropathies in light of a new theory of autoimmunity. Lancet 1986;2:251-252.

Wharton M, Cochi SL, Hutcheson RH, Bistowish JM, Schaffner W. A large outbreak of mumps in a postvaccine era. Journal of Infectious Diseases 1988;158:1253-1260.

White CC, Koplan JP, Orenstein WA. Benefits, risks and costs of immunization for measles, mumps and rubella. American Journal of Public Health 1985;75:739-744.

White F. Measles vaccine associated encephalitis in Canada (letter). Lancet 1983;2:683-684.

White WG. Reactions after plain and adsorbed tetanus vaccines (letter). Lancet 1980;1:42.

White WG, Barnes GM, Barker E, Gall D, Knight P, Griffith AH et al. Reactions to tetanus toxoid. Journal of Hygiene 1973;71:283-297.

Whittingham HE. Anaphylaxis following administration of tetanus toxoid. British Medical Journal 1940;1:292-293.

Whittle E, Roberton NR. Transverse myelitis after diphtheria, tetanus, and polio immunisation. British Medical Journal 1977;1:1450.

Whittle H, Hanlon P, O'Neill K, Hanlon L, Marsh V, Jupp E et al. Trial of high-dose Edmonston-Zagreb measles vaccine in the Gambia: antibody response and side-effects. Lancet 1988;2:811-814.

WHO Consultative Group. The relation between acute persisting spinal paralysis and poliomyelitis vaccine: results of a ten-year enquiry. Bulletin of the World Health Organization 1982;60:231-242.

Wiechers DO. New concepts of the reinnervated motor unit revealed by vaccine-associated poliomyelitis. Muscle and Nerve 1988;11:356-364.

Wiechers DO. Reinnervation after acute poliomyelitis. Birth Defects 1987;23:213-221.

Wiersbitzky S, Bruns R. [Bacterial meningitis following Hib-vaccination: a causal connection?] Meningitis purulenta nach Hib-Schutzimpfung: Kausaler zusammenhang? Kinderarztliche Praxis 1992;60:27.

Wiersbitzky S, Bruns R. [Hib vaccinations and complications?] Schwere Gastroenteritis nach Hib-Schutzimpfung? Kinderarztliche Praxis 1992;60:102.

Wiersbitzky S, Bruns R. Safety of vaccines in childhood. Lancet 1993;341:379.

Wiersbitzky S, Bruns R, Beyer B. [Incubation vaccination ("post-exposure vaccination") with MMR vaccine during a mumps epidemic? The Pediatric Vaccine Counseling Unit] Inkubationsimpfung ("Riegelungsimpfung") mit MMR-Vakzine wahrend einer Mumpsepidemie? Die padiatrische Impfberatungsstelle. Kinderarztliche Praxis 1992;60:207-208.

Wiersbitzky S, Bruns R, Griefahn B, Wiersbitzky H. [Near-miss sudden infant death (nearly sudden infant death syndrome/NSIDS) following second DPT vaccination?] Beinahe plotzlicher Kindstod (Nearly Sudden Infant Death Syndrome/NSIDS) nach der 2. DPT-Impfung? Kinderarztliche Praxis 1992;60:246-248.

Wiersbitzky S, Bruns R, Peters A, Mentel R. [Encephalitis, meningitis serosa and parotitis after MMR preventive vaccination? The Pediatric Vaccination Counseling Unit] Enzephalitis, Meningitis serosa und Parotitis nach MMR-Schutzimpfung? Die padiatrische Impfberatungsstelle. Kinderarztliche Praxis 1992;60:203-205.

Wiersbitzky S, Bruns R, Schroder C, Warmuth M. [Thrombocytopenic purpura following immunization with a live vaccine (mumps-measles-rubella vaccination)?] Thrombozytopenische Purpura nach Impfung mit Lebendvakzine (Mumps-Masern-Roteln-Schutzimpfung)? Kinderarztliche Praxis 1992;60:28-29.

Wiersbitzky S, Bruns R, Wiersbitzky H. [Hyperpyretic reaction following combined vaccination DPT, Hib and oral polio in an infant] Hyperpyretische Reaktion nach kombinierter Hib-, DPT- und oraler Polio-Schutzimpfung bei einem Saugling? Kinderarztliche Praxis 1992;60:304-305.

Wiesmann E, Keller HP, Steiner P. [Diphtheria vaccination of adults] Die Diphtherieimpfung Erwachsener. Schweizerische Medizinische Wochenschrift 1972;102:41-43.

Wiggins CA, Dykewicz MS, Patterson R. Idiopathic anaphylaxis: a review. Annals of Allergy 1989;62:1-4.

Wilfert CM. Epidemiology of *Haemophilus influenzae* type b infections. Pediatrics 1990;85(4 Pt 2):631-635.

Wilhelm DJ, Paegle RD. Thrombocytopenic purpura and pneumonia following measles vaccination. American Journal of Diseases of Children 1967;113:534-537.

Wilkinson JR. Measles immunisation: contraindications perceived by general practitioners in one health district. Public Health 1986;100:144-148.

Williamson S. Anti-vaccination leagues. Archives of Disease in Childhood 1984;59:1195-1196.

Willinger M, James LS, Catz C et al. Defining the sudden infant death syndrome (SIDS): deliberations of an expert panel convened by the National Institute of Child Health and Human Development. Pediatric Pathology 1991;11:677-684.

Wilson GS. The Hazards of Immunization. London and New York: Oxford University Press (Athlone); 1967.

Wilson J, Robinson R. Poliomyelitis after contact with recently vaccinated infant (letter). British Medical Journal 1974;2:53.

Wilson LM. Some aspects of epidemiology in paediatric oncology. Proceedings of the Royal Society of Medicine 1975;68:657-659.

Wilson S, Aprile MA. Sensitizing versus immunizing properties of inactivated measles vaccine. Progress in Immunobiological Standardization 1970;4:657-660.

Winer JB, Hughes RA, Anderson MJ, Jones DM, Kangro J, Watkins RP. A prospective study of acute idiopathic neuropathy. II. Antecedent events. Journal of Neurology, Neurosurgery and Psychiatry 1988;51:613-618.

Winner SJ, Evans G. Age-specific incidence of Guillain-Barre syndrome in Oxfordshire. Quarterly Journal of Medicine 1990;77(New Series):1297-1304.

Wolters KL, Dehmel H. Abschliessende untersuchungen uber die Tetanus Prophylaxe durch active Immunisierung. Zeitschrift fur Hygeitschrift 1942;124:326-332.

Wong S, Dykewicz MS, Patterson R. Idiopathic anaphylaxis: a clinical summary of 175 patients. Archives of Internal Medicine 1974;150:1323-1328.

Wong VC, Ip HM, Reesink HW. Prevention of the HBsAg carrier state in newborn infants of mothers who are chronic carriers of HBsAg and HBeAg by administration of hepatitis B vaccine and hepatitis B immunoglobulin: double-blind randomised placebo-controlled study. Lancet 1984;1:921-926.

Wong WK, Tan C, Ng SK, Goh CL. Thimerosal allergy and its relevance in Singapore. Contact Dermatitis 1992;26:195-196.

Woods DR, Mason DD. Six areas lead national early immunization drive. Public Health Reports 1992;107:252-256.

Woolling KR, Ruston JG. Serum neuritis: report of two cases and brief review of the syndrome. Archives of Neurology and Psychiatry 1950;64:568-573.

World Health Organization. Measles Vaccines, Technical Report No. 263. World Health Organization: Geneva; 1963.

WRC-TV. DPT: Vaccine Roulette. Washington DC: WRC-TV, 1982.

Wright PF, Hatch MH, Kasselberg AG, Lowry SP, Wadlington WB, Karzon DT. Vaccine-associated poliomyelitis in a child with sex-linked agammaglobulinemia. Journal of Pediatrics 1977;91:408-412.

Wright PF, Kim-Farley RJ, de Quadros CA, Robertson SE, Scott RM, Ward NA et al. Strategies for the global eradication of poliomyelitis by the year 2000. New England Journal of Medicine 1991;325:1774-1779.

Wutzler P, Sprossig M, Schneider J et al. [A complication after oral protective immunisation against poliomyelitis] Komplikation nach oraler Poliomyelitis-Schutzimpfung. Padiatrie und Grenzgebiete 1984;23:289-297.

Wyatt G. Planning an immunisation schedule. Practitioner 1992;236:479-480, 482.

Wyatt HV. Poliomyelitis in hypogammaglobulinemics. Journal of Infectious Diseases 1973;128:802-806.

Wyatt HV. Provocation poliomyelitis: neglected clinical observations from 1914 to 1950. Bulletin of the History of Medicine 1981;55:543-557.

Wyatt HV. Did thalidomide promote poliomyelitis following oral poliovirus vaccination in West Berlin in 1960? Perspectives in Biology and Medicine 1983;27:93-106.

Wyatt HV. Injections cripple, injections kill (letter). Journal of the Indian Medical Association 1986;84:193-194.

Wyatt HV. Injections and poliomyelitis: what are the risks of vaccine associated paralysis? Developments in Biological Standardization 1986;65:123-128.

Wyatt HV. Poliovaccination in the Gambia (letter). Lancet 1987;2:43.

Wyatt HV. Incubation of poliomyelitis as calculated from the time of entry into the central nervous system via the peripheral nerve pathways. Reviews of Infectious Diseases 1990;12:547-556.

Wyatt HV. Provocation paralysis (letter). Lancet 1993;341:61-62.

Xu ZY, Margolis HS. Determinants of hepatitis B vaccine efficacy and implications for vaccination strategies. Viral Hepatitis in China: Problems and Control Strategies. Monographs in Virology 1992;19:87-98.

Yamada A, Takeuchi K, Tanabayashi K, Hishiyama M, Takahashi Y, Sugiura A. Differentiation of the mumps vaccine strains from the wild viruses by the nucleotide sequences of the P gene. Vaccine 1990;8:553-557.

Yamauchi T, Wilson C, St. Geme JW. Transmission of live, attenuated mumps virus to the human placenta. New England Journal of Medicine 1974;290:710-712.

Yanagi Y, Cubitt BA, Oldstone MB A. Measles virus inhibits mitogen-induced T cell proliferation but does not directly perturb the T cell activation process inside the cell. Virology 1992;187:280-289.

Yap I, Guan R, Chan SH. Recombinant DNA hepatitis B vaccine containing Pre-S components of the HBV coat protein—a preliminary study on immunogenicity. Vaccine 1992;10:439-442.

Yeoh EK, Chang WK, Ip P, Chan KH, Chan E, Fung C. Efficacy and safety of recombinant hepatitis B vaccine in infants born to HBsAg-positive mothers. Journal of Infection 1986;13(Suppl. A):15-18.

Yogev R, Arditi M, Chadwick EG, Amer MD, Sroka PA. Haemophilus influenzae type b conjugate vaccine (meningococcal protein conjugate): immunogenicity and safety at various doses. Pediatrics 1990;85(4 Pt 2):690-693.

Yohannan MD, Ramia S, al Frayh AR. Acute paralytic poliomyelitis presenting as Guillain-Barre syndrome. Journal of Infection 1991;22:129-133.

Yoon JW, Austin M, Onodera T, Notkins AL. Virus-induced diabetes mellitus. New England Journal of Medicine 1979;300:1173-1179.

Yoon JW, Eun HM, Essani K, Roncari DA, Bryan LE et al. Possible mechanisms in the pathogenesis of virus-induced diabetes mellitus. [Clinical and Investigative Medicine] Medecine Clinique et Experimentale 1987;10:450-456.

Yoon JW, Kim CJ, Pak CY, McArthur RG et al. Effects of environmental factors on the development of insulin-dependent diabetes mellitus. [Clinical and Investigative Medicine] Medecine Clinique et Experimentale 1987;10:457-469.

Yoon JW, Onodera T, Notkins AL. Virus-induced diabetes mellitus: XV. Beta cell damage and insulin-dependent hyperglycemia in mice infected with coxsackie virus B-4. Journal of Experimental Medicine 1978;148:1068-1080.

Yoon JW, Ray UR et al. Perspectives on the role of viruses in insulin-dependent diabetes. Diabetes Care 1985;8(Suppl. 1):39-44.

Yu DT, Winchester RJ, Fu SM, Gibofsky A, Ko HS, Kunkel HG. Peripheral blood Ia-positive T cells: increases in certain diseases and after immunization. Journal of Experimental Medicine 1980;151:91-100.

Yunginger JW. Anaphylaxis. Current Problems in Pediatrics 1992;22:130-147.

Zajac BA, West DJ, McAleer WJ, Scolnick EM. Overview of clinical studies with hepatitis B vaccine made by recombinant DNA. Journal of Infection 1986;13(Suppl. A):39-45.

Zaloga GP, Chernow B. Life-threatening anaphylactic reaction to tetanus toxoid. Annals of Allergy 1982;49:107-108.

Zevakov VF, Semak SY, Titarenko VI, Andreichenko NV, Gedzul OV. Poliomyelitis viruses in the etiology of aseptic meningitides in Odessa, 1979-1983. Voprosy Virusologii 1987;32:458-464.

Zieger B, Basener G, Berdrow J et al. [Vaccinations and complications after vaccination in travellers] Impfungen und Impfkomplikationen bei Auslandsreisenden. Deutsche Gesundheitswesen 1976;31:1956-1958.

Zilber N, Rannon L, Alter M, Kahana E. Measles, measles vaccination, and risk of subacute sclerosing panencephalitis (SSPE). Neurology 1983;33:1558-1564.

Zimmerman B, Gold R, Lavi S. Adverse effects of immunization: is prevention possible? Postgraduate Medicine 1987;82:225-229, 232.

Zimmerman RK, Giebink GS. Childhood immunizations: a practical approach for clinicians. American Family Physician 1992;45:1759-1772.

Zingher A, Park HW. Immunity results obtained in school children with diphtheria toxoid (modified toxin) with 1/10 L+ mixtures of toxin-antitoxin. Proceedings of the Society for Experimental Biology and Medicine 1923;21:383-385.

Zoltowska A. Immunomorphologic patterns in intensively immunized guinea pigs. Archivum Immunologiae et Therapiae Experimentalis 1971;19:417-429.

Zoltowska A. Sarcoidal reactions in animals intensively immunized with tetanus vaccine. Archivum Immunologiae et Therapiae Experimentalis 1974;22:341-347.

Zwemer R, Hodge S, Owen LG, Fliegelman MT. Persistent toxic erythema and chronic urticaria: possible association with the use of measles virus vaccine. Archives of Dermatology 1971;104:390-392.

Index